Methods in Molecular Biology

Series Editor
John M. Walker
School of Life and Medical Sciences
University of Hertfordshire
Hatfield, Hertfordshire, AL10 9AB, UK

For further volumes:
http://www.springer.com/series/7651

Fibrosis

Methods and Protocols

Edited by

Laure Rittié

Department of Dermatology, University of Michigan Medical School, Ann Arbor, MI, USA; Dermatology Therapeutic Area, GlaxoSmithKline, Collegeville, PA, USA

Humana Press

Editor
Laure Rittié
Department of Dermatology
University of Michigan Medical School
Ann Arbor, MI, USA

Dermatology Therapeutic Area
GlaxoSmithKline
Collegeville, PA, USA

ISSN 1064-3745 ISSN 1940-6029 (electronic)
Methods in Molecular Biology
ISBN 978-1-4939-7112-1 ISBN 978-1-4939-7113-8 (eBook)
DOI 10.1007/978-1-4939-7113-8

Library of Congress Control Number: 2017940794

Printed on acid-free paper

This Humana Press imprint is published by Springer Nature
The registered company is Springer Science+Business Media LLC
The registered company address is: 233 Spring Street, New York, NY 10013, U.S.A.

Preface

The term "fibrosis" designates the formation of excess fibrous connective tissue that can affect a plethora of tissues and organs. Extracellular matrix (ECM) deposition is typically a normal reaction to injury that allows tissue repair and restoration of tissue strength. However, when the response turns awry, ECM deposition becomes pathogenic and results in thickened extracellular environment that hampers tissue properties and may lead to organ failure.

Fibrosis' prevalence within so many organs makes it quite complex to study. Researchers thereby rely on multiple in vitro, ex vivo, and in vivo models aimed at recapitulating one of several aspects of the fibrotic reaction. *Fibrosis: Methods and Protocols* was crafted with the objective of creating a "bench manual" for scientists concentrating on fibrosis research. This volume compiles a collection of state-of-the-art protocols that will serve not only as recipes for bench scientists but also as accepted methods for the field. For each chapter, experts in their respective field present their routinely used method to study one aspect of fibrosis and, maybe most importantly, their most helpful tips, organized in "Notes." They also detail, in the "Introduction" section, the advantages and limitations of their method. Lastly, most chapters are illustrated with examples of experimental settings, screenshots, or typical results, meant to ensure a detailed comprehension of the method for accurate execution and replication.

In this volume, the reader will first find a thorough perspective encompassing the clinical scope of fibrosis, an up-to-date review of the molecular mechanisms leading to the development of tissue fibrosis, and an overview of the current challenges of fibrosis research. This perspective will serve as the introduction of *Fibrosis: Methods and Protocols*, which is organized in four parts. Part I focuses on animal models of fibrosis. Nine chapters will provide detailed protocols on how to mimic fibrosis in the lung, the skin, the liver, the cornea, and the heart, and how to generate transgenic mouse models overexpressing a gene of interest in fibroblasts, predominant mesenchymal cells activated during fibrosis.

Part II focuses on cell culture systems. Four chapters provide detailed methods for studying the cell types that are increasingly viewed as important for the development of fibrosis, i.e., hepatic stellate cells, adipose-derived stromal cells, dermal cell populations, and peripheral tissues' mast cells. Four additional chapters will concentrate on cell culture models aimed at studying the biomechanical influence that the ECM exerts on cells: the cell-populated collagen lattice model, the deformable microposts model, the hydrogels, and the decellularized lung matrices model.

Part III focuses on the purification, quantification, and analysis of the ultimate architects of fibrosis: the ECM proteins. The reader will find protocols to isolate type I collagen and fibronectin for in vitro experimentation purposes, to isolate and quantify transcripts from laser capture-microdissected tissue, to quantify collagen I, TGFβ, and elastin proteins in tissues, to study collagen assembly in vitro, and to specifically identify fibrillar collagens in tissue samples by picro-Sirius red staining or by second harmonic generation (SHG) imaging (a stain- and dye-free imaging technique specific for collagen).

Lastly, Part IV focuses on the more modern optical and computational methods. The reader will find tremendously useful protocols describing computer-assisted methods for quantifying fibrillar collagen alignment, exploring the nano-surface of collagen with atomic force microscopy (AFM), for enhancing the quality of multiplex staining using spectral unmixing, and for interrogating the increasingly abundant deposited gene expression datasets commonly seen as intimidating for the non-bioinformatician, but no longer intimidating after reading this chapter.

In all, *Fibrosis: Methods and Protocols* was crafted by 94 scientists and physicians (40% female) dispersed on thirteen countries and four continents. I wish to thank each of them for their tremendous contribution: be rewarded in that each chapter will undoubtedly be very useful to many investigators around the world. It has been my pleasure to work with you and bring our readers a volume that I believe will make a difference in ascertaining quality and repeatability of research experiments in the fibrosis field. Readers, please share your appreciation by citing the chapter(s) you used for your experiments. I would also like to thank the Series editor, John Walker, for his guidance during the process of compiling this volume and acknowledge the executive staff at Springer for their logistical help and support. Nurturing this book has been a great journey. I learned a lot, and I encourage scientists at all levels to do the same and jump in the adventure of becoming an ad hoc editor.

Ann Arbor, MI, USA
Collegeville, PA, USA

Laure Rittié

Contents

Contributors

JOHANN BAUERSACHS • *Department of Cardiology and Angiology, Medical School Hannover, Hannover, Germany*

GEORGE BOU-GHARIOS • *Department of Musculoskeletal Biology, Institute of Ageing and Chronic Disease, University of Liverpool, Liverpool, UK*

SCOTT N. BYRNE • *Cellular Photoimmunology Group, Discipline of Infectious Diseases and Immunology, Sydney Medical School at The Charles Perkins Centre, University of Sydney, Sydney, NSW, Australia*

HÉCTOR CAPELLA-MONSONÍS • *Regenerative, Modular & Developmental Engineering Laboratory (REMODEL), National University of Ireland Galway, Galway, Ireland; Science Foundation Ireland Centre for Research in Medical Devices (CÚRAM), National University of Ireland Galway, Galway, Ireland*

GRACE CHU • *Department of Musculoskeletal Biology, Institute of Ageing and Chronic Disease, University of Liverpool, Liverpool, UK*

RICCARDO CICCHI • *National Institute of Optics, National Research Council (INO-CNR), Sesto Fiorentino, Italy; European Laboratory for Non-linear Spectroscopy (LENS), University of Florence, Sesto Fiorentino, Italy*

JOÃO QUINTAS COENTRO • *Regenerative, Modular & Developmental Engineering Laboratory (REMODEL), National University of Ireland Galway, Galway, Ireland; Science Foundation Ireland Centre for Research in Medical Devices (CÚRAM), National University of Ireland Galway, Galway, Ireland*

ELAINE C. DAVIS • *Department of Anatomy and Cell Biology, McGill University, Montreal, QC, Canada*

BENOIT DE CROMBRUGGHE • *MD Anderson Cancer Center, The University of Texas, Houston, TX, USA*

RODNEY J. DILLEY • *Ear Science Institute Australia, Perth, Western Australia, Australia; School of Surgery (M509), University of Western Australia, Perth, Western Australia, Australia; Center for Cell Therapy and Regenerative Medicine, University of Western Australia, Perth, Western Australia, Australia*

JIE DING • *Wound Healing Research Group, Division of Plastic and Reconstructive Surgery, Department of Surgery, University of Alberta, Edmonton, AB, Canada*

COLE R. DRIFKA • *Laboratory for Optical and Computational Instrumentation, University of Wisconsin, Madison, WI, USA; Department of Biomedical Engineering, University of Wisconsin, Madison, WI, USA; Morgridge Institute for Research, Madison, WI, USA*

BEATE ECKES • *Department of Dermatology, University of Cologne, Cologne, Germany*

KEVIN W. ELICEIRI • *Laboratory for Optical and Computational Instrumentation, University of Wisconsin, Madison, WI, USA; Department of Biomedical Engineering, University of Wisconsin, Madison, WI, USA; Morgridge Institute for Research, Madison, WI, USA*

FARZAD FEREIDOUNI • *Department of Pathology and Laboratory Medicine, University of California-Davis Medical Center, Sacramento, CA, USA*

GARY J. FISHER • *Department of Dermatology, University of Michigan Medical School, Ann Arbor, MI, USA*
DANIELA FRACCAROLLO • *Department of Cardiology and Angiology, Medical School Hannover, Hannover, Germany*
PAOLO GALUPPO • *Department of Cardiology and Angiology, Medical School Hannover, Hannover, Germany*
AZIZ GHAHARY • *BC Professional Firefighters' Burn and Wound Healing Laboratory, Department of Surgery, Division of Plastic Surgery, University of British Columbia, Vancouver, BC, Canada*
VASILIKI GKRETSI • *Cancer Biophysics Laboratory, Department of Mechanical and Manufacturing Engineering, University of Cyprus, Nicosia, Cyprus, Greece*
FRANCINA GONZALEZ DE LOS SANTOS • *Department of Pathology, University of Michigan Medical School, Ann Arbor, MI, USA*
VALERIA GRACEFFA • *Regenerative, Modular & Developmental Engineering Laboratory (REMODEL), National University of Ireland Galway, Galway, Ireland; Science Foundation Ireland Centre for Research in Medical Devices (CÚRAM), National University of Ireland Galway, Galway, Ireland*
YANG GUO • *Department of Chemistry, University of Michigan, Ann Arbor, MI, USA*
ZACHARY T. HARMANY • *Department of Pathology and Laboratory Medicine, University of California-Davis Medical Center, Sacramento, CA, USA*
J. ROBIN HARRIS • *Institute of Zoology, University of Mainz, Mainz, Germany*
JAMAR HAWKINS • *Department of Mechanical and Industrial Engineering, University of Massachusetts, Amherst, MA, USA*
JULIA HOFFMANN • *Ludwig Boltzmann Institute for Lung Vascular Research, Graz, Austria*
AMY L. HORWELL • *Department of Musculoskeletal Biology, Institute of Ageing and Chronic Disease, University of Liverpool, Liverpool, UK*
MICHAEL S. HU • *Hagey Laboratory for Pediatric Regenerative Medicine, Division of Plastic and Reconstructive Surgery, Department of Surgery, School of Medicine, Stanford University, Stanford, CA, USA; Institute for Stem Cell Biology and Regenerative Medicine, Stanford University, Stanford, CA, USA; Department of Surgery, John A. Burns School of Medicine, University of Hawai'i, Honolulu, HI, USA*
AUDREY E.K. HUTCHEON • *Schepens Eye Research Institute/MEE and Department of Ophthalmology, Harvard Medical School, Boston, MA, USA*
GISLI JENKINS • *Division of Respiratory Medicine, School of Medicine, Nottingham City Hospital, University of Nottingham, Nottingham, UK*
SERGIO A. JIMENEZ • *The Joan and Joel Rosenbloom Center for Fibrotic Diseases and The Jefferson Institute of Molecular Medicine, Thomas Jefferson University, Philadelphia, PA, USA*
ALISON E. JOHN • *Division of Respiratory Medicine, School of Medicine, Nottingham City Hospital, University of Nottingham, Nottingham, UK*
ADIB KEIKHOSRAVI • *Laboratory for Optical and Computational Instrumentation, University of Wisconsin, Madison, WI, USA; Department of Biomedical Engineering, University of Wisconsin, Madison, WI, USA*
SABINE KLEIN • *Laboratory for Liver Fibrosis and Portal Hypertension, Department of Internal Medicine I, University of Clinic Bonn, Bonn, Germany*
GRAZYNA KWAPISZEWSKA • *Ludwig Boltzmann Institute for Lung Vascular Research, Graz, Austria; Institute of Physiology, Medical University of Graz, Graz, Austria*

TRIPP LEAVITT • *Hagey Laboratory for Pediatric Regenerative Medicine, Division of Plastic and Reconstructive Surgery, Department of Surgery, School of Medicine, Stanford University, Stanford, CA, USA; Boston University School of Medicine, Boston, MA, USA*

RICHARD M. LEVENSON • *Department of Pathology and Laboratory Medicine, University of California-Davis Medical Center, Sacramento, CA, USA*

IAN M.H. LI • *Department of Musculoskeletal Biology, Institute of Ageing and Chronic Disease, University of Liverpool, Liverpool, UK*

LING LI • *Department of Anatomy and Cell Biology, McGill University, Montreal, QC, Canada*

LAWRENCE J. LIEW • *Ear Science Institute Australia, Perth, Western Australia, Australia; School of Surgery (M509), University of Western Australia, Perth, Western Australia, Australia*

YUMING LIU • *Laboratory for Optical and Computational Instrumentation, University of Wisconsin, Madison, WI, USA*

TIANJU LIU • *Department of Pathology, University of Michigan Medical School, Ann Arbor, MI, USA*

MICHAEL T. LONGAKER • *Hagey Laboratory for Pediatric Regenerative Medicine, Division of Plastic and Reconstructive Surgery, Department of Surgery, School of Medicine, Stanford University, Stanford, CA, USA; Institute for Stem Cell Biology and Regenerative Medicine, Stanford University, Stanford, CA, USA*

EDWARD MACARAK • *The Joan and Joel Rosenbloom Center for Fibrotic Diseases and The Jefferson Institute of Molecular Medicine, Thomas Jefferson University, Philadelphia, PA, USA*

GUNEET S. MEHTA • *Laboratory for Optical and Computational Instrumentation, University of Wisconsin, Madison, WI, USA; Department of Biomedical Engineering, University of Wisconsin, Madison, WI, USA*

ANNE MARIA MULLEN • *Teagasc Research CentreAshtown, Dublin, Ireland*

LAYLA NABAI • *BC Professional Firefighters' Burn and Wound Healing Laboratory, Department of Surgery, Division of Plastic Surgery, University of British Columbia, Vancouver, BC, Canada*

GIULIA NOBILE • *Unit of Biochemistry, Department of Molecular Medicine, University of Pavia, Pavia, Italy*

HUAN TING ONG • *Ear Science Institute Australia, Perth, Western Australia, Australia*

COSTAS S. PATRICKIOS • *Department of Chemistry, University of Cyprus, Nicosia, Cyprus, Greece*

FRANCESCO S. PAVONE • *European Laboratory for Non-linear Spectroscopy (LENS), University of Florence, Sesto Fiorentino, Italy; Department of Physics, University of Florence, Sesto Fiorentino, Italy*

SEM H. PHAN • *Department of Pathology, University of Michigan Medical School, Ann Arbor, MI, USA*

SONSOLES PIERA-VELAZQUEZ • *The Joan and Joel Rosenbloom Center for Fibrotic Diseases and The Jefferson Institute of Molecular Medicine, Thomas Jefferson University, Philadelphia, PA, USA*

GIAMPIERO PIETROCOLA • *Unit of Biochemistry, Department of Molecular Medicine, University of Pavia, Pavia, Italy*

BARTOSZ PILECKI • *Institute of Molecular Medicine, University of Southern Denmark, Odense C, Denmark*

JOANNE PORTE • *Division of Respiratory Medicine, School of Medicine, Nottingham City Hospital, University of Nottingham, Nottingham, UK*
NAHUM PUEBLA-OSORIO • *Department of Lymphoma/Myeloma, The University of Texas M.D. Anderson Cancer Center, Houston, TX, USA*
MICHAEL RAGHUNATH • *Centre for Cell Biology & Tissue Engineering, Competence Centre Tissue Engineering for Drug Development (TEDD), Department Life Sciences and Facility Management, Institute for Chemistry and Biotechnology (ICBT), Zürich University of Applied Sciences, Wädenswil, Switzerland*
SIMONETTA RINDI • *Unit of Biochemistry, Department of Molecular Medicine, University of Pavia, Pavia, Italy*
LAURE RITTIÉ • *Department of Dermatology, University of Michigan Medical School, Ann Arbor, MI, USA; Dermatology Therapeutic Area, GlaxoSmithKline, Collegeville, PA, USA*
JOEL ROSENBLOOM • *The Joan and Joel Rosenbloom Center for Fibrotic Diseases and The Jefferson Institute of Molecular Medicine, Thomas Jefferson University, Philadelphia, PA, USA*
SERI N.E. SARCHIO • *Cellular Photoimmunology Group, Discipline of Infectious Diseases and Immunology, Sydney Medical School at The Charles Perkins Centre, University of Sydney, Sydney, NSW, Australia; Faculty of Medicine and Health Sciences, Universiti Putra MalaysiaMalaysia, Malaysia*
SIBILLE SAUER-LEHNEN • *Institute of Molecular Pathobiochemistry, Experimental Gene Therapy and Clinical Chemistry, RWTH University Hospital Aachen, Aachen, Germany*
GABRIELE SCHERR • *Department of Dermatology, University of Cologne, Cologne, Germany*
ROBERT SCHIERWAGEN • *European Foundation for the Study of Chronic Liver Failure, Barcelona, Spain*
GRITH LYKKE SØRENSEN • *Institute of Molecular Medicine, University of Southern Denmark, Odense C, Denmark*
PIETRO SPEZIALE • *Unit of Biochemistry, Department of Molecular Medicine, University of Pavia, Pavia, Italy*
TRIANTAFYLLOS STYLIANOPOULOS • *Cancer Biophysics Laboratory, Department of Mechanical and Manufacturing Engineering, University of Cyprus, Nicosia, Cyprus, Greece*
ANDREAS STYLIANOU • *Cancer Biophysics Laboratory, Department of Mechanical and Manufacturing Engineering, University of Cyprus, Nicosia, Cyprus, Greece*
YUBING SUN • *Department of Mechanical and Industrial Engineering, University of Massachusetts, Amherst, MA, USA*
FRANK TACKE • *Department of Internal Medicine III, RWTH University Hospital Aachen, Aachen, Germany*
CARMEN G. TAG • *Institute of Molecular Pathobiochemistry, Experimental Gene Therapy and Clinical Chemistry, RWTH University Hospital Aachen, Aachen, Germany*
AMANDA L. TATLER • *Division of Respiratory Medicine, School of Medicine, Nottingham City Hospital, University of Nottingham, Nottingham, UK*
RICHARD TOWNSEND • *Biotechnology, Henry Ford College, Dearborn, MI, USA*
JONEL TREBICKA • *Institute for Bioengineering of Catalonia, Barcelona, Spain*
EDWARD E. TREDGET • *Wound Healing Research Group, Division of Plastic and Reconstructive Surgery, Department of Surgery, University of Alberta, Edmonton, AB, Canada; Division of Critical Care Medicine, Department of Surgery, University of Alberta, Edmonton, AB, Canada*

LAM C. TSOI • *Department of Dermatology, University of Michigan, Ann Arbor, MI, USA; Department of Computational Medicine & Bioinformatics, University of Michigan, Ann Arbor, MI, USA; Department of Biostatistics, University of Michigan, Ann Arbor, MI, USA*

FRANZISKA E. UHL • *Department of Med-Pulmonary, College of Medicine, University of Vermont, Burlington, VT, USA*

STEPHEN E. ULLRICH • *Department of Immunology and the Center for Cancer Immunology Research, The University of Texas M.D. Anderson Cancer Center, Houston, TX, USA*

FRANK ERHARD USCHNER • *Faculty of Health Sciences, University of Southern Denmark, Odense, Denmark*

DARCY E. WAGNER • *Comprehensive Pneumology Center, Lung Repair and Regeneration, Helmholtz Zentrum München and University Hospital of the Ludwig Maximilians Universität, Member of the German Center for Lung Research (DZL), Munich, Germany*

FANG WANG • *Department of Dermatology, University of Cologne, Cologne, Germany*

SABINE WEISKIRCHEN • *Institute of Molecular Pathobiochemistry, Experimental Gene Therapy and Clinical Chemistry, RWTH University Hospital Aachen, Aachen, Germany*

RALF WEISKIRCHEN • *Institute of Molecular Pathobiochemistry, Experimental Gene Therapy and Clinical Chemistry, RWTH University Hospital Aachen, Aachen, Germany*

DANIEL J. WEISS • *Department of Med-Pulmonary, College of Medicine, University of Vermont, Burlington, VT, USA*

JOCHEN WILHELM • *Department of Internal Medicine, Justus-Liebig-University, Giessen, Germany; Universities of Giessen and Marburg Lung Center (UGMLC), Giessen, Germany*

CHRISTAL A. WORTHEN • *Department of Dermatology, University of Michigan Medical School, Ann Arbor, MI, USA*

ZHUNING WU • *Regenerative, Modular & Developmental Engineering Laboratory (REMODEL), National University of Ireland Galway, Galway, Ireland; Science Foundation Ireland Centre for Research in Medical Devices (CÚRAM), National University of Ireland Galway, Galway, Ireland*

TIANFA XIE • *Department of Mechanical and Industrial Engineering, University of Massachusetts, Amherst, MA, USA*

TOSHIYUKI YAMAMOTO • *Department of Dermatology, Fukushima Medical University, Fukushima, Japan*

DIMITRIOS I. ZEUGOLIS • *Regenerative, Modular & Developmental Engineering Laboratory (REMODEL), National University of Ireland Galway, Galway, Ireland; Science Foundation Ireland Centre for Research in Medical Devices (CÚRAM), National University of Ireland Galway, Galway, Ireland*

JAMES D. ZIESKE • *Schepens Eye Research Institute/MEE and Department of Ophthalmology, Harvard Medical School, Boston, MA, USA*

PAOLA ZIGRINO • *Department of Dermatology, University of Cologne, Cologne, Germany*

Chapter 1

Human Fibrotic Diseases: Current Challenges in Fibrosis Research

Joel Rosenbloom, Edward Macarak, Sonsoles Piera-Velazquez, and Sergio A. Jimenez

Abstract

Human fibrotic diseases constitute a major health problem worldwide owing to the large number of affected individuals, the incomplete knowledge of the fibrotic process pathogenesis, the marked heterogeneity in their etiology and clinical manifestations, the absence of appropriate and fully validated biomarkers, and, most importantly, the current void of effective disease-modifying therapeutic agents. The fibrotic disorders encompass a wide spectrum of clinical entities including systemic fibrotic diseases such as systemic sclerosis (SSc), sclerodermatous graft vs. host disease, and nephrogenic systemic fibrosis, as well as numerous organ-specific disorders including radiation-induced fibrosis and cardiac, pulmonary, liver, and kidney fibrosis. Although their causative mechanisms are quite diverse and in several instances have remained elusive, these diseases share the common feature of an uncontrolled and progressive accumulation of fibrotic tissue in affected organs causing their dysfunction and ultimate failure. Despite the remarkable heterogeneity in the etiologic mechanisms responsible for the development of fibrotic diseases and in their clinical manifestations, numerous studies have identified activated myofibroblasts as the common cellular element ultimately responsible for the replacement of normal tissues with nonfunctional fibrotic tissue. Critical signaling cascades, initiated primarily by transforming growth factor-β (TGF-β), but also involving numerous cytokines and signaling molecules which stimulate profibrotic reactions in myofibroblasts, offer potential therapeutic targets. Here, we briefly review the current knowledge of the molecular mechanisms involved in the development of tissue fibrosis and point out some of the most important challenges to research in the fibrotic diseases and to the development of effective therapeutic approaches for this often fatal group of disorders. Efforts to further clarify the complex pathogenetic mechanisms of the fibrotic process should be encouraged to attain the elusive goal of developing effective therapies for these serious, untreatable, and often fatal disorders.

Key words Fibrotic disease, Fibrosis, Transforming growth factor-β (TGF-β), Myofibroblasts, Extracellular matrix, Collagen, Systemic sclerosis, Idiopathic pulmonary fibrosis

1 Introduction

Virtually every organ in the human body can be affected by physiologic and pathologic fibrotic reactions. Under homeostatic conditions, these reactions are self-limited and constitute an

Laure Rittié (ed.), *Fibrosis: Methods and Protocols*, Methods in Molecular Biology, vol. 1627,
DOI 10.1007/978-1-4939-7113-8_1, © Springer Science+Business Media LLC 2017

important reparative process aimed at the restoration of the functional integrity of injured tissues through a complex sequence of events known as normal tissue repair. However, under pathologic circumstances, the normal tissue repair reaction escapes the homeostatic regulatory mechanisms and evolves into an uncontrolled fibrotic process characterized by the progressive and uncontrolled accumulation of exaggerated amounts of fibrotic tissue which disrupts the normal organ architecture and ultimately leads to organ failure [1–3]. These reactions cause multi-system diseases such as systemic sclerosis (SSc) [4–6] and nephrogenic systemic fibrosis [7, 8], as well as fibrotic disorders affecting individual organs including the pulmonary, kidney, liver, cardiac, and bladder. The most common systemic and organ-specific fibrotic disorders are listed in Table 1. Owing to the widespread and multi-organ occurrence of fibrotic diseases, it is difficult to determine their total incidence, although it has been estimated that as high as 45% of the mortality in Western developed countries is caused by their collective occurrence [1]. Despite considerable understanding of the pathogenesis of the fibrotic process attained recently [1–3, 10–15], there remains no effective disease-modifying therapy for these serious and often fatal diseases.

Although the causative mechanisms of the fibrotic diseases are quite diverse, they all share common molecular alterations that result in the exaggerated and uncontrolled accumulation of extracellular matrix (ECM) macromolecules in the affected tissues and in the replacement of normal tissues with nonfunctional fibrotic tissue [1–3, 10–15]. Such replacement is responsible for their extensive morbidity and high mortality. At the cellular level, it is broadly accepted that myofibroblasts are the cells ultimately responsible for the pathologic fibrotic process in the fibrotic disorders [16–21]. Myofibroblasts comprise a distinctive population of mesenchymal cells expressing α-smooth muscle actin (α-SMA) and displaying a marked increase in the production of fibrillar collagens (types I, III, V, and VI) and other ECM macromolecules coupled with an increase in TIMP production leading to inhibition of ECM-degradative enzymes [22–25]. Furthermore, myofibroblasts induce changes in the biomechanical properties of the affected tissues causing a progressive increase in tissue stiffness, a newly recognized extremely potent profibrotic stimulus [26–30].

The origin of myofibroblasts may vary depending upon the organ affected and the particular fibrotic reaction [18, 19, 31]. There are several potential sources including (1) recruitment of fibroblast precursor cells (fibrocytes) from the bone marrow; (2) transdifferentiation of various differentiated cell types including pericytes, adipocytes, and epithelial, mesothelial, and endothelial cells into a mesenchymal phenotype; and (3) proliferation and activation of quiescent tissue-resident fibroblasts into a myofibroblast phenotype. The current preponderance of opinion is that the

Table 1
Systemic and organ specific of human fibrotic diseases [Adapted from ref. 9]

A. Systemic fibrotic diseases
• Systemic sclerosis
• Multifocal fibrosclerosis (IgG_4-associated fibrosis)
• Nephrogenic systemic fibrosis
• Sclerodermatous graft vs. host disease
B. Organ-specific fibrotic diseases
Cardiac fibrosis
• Hypertension-associated cardiac fibrosis
• Post-myocardial infarction
• Chagas disease-induced myocardial fibrosis
Kidney fibrosis
• Diabetic and hypertensive nephropathy
• Urinary tract obstruction-induced kidney fibrosis
• Inflammatory/autoimmune-induced kidney fibrosis
• Aristolochic acid nephropathy
• Polycystic kidney disease
Pulmonary fibrosis
• Idiopathic pulmonary fibrosis
• Silica-induced pneumoconiosis (silicosis)
• Asbestos-induced pulmonary fibrosis (asbestosis)
• Chemotherapeutic agent-induced pulmonary fibrosis
Liver and portal vein fibrosis
• Alcoholic and nonalcoholic liver fibrosis
• Hepatitis C-induced liver fibrosis
• Primary biliary cirrhosis
• Parasite-induced liver fibrosis (schistosomiasis)
C. Other organ-specific fibrotic diseases
• Radiation-induced fibrosis (various organs)
• Bladder fibrosis
• Intestinal fibrosis
• Peritoneal sclerosis

(continued)

Table 1
(continued)

• Diffuse fasciitis
• Localized scleroderma, keloids
• Dupuytren's disease
• Peyronie's disease
• Myelofibrosis
• Oral submucous fibrosis

activation of tissue-resident fibroblasts is the major source of activated myofibroblasts, although epithelial to mesenchymal transition (EMT), endothelial to mesenchymal transition (EndoMT), or pericyte to myofibroblast transition may play a role under specific circumstances [9, 18, 31, 32]. Besides the transdifferentiation of these cells, recent studies have demonstrated that Gli1+ progenitor mesenchymal stem-like cells with preferential perivascular localization represent an important source for the generation of myofibroblasts in renal fibrotic diseases [33–35] and that the majority of dermal myofibroblasts in SSc-induced cutaneous fibrosis arise from adiponectin-positive progenitor adipocytes [36–38] in a process mediated by FIZZ1 [39]. It should be emphasized, however, that even though the transdifferentiation of various cell types may not be a predominant source of myofibroblasts during fibrotic disorders, the alterations in the phenotype of the transdifferentiated cells may result in the production and secretion of profibrotic factors, including TGF-β, playing an important role in the fibrotic process. Furthermore, these phenotypically modified cells may produce numerous macromolecules which may enhance the fibrotic response such as the EDA form of fibronectin (Fn^{EDA}) and other ECM components including proteoglycans and several matricellular molecules [40–42].

2 Targeting Myofibroblast Activation for Inhibition of Tissue Fibrosis

There are multiple potential levels that could be targeted for inhibition of the fibrotic response, including elimination of the primary cause such as by treatment of viral hepatitis, diminution of the immunologic and inflammatory responses in SSc and idiopathic pulmonary fibrosis (IPF), and elimination of the untoward profibrotic activities of myofibroblasts. Regrettably, owing to the lack of a comprehensive understanding of the etiologic mechanisms in the majority of the fibrotic disorders, opportunities for elimination of the originating cause of the fibrotic reaction are rare, and reduction of the immunologic and inflammatory responses has proven to be generally ineffective in abrogating pathologic fibrotic processes. Thus, modulation of the deleterious profibrotic activity of myofibroblasts remains the most attractive therapeutic approach. This, in turn, requires that the control of molecular reactions most important in generating the excessive ECM by the myofibroblast be precisely understood, as discussed recently [43]. In the following sections, the molecular pathways involved in myofibroblast activation and in the expression of their potent profibrotic effects will be briefly reviewed.

3 The Transforming Growth Factor-β (TGF-β) Pathways

The TGF-β family of proteins comprises several pleiotropic growth factors that play crucial roles in numerous physiological processes including embryogenesis, cellular development and differentiation, immunologic system development, inflammatory response functions, and wound repair [44–48]. Furthermore, numerous studies have shown that the three TGF-β isoforms are potent inducers of myofibroblasts either through activation of quiescent fibroblasts or through the phenotypic conversion of various cell types into activated myofibroblasts [49–51]. The TGF-βs are the most potent inducers of profibrotic cellular effects, and owing to their potent profibrotic activities, they have been implicated in the pathogenesis of various fibrotic human diseases [52–57]. The profibrogenic effects of TGF-β are mediated by the transcriptional stimulation of the expression of critical genes involved in the fibrotic process as well as by several important posttranslational epigenetic regulatory mechanisms [58].

TGF-β is initially produced as an inactive homodimeric peptide which is secreted into the extracellular space as a large latent complex. This complex consists of latent TGF-β-binding protein covalently bound to a small latency complex which in turn is formed by a homodimer of TGF-β bound to an arginine-glycine-aspartate (RGD) containing N-terminal latency associated binding peptide [59–62]. TGF-β can undergo several alternative proteolytic or conformational activating events. Once activated TGF-β binds to a serine/threonine transmembrane receptor kinase known as TGF-β receptor II (TβRII). The intracellular transduction pathways following TGF-β binding to its cognate receptors are complex and involve both Smad-mediated pathways referred to as canonical and non-Smad pathways referred to as noncanonical [63–65]. These pathways are diagrammatically illustrated in Fig. 1. In the canonical pathway, the ligand-bound TβRII recruits and phosphorylates a TGF-β receptor I (TβRI). There are several TβRI which are known as activin-like kinases (ALKs), with ALK-5 being the most

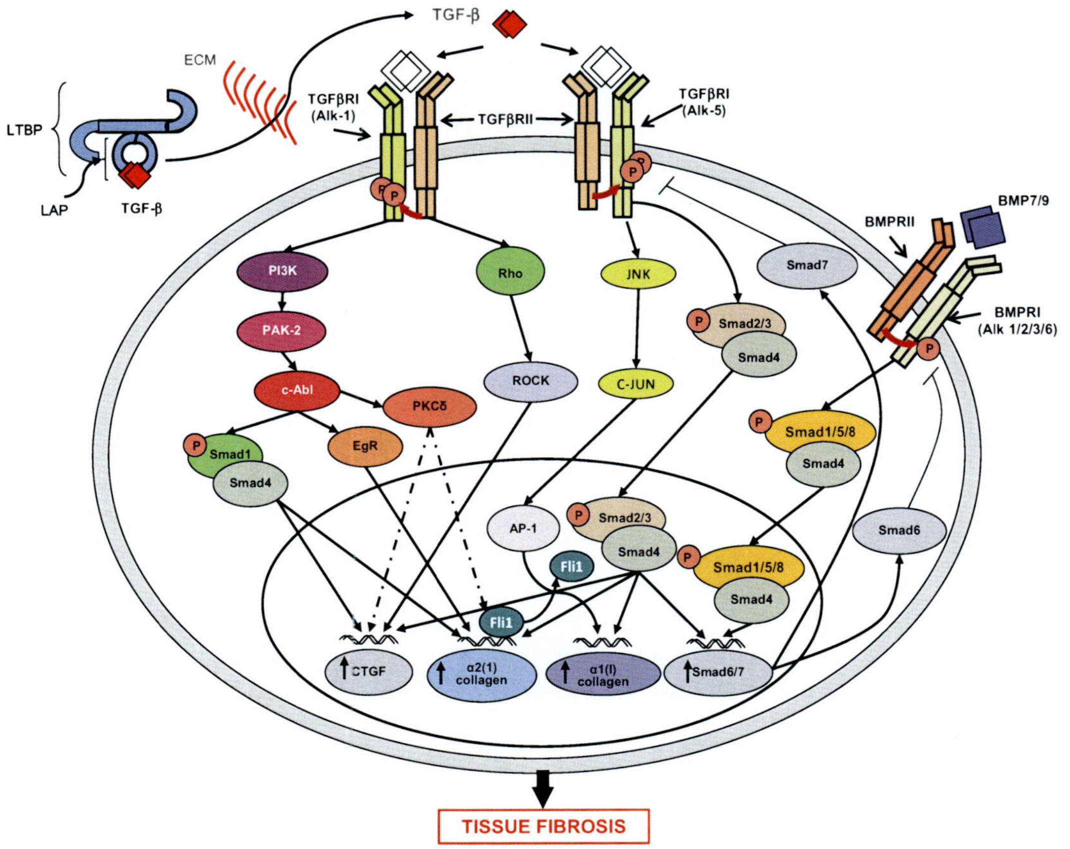

Fig. 1 TGF-β and BMP-signaling pathways critical for the fibrotic response. Following TGF-β binding, the TGFβRII receptor recruits a TGFβRI, either activin-like kinase (Alk)-1 or Alk-5 and activates it by phosphorylation. Alk-5 then specifically phosphorylates receptor-regulated Smad2 and Smad3 which then complex with Co-Smad4 resulting in their transport to the nucleus where they interact with various co-activators or co-repressors to regulate transcription of critical genes, here represented by connective tissue growth factor (CTGF/CCN2) and COL1A1 and COL1A2 genes. Also illustrated are several TGF-β signaling noncanonical pathways. An important one involves the phosphorylation and activation of the cellular c-Abelson kinase (c-Abl) non-receptor resulting in activation of several downstream critical factors including Smad1, early growth response protein (Egr-1), and protein kinase C delta (PKC-δ), all of which contribute to the fibrotic response. The pathways mediating the anti-fibrotic effects of BMP involve binding to specific BMP receptors with subsequent phosphorylation of the type I receptor and activation of Smads 1/5/8 forming a heterotrimeric complex that enters the nucleus and stimulates the expression of genes encoding the inhibitory Smads 6 and 7. Increased production of these inhibitory Smads results in important anti-fibrotic effects mediated at least in part by inhibition of TGF-β and BMP receptor activation. [Adapted from ref. 11]

important in the context of the fibrotic process. ALK-5 is phosphorylated by TβRII, and signaling from the phosphorylated TβRI to the nucleus occurs through the receptor-activated R-Smads, Smad2, and Smad3, which are phosphorylated by TβR1. The phosphorylated Smad2/Smad3 then bind to the co-Smad, Smad4, forming a complex that translocates across the nuclear membrane. The Smad complex within the nucleus in association with various transcription factors, co-activators, and co-repressors modulates the expression of target genes [58, 64]. Noncanonical TGF-β-initiated signaling cascades are independent of R-Smads. These noncanonical pathways can be activated in a cell-specific and context-dependent manner and mediate important TGF-β profibrotic effects [63, 65]. For example, TGF-β stimulation leads to the activation of PI3K, which in turn activates two important profibrotic pathways: p21-activated kinase (PAK2)/c-Abelson kinase (c-Abl) and Akt-mTORC1 [66]. Downstream targets of c-Abl include several mediators involved in the fibrotic response. Activated c-Abl phosphorylates protein kinase C-δ (PKC-δ), a potent profibrotic mediator recently shown to upregulate collagen gene transcription in SSc dermal fibroblasts [67]. Phosphorylated PKC-δ has also been shown to in turn phosphorylate the transcription factor Fli1, reversing its inhibitory effect on collagen gene expression [68]. Another important non-Smad-signaling pathway is through activation of c-Jun-N-terminal kinase (JNK) resulting in the activation of c-Jun, a critical profibrotic transcription factor [63, 65]. Besides serine/threonine phosphorylation, TβRII can also be phosphorylated on tyrosine residues in response to TGF-β [69, 70] leading to activation of ERK1/2 MAPK which plays an important role by regulating myofibroblast formation as well as ECM synthesis [71, 72].

One of the important aspects of TGF-β action is the stimulation of other mediators having fibrogenic potential. These include, but are not limited to, connective tissue growth factor (CTGF or CCN2; see Subheading 5.3), platelet-derived growth factor (PDGF), and epidermal growth factor (EGF/ErbB) ligands. For example, it has been demonstrated that TGF-β-induced ErbB activation was achieved by upregulation of ErbB ligands through autocrine signaling from the PDGF receptor (PDGFR) via MEK/ERK [73]. It is obvious from the above that the molecular changes initiated by TGF-β are complex. Nevertheless, although challenging, approaches with therapeutic agents can be carefully designed to take advantage of specific points within critical pathways to abrogate their deleterious profibrotic effects.

4 Bone Morphogenetic Protein (BMP) Signaling in Fibrosis

The BMPs comprise several proteins that are members of the TGF-β superfamily of growth factors. The BMPs were originally described for their ability to induce de novo formation of bone tissue in vivo; however, numerous studies have shown that these proteins have a variety of other important biological activities [74, 75]. Among their pleiotropic effects, recent studies have demonstrated that some BMPs may also participate in the pathogenesis of fibrosis [76, 77]. In contrast to the TGF-βs, however, several BMPs including BMP-6, BMP-7, and BMP-9 exert anti-fibrotic effects and have been considered to represent a counterbalance mechanism to modulate the profibrotic effects of the TGF-βs. BMP-7 and BMP-9 are the most extensively studied BMPs in the context of tissue fibrotic reactions [78–80]. The BMP signaling pathways are highly similar to those involved in TGF-β profibrotic signaling [81–83]. BMPs bind to their specific membrane-associated receptors (BMPRs) inducing the phosphorylation of the type I BMP receptor and, as a result, activating and phosphorylating Smads 1, 5, and 8. Phosphorylated Smads1/5/8 form heteromeric complexes with Smad4 that translocate into the nucleus to induce specific gene transcriptional effects [84, 85], as shown in Fig. 1.

The mechanisms involved in the anti-fibrotic effects of the BMPs are complex and have not been fully elucidated, although it has become apparent that some of these effects are mediated through the induction of expression and the production of inhibitory Smad proteins 6 and 7. Smad 6 and 7 block the TGF-β signaling pathways at the TGF-β receptor activation level and very likely also at the transcriptional level abrogating the effects mediated by the receptor-activated Smad pathways [86–88]. BMP-7 has also been shown to block the activation of Smad-dependent as well as Smad-independent pathways', such as p38, ERK, and MAPKs, effects mediated by the activation of Smads 1 and 5 opposing TGF-β/Smad3 activation [87, 89]. BMP-7 also antagonizes TGF-β1-induced suppression of matrix degradation by abrogating TGF-β1-induced inactivation of MMP-2 [90]. Although the anti-fibrotic role of BMPs has been demonstrated in numerous in vitro and in vivo studies and it has been shown that BMP-6 and BMP-7 play a protective role in some forms of liver and kidney fibrosis [77, 91–93], some other studies have indicated that BMP-9 may stimulate the production of certain proteins that have been implicated in liver fibrosis [76].

5 Other Molecular Pathways Involved in the Fibrotic Process

The generation of excessive amounts of ECM and the abnormal deposition of these molecules during the establishment and progression of the fibrotic process are extremely complex, and although the TGF-β family of growth factors play the most important role, there are numerous other molecular pathways that also participate depending on the specific trigger initiating the fibrotic process and the tissues or organs involved. Although the diverse mechanisms mediated by these pathways result in an extremely intricate picture, the detailed understanding of their components and of their interactions during the establishment and progression of the fibrotic process may provide novel therapeutic targets to modify the

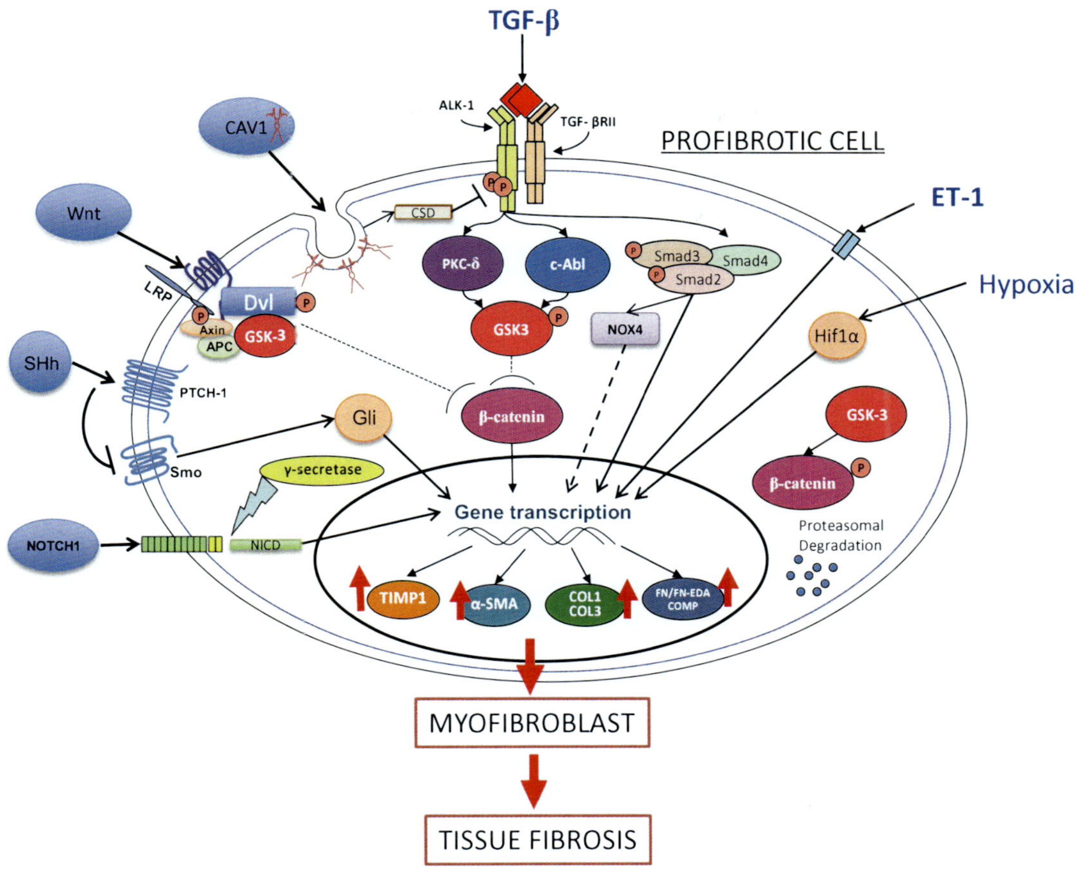

Fig. 2 Molecular mechanisms of tissue fibrotic reactions. The diagram shows the TGF-β, ET-1, NOTCH, CAV-1, WNT, NOX4, and HIF-1α pathways that may participate in the development of tissue fibrotic reactions. The central pathway is initiated following TGF-β binding and subsequent activation of Smad-dependent and Smad-independent TGF-β intracellular signaling. Most of the other pathways have been shown to interact or to modulate the TGF-β-mediated cascades. The ultimate effect of these complex intracellular signaling events is the activation of a profibrotic transcriptional gene regulation program leading to pathological tissue fibrosis caused by the activation of myofibroblasts and their increased production of various myofibroblast-specific and profibrotic macromolecules including α-SMA, COL1, COL3, FN, FN-EDA, COMP, and MMP inhibitor TIMP. [Adapted from ref. 9]

devastating effects of the fibrotic diseases. Some of these pathways are illustrated in Fig. 2 and will be briefly reviewed in the following sections.

5.1 Matrix Stiffness and Rho-Associated Kinases

While activation of myofibroblasts and stimulation of ECM production by TGF-β and other cytokines are complex and incompletely understood, recent studies have focused on the roles of reorganization of the actin cytoskeleton. In this regard, there is increasing interest in the mechanical properties of the ECM, particularly of the effect of tissue stiffness on the behavior of resident fibroblasts with respect to their biosynthetic activities [27–30, 94, 95]. Although the exact mechanisms whereby increased matrix stiffness stimulates production of polymerized α-SMA remain to be elucidated, this effect can result in nuclear translocation of megakaryoblastic leukemia factor (MKL)-1, a transcription factor that plays a critical role in the stimulation of expression of fibrotic genes [95]. Furthermore, stiffening can promote RhoA production and activation, resulting in increased ROCK activity and enhanced fibroblast contractility. In addition, there may be cross talk between the MAP kinase ERK 1/2, a potential downstream target of ROCK, and TGF-β [96]. All these findings suggest that as the fibrotic process proceeds and tissues become increasingly stiff, a vicious cycle gets established in which the matrix stiffness itself promotes further ECM production.

5.2 Endothelin-1

Endothelin-1 (ET-1) is a polypeptide with potent vasoconstrictive activity and is a major factor in the pathophysiology of pulmonary arterial hypertension [97, 98]. Extensive experimental evidence indicates that ET-1 may also have profibrotic activity and play a role in organ fibrosis [99–101]. Indeed, it has been demonstrated that ET-1 not only can increase the production of ECM macromolecules such as collagen types I and III, but also it has been shown that ET-1 inhibits production of matrix metalloproteinase-1 in normal human fibroblasts [102]. Furthermore, increased levels of ET-1 have been found in several fibrotic diseases and in experimental pulmonary fibrosis [100, 103, 104]. Additionally, ET-1 may have a potential role in the generation of myofibroblasts through EMT or EndoMT, effects possibly mediated through the endothelin A receptor [105, 106] and through the synergistic stimulation of TGF-β induced EndoMT [107, 108]. These findings, collectively, strongly suggest that ET-1 may play an important role in the pathophysiology of human fibrotic diseases.

5.3 Connective Tissue Growth Factor (CTGF/ CCN2)

CTGF, also known as CCN2, a growth factor with multiple effects, is now regarded as an important effector in both normal and pathologic fibrotic responses [109–112]. CTGF provokes a potent profibrotic response when added to cultured fibroblasts, and elevated CTGF levels have been found in a variety of experimental fibrotic models in mice [109–114]. TGF-β stimulates CTGF synthesis in a variety of cell types, and CTGF can act as a downstream mediator to enhance the profibrotic activity of TGF-β by stimulating the production of ECM components including type I collagen and fibronectin [110, 112]. Importantly, imatinib mesylate, an inhibitor of c-Abl, blocked activation of the Smad1 pathway when normal fibroblasts were stimulated with TGF-β and inhibited stimulation of CTGF expression in SSc fibroblasts [71].Therefore, at least in some circumstances, c-Abl appears to be required for Smad1 activation. Furthermore, CTGF expression can be stimulated through the RhoA/ROCK pathway [115].

5.4 Platelet-Derived Growth Factor

The PDGF family consists of four different polypeptides (PDGF-A, PDGF-B, PDGF-C, PDGF-D) which form disulfide-bonded dimers such as PDGF-AA and PDGF-BB as well as PDGF-AB heterodimers [116].Two structurally related tyrosine kinase receptors, PDGFRα and PDGFRβ, bind PDGF ligands which leads to receptor homo- or hetero-dimerization and autophosphorylation of specific tyrosine residues within the receptor cytoplasmic domain [116–118]. This receptor activation initiates multiple signal translocation pathways including PI3K, Ras-MAPK, Src family kinases, and phospholipase Cγ (PLCγ) resulting in important cellular responses including proliferation, chemotaxis, and actin reorganization. It is now clear that PDGF can be involved in fibrotic reactions affecting multiple organs, including pulmonary, renal, and hepatic fibrosis, as well as SSc [119]. Fibroblasts can be regarded as both a major source and target since they secrete PDGF-A as well as express PDGFRα on their cell surface [120–122]. Thus, a PDGF-A-/PDGFRα-signaling loop can stimulate fibroblasts to synthesize ECM and release profibrotic mediators. Since PDGF-B is released primarily by macrophages and hepatic stellate cells, this suggests a major role for PDGF-B/PDGFRβ signaling in liver fibrosis [123, 124]. PDGF signaling becomes activated upon tissue injury to promote wound closure and is turned off when the repair processes are completed [125]. However, excessive scar formation and tissue fibrosis can result if PDGF signaling is not terminated.

5.5 Wnt-Signaling

While the Wnt proteins, consisting of a multigene family of secreted glycoproteins, play crucial roles in embryogenesis, numerous studies have shown that the Wnt/β-catenin pathway is involved in several profibrotic processes including myofibroblast activation via Smad-dependent autocrine TGF-β signaling [126–131]. Besides its structural role, β-catenin plays a critical role in canonical Wnt signaling. In the absence of Wnt signals, β-catenin is phosphorylated by a complex consisting of adenomatous polyposis coli (APC), axin, glycogen synthase kinase-3β (GSK-3β), and casein kinase which promotes subsequent ubiquitin-mediated β-catenin degradation. When secreted Wnt proteins bind to cell-surface Frizzled (FZD) receptors and lower density lipoprotein receptor-related protein co-receptor (LRP5/6), the degradation complex is disrupted resulting in the stabilization of β-catenin which translocates to the nucleus where it binds to T-cell factor/lymphoid enhancer-binding factor (Tcf/Lef) to induce target gene transcription [132, 133]. Aberrant canonical Wnt signaling has been implicated in SSc [126, 127, 130, 131] as well as in pulmonary, renal, dermal, and liver fibrosis, in addition to scarring following myocardial infarction and fibrosis accompanying muscular dystrophy [134–138]. Under homeostatic conditions, Wnt signaling must be tightly controlled. Indeed, an array of potent negative regulators has been identified, among which the Dickkopf proteins (DKK 1–4) play key roles. DKK-1 is the best studied of them, and it functions as a natural antagonist of Wnt signaling [139, 140].

5.6 Hedgehog Signaling

Three different mammalian orthologs of the *Drosophila melanogaster* hedgehog (Hh) morphogen have been identified in humans. They are highly hydrophobic-secreted peptides called sonic hedgehog (Shh), Indian hedgehog, and desert hedgehog with Shh being the most important in the present context [141]. Patched (Ptc), a 12-pass transmembrane protein, binds Hh ligands, but in the absence of ligand, Ptc interacts with and inhibits Smoothened (Smo), a seven-pass transmembrane protein [142]. However, binding of Shh to Ptc induces conformational changes that prevent Ptc from inhibiting Smo, which initiates signaling events resulting in stabilization of Gli family zinc finger transcription factors resulting in enhanced expression of Hh target genes [143]. While Hh signaling is critical during embryonic development, inappropriate activation in adults has been implicated in the pathogenesis of various diseases, including malignancies [144–146]. In SSc-cultured fibroblasts, overexpression of Shh causes accumulation of Gli-2 and increases expression of Hh target genes [147]. An extensive immunofluorescence analysis of affected SSc skin demonstrated intense staining in dermal fibroblasts and endothelial cells. Other results from this study found that TGF-β increased expression of Shh and that Shh induced strong stimulation of fibroblast to myofibroblast transition in normal dermal fibroblasts comparable to that caused by TGF-β [147]. In addition to causing a potent stimulation of the production of collagen, overexpression of Shh in the skin of mice induced fibrosis, and mice lacking one allele of the inhibitor receptor Ptc 1 gene were more sensitive to experimentally induced fibrosis [147].

5.7 Notch Signaling

Also first discovered in *Drosophila*, Notch signaling is initiated by binding of members of two ligand families, Jagged and Delta-like to Notch receptors, which results in cleavage of these receptors by the secretase complex and release of the active Notch intracellular domain (NICD) [148, 149]. Translocation of the NCID into the nucleus activates transcription of multiple target genes such as Hairy/Enhancer of Split (Hes) [150]. As with hedgehog, Notch signaling is crucial during embryonic development and is highly regulated in the adult. There is accumulating evidence for the participation of Notch signaling in fibrotic diseases, although the molecular mechanisms involved in fibroblast activation and enhanced ECM production need further determination [151–154].

5.8 Role of Hypoxia and Oxidative Stress

5.8.1 Hypoxia

In a variety of fibrotic diseases including SSc and kidney and cardiac fibrosis, hypoxia has been shown to play an important pathogenic role [155–158]. The critical cellular and molecular responses to hypoxia are mediated by HIF-1α, the key regulatory molecule. The fibrotic reaction induced by HIF-1α involves the activation of profibrotic genes [159] and the synergistic interaction of HIF-1α with profibrotic growth factors such as TGF-β and VEGF [160].

Significantly, genetic manipulation of HIF-1α in a murine proximal tubule epithelial cell model demonstrated that HIF-1α enhanced EMT in vitro and in vivo [161].

5.8.2 Oxidative Stress

Reciprocal interactions between TGF-β and reactive oxygen species (ROS) have recently been recognized as a potentially important pathway in the pathogenesis of fibrotic processes [162, 163]. Normal fibroblasts as well as other cells produce ROS which are involved in numerous essential physiological reactions. However, deleterious production of ROS can participate in the pathogenesis of fibrotic disorders including SSc, IPF, and liver fibrosis [164–166]. Although intracellular ROS can be produced by several reactions, activation of the NADPH oxidase system is responsible for most of the ROS production. There are seven NADPH oxidase isoforms, but NOX4 unlike all other members of the NOX family is constitutively active, and, therefore, its regulation occurs mainly at the expression level. The participation of NOX4 as an important downstream effector of TGF-β-induced myofibroblast generation and profibrotic effects and its role in the pathogenesis of various fibrotic disorders such as IPF and liver fibrosis have been demonstrated [167–176]. Our group recently found increased levels of NOX4 in affected SSc skin and increased expression of NOX4 transcripts in cultured SSc dermal fibroblasts. Furthermore, in confirmation of previous studies, we showed that TGF-β caused a potent stimulation of NOX4 gene expression and NOX4 protein levels and that inhibition of NOX4 by a potent and highly selective NOX4 inhibitor modified the profibrotic effects of TGF-β1 [175].

5.9 MicroRNA Involved in Tissue Fibrosis

MicroRNAs (miRNAs) are small noncoding RNA that modulate the expression of a large number of protein-coding genes at the posttranscriptional level [177]. Recent interest has been devoted to elucidating their participation in tissue fibrosis, and numerous miRNA have been shown to be involved in the fibrotic process exerting either profibrotic or anti-fibrotic effects. These effects are mediated by their ability to target a large number of translated mRNAs coded by genes involved in ECM structure, function, and homeostasis, such as those encoding collagens, matrix metalloproteinases, Smad-signaling proteins, and even TGF-β itself [178–180]. Furthermore, numerous miRNAs have been shown to play important roles in the pathogenesis of SSc and other cutaneous fibrotic disorders [181, 182], IPF [183] and cardiac, liver, and kidney fibrosis [184–186].

5.10 Role of Caveolin-1

Caveolin-1 (CAV1), the main protein component of caveolae, plays an important role in the internalization, trafficking, and degradation of TGF-β receptors and, therefore, is involved in the regulation of TGF-β signaling and TGF-β-mediated fibrotic responses [187–189]. Knockout of *Cav1* in mice (*Cav1*$^{-}$/$^{-}$) resulted in extensive skin and lung fibrosis [187, 190]. Subsequent investigation demonstrated that CAV1 protein and gene expression were markedly decreased in affected tissues from patients with SSc and IPF [190–192] and that restoration of CAV1 levels in vitro by administration of CAV1 functional domains corrected the profibrotic phenotype of these cells [192, 193]. Another important profibrotic role of CAV1 was recently shown employing immune endothelial cells isolated from lungs of *Cav1*$^{-}$/$^{-}$ mice [194]. The results demonstrated that in *Cav1*$^{-}$/$^{-}$ mice, CAV1 deficiency participates in the development and progression of tissue fibrosis and fibrotic diseases mediated by the generation of activated myofibroblasts through the establishment of EndoMT.

6 Current Challenges for Fibrosis Research

6.1 Scope of Problem

Fibrotic diseases constitute a major worldwide health problem, and although there is an increasing appreciation of their immense scope and health-related and economic impact, resources devoted to research studies in these disorders remain quite inadequate in relation to their need.

6.2 Complexity of Pathogenesis

Although substantial progress has been accomplished regarding the pathogenesis of fibrotic diseases, they still remain a major challenge, not only because of the variety and multiplicity of initiating events but also because of the large number of profibrotic mediators involved. While TGF-β is considered the primary fibrotic effector, many other cytokines and signaling molecules are involved in fibrotic reactions creating a highly complex network of redundant signaling pathways that must be considered when attempting to develop effective anti-fibrotic therapies.

6.3 Difficulty in Determination of Disease Progression

Another important challenge for research studies in the fibrotic diseases is related to severe hurdles in assessment and longitudinal evaluation of their course and progression. Several features of the fibrotic diseases pose difficulties in monitoring disease progression. (1) For the most part, these diseases are chronic in nature, extending in time for months and frequently for years; (2) while, in some instances, physiologic or radiographic tests can monitor disease progression, they are limited in scope; (3) there are no validated noninvasive biomarkers or endpoints, and (4) even within a given disease diagnosis, such as SSc or IPF, patient variability is substantial, and stratification is difficult. The end result of these difficulties is that clinical trials must extend over long periods of time, require large numbers of patients to achieve statistical power, and are exceedingly expensive. Therefore, substantial effort should be devoted to identify and prove the validity of biomarkers whose use can address the above current limitations.

6.4 Therapeutic Approaches

Currently, therapeutic interventions for the fibrotic diseases are quite limited. For example, only two drugs, pirfenidone and nintedanib, have been approved for IPF, and no disease-modifying drug has been approved for SSc or other fibrotic diseases. Because of the complex pathogenesis and the extreme redundancy of the pathways involved, it is unlikely that any single drug will be successful in arresting or modifying the progression of major fibrotic diseases. Thus, it is highly likely that simultaneous administration of several drugs will be required, a situation that presents a tremendous challenge in the design and execution of clinical trials.

Acknowledgments

Partially supported by NIH grant AR 19616 to SAJ. We thank the expert assistance of Alana Pagano and Carol Kelly in the preparation of the manuscript.

References

1. Wynn TA (2008) Cellular and molecular mechanisms of fibrosis. J Pathol 214(2):199–210. doi:10.1002/path.2277
2. Rosenbloom J, Castro SV, Jimenez SA (2010) Narrative review: fibrotic diseases: cellular and molecular mechanisms and novel therapies. Ann Intern Med 152(3):159–166. doi:10.7326/0003-4819-152-3-201002020-00007
3. Rockey DC, Bell PD, Hill JA (2015) Fibrosis – a common pathway to organ injury and failure. N Engl J Med 373(1):96. doi:10.1056/NEJMc1504848
4. Varga J, Abraham D (2007) Systemic sclerosis: a prototypic multisystem fibrotic disorder. J Clin Invest 117(3):557–567. doi:10.1172/jci31139
5. Gabrielli A, Avvedimento EV, Krieg T (2009) Scleroderma. N Engl J Med 360(19):1989–2003. doi:10.1056/NEJMra0806188
6. Ho YY, Lagares D, Tager AM et al (2014) Fibrosis – a lethal component of systemic sclerosis. Nat Rev Rheumatol 10(7):390–402. doi:10.1038/nrrheum.2014.53
7. Cowper SE, Su LD, Bhawan J et al (2001) Nephrogenic fibrosing dermopathy. Am J Dermatopathol 23(5):383–393. doi:10.1111/j.0303-6987.2005.0320e.x
8. Mendoza FA, Artlett CM, Sandorfi N et al (2006) Description of 12 cases of nephrogenic fibrosing dermopathy and review of the literature. Semin Arthritis Rheum 35(4):238–249. doi:10.1016/j.semarthrit.2005.08.002
9. Piera-Velazquez S, Mendoza FA, Jimenez SA (2016) Endothelial to mesenchymal transition (EndoMT) in the pathogenesis of human fibrotic diseases. J Clin Med 5(4). doi:10.3390/jcm5040045
10. Jimenez SA, Hitraya E, Varga J (1996) Pathogenesis of scleroderma. Collagen. Rheum Dis Clin N Am 22(4):647–674
11. Rosenbloom J, Mendoza FA, Jimenez SA (2013) Strategies for anti-fibrotic therapies. Biochim Biophys Acta 1832(7):1088–1103. doi:10.1016/j.bbadis.2012.12.007
12. Castelino FV, Varga J (2014) Emerging cellular and molecular targets in fibrosis: implications for scleroderma pathogenesis and targeted therapy. Curr Opin Rheumatol 26(6):607–614. doi:10.1097/bor.0000000000000110
13. Thannickal VJ, Henke CA, Horowitz JC et al (2014) Matrix biology of idiopathic pulmonary fibrosis: a workshop report of the National Heart, Lung, and Blood Institute. Am J Pathol 184(6):1643–1651. doi:10.1016/j.ajpath.2014.02.003
14. Karsdal MA, Manon-Jensen T, Genovese F et al (2015) Novel insights into the function and dynamics of extracellular matrix in liver fibrosis. Am J Physiol Gastrointest Liver Physiol 308(10):G807–G830. doi:10.1152/ajpgi.00447.2014
15. Denton CP (2015) Systemic sclerosis: from pathogenesis to targeted therapy. Clin Exp Rheumatol 33(4 Suppl 92):S3–S7

16. Gabbiani G (1981) The myofibroblast: a key cell for wound healing and fibrocontractive diseases. Prog Clin Biol Res 54:183–194
17. Desmouliere A (1995) Factors influencing myofibroblast differentiation during wound healing and fibrosis. Cell Biol Int 19(5):471–476. doi:10.1006/cbir.1995.1090
18. McAnulty RJ (2007) Fibroblasts and myofibroblasts: their source, function and role in disease. Int J Biochem Cell Biol 39(4):666–671. doi:10.1016/j.biocel.2006.11.005
19. Hinz B, Phan SH, Thannickal VJ et al (2007) The myofibroblast: one function, multiple origins. Am J Pathol 170(6):1807–1816. doi:10.2353/ajpath.2007.070112
20. Hinz B, Phan SH, Thannickal VJ et al (2012) Recent developments in myofibroblast biology: paradigms for connective tissue remodeling. Am J Pathol 180(4):1340–1355. doi:10.1016/j.ajpath.2012.02.004
21. Hu B, Phan SH (2013) Myofibroblasts. Curr Opin Rheumatol 25(1):71–77. doi:10.1097/BOR.0b013e32835b1352
22. Kirk TZ, Mark ME, Chua CC et al (1995) Myofibroblasts from scleroderma skin synthesize elevated levels of collagen and tissue inhibitor of metalloproteinase (TIMP-1) with two forms of TIMP-1. J Biol Chem 270(7):3423–3428
23. Abraham DJ, Eckes B, Rajkumar V et al (2007) New developments in fibroblast and myofibroblast biology: implications for fibrosis and scleroderma. Curr Rheumatol Rep 9(2):136–143. doi:10.1007/s11926-007-0008-z
24. Gilbane AJ, Denton CP, Holmes AM (2013) Scleroderma pathogenesis: a pivotal role for fibroblasts as effector cells. Arthritis Res Ther 15(3):215. doi:10.1186/ar4230
25. Kendall RT, Feghali-Bostwick CA (2014) Fibroblasts in fibrosis: novel roles and mediators. Front Pharmacol 5:123. doi:10.3389/fphar.2014.00123
26. Laurent GJ, Chambers RC, Hill MR et al (2007) Regulation of matrix turnover: fibroblasts, forces, factors and fibrosis. Biochem Soc Trans 35(Pt 4):647–651. doi:10.1042/bst0350647
27. Wells RG, Discher DE (2008) Matrix elasticity, cytoskeletal tension, and TGF-beta: the insoluble and soluble meet. Sci Signal 1(10):pe13. doi:10.1126/stke.110pe13
28. Hinz B (2009) Tissue stiffness, latent TGF-beta1 activation, and mechanical signal transduction: implications for the pathogenesis and treatment of fibrosis. Curr Rheumatol Rep 11(2):120–126
29. Parker MW, Rossi D, Peterson M et al (2014) Fibrotic extracellular matrix activates a profibrotic positive feedback loop. J Clin Invest 124(4):1622–1635. doi:10.1172/jci71386
30. Rittié L (2015) Another dimension to the importance of the extracellular matrix in fibrosis. J Cell Commun Signal 9(1):99–100. doi:10.1007/s12079-015-0282-x
31. Postlethwaite AE, Shigemitsu H, Kanangat S (2004) Cellular origins of fibroblasts: possible implications for organ fibrosis in systemic sclerosis. Curr Opin Rheumatol 16(6):733–738
32. Humphreys BD, Lin SL, Kobayashi A et al (2010) Fate tracing reveals the pericyte and not epithelial origin of myofibroblasts in kidney fibrosis. Am J Pathol 176(1):85–97. doi:10.2353/ajpath.2010.090517
33. Duffield JS (2014) Cellular and molecular mechanisms in kidney fibrosis. J Clin Invest 124(6):2299–2306. doi:10.1172/JCI72267
34. Kramann R, Humphreys BD (2014) Kidney pericytes: roles in regeneration and fibrosis. Semin Nephrol 34(4):374–383. doi:10.1016/j.semnephrol.2014.06.004
35. Kramann R, Schneider RK, DiRocco DP et al (2015) Perivascular Gli1+ progenitors are key contributors to injury-induced organ fibrosis. Cell Stem Cell 16(1):51–66. doi:10.1016/j.stem.2014.11.004
36. Onuora S (2015) Connective tissue diseases: adipocyte-myofibroblast transition: linking intradermal fat loss to skin fibrosis in SSc. Nat Rev Rheumatol 11(2):63. doi:10.1038/nrrheum.2014.223
37. Marangoni RG, Korman BD, Wei J et al (2015) Myofibroblasts in murine cutaneous fibrosis originate from adiponectin-positive intradermal progenitors. Arthritis Rheumatol 67(4):1062–1073. doi:10.1002/art.38990
38. Kruglikov IL, Scherer PE (2016) Dermal adipocytes: from irrelevance to metabolic targets? Trends Endocrinol Metab 27(1):1–10. doi:10.1016/j.tem.2015.11.002
39. Martins V, Gonzalez De Los Santos F, Wu Z et al (2015) FIZZ1-induced myofibroblast transdifferentiation from adipocytes and its potential role in dermal fibrosis and lipoatrophy. Am J Pathol 185(10):2768–2776. doi:10.1016/j.ajpath.2015.06.005
40. Resovi A, Pinessi D, Chiorino G et al (2014) Current understanding of the thrombospondin-1 interactome. Matrix Biol 37:83–91. doi:10.1016/j.matbio.2014.01.012
41. Murphy-Ullrich JE, Sage EH (2014) Revisiting the matricellular concept. Matrix Biol 37:1–14. doi:10.1016/j.matbio.2014.07.005
42. Iozzo RV, Schaefer L (2015) Proteoglycan form and function: a comprehensive nomenclature of proteoglycans. Matrix Biol 42:11–55. doi:10.1016/j.matbio.2015.02.003

43. Kramann R, DiRocco DP, Humphreys BD (2013) Understanding the origin, activation and regulation of matrix-producing myofibroblasts for treatment of fibrotic disease. J Pathol 231(3):273–289
44. Roberts AB, Sporn MB, Assoian RK et al (1986) Transforming growth factor type beta: rapid induction of fibrosis and angiogenesis in vivo and stimulation of collagen formation in vitro. Proc Natl Acad Sci U S A 83(12):4167–4171
45. Sporn MB, Roberts AB (1989) Transforming growth factor-beta. Multiple actions and potential clinical applications. JAMA 262(7):938–941
46. Santibanez JF, Quintanilla M, Bernabeu C (2011) TGF-beta/TGF-beta receptor system and its role in physiological and pathological conditions. Clin Sci (Lond) 121(6):233–251. doi:10.1042/cs20110086
47. Moses HL, Roberts AB, Derynck R (2016) The discovery and early days of TGF-beta: a historical perspective. Cold Spring Harb Perspect Biol 8(7). doi:10.1101/cshperspect.a021865
48. Fujio K, Komai T, Inoue M et al (2016) Revisiting the regulatory roles of the TGF-beta family of cytokines. Autoimmun Rev 15(9):917–922. doi:10.1016/j.autrev.2016.07.007
49. Goumans MJ, Liu Z, ten Dijke P (2009) TGF-beta signaling in vascular biology and dysfunction. Cell Res 19(1):116–127. doi:10.1038/cr.2008.326
50. Medici D, Potenta S, Kalluri R (2011) Transforming growth factor-beta2 promotes Snail-mediated endothelial-mesenchymal transition through convergence of Smad-dependent and Smad-independent signalling. Biochem J 437(3):515–520. doi:10.1042/bj20101500
51. van Meeteren LA, ten Dijke P (2012) Regulation of endothelial cell plasticity by TGF-beta. Cell Tissue Res 347(1):177–186. doi:10.1007/s00441-011-1222-6
52. Border WA, Noble NA (1994) Transforming growth factor beta in tissue fibrosis. N Engl J Med 331(19):1286–1292. doi:10.1056/nejm199411103311907
53. Pohlers D, Brenmoehl J, Loffler I et al (2009) TGF-beta and fibrosis in different organs – molecular pathway imprints. Biochim Biophys Acta 1792(8):746–756. doi:10.1016/j.bbadis.2009.06.004
54. Varga J, Whitfield ML (2009) Transforming growth factor-beta in systemic sclerosis (scleroderma). Front Biosci (Schol Ed) 1:226–235
55. Jimenez SA, Castro SV, Piera-Velazquez S (2010) Role of growth factors in the pathogenesis of tissue fibrosis in systemic sclerosis. Curr Rheumatol Rev 6(4):283–294
56. Biernacka A, Dobaczewski M, Frangogiannis NG (2011) TGF-beta signaling in fibrosis. Growth Factors 29(5):196–202. doi:10.3109/08977194.2011.595714
57. Lafyatis R (2014) Transforming growth factor beta – at the centre of systemic sclerosis. Nat Rev Rheumatol 10(12):706–719. doi:10.1038/nrrheum.2014.137
58. Meng XM, Nikolic-Paterson DJ, Lan HY (2016) TGF-beta: the master regulator of fibrosis. Nat Rev Nephrol 12(6):325–338. doi:10.1038/nrneph.2016.48
59. Miyazono K, Olofsson A, Colosetti P et al (1991) A role of the latent TGF-beta 1-binding protein in the assembly and secretion of TGF-beta 1. EMBO J 10(5):1091–1101
60. Taipale J, Miyazono K, Heldin CH et al (1994) Latent transforming growth factor-beta 1 associates to fibroblast extracellular matrix via latent TGF-beta binding protein. J Cell Biol 124(1–2):171–181
61. Murphy-Ullrich JE, Poczatek M (2000) Activation of latent TGF-beta by thrombospondin-1: mechanisms and physiology. Cytokine Growth Factor Rev 11(1–2):59–69
62. Sheppard D (2005) Integrin-mediated activation of latent transforming growth factor beta. Cancer Metastasis Rev 24(3):395–402. doi:10.1007/s10555-005-5131-6
63. Derynck R, Zhang YE (2003) Smad-dependent and Smad-independent pathways in TGF-beta family signalling. Nature 425(6958):577–584. doi:10.1038/nature02006
64. ten Dijke P, Hill CS (2004) New insights into TGF-beta-Smad signalling. Trends Biochem Sci 29(5):265–273. doi:10.1016/j.tibs.2004.03.008
65. Moustakas A, Heldin CH (2005) Non-Smad TGF-beta signals. J Cell Sci 118(Pt 16):3573–3584. doi:10.1242/jcs.02554
66. Wilkes MC, Leof EB (2006) Transforming growth factor beta activation of c-Abl is independent of receptor internalization and regulated by phosphatidylinositol 3-kinase and PAK2 in mesenchymal cultures. J Biol Chem 281(38):27846–27854. doi:10.1074/jbc.M603721200
67. Jimenez SA, Gaidarova S, Saitta B et al (2001) Role of protein kinase C-delta in the regulation of collagen gene expression in scleroderma fibroblasts. J Clin Invest 108(9):1395–1403. doi:10.1172/jci12347
68. Bujor AM, Asano Y, Haines P et al (2011) The c-Abl tyrosine kinase controls protein kinase C delta-induced Fli-1 phosphorylation in human dermal fibroblasts. Arthritis Rheum 63(6):1729–1737. doi:10.1002/art.30284

69. Lawler S, Feng XH, Chen RH et al (1997) The type II transforming growth factor-beta receptor autophosphorylates not only on serine and threonine but also on tyrosine residues. J Biol Chem 272(23):14850–14859
70. Galliher AJ, Schiemann WP (2007) Src phosphorylates Tyr284 in TGF-beta type II receptor and regulates TGF-beta stimulation of p38 MAPK during breast cancer cell proliferation and invasion. Cancer Res 67(8):3752–3758. doi:10.1158/0008-5472.can-06-3851
71. Pannu J, Asano Y, Nakerakanti S et al (2008) Smad1 pathway is activated in systemic sclerosis fibroblasts and is targeted by imatinib mesylate. Arthritis Rheum 58(8):2528–2537. doi:10.1002/art.23698
72. Caraci F, Gili E, Calafiore M et al (2008) TGF-beta1 targets the GSK-3 beta/beta-catenin pathway via ERK activation in the transition of human lung fibroblasts into myofibroblasts. Pharmacol Res 57(4):274–282. doi:10.1016/j.phrs.2008.02.001
73. Andrianifahanana M, Wilkes MC, Gupta SK et al (2013) Profibrotic TGFbeta responses require the cooperative action of PDGF and ErbB receptor tyrosine kinases. FASEB J 27(11):4444–4454. doi:10.1096/fj.12-224907
74. Chen D, Zhao M, Mundy GR (2004) Bone morphogenetic proteins. Growth Factors 22(4):233–241. doi:10.1080/08977190412331279890
75. Mulloy B, Rider CC (2015) The bone morphogenetic proteins and their antagonists. Vitam Horm 99:63–90. doi:10.1016/bs.vh.2015.06.004
76. Bi J, Ge S (2014) Potential roles of BMP9 in liver fibrosis. Int J Mol Sci 15(11):20656–20667. doi:10.3390/ijms151120656
77. Li RX, Yiu WH, Tang SC (2015) Role of bone morphogenetic protein-7 in renal fibrosis. Front Physiol 6:114. doi:10.3389/fphys.2015.00114
78. Zeisberg M, Hanai J, Sugimoto H et al (2003) BMP-7 counteracts TGF-beta1-induced epithelial-to-mesenchymal transition and reverses chronic renal injury. Nat Med 9(7):964–968. doi:10.1038/nm888
79. Weiskirchen R, Meurer SK, Gressner OA et al (2009) BMP-7 as antagonist of organ fibrosis. Front Biosci (Landmark Ed) 14:4992–5012
80. Weiskirchen R, Meurer SK (2013) BMP-7 counteracting TGF-beta1 activities in organ fibrosis. Front Biosci (Landmark Ed) 18:1407–1434
81. Miyazono K, Kusanagi K, Inoue H (2001) Divergence and convergence of TGF-beta/BMP signaling. J Cell Physiol 187(3):265–276. doi:10.1002/jcp.1080
82. Miyazawa K, Shinozaki M, Hara T et al (2002) Two major Smad pathways in TGF-beta superfamily signalling. Genes Cells 7(12):1191–1204
83. Meng XM, Chung AC, Lan HY (2013) Role of the TGF-beta/BMP-7/Smad pathways in renal diseases. Clin Sci (Lond) 124(4):243–254. doi:10.1042/CS20120252
84. Miyazono K, Kamiya Y, Morikawa M (2010) Bone morphogenetic protein receptors and signal transduction. J Biochem 147(1):35–51. doi:10.1093/jb/mvp148
85. Mueller TD, Nickel J (2012) Promiscuity and specificity in BMP receptor activation. FEBS Lett 586(14):1846–1859. doi:10.1016/j.febslet.2012.02.043
86. Bai S, Shi X, Yang X et al (2000) Smad6 as a transcriptional corepressor. J Biol Chem 275(12):8267–8270
87. Wang S, Hirschberg R (2004) Bone morphogenetic protein-7 signals opposing transforming growth factor beta in mesangial cells. J Biol Chem 279(22):23200–23206. doi:10.1074/jbc.M311998200
88. Yan X, Liu Z, Chen Y (2009) Regulation of TGF-beta signaling by Smad7. Acta Biochim Biophys Sin Shanghai 41(4):263–272
89. Motazed R, Colville-Nash P, Kwan JT et al (2008) BMP-7 and proximal tubule epithelial cells: activation of multiple signaling pathways reveals a novel anti-fibrotic mechanism. Pharm Res 25(10):2440–2446. doi:10.1007/s11095-008-9551-1
90. Wang S, Hirschberg R (2003) BMP7 antagonizes TGF-beta-dependent fibrogenesis in mesangial cells. Am J Physiol Renal Physiol 284(5):F1006–F1013. doi:10.1152/ajprenal.00382.2002
91. Wang SN, Lapage J, Hirschberg R (2001) Loss of tubular bone morphogenetic protein-7 in diabetic nephropathy. J Am Soc Nephrol 12(11):2392–2399
92. Wang S, de Caestecker M, Kopp J et al (2006) Renal bone morphogenetic protein-7 protects against diabetic nephropathy. J Am Soc Nephrol 17(9):2504–2512. doi:10.1681/ASN.2006030278
93. Munoz-Felix JM, Gonzalez-Nunez M, Martinez-Salgado C et al (2015) TGF-beta/BMP proteins as therapeutic targets in renal fibrosis. Where have we arrived after 25 years of trials and tribulations? Pharmacol Ther 156:44–58. doi:10.1016/j.pharmthera.2015.10.003
94. Kessler D, Dethlefsen S, Haase I et al (2001) Fibroblasts in mechanically stressed collagen lattices assume a "synthetic" phenotype. J Biol Chem 276(39):36575–36585. doi:10.1074/jbc.M101602200

95. Huang X, Yang N, Fiore VF et al (2012) Matrix stiffness-induced myofibroblast differentiation is mediated by intrinsic mechanotransduction. Am J Respir Cell Mol Biol 47(3):340–348. doi:10.1165/rcmb.2012-0050OC
96. Hayashida T, Decaestecker M, Schnaper HW (2003) Cross-talk between ERK MAP kinase and Smad signaling pathways enhances TGF-beta-dependent responses in human mesangial cells. FASEB J 17(11):1576–1578. doi:10.1096/fj.03-0037fje
97. Thorin E, Clozel M (2010) The cardiovascular physiology and pharmacology of endothelin-1. Adv Pharmacol 60:1–26. doi:10.1016/b978-0-12-385061-4.00001-5
98. Kawanabe Y, Nauli SM (2011) Endothelin. Cell Mol Life Sci 68(2):195–203. doi:10.1007/s00018-010-0518-0
99. Shi-Wen X, Denton CP, Dashwood MR et al (2001) Fibroblast matrix gene expression and connective tissue remodeling: role of endothelin-1. J Invest Dermatol 116(3):417–425. doi:10.1046/j.1523-1747.2001.01256.x
100. Xu SW, Howat SL, Renzoni EA et al (2004) Endothelin-1 induces expression of matrix-associated genes in lung fibroblasts through MEK/ERK. J Biol Chem 279(22):23098–23103. doi:10.1074/jbc.M311430200
101. Jing J, Dou TT, Yang JQ et al (2015) Role of endothelin-1 in the skin fibrosis of systemic sclerosis. Eur Cytokine Netw 26(1):10–14. doi:10.1684/ecn.2015.0360
102. Abraham D, Ponticos M, Nagase H (2005) Connective tissue remodeling: cross-talk between endothelins and matrix metalloproteinases. Curr Vasc Pharmacol 3(4):369–379. doi:10.2174/157016105774329480
103. Park SH, Saleh D, Giaid A et al (1997) Increased endothelin-1 in bleomycin-induced pulmonary fibrosis and the effect of an endothelin receptor antagonist. Am J Respir Crit Care Med 156(2 Pt 1):600–608. doi:10.1164/ajrccm.156.2.9607123
104. Ross B, D'Orleans-Juste P, Giaid A (2010) Potential role of endothelin-1 in pulmonary fibrosis: from the bench to the clinic. Am J Respir Cell Mol Biol 42(1):16–20. doi:10.1165/rcmb.2009-0175TR
105. Kim KK, Chapman HA (2007) Endothelin-1 as initiator of epithelial-mesenchymal transition: potential new role for endothelin-1 during pulmonary fibrosis. Am J Respir Cell Mol Biol 37(1):1–2. doi:10.1165/rcmb.2007-0001ED
106. Widyantoro B, Emoto N, Nakayama K et al (2010) Endothelial cell-derived endothelin-1 promotes cardiac fibrosis in diabetic hearts through stimulation of endothelial-to-mesenchymal transition. Circulation 121(22):2407–2418. doi:10.1161/circulationaha.110.938217
107. Cipriani P, Di Benedetto P, Ruscitti P et al (2015) The endothelial-mesenchymal transition in systemic sclerosis is induced by endothelin-1 and transforming growth factor-beta and may be blocked by macitentan, a dual endothelin-1 receptor antagonist. J Rheumatol 42(10):1808–1816. doi:10.3899/jrheum.150088
108. Wermuth PJ, Li Z, Jimenez SA (2016) Stimulation of TGF-β1-induced endothelial-to-mesenchymal transition and tissue fibrosis by endothelin-1 (ET-1): a novel profibrotic effect of ET-1. PLoS One 11(9):e0161988. doi:10.1371/journal.pone.0161988
109. Igarashi A, Nashiro K, Kikuchi K et al (1995) Significant correlation between connective tissue growth factor gene expression and skin sclerosis in tissue sections from patients with systemic sclerosis. J Invest Dermatol 105(2):280–284
110. Grotendorst GR (1997) Connective tissue growth factor: a mediator of TGF-beta action on fibroblasts. Cytokine Growth Factor Rev 8(3):171–179
111. Sato S, Nagaoka T, Hasegawa M et al (2000) Serum levels of connective tissue growth factor are elevated in patients with systemic sclerosis: association with extent of skin sclerosis and severity of pulmonary fibrosis. J Rheumatol 27(1):149–154
112. Leask A, Abraham DJ (2003) The role of connective tissue growth factor, a multifunctional matricellular protein, in fibroblast biology. Biochem Cell Biol 81(6):355–363. doi:10.1139/o03-069
113. Shi-Wen X, Leask A, Abraham D (2008) Regulation and function of connective tissue growth factor/CCN2 in tissue repair, scarring and fibrosis. Cytokine Growth Factor Rev 19(2):133–144. doi:10.1016/j.cytogfr.2008.01.002
114. Ponticos M, Holmes AM, Shi-wen X et al (2009) Pivotal role of connective tissue growth factor in lung fibrosis: MAPK-dependent transcriptional activation of type I collagen. Arthritis Rheum 60(7):2142–2155. doi:10.1002/art.24620
115. Ruperez M, Rodrigues-Diez R, Blanco-Colio LM et al (2007) HMG-CoA reductase inhibitors decrease angiotensin II-induced vascular fibrosis: role of RhoA/ROCK and MAPK pathways. Hypertension 50(2):377–383. doi:10.1161/hypertensionaha.107.091264
116. Betsholtz C (2003) Biology of platelet-derived growth factors in development. Birth Defects Res C Embryo Today 69(4):272–285. doi:10.1002/bdrc.10030

117. Alvarez RH, Kantarjian HM, Cortes JE (2006) Biology of platelet-derived growth factor and its involvement in disease. Mayo Clin Proc 81(9):1241–1257. doi:10.4065/81.9.1241
118. Farooqi AA, Waseem S, Riaz AM et al (2011) PDGF: the nuts and bolts of signalling toolbox. Tumour Biol 32(6):1057–1070. doi:10.1007/s13277-011-0212-3
119. Bonner JC (2004) Regulation of PDGF and its receptors in fibrotic diseases. Cytokine Growth Factor Rev 15(4):255–273. doi:10.1016/j.cytogfr.2004.03.006
120. Yamakage A, Kikuchi K, Smith EA et al (1992) Selective upregulation of platelet-derived growth factor alpha receptors by transforming growth factor beta in scleroderma fibroblasts. J Exp Med 175(5): 1227–1234
121. Tallquist M, Kazlauskas A (2004) PDGF signaling in cells and mice. Cytokine Growth Factor Rev 15(4):205–213. doi:10.1016/j.cytogfr.2004.03.003
122. Olson LE, Soriano P (2009) Increased PDGFR alpha activation disrupts connective tissue development and drives systemic fibrosis. Dev Cell 16(2):303–313. doi:10.1016/j.devcel.2008.12.003
123. Czochra P, Klopcic B, Meyer E et al (2006) Liver fibrosis induced by hepatic overexpression of PDGF-B in transgenic mice. J Hepatol 45(3):419–428. doi:10.1016/j.jhep.2006.04.010
124. Ogawa S, Ochi T, Shimada H et al (2010) Anti-PDGF-B monoclonal antibody reduces liver fibrosis development. Hepatol Res 40(11):1128–1141. doi:10.1111/j.1872-034X.2010.00718.x
125. Heldin CH, Westermark B (1999) Mechanism of action and in vivo role of platelet-derived growth factor. Physiol Rev 79(4):1283–1316
126. Lam AP, Flozak AS, Russell S et al (2011) Nuclear beta-catenin is increased in systemic sclerosis pulmonary fibrosis and promotes lung fibroblast migration and proliferation. Am J Respir Cell Mol Biol 45(5):915–922. doi:10.1165/rcmb.2010-0113OC
127. Beyer C, Schramm A, Akhmetshina A et al (2012) Beta-catenin is a central mediator of pro-fibrotic Wnt signaling in systemic sclerosis. Ann Rheum Dis 71(5):761–767. doi:10.1136/annrheumdis-2011-200568
128. Niehrs C (2012) The complex world of WNT receptor signalling. Nat Rev Mol Cell Biol 13(12):767–779. doi:10.1038/nrm3470
129. Clevers H, Nusse R (2012) Wnt/beta-catenin signaling and disease. Cell 149(6):1192–1205. doi:10.1016/j.cell.2012.05.012
130. Wei J, Fang F, Lam AP et al (2012) Wnt/beta-catenin signaling is hyperactivated in systemic sclerosis and induces Smad-dependent fibrotic responses in mesenchymal cells. Arthritis Rheum 64(8):2734–2745. doi:10.1002/art.34424
131. Bergmann C, Distler JH (2016) Canonical Wnt signaling in systemic sclerosis. Lab Investig 96(2):151–155. doi:10.1038/labinvest.2015.154
132. Nusse R (2005) Wnt signaling in disease and in development. Cell Res 15(1):28–32. doi:10.1038/sj.cr.7290260
133. Huang H, He X (2008) Wnt/beta-catenin signaling: new (and old) players and new insights. Curr Opin Cell Biol 20(2):119–125. doi:10.1016/j.ceb.2008.01.009
134. Konigshoff M, Balsara N, Pfaff EM et al (2008) Functional Wnt signaling is increased in idiopathic pulmonary fibrosis. PLoS One 3(5):e2142. doi:10.1371/journal.pone.0002142
135. He W, Dai C, Li Y et al (2009) Wnt/beta-catenin signaling promotes renal interstitial fibrosis. J Am Soc Nephrol 20(4):765–776. doi:10.1681/asn.2008060566
136. He W, Zhang L, Ni A et al (2010) Exogenously administered secreted frizzled related protein 2 (Sfrp2) reduces fibrosis and improves cardiac function in a rat model of myocardial infarction. Proc Natl Acad Sci U S A 107(49):21110–21115. doi:10.1073/pnas.1004708107
137. Trensz F, Haroun S, Cloutier A et al (2010) A muscle resident cell population promotes fibrosis in hind limb skeletal muscles of mdx mice through the Wnt canonical pathway. Am J Physiol Cell Physiol 299(5):C939–C947. doi:10.1152/ajpcell.00253.2010
138. Wei J, Melichian D, Komura K et al (2011) Canonical Wnt signaling induces skin fibrosis and subcutaneous lipoatrophy: a novel mouse model for scleroderma? Arthritis Rheum 63(6):1707–1717. doi:10.1002/art.30312
139. Bafico A, Liu G, Yaniv A et al (2001) Novel mechanism of Wnt signalling inhibition mediated by Dickkopf-1 interaction with LRP6/arrow. Nat Cell Biol 3(7):683–686. doi:10.1038/35083081
140. Pinzone JJ, Hall BM, Thudi NK et al (2009) The role of Dickkopf-1 in bone development, homeostasis, and disease. Blood 113(3):517–525. doi:10.1182/blood-2008-03-145169
141. Echelard Y, Epstein DJ, St-Jacques B et al (1993) Sonic hedgehog, a member of a family of putative signaling molecules, is implicated in the regulation of CNS polarity. Cell 75(7):1417–1430. doi:10.1016/0092-8674(93)90627-3
142. Rohatgi R, Milenkovic L, Corcoran RB et al (2009) Hedgehog signal transduction by Smoothened: pharmacologic evidence for a

2-step activation process. Proc Natl Acad Sci U S A 106(9):3196–3201. doi:10.1073/pnas.0813373106
143. Rohatgi R, Scott MP (2007) Patching the gaps in hedgehog signalling. Nat Cell Biol 9(9):1005–1009. doi:10.1038/ncb435
144. Xie J, Murone M, Luoh SM et al (1998) Activating Smoothened mutations in sporadic basal-cell carcinoma. Nature 391(6662):90–92. doi:10.1038/34201
145. Dahmane N, Sanchez P, Gitton Y et al (2001) The sonic hedgehog-Gli pathway regulates dorsal brain growth and tumorigenesis. Development 128(24):5201–5212
146. Thayer SP, di Magliano MP, Heiser PW et al (2003) Hedgehog is an early and late mediator of pancreatic cancer tumorigenesis. Nature 425(6960):851–856. doi:10.1038/nature02009
147. Horn A, Palumbo K, Cordazzo C et al (2012) Hedgehog signaling controls fibroblast activation and tissue fibrosis in systemic sclerosis. Arthritis Rheum 64(8):2724–2733. doi:10.1002/art.34444
148. D'Souza B, Miyamoto A, Weinmaster G (2008) The many facets of Notch ligands. Oncogene 27(38):5148–5167. doi:10.1038/onc.2008.229
149. Fortini ME (2009) Notch signaling: the core pathway and its posttranslational regulation. Dev Cell 16(5):633–647. doi:10.1016/j.devcel.2009.03.010
150. Borggrefe T, Liefke R (2012) Fine-tuning of the intracellular canonical Notch signaling pathway. Cell Cycle 11(2):264–276. doi:10.4161/cc.11.2.18995
151. Dees C, Tomcik M, Zerr P et al (2011) Notch signalling regulates fibroblast activation and collagen release in systemic sclerosis. Ann Rheum Dis 70(7):1304–1310. doi:10.1136/ard.2010.134742
152. Kavian N, Servettaz A, Weill B et al (2012) New insights into the mechanism of notch signalling in fibrosis. Open Rheumatol J 6:96–102. doi:10.2174/1874312901206010096
153. Louvi A, Artavanis-Tsakonas S (2012) Notch and disease: a growing field. Semin Cell Dev Biol 23(4):473–480. doi:10.1016/j.semcdb.2012.02.005
154. Distler A, Lang V, Del Vecchio T et al (2014) Combined inhibition of morphogen pathways demonstrates additive antifibrotic effects and improved tolerability. Ann Rheum Dis 73(6):1264–1268. doi:10.1136/annrheumdis-2013-204221
155. Beyer C, Schett G, Gay S et al (2009) Hypoxia. Hypoxia in the pathogenesis of systemic sclerosis. Arthritis Res Ther 11(2):220. doi:10.1186/ar2598
156. Haase VH (2009) Pathophysiological consequences of HIF activation: HIF as a modulator of fibrosis. Ann N Y Acad Sci 1177:57–65. doi:10.1111/j.1749-6632.2009.05030.x
157. Semenza GL (2012) Hypoxia-inducible factors in physiology and medicine. Cell 148(3):399–408. doi:10.1016/j.cell.2012.01.021
158. Lokmic Z, Musyoka J, Hewitson TD et al (2012) Hypoxia and hypoxia signaling in tissue repair and fibrosis. Int Rev Cell Mol Biol 296:139–185. doi:10.1016/b978-0-12-394307-1.00003-5
159. Distler JH, Jungel A, Pileckyte M et al (2007) Hypoxia-induced increase in the production of extracellular matrix proteins in systemic sclerosis. Arthritis Rheum 56(12):4203–4215. doi:10.1002/art.23074
160. Sanchez-Elsner T, Botella LM, Velasco B et al (2001) Synergistic cooperation between hypoxia and transforming growth factor-beta pathways on human vascular endothelial growth factor gene expression. J Biol Chem 276(42):38527–38535. doi:10.1074/jbc.M104536200
161. Higgins DF, Kimura K, Bernhardt WM et al (2007) Hypoxia promotes fibrogenesis in vivo via HIF-1 stimulation of epithelial-to-mesenchymal transition. J Clin Invest 117(12):3810–3820. doi:10.1172/jci30487
162. Liu RM, Desai LP (2015) Reciprocal regulation of TGF-beta and reactive oxygen species: a perverse cycle for fibrosis. Redox Biol 6:565–577. doi:10.1016/j.redox.2015.09.009
163. Richter K, Konzack A, Pihlajaniemi T et al (2015) Redox-fibrosis: impact of TGFbeta1 on ROS generators, mediators and functional consequences. Redox Biol 6:344–352. doi:10.1016/j.redox.2015.08.015
164. Kliment CR, Oury TD (2010) Oxidative stress, extracellular matrix targets, and idiopathic pulmonary fibrosis. Free Radic Biol Med 49(5):707–717. doi:10.1016/j.freeradbiomed.2010.04.036
165. Siani A, Tirelli N (2014) Myofibroblast differentiation: main features, biomedical relevance, and the role of reactive oxygen species. Antioxid Redox Signal 21(5):768–785. doi:10.1089/ars.2013.5724
166. Bourji K, Meyer A, Chatelus E et al (2015) High reactive oxygen species in fibrotic and nonfibrotic skin of patients with diffuse cutaneous systemic sclerosis. Free Radic Biol Med 87:282–289. doi:10.1016/j.freeradbiomed.2015.07.002
167. Cucoranu I, Clempus R, Dikalova A et al (2005) NAD(P)H oxidase 4 mediates transforming growth factor-beta1-induced differentiation of cardiac fibroblasts into myofibroblasts.

Circ Res 97(9):900–907. doi:10.1161/01.res.0000187457.24338.3d
168. Hecker L, Vittal R, Jones T et al (2009) NADPH oxidase-4 mediates myofibroblast activation and fibrogenic responses to lung injury. Nat Med 15(9):1077–1081. doi:10.1038/nm.2005
169. Amara N, Goven D, Prost F et al (2010) NOX4/NADPH oxidase expression is increased in pulmonary fibroblasts from patients with idiopathic pulmonary fibrosis and mediates TGFbeta1-induced fibroblast differentiation into myofibroblasts. Thorax 65(8):733–738. doi:10.1136/thx.2009.113456
170. Barnes JL, Gorin Y (2011) Myofibroblast differentiation during fibrosis: role of NAD(P)H oxidases. Kidney Int 79(9):944–956. doi:10.1038/ki.2010.516
171. Crestani B, Besnard V, Boczkowski J (2011) Signalling pathways from NADPH oxidase-4 to idiopathic pulmonary fibrosis. Int J Biochem Cell Biol 43(8):1086–1089. doi:10.1016/j.biocel.2011.04.003
172. Sancho P, Mainez J, Crosas-Molist E et al (2012) NADPH oxidase NOX4 mediates stellate cell activation and hepatocyte cell death during liver fibrosis development. PLoS One 7(9):e45285. doi:10.1371/journal.pone.0045285
173. Jiang F, Liu GS, Dusting GJ et al (2014) NADPH oxidase-dependent redox signaling in TGF-beta-mediated fibrotic responses. Redox Biol 2:267–272. doi:10.1016/j.redox.2014.01.012
174. Paik YH, Kim J, Aoyama T et al (2014) Role of NADPH oxidases in liver fibrosis. Antioxid Redox Signal 20(17):2854–2872. doi:10.1089/ars.2013.5619
175. Piera-Velazquez S, Makul A, Jimenez SA (2015) Increased expression of NAPDH oxidase 4 in systemic sclerosis dermal fibroblasts: regulation by transforming growth factor beta. Arthritis Rheumatol 67(10):2749–2758. doi:10.1002/art.39242
176. Spadoni T, Svegliati Baroni S, Amico D et al (2015) A reactive oxygen species-mediated loop maintains increased expression of NADPH oxidases 2 and 4 in skin fibroblasts from patients with systemic sclerosis. Arthritis Rheumatol 67(6):1611–1622. doi:10.1002/art.39084
177. Wang Y, Stricker HM, Gou D et al (2007) MicroRNA: past and present. Front Biosci 12:2316–2329
178. Jiang X, Tsitsiou E, Herrick SE et al (2010) MicroRNAs and the regulation of fibrosis. FEBS J 277(9):2015–2021. doi:10.1111/j.1742-4658.2010.07632.x
179. Bowen T, Jenkins RH, Fraser DJ (2013) MicroRNAs, transforming growth factor beta-1, and tissue fibrosis. J Pathol 229(2):274–285. doi:10.1002/path.4119
180. Rutnam ZJ, Wight TN, Yang BB (2013) miRNAs regulate expression and function of extracellular matrix molecules. Matrix Biol 32(2):74–85. doi:10.1016/j.matbio.2012.11.003
181. Zhu H, Luo H, Zuo X (2013) MicroRNAs: their involvement in fibrosis pathogenesis and use as diagnostic biomarkers in scleroderma. Exp Mol Med 45:e41. doi:10.1038/emm.2013.71
182. Babalola O, Mamalis A, Lev-Tov H et al (2013) The role of microRNAs in skin fibrosis. Arch Dermatol Res 305(9):763–776. doi:10.1007/s00403-013-1410-1
183. Pandit KV, Milosevic J (2015) MicroRNA regulatory networks in idiopathic pulmonary fibrosis. Biochem Cell Biol 93(2):129–137. doi:10.1139/bcb-2014-0101
184. He Y, Huang C, Zhang SP et al (2012) The potential of microRNAs in liver fibrosis. Cell Signal 24(12):2268–2272. doi:10.1016/j.cellsig.2012.07.023
185. Srivastava SP, Koya D, Kanasaki K (2013) MicroRNAs in kidney fibrosis and diabetic nephropathy: roles on EMT and EndMT. Biomed Res Int 2013:125469. doi:10.1155/2013/125469
186. Thum T (2014) Noncoding RNAs and myocardial fibrosis. Nat Rev Cardiol 11(11):655–663. doi:10.1038/nrcardio.2014.125
187. Razani B, Zhang XL, Bitzer M et al (2001) Caveolin-1 regulates transforming growth factor (TGF)-beta/SMAD signaling through an interaction with the TGF-beta type I receptor. J Biol Chem 276(9):6727–6738. doi:10.1074/jbc.M008340200
188. Del Galdo F, Lisanti MP, Jimenez SA (2008) Caveolin-1, transforming growth factor-beta receptor internalization, and the pathogenesis of systemic sclerosis. Curr Opin Rheumatol 20(6):713–719
189. Gvaramia D, Blaauboer ME, Hanemaaijer R et al (2013) Role of caveolin-1 in fibrotic diseases. Matrix Biol 32(6):307–315. doi:10.1016/j.matbio.2013.03.005
190. Del Galdo F, Sotgia F, de Almeida CJ et al (2008) Decreased expression of caveolin 1 in patients with systemic sclerosis: crucial role in the pathogenesis of tissue fibrosis. Arthritis Rheum 58(9):2854–2865. doi:10.1002/art.23791
191. Wang XM, Zhang Y, Kim HP et al (2006) Caveolin-1: a critical regulator of lung fibrosis in idiopathic pulmonary fibrosis. J Exp Med 203(13):2895–2906. doi:10.1084/jem.20061536

192. Tourkina E, Richard M, Gooz P et al (2008) Antifibrotic properties of caveolin-1 scaffolding domain in vitro and in vivo. Am J Physiol Lung Cell Mol Physiol 294(5):L843–L861. doi:10.1152/ajplung.00295.2007
193. Jasmin JF, Mercier I, Dupuis J et al (2006) Short-term administration of a cell-permeable caveolin-1 peptide prevents the development of monocrotaline-induced pulmonary hypertension and right ventricular hypertrophy. Circulation 114(9):912–920. doi:10.1161/circulationaha.106.634709
194. Li Z, Wermuth PJ, Benn BS et al (2013) Caveolin-1 deficiency induces spontaneous endothelial-to-mesenchymal transition in murine pulmonary endothelial cells in vitro. Am J Pathol 182(2):325–331. doi:10.1016/j.ajpath.2012.10.022

Part I

Animal Models of Fibrosis

Chapter 2

The Bleomycin Model of Pulmonary Fibrosis

Tianju Liu, Francina Gonzalez De Los Santos, and Sem H. Phan

Abstract

Interstitial lung disease (ILD) comprises a large number of chronic lung disease characterized by varying degrees of inflammation and fibrosis. Mostly they are idiopathic including idiopathic pulmonary fibrosis (IPF), which is a specific disorder characterized by progressive fibrosis leading commonly to end-stage lung disease, respiratory failure, and fatal outcome. IPF and many of these fibrotic ILDs lack effective therapy despite recent approval of two drugs to slow progression in certain IPF patients. Because there are no natural models for IPF, the use of animal models that reproduce key known features of the disease is warranted. Thus, different animal models have been developed to investigate key mechanisms underlying pathogenesis of pulmonary fibrosis and identify potential therapeutic targets for IPF. While no animal model can recapitulate all features of human disease, several are available to address select features of IPF and other fibrotic ILDs. Historically, among the first to be developed and used widely is the bleomycin model, which is the best-characterized and currently most extensively used animal model due to its ability to reproduce many aspects of IPF and other fibrotic ILDs, good reproducibility, and ease of induction. Studies using the bleomycin model have identified many of the cellular and molecular mechanisms now recognized as being important in pathogenesis of IPF and other fibrotic ILDs, as well as novel therapies for these diseases, including two recent drugs approved for treatment of IPF. This chapter will describe commonly used techniques for induction of the model by endotracheal administration of bleomycin through surgical and nonsurgical (transoral instillation).

Key words Bleomycin, Idiopathic pulmonary fibrosis, Mouse, Endotracheal instillation

1 Introduction

1.1 General Considerations

Chronic fibrosis is often associated with many ILDs, and for many in the idiopathic category, there is currently no effective therapy due in part to lack of known etiology and adequate knowledge of their natural history and/or pathogenic mechanisms. In IPF this is characterized by alveolar epithelial cell damage, subsequent release of pro-inflammatory and pro-fibrotic cytokines and other mediators, accumulation of activated fibroblasts and myofibroblasts in the fibrotic foci, and the excessive abnormal deposition of extracellular matrix proteins. Inexorable progression of fibrosis results in loss of normal lung architecture, end-stage lung disease,

Laure Rittié (ed.), *Fibrosis: Methods and Protocols*, Methods in Molecular Biology, vol. 1627,
DOI 10.1007/978-1-4939-7113-8_2,

respiratory failure, and eventual fatal outcome [1–3]. IPF is characterized by the histological pattern of usual interstitial pneumonia [4]. Although no single animal model of pulmonary fibrosis recapitulates all features of the human disease, use of animal models has led to reproduction of many of the manifestations of IPF. Among the various animal models of pulmonary fibrosis (bleomycin, FITC, silica, radiation, etc.), the bleomycin model is the most extensively used and best-characterized murine model in use today [5, 6].

Bleomycin is a family of complex glycopeptides [7] with antineoplastic properties, initially isolated from a strain of actinobacteria, *Streptomyces verticillus* [8]. Its primary clinical use is as an antitumor antibiotic for various carcinomas and lymphomas [9–11]. Bleomycin-induced toxicity occurs predominantly in the organs of the lung, skin, and mucous membranes due to the lack of the bleomycin-inactivating enzyme, bleomycin hydrolase in those tissues [9, 12, 13]. Intradermal injections of bleomycin can be used to exclusively model skin fibrosis (method detailed in Chap. 3). Pulmonary fibrosis is a well-known side effect of bleomycin, because the lung expresses very low levels of this enzyme. This enables persistence of the compound with consequent greater susceptibility to bleomycin-induced lung injury relative to other organs [13–17]. The use of bleomycin is limited by the development of pulmonary fibrosis in 3–5% of patients receiving this chemotherapeutic agent [5]. This notable and undesirable side effect of bleomycin leads to its use in animal models studying mechanisms of pulmonary fibrosis of relevance to IPF. Bleomycin as an agent to induce experimental lung fibrosis is first described in dogs and subsequently in mice, hamsters, rats, and sheep [18–22]. Eventually, it becomes an established model in rodents for the study of pathogenic mechanisms involved in both acute and chronic stages of fibrotic lung diseases and for identification of novel therapeutic targets followed by evaluation of relevant potential therapies [21, 23].

Delivery of bleomycin to the lung causes pulmonary injury, inflammation, and subsequent fibrosis [5]. In the presence of iron and oxygen, bleomycin can generate reactive oxygen species (ROS) and cause DNA strand scission, which is thought to be the basis for its antitumor activity and presumed mechanism for causing cytotoxicity and tissue injury [5, 24, 25]. However, the doses used in the rodent model of fibrosis appear not to cause significant DNA damage [26], thus making it unclear if this is the basis for the injury in this model. However the ROS produced in response to bleomycin can also cause lipid peroxidation and protein oxidation, which may be involved in the mechanism driving fibrosis in this model [5].

1.2 Advantages and Disadvantages of the Bleomycin Model

Due to its early historical introduction and thus more extensive experience with it, the bleomycin model is best characterized in many important aspects of pulmonary fibrosis with limited relevance to IPF. These include in vivo mechanisms of TGF-β activation, epithelial cell injury and basement membrane damage, and interstitial and intra-alveolar fibrosis with dense collagen deposition [27–29]. The model has provided useful information encompassing both acute and chronic lung injury along with the reparative stage of the fibrotic process. Some of the molecular signatures as well as some histopathological hallmarks at distinct stages of bleomycin-induced lung fibrosis resemble those encountered in human fibrotic lung diseases, including IPF. In this regard, it is noteworthy that the preclinical development of two drugs, pirfenidone and nintedanib, recently approved for slowing progression of certain subsets of IPF patients, has been done using the bleomycin model [30–32]. Moreover with respect to pirfenidone, its effectiveness was first discovered using the bleomycin model [33]. The acute injury stage of the response to bleomycin has also been exploited as a model of acute lung injury, such as in acute respiratory distress syndrome (ARDS) as well as potential utility as a model of acute exacerbation in IPF [34, 35]. Thus in addition to its utility as a model of chronic fibrotic lung disease, it is useful as well for modeling more acute stages of lung injury that can lead to fibrosis. The murine model is also particularly useful for elucidation of the role of genetic background in influencing susceptibility to IPF and other fibrotic ILDs because of the strain differences in responsiveness to bleomycin-induced pulmonary fibrosis [36–38]. Recent studies have also exploited the model for studying the role of aging in increased susceptibility to IPF [39]. Thus, despite its imperfections as a model of human chronic progressive lung disease, the bleomycin model has been quite useful for elucidating mechanistic insight and drug discovery, perhaps in a more limited fashion. It has certainly been useful for evaluation of the in vivo fibrogenic significance of descriptive observations emanating from clinical studies of IPF and other fibrotic ILDs.

A key additional advantage of the bleomycin model of pulmonary fibrosis is the ease of induction depending on the method chosen and its good reproducibility. It can be delivered locally or systemically, including endotracheal, intranasal, intravenous, and intraperitoneal routes. Using the local approach, administration of a single dose of bleomycin produces a rapid development of injury and acute inflammation followed by a chronic inflammatory phase with the development of fibrosis over the subsequent weeks. More severe fibrosis is noted from repetitive drug dosing; however, key molecular signatures are similar between single vs. repetitive dosing [40–42]. Depending on the dose of bleomycin and/or the murine strain used, this time course of events and intensity of injury or fibrosis can vary significantly, thus enabling modeling of select stages of disease (e.g., early vs. late, acute exacerbation vs. normal progression, etc.) and/or type of disease (e.g., ARDS vs. IPF). A significant advantage is that the development of fibrosis is relatively quick with the peak fibrotic response occurring at around

3–4 weeks after a single dose of drug via endotracheal delivery. The shorter time frame and reproducibility also mean reduced costs associated with animal purchase and husbandry. Thus, in addition to being economical (especially the single-dose model), the strengths of the bleomycin model lie in its relative ease of induction, reproducibility, and versatility [43].

A key criticism, hence disadvantage, of the bleomycin model is the self-limiting nature of the fibrosis, which contrasts with the progressive chronic fibrosis typical of the known natural history of human IPF [6, 44, 45]. There is a suggestion that repetitive bleomycin dosing may ameliorate some of this criticism with respect to modeling of human IPF [40]. The claim of spontaneous resolution of fibrosis in the bleomycin model represents another potential disadvantage since the unending progression of fibrosis in IPF usually ends in end-stage lung with honeycombing and certainly no evidence of spontaneous resolution of fibrosis [44, 46]. However, this is not universally observed since there are reports showing the persistence of fibrosis in the bleomycin model up to 3–6 months [6, 47]. The basis for this discrepancy is unclear but may be related to the dosing of bleomycin and/or murine strain used in the different studies. Another common criticism is the role of inflammation in the model. As noted in the time course of events after bleomycin treatment, significant chronic inflammation is evident and appears to be important for the developing fibrosis, which appears not to be the case in IPF based on lack of responsiveness to anti-inflammatory steroid treatment and dearth of inflammatory cells in IPF lung tissue [44, 45, 48]. Some studies however indicate only limited, if any, dependence of fibrosis on the inflammation noted in the model [49]. A way to demonstrate this has been to separate the fibrosis from the inflammation by examining the effects of interventions during the fibrotic phase of the model (usually days 14–28 after model induction) when the inflammation is starting to wane [50]. Recent studies have attempted to tweak the model in such a way as to highlight certain more limited phases of fibrogenesis observed in IPF. These modifications or modified use of the model have reduced but not eliminated many of the noted limitations. Nevertheless despite these limitations, the many significant advantages of the model and its track record for elucidating in vivo mechanisms plus utility for drug discovery make the bleomycin model a valuable asset for preclinical and mechanistic studies. It certainly remains as one of the most widely used model for studies of chronic progressive lung diseases today and arguably the best available experimental model in this regard.

1.3 Model Progression

The development or progression of lung injury/fibrosis in various bleomycin animal models is quite similar regardless of species and routes of administration. The lung injury progresses through three stages. (1) Acute injury and inflammatory phase (1–7 days post-endotracheal injection of bleomycin) are characterized by influx of inflammatory cells with activation and elaboration of a multitude of inflammatory mediators due to widespread damage to the epithelium, combined with vascular leak, upregulation of pro-inflammatory cytokines, and chemokines [6]. (2) Transition phase from inflammation to active fibrosis (7–14 days post of bleomycin) shows gradual subsidence of the inflammatory response with accompanying increase in fibroproliferation, initiation of myofibroblast emergence, and interstitial collagen gene expression peaking toward the end of this phase and beginning of the next [50]. (3) After the third week post-bleomycin is the chronic fibrosis stage when intra-alveolar and septal fibrosis becomes morphologically evident. This phase is characterized by the expansion of the myofibroblast population and increased deposition of extracellular matrix. Lung collagen synthesis remains elevated along with production of other extracellular matrix components as part of the attempted repair process. The increased deposition of lung collagen usually peaks at about 28 days post-bleomycin treatment [6, 51–53]. The development of fibrosis in this model can be assessed histologically and biochemically by measurement of lung hydroxyproline content to estimate total lung collagen content. Some reports show that the fibrotic lesions resolve after day 21–28 [6, 45], while other recent studies indicate persistence of fibrosis, albeit with less inflammation as long as 6 months after a single or repetitive bleomycin treatment(s) [40, 47]. Moreover, these studies show that the bleomycin model has many similarities with human IPF. Despite this discrepancy regarding resolution of fibrosis, there is agreement with respect to the lack of progression beyond the first month after bleomycin treatment, namely, active fibrosis wanes, and no further increase in fibrotic lesions are noted. Figure 1 shows the characteristic pathology of lung fibrosis caused by a single dose of bleomycin through transoral instillation. Fibrosis is fully developed with extensive and diffuse involvement of the lung at the third week (Fig. 1b), with persistence of the developed fibrotic lesions at 8 (Fig. 1c) and 12 (Fig. 1d) weeks after bleomycin instillation. However no progression or extension of fibrotic lesion areas is noted beyond the third week. Repetitive dosing with bleomycin results in similar fibrotic outcome without significant differences in key fibrotic parameters [40].

1.4 Experimental Design

The detailed protocols in this chapter are designed for the bleomycin mouse model induced by endotracheal administration via non-surgical transoral instillation or direct injection into the trachea. The approach can also be modified for the repetitive model by adjusting to a lower dose of bleomycin (e.g., 50% of the single instillation dose) using the transoral route of administration at the desired frequency and intervals in between treatments. It can also be adapted for the rat model by increasing the drug dose/volume, adjusted accordingly for this species and based on the body weight.

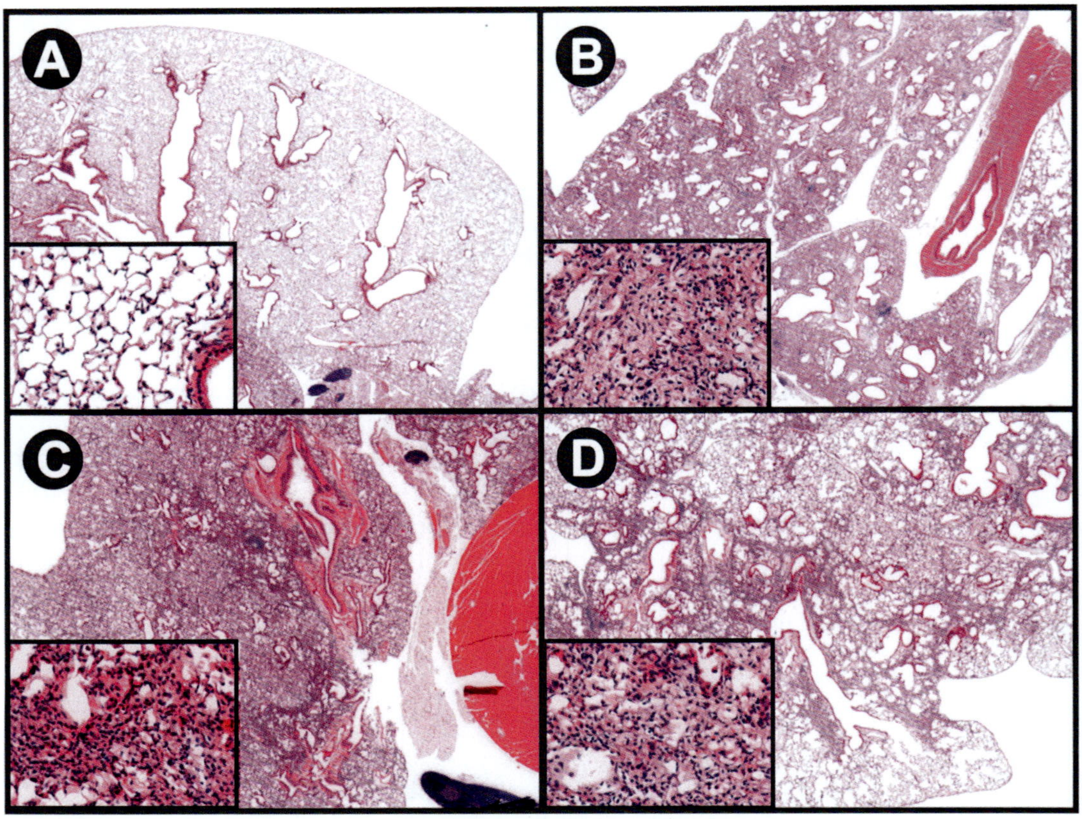

Fig. 1 Lung histopathology after single dose of bleomycin treatment. Bleomycin (2 U/kg) was administered into an 8-week-old female C57BL/6 mice by transoral instillation at day 0. Representative hematoxylin- and eosin-stained lung tissue sections are shown. The mice were sacrificed at 3 (**a** and **b**), 6 (**c**), and 12 (**d**) weeks after bleomycin instillation. Except for the PBS control (**a**), all panels showed lung section from bleomycin-treated mice. The lungs were inflated with 10% buffered formaldehyde. Original magnification, 20X; *insets*: 200X

Several factors should be considered before selecting the appropriate bleomycin model to use, including the route for delivery, dose, dosing frequency, animal gender, and genetic or strain background.

1.4.1 Route of Administration

Although recent findings suggest that repetitive endotracheal administration of bleomycin mimics the chronic aspect of pulmonary fibrosis [54, 55], other studies show little difference between the repetitive dosing vs. single endotracheal dosing with respect to the development of fibrosis [41, 47]. The method of delivery is similar although the dosing per treatment in the repetitive model is reduced [40]. A significant disadvantage of the repetitive model is the greater length of time needed for fibrosis to be fully developed, and thus the increased cost of both bleomycin and animal husbandry. In the more widely used model, bleomycin is usually given by a single dose in weight-adjusted dosages. The routes of drug delivery include direct endotracheal injection or via transoral instillation and systemically via intravenous or intraperitoneal injections. The direct endotracheal delivery of bleomycin is more widely used than systemic approaches because of relative ease of induction and is more economical since lower and less frequent dosing is required, plus the shorter time course of the study. Systemic administration is thought to cause more diffuse disease with a slower time course for development of fibrosis, which may be more representative of events in IPF and also may be useful to mimic the usual delivery route in clinical application as a chemotherapeutic agent [46]. A significant disadvantage is the length of time needed and the requirement for higher and repeated doses of bleomycin. Traditional endotracheal delivery of bleomycin is performed by a surgical procedure. Trachea of the mouse under anesthesia is exposed by surgical incision, and bleomycin is then directly injected into the trachea [44, 56]. This endotracheal delivery method has since been modified by use of a transoral approach and is now more widely used [5, 47, 57]. Transoral instillation is quicker and noninvasive since no surgery is required, thus allowing more rapid recovery, and postsurgical monitoring is eliminated. It may also produce a more uniform distribution due to gravity and natural inhalation by the mouse [5, 48]. The protocol described in this chapter is focused on this transoral instillation approach for its ease, efficient, and reproducible use.

1.4.2 Genetic and Gender Variation

The role of gender in animal model studies of pulmonary fibrosis is controversial. In rats, females exhibit greater sensitivity to bleomycin with higher levels of fibrosis compared to males, which is abolished by ovariectomy [58]. Moreover estrogen treatment of male rats enhances their response to bleomycin. In contrast studies in mice reveal either no significant difference or a greater male responsiveness in bleomycin-induced pulmonary fibrosis, although males exhibit greater decline in lung function [5]. The genetic susceptibility to bleomycin is a heritable trait controlled by a few genetic loci, and X-linked factor may be associated fibrosis phenotype [38]. The susceptibility to bleomycin in mice is strain and genetic background dependent with C57BL/6 mice being high responders and DBA/2 mice being intermediate, while BALB/c mice are relatively bleomycin resistant [52]. The basis for the noted differences is not entirely clear but is likely due to different expression levels of bleomycin hydrolase, as well as expression patterns of cytokines and proteases/antiproteases [36–38].

1.4.3 Dosage of Bleomycin

A wide range of doses of bleomycin for model induction is reported in the literature. In part this could be due to the fact that the potency of bleomycin may vary between companies and their lot numbers. The response to the drug is also mouse strain dependent. Thus, an optimal dose for the desired effect has to be determined in preliminary studies for each batch of bleomycin. The commonly used doses through direct endotracheal administration into the lung are CBA/J mice, 1 U/kg; C57BL/6, 2 U/kg; BALB/c, 10 U/kg; and Fisher 344 rat, 7.5 U/kg [56, 57, 59]. Mortality is usually minimal at these doses, while increasing the dose can significantly increase mortality in most of these animals, often during the acute injury phase and before chronic fibrosis is fully developed. For systemic administration the dose is generally 10–20 times higher, while in repetitive dosing, the dose is usually half the single-dose protocol.

1.4.4 Selection of Time Point for Analysis

Choosing the appropriate endpoint in the bleomycin model depends on the specific parameter of the injury and fibrotic process that needs to be evaluated. Analyses during the first 3 days will reflect the acute injury and inflammatory response to bleomycin. Bronchoalveolar lavage fluid (BALF) is often analyzed for changes in total and differential cell counts. The fibroproliferative response manifested by increasing numbers of fibroblasts and myofibroblasts usually occurs 2 weeks after local delivery of bleomycin, so this is an appropriate time point to study mesenchymal cell proliferation. To evaluate established fibrosis in lung tissue, 3–4 weeks after drug treatment should be considered because the peak of collagen deposition appears at this time point [5]. Semiquantitative histological analysis, quantification of total collagen content by hydroxyproline analysis, as well as the assessment of lung myofibroblast differentiation as measured by α-smooth muscle actin expression may be conducted during this period [5, 60].

1.4.5 Therapeutic Intervention

The bleomycin model has been extensively used in drug discovery studies for identification of novel therapeutic targets, evaluation of potential efficacy of the compound directed at the identified target, preclinical evaluation, and in proof of concept studies. It is almost routinely used along with another model for demonstration of efficacy. For use in such studies, it is important to distinguish between anti-inflammatory and anti-fibrotic drug effects since the bleomycin model has both acute injury and inflammatory phase with a subsequent fibrotic phase. Thus for evaluation of anti-fibrotic therapy, delayed initiation (e.g., >day 12–14 after bleomycin treatment) of treatment with the test compound should be considered [4, 61, 62]. This approach will obviate effects on inflammation that may make it difficult to distinguish an anti-inflammatory effect resulting in subsequent inhibition of fibrosis vs. a purely anti-fibrotic effect independent of effects on inflammation.

2 Materials

2.1 Transoral Instillation of Bleomycin in Mice

1. Mice, 6–8 weeks old, that have been acclimated for a week in the local facility (*see* **Note 1**).
2. Phosphate buffer saline (PBS).

3. Bleomycin (we use the one from APP Pharmaceuticals LLC, Schaumburg, IL). Reconstitute bleomycin dry powder with sterile PBS to the desired unit concentration (2–10 U/mL, 1 Unit = 1 mg). Small aliquots of a concentrated stock solution can be stored at −80 °C up to a year for future use (*see* **Notes 2** and **3**).
4. Ketamine.
5. Xylazine.
6. 1 mL syringe with 26 ½ G needle.
7. Ophthalmic ointment.
8. Forceps.
9. Heat lamp.
10. Disposable underpads.
11. Surgery board with an approximately 70° angle (from horizontal) with looped surgical suture thread attached at the top (Fig. 2).
12. Scale.
13. Alcohol pre pad.
14. 70% ethanol (v/v, in water).
15. 10 mL syringe with 22½ G needles.
16. Paper towels.

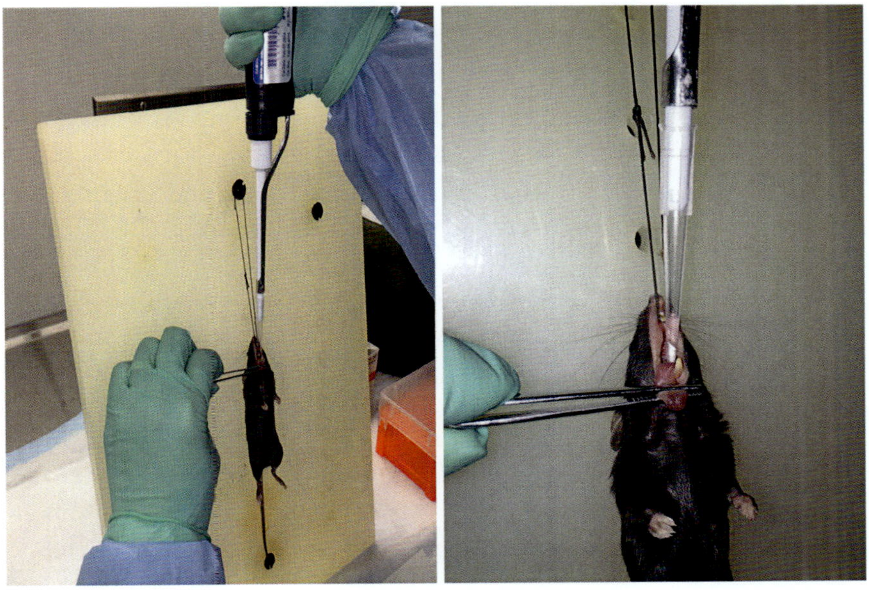

Fig. 2 Nonsurgical transoral instillation of bleomycin into mouse lung. The mouse is anesthetized with ketamine/xylazine and suspended on an approximately 70° angled surgery board. Bleomycin is delivered through transoral instillation by using a 200 μL pipet as described in text. An apparatus for the procedure is shown on the *left*, and a view of exposed oral cavity is shown on the *right*

17. 23½ G needles.
18. 15 mL tubes.

2.2 Additional Materials Needed for Direct Endotracheal Injection of Bleomycin

These materials are in addition of the ones listed in Subheading 2.1.

1. Betadine.
2. Sterile scissors.
3. Auto-suture clips 9 mm.
4. Scalpel blades.
5. Electric shaver.
6. Ethanol swabs.

3 Methods

3.1 Transoral Instillation of Bleomycin in Mice

1. Prepare the desire dilution of bleomycin to administer based on body weight.
2. To anesthetize mice using a combination of ketamine/ xylazine: weigh each mouse, and calculate ketamine/xylazine dose per kg body weight (*see* **Note 4**); restrain the mouse by grasping it by the scruff, and inject 200 μL of ketamine/xylazine solution intraperitoneally (IP) using a 1 mL syringe with 26½ G needle. The duration of anesthesia is 20–30 min.
3. Within 5 min of injection of anesthetic, the mouse will settle down and stop moving. Verify sedation by lack of withdrawal upon firmly pinching a toe, and proceed with the next steps if sedation is achieved.
4. Apply to prevent eyes from drying.
5. Load the required volume of bleomycin or sterile PBS into a sterile 200 μL pipet tip.
6. Place mouse on the surgery board, and suspend via the upper incisors using the surgical thread loop (Fig. 2). Ensure adequate lighting is available for visualization of vocal cords.
7. Pull and extend the tongue gently using sterile padded forceps to one side, toward the mandible to visualize the vocal cords; then, lower the pipet tip loaded with bleomycin into the back of the oral cavity to deliver the liquid through the vocal cords during inspiration (Fig. 2). Wait to hear a gasp, which confirms endotracheal delivery of the liquid. Control animals receive an equal volume of sterile PBS instead of the bleomycin solution.
8. Release the tongue and carefully dislodge the upper incisors from the suspension thread. Place the mouse under a heating lamp or pad until it recovers from the anesthesia, commonly within an hour after injection of anesthetic.

9. Clean the forceps with alcohol pad before and after each use.
10. Monitor the mice daily until they are euthanized for analysis. Body weights and other parameters can be evaluated and recorded daily or as needed.
11. Euthanized the animals at the time points of interest: inject the mice with an overdose of ketamine/xylazine solution based on body weight (1.5 times the dose for regular anesthesia).
12. After 5 min verify sedation by lack of withdrawal upon firmly pinching a toe.
13. Lay mouse in supine position and pin down arms and legs with 22½ G needles.
14. Load 10 mL PBS into a 10 mL syringe with a 22½ G needle.
15. Dampen the abdomen and chest area with 70% ethanol spray.
16. With forceps, pull up the skin of the lower abdomen and using scissors, make a transverse incision to create a small opening into the abdominal cavity, and then make a midline incision in a cranial direction up to the level of the diaphragm.
17. Extend the midline incision cranially up to the neck, followed by lateral incisions (both directions) at the level of the clavicles and also at the level of the diaphragm after carefully separating it from the body wall. Expose the ribcage by setting aside the body wall flaps created by these incisions. Using scissors carefully cut along the sternum while angling upwards to avoid damaging the lungs and heart, followed by cutting of the ribcage along both sides of the chest to fully expose the lungs and heart.
18. Optional: For blood collection, use a 1 mL insulin syringe with a 26½ G needle to withdraw 0.4–1 mL of blood from the left ventricle (which should still be contracting).
19. Move the intestines gently to the right side (of the mouse) to expose the abdominal aorta. Transect the aorta to exsanguinate and absorb the blood with paper towels (there will be less blood after blood collection).
20 To remove blood from the lung vasculature, use forceps to hold on to the heart apex, and insert the 22½ G needle of the 10 mL syringe loaded with PBS (**step 14**) into the right ventricle of the heart, and inject the PBS until the lungs are maximally blanched.
21. If the heart is not contracting, it can be gently massaged using the forceps to assist perfusion of the lungs with the PBS.
22. Cut off the apex of the heart to drain the blood and prevent any blood from returning to the lung.
23. Optional: Lung lavage can be performed and BALF collected before removing the lungs by following the next six steps. If there is no need to collect either one, directly proceed to **step 30**.

24. To collect BALF, expose the trachea in the neck area and separate it from surrounding tissues using a surgical probe.
25. Insert the probe dorsal of the trachea to further separate it from the rest of the neck muscles, and lift it up to thread suture underneath the trachea.
26. After stabilizing the trachea with the suture, puncture it with a 22½ G needle directed caudally at a 45° angle (be careful not to puncture the dorsal wall of the trachea).
27. Insert an 18 G blunt-end needle or catheter through the opening made by the 22½ G needle in the trachea, and tie the surgical suture on the needle tip/trachea to hold it in place.
28. Fill a 1 mL syringe with 1 mL PBS, and attach it to the needle inserted in the trachea.
29. Lavage the lungs five times with 1 mL of PBS each time, and collect the BALF in a 15 mL tube. Promptly place on ice for further processing.
30. Promptly remove the lungs and place them on ice for further processing (*see* **Note 5**). The procedures after exsanguination should be undertaken as rapidly as possible to maximize recovery of intact mRNA and viable cells for further analysis.

3.2 Direct Endotracheal Injection of Bleomycin in Mice

1. The mice are anesthetized with a combination of ketamine and xylazine solution as described in Subheading 3.1 (**step 2**).
2. Shave the neck area and sterilize using betadine and alcohol swabs. Lay the mouse on the surgery board, and immobilize the tail and arms of the mouse with adhesive tape.
3. Using sterile forceps, pull up the skin in the sterilized neck area, and carefully make a 1 cm midline incision with sterile scissors taking care not to cut into underlying tissues. Expose the trachea through the incision using a sterile surgical probe.
4. Load a 1 mL syringe fitted with a 26 G needle with the appropriate amount of pre-diluted bleomycin or an equal volume of sterile PBS for controls. While directed caudally and at an oblique angle, carefully insert the needle into the visualized trachea; taking care not to go through to the dorsal wall of the trachea, rapidly inject the bleomycin solution during a single inspiration.
5. After withdrawing the needle, close the incision with an auto suture clip.
6. Place the animal on warmer pads to stabilize body temperature and allow recovery. Monitor until fully awake, commonly within an hour after induction of anesthesia.
7. Euthanize the mice for desired analysis at the time points of interest following the steps described in Subheading 3.1.

4 Notes

1. The C57BL/6 strain is commonly used because of its good responsiveness to bleomycin. Moreover abundant transgenic strains have this background. The doses in these protocols are based on usage of this strain. Older mice (>12–18 months) can be used in studies of age-dependent fibrosis, which would correspond to 60–70-year-old humans [63, 64]. The effects of bleomycin on gender are not clear and should be carefully considered. In general, the use of females may be advantageous for bleomycin studies because they do not cannibalize their sick littermates, and there is less fighting among the litter. However other considerations may trump this advantage.
2. Bleomycin is known to cause acute lung injury and subsequent fibrosis. Avoid inhalation of both the lyophilized and solubilized forms of bleomycin.
3. Because bleomycin is highly hygroscopic, it is recommended that the entire vial of lyophilized bleomycin be reconstituted at once to prevent the potential error of measurement.
4. Concentrations of anesthetic agents: dose ranges: ketamine (anesthetic) 80–120 mg/kg, xylazine 5–15 mg/kg. Mice and rats with different ages, genders, or genetic backgrounds have different responses to anesthetic drugs. The anesthetic dosages need to be optimized accordingly. The recommended doses of ketamine and xylazine used in C57BL/6 mice are 87 and 13 mg/kg, respectively.
5. Lungs can be inflated with fixative (e.g., 10% buffered formaldehyde) through the trachea before removing the lungs for further processing and use in histopathological examination, immunostaining, etc.

Acknowledgments

This work was supported by NIH grants HL052285 and HL112880. We thank Zhe Wu and Lisa Riggs for their excellent technical assistances.

References

1. Gross TJ, Hunninghake GW (2001) Idiopathic pulmonary fibrosis. N Engl J Med 345(7):517–525. doi:10.1056/NEJMra003200
2. Phan SH (2003) Fibroblast phenotypes in pulmonary fibrosis. Am J Respir Cell Mol Biol 29(3 Suppl):S87–S92
3. Hinz B, Phan SH, Thannickal VJ et al (2007) The myofibroblast: one function, multiple origins. Am J Pathol 170(6):1807–1816. doi:10.2353/ajpath.2007.070112
4. Moeller A, Ask K, Warburton D et al (2008) The bleomycin animal model: a useful tool to

investigate treatment options for idiopathic pulmonary fibrosis? Int J Biochem Cell Biol 40(3):362–382. doi:10.1016/j.biocel.2007.08.011

5. Walters DM, Kleeberger SR (2008) Mouse models of bleomycin-induced pulmonary fibrosis. Curr Protoc Pharmacol Chapter 5:Unit 5.46. doi:10.1002/0471141755.ph0546s40
6. Moore BB, Hogaboam CM (2008) Murine models of pulmonary fibrosis. Am J Physiol Lung Cell Mol Physiol 294(2):L152–L160. doi:10.1152/ajplung.00313.2007
7. Umezawa H, Ishizuka M, Maeda K et al (1967) Studies on bleomycin. Cancer 20(5):891–895
8. Umezawa H, Maeda K, Takeuchi T et al (1966) New antibiotics, bleomycin A and B. J Antibiot (Tokyo) 19(5):200–209
9. Yagoda A, Mukherji B, Young C et al (1972) Bleomycin, an antitumor antibiotic. Clinical experience in 274 patients. Ann Intern Med 77(6):861–870
10. Blum RH, Carter SK, Agre K (1973) A clinical review of bleomycin – a new antineoplastic agent. Cancer 31(4):903–914
11. Umezawa H (1974) Chemistry and mechanism of action of bleomycin. Fed Proc 33(11):2296–2302
12. Rudders RA, Hensley GT (1973) Bleomycin pulmonary toxicity. Chest 63(4):627–628
13. Sostman HD, Matthay RA, Putman CE (1977) Cytotoxic drug-induced lung disease. Am J Med 62(4):608–615
14. Onuma T, Holland JF, Masuda H et al (1974) Microbiological assay of bleomycin: inactivation, tissue distribution, and clearance. Cancer 33(5):1230–1238
15. Phan SH, Thrall RS, Ward PA (1980) Bleomycin-induced pulmonary fibrosis in rats: biochemical demonstration of increased rate of collagen synthesis. Am Rev Respir Dis 121(3):501–506. doi:10.1164/arrd.1980.121.3.501
16. Phan SH, Thrall RS, Williams C (1981) Bleomycin-induced pulmonary fibrosis. Effects of steroid on lung collagen metabolism. Am Rev Respir Dis 124(4):428–434. doi:10.1164/arrd.1981.124.4.428
17. Phan SH, Thrall RS (1982) The role of soluble factors in bleomycin-induced pulmonary fibrosis. Am J Pathol 106(2):156–164
18. Fleischman RW, Baker JR, Thompson GR et al (1971) Bleomycin-induced interstitial pneumonia in dogs. Thorax 26(6):675–682
19. Adamson IY, Bowden DH (1974) The pathogenesis of bleomycin-induced pulmonary fibrosis in mice. Am J Pathol 77(2):185–197
20. Snider GL, Hayes JA, Korthy AL (1978) Chronic interstitial pulmonary fibrosis produced in hamsters by endotracheal bleomycin: pathology and stereology. Am Rev Respir Dis 117(6):1099–1108. doi:10.1164/arrd.1978.117.6.1099
21. Thrall RS, McCormick JR, Jack RM et al (1979) Bleomycin-induced pulmonary fibrosis in the rat: inhibition by indomethacin. Am J Pathol 95(1):117–130
22. Organ L, Bacci B, Koumoundouros E et al (2015) Structural and functional correlations in a large animal model of bleomycin-induced pulmonary fibrosis. BMC Pulm Med 15:81. doi:10.1186/s12890-015-0071-6
23. Chandler DB, Hyde DM, Giri SN (1983) Morphometric estimates of infiltrative cellular changes during the development of bleomycin-induced pulmonary fibrosis in hamsters. Am J Pathol 112(2):170–177
24. Lown JW, Sim SK (1977) The mechanism of the bleomycin-induced cleavage of DNA. Biochem Biophys Res Commun 77(4):1150–1157. doi:10.1016/S0006-291X(77)80099-5
25. Claussen CA, Long EC (1999) Nucleic acid recognition by metal complexes of bleomycin. Chem Rev 99(9):2797–2816. doi:10.1002/chin.199948318
26. Liu T, Chung MJ, Ullenbruch M et al (2007) Telomerase activity is required for bleomycin-induced pulmonary fibrosis in mice. J Clin Invest 117(12):3800–3809. doi:10.1172/JCI32369
27. Usuki J, Fukuda Y (1995) Evolution of three patterns of intra-alveolar fibrosis produced by bleomycin in rats. Pathol Int 45(8):552–564. doi:10.1111/j.1440-1827.1995.tb03503.x
28. Munger JS, Huang X, Kawakatsu H et al (1999) The integrin alpha v beta 6 binds and activates latent TGF beta 1: a mechanism for regulating pulmonary inflammation and fibrosis. Cell 96(3):319–328. S0092-8674(00)80545-0 [pii]
29. Bauer Y, Tedrow J, de Bernard S et al (2015) A novel genomic signature with translational significance for human idiopathic pulmonary fibrosis. Am J Respir Cell Mol Biol 52(2):217–231. doi:10.1165/rcmb.2013-0310OC
30. Wollin L, Wex E, Pautsch A et al (2015) Mode of action of nintedanib in the treatment of idiopathic pulmonary fibrosis. Eur Respir J 45(5):1434–1445. doi:10.1183/09031936.00174914
31. King CS, Nathan SD (2015) Practical considerations in the pharmacologic treatment of idiopathic pulmonary fibrosis. Curr Opin Pulm Med 21(5):479–489. doi:10.1097/MCP.0000000000000190

32. Grimminger F, Gunther A, Vancheri C (2015) The role of tyrosine kinases in the pathogenesis of idiopathic pulmonary fibrosis. Eur Respir J 45(5):1426–1433. doi:10.1183/09031936.00149614

33. Iyer SN, Wild JS, Schiedt MJ et al (1995) Dietary intake of pirfenidone ameliorates bleomycin-induced lung fibrosis in hamsters. J Lab Clin Med 125(6):779–785

34. Mackinnon AC, Gibbons MA, Farnworth SL et al (2012) Regulation of transforming growth factor-beta1-driven lung fibrosis by galectin-3. Am J Respir Crit Care Med 185(5):537–546. doi:10.1164/rccm.201106-0965OC

35. Peters DM, Vadasz I, Wujak L et al (2014) TGF-beta directs trafficking of the epithelial sodium channel ENaC which has implications for ion and fluid transport in acute lung injury. Proc Natl Acad Sci U S A 111(3):E374–E383. doi:10.1073/pnas.1306798111

36. Sebti SM, Mignano JE, Jani JP et al (1989) Bleomycin hydrolase: molecular cloning, sequencing, and biochemical studies reveal membership in the cysteine proteinase family. Biochemistry 28(16):6544–6548

37. Phan SH, Kunkel SL (1992) Lung cytokine production in bleomycin-induced pulmonary fibrosis. Exp Lung Res 18(1):29–43. doi:10.3109/01902149209020649

38. Haston CK, Amos CI, King TM et al (1996) Inheritance of susceptibility to bleomycin-induced pulmonary fibrosis in the mouse. Cancer Res 56(11):2596–2601

39. Thannickal VJ (2013) Mechanistic links between aging and lung fibrosis. Biogerontology 14(6):609–615. doi:10.1007/s10522-013-9451-6

40. Degryse AL, Tanjore H, XC X et al (2010) Repetitive intratracheal bleomycin models several features of idiopathic pulmonary fibrosis. Am J Physiol Lung Cell Mol Physiol 299(4):L442–L452. doi:10.1152/ajplung.00026.2010

41. Peng R, Sridhar S, Tyagi G et al (2013) Bleomycin induces molecular changes directly relevant to idiopathic pulmonary fibrosis: a model for "active" disease. PLoS One 8(4):e59348. doi:10.1371/journal.pone.0059348

42. Williamson JD, Sadofsky LR, Hart SP (2015) The pathogenesis of bleomycin-induced lung injury in animals and its applicability to human idiopathic pulmonary fibrosis. Exp Lung Res 41(2):57–73. doi:10.3109/01902148.2014.979516

43. Chua F, Gauldie J, Laurent GJ (2005) Pulmonary fibrosis: searching for model answers. Am J Respir Cell Mol Biol 33(1):9–13. doi:10.1165/rcmb.2005-0062TR

44. Borzone G, Moreno R, Urrea R et al (2001) Bleomycin-induced chronic lung damage does not resemble human idiopathic pulmonary fibrosis. Am J Respir Crit Care Med 163(7):1648–1653. doi:10.1164/ajrccm.163.7.2006132

45. Lawson WE, Polosukhin VV, Stathopoulos GT et al (2005) Increased and prolonged pulmonary fibrosis in surfactant protein C-deficient mice following intratracheal bleomycin. Am J Pathol 167(5):1267–1277. doi:10.1016/S0002-9440(10)61214-X

46. Della Latta V, Cecchettini A, Del Ry S et al (2015) Bleomycin in the setting of lung fibrosis induction: from biological mechanisms to counteractions. Pharmacol Res 97:122–130. doi:10.1016/j.phrs.2015.04.012

47. Limjunyawong N, Mitzner W, Horton MR (2014) A mouse model of chronic idiopathic pulmonary fibrosis. Physiol Rep 2(2):e00249. doi:10.1002/phy2.249

48. Foster WM, Walters DM, Longphre M et al (2001) Methodology for the measurement of mucociliary function in the mouse by scintigraphy. J Appl Physiol (1985) 90(3):1111–1117

49. Hu B, Wu Z, Nakashima T et al (2012) Mesenchymal-specific deletion of C/EBPbeta suppresses pulmonary fibrosis. Am J Pathol 180(6):2257–2267. doi:10.1016/j.ajpath.2012.02.010

50. Chaudhary NI, Schnapp A, Park JE (2006) Pharmacologic differentiation of inflammation and fibrosis in the rat bleomycin model. Am J Respir Crit Care Med 173(7):769–776. doi:10.1164/rccm.200505-717OC

51. Phan SH, Armstrong G, Sulavik MC et al (1983) A comparative study of pulmonary fibrosis induced by bleomycin and an O2 metabolite producing enzyme system. Chest 83(5 Suppl):44S–45S. doi:10.1378/chest.83.5.44S

52. Schrier DJ, Kunkel RG, Phan SH (1983) The role of strain variation in murine bleomycin-induced pulmonary fibrosis. Am Rev Respir Dis 127(1):63–66. doi:10.1164/arrd.1983.127.1.63

53. Scotton CJ, Chambers RC (2010) Bleomycin revisited: towards a more representative model of IPF? Am J Physiol Lung Cell Mol Physiol 299(4):L439–L441. doi:10.1152/ajplung.00258.2010

54. Mouratis MA, Aidinis V (2011) Modeling pulmonary fibrosis with bleomycin. Curr Opin Pulm Med 17(5):355–361. doi:10.1097/MCP.0b013e328349ac2b

55. Degryse AL, Lawson WE (2011) Progress toward improving animal models for idiopathic pulmonary fibrosis. Am J Med Sci 341(6):444–449. doi:10.1097/MAJ.0b013e31821aa000

56. Gharaee-Kermani M, Ullenbruch M, Phan SH (2005) Animal models of pulmonary fibrosis. Methods Mol Med 117:251–259. doi:10.1385/1-59259-940-0:251

57. Liu T, Dhanasekaran SM, Jin H et al (2004) FIZZ1 stimulation of myofibroblast differentiation. Am J Pathol 164(4):1315–1326. doi:10.1016/S0002-9440(10)63218-X

58. Gharaee-Kermani M, Hatano K, Nozaki Y et al (2005) Gender-based differences in bleomycin-induced pulmonary fibrosis. Am J Pathol 166(6):1593–1606. doi:10.1016/S0002-9440(10)62470-4

59. Liu T, Jin H, Ullenbruch M et al (2004) Regulation of found in inflammatory zone 1 expression in bleomycin-induced lung fibrosis: role of IL-4/IL-13 and mediation via STAT-6. J Immunol 173(5):3425–3431. doi:10.4049/jimmunol.173.5.3425

60. Liu T, Yu H, Ding L et al (2015) Conditional knockout of telomerase reverse transcriptase in mesenchymal cells impairs mouse pulmonary fibrosis. PLoS One 10(11):e0142547. doi:10.1371/journal.pone.0142547

61. Choi JE, Lee SS, Sunde DA et al (2009) Insulin-like growth factor-I receptor blockade improves outcome in mouse model of lung injury. Am J Respir Crit Care Med 179(3):212–219. doi:10.1164/rccm.200802-228OC

62. Koh RY, Lim CL, Uhal BD et al (2015) Inhibition of transforming growth factor-beta via the activin receptor-like kinase-5 inhibitor attenuates pulmonary fibrosis. Mol Med Rep 11(5):3808–3813. doi:10.3892/mmr.2015.3193

63. Huang WT, Akhter H, Jiang C et al (2015) Plasminogen activator inhibitor 1, fibroblast apoptosis resistance, and aging-related susceptibility to lung fibrosis. Exp Gerontol 61:62–75. doi:10.1016/j.exger.2014.11.018

64. Dutta S, Sengupta P (2016) Men and mice: relating their ages. Life Sci 152:244–248. doi:10.1016/j.lfs.2015.10.025

Chapter 3

Intradermal Injections of Bleomycin to Model Skin Fibrosis

Toshiyuki Yamamoto

Abstract

Systemic sclerosis (scleroderma) is a fibrotic condition characterized by immunologic abnormalities, vascular injury, and increased accumulation of extracellular matrix proteins in the affected organs. Although the etiology of scleroderma has not yet been fully elucidated, a growing body of evidence suggests that extracellular matrix overproduction by activated fibroblasts results from a complex interaction among endothelial cells, immunocytes, and fibroblasts, involving a number of mediators such as cytokines, chemokines, growth factors, and their receptors. For a better understanding of the pathophysiology of scleroderma, animal models are important tools. They reproduce several histological as well as biochemical aspects resembling human scleroderma, and we can learn lots of new findings through animal studies. On the other hand, it must be emphasized that there are no animal models so far exhibiting all the aspects of human scleroderma, and studying animal models cannot answer all the problems of human scleroderma. This paper introduces current concepts of various animal models for scleroderma and discusses their advantages/disadvantages, contribution to our understanding of the pathogenesis, and therapeutic approach for human scleroderma.

Key words Scleroderma, Animal model, Bleomycin

1 Introduction

Systemic sclerosis (SSc) is a connective tissue disease which shows fibrogenesis and vasculogenesis. Although the pathogenesis of SSc has not been fully elucidated yet, it is characterized by the excessive accumulation of extracellular matrix (ECM) proteins in the skin and various internal organs, vascular injury, and immunological abnormalities [1]. In early stages of SSc, activated fibroblasts in the affected areas produce high amounts of collagen. Histological analysis of the initial stage of scleroderma reveals perivascular infiltrates of mononuclear cells in the dermis, which is associated with increased collagen synthesis in the surrounding fibroblasts. A number of studies have demonstrated the crucial role of several fibrogenic cytokines released from immunocytes in initiating the sequence of events leading to fibrosis. Animal models are useful in providing clues for the study of various human diseases and for the

Laure Rittié (ed.), *Fibrosis: Methods and Protocols*, Methods in Molecular Biology, vol. 1627,
DOI 10.1007/978-1-4939-7113-8_3,

exploration of new treatments. Although animal models which exhibit all the aspects of SSc are not currently available, several experimental animal models, such as tight skin (Tsk) mice, Tsk2 mice, bleomycin-induced murine scleroderma, sclerodermatous graft-versus-host disease (Scl GVHD) mice, exogenous injections of transforming growth factor-β (TGF-β)/connective tissue growth factor (CTGF)-induced murine fibrosis model, and UCD 200 chicken, Fli-1-deficient mice, as well as several transgenic or knockout mice, have been examined so far [2]. Among them, bleomycin-induced murine model is established because of the simple method, reproducibility, and independence of mice strain.

Bleomycin was originally isolated from the fungus *Streptomyces verticillus* and is frequently used as an antitumor agent for the treatment of various kinds of malignancy. In addition, bleomycin is used by dermatologists as a treatment for recalcitrant warts, hypertrophic scars, and keloid [3]. Bleomycin hydrolase inactivates bleomycin by hydrolyzing the amide bond in the β-aminoalanineamide moiety. Due to the deficiency of the enzyme in the lungs and the skin, bleomycin-induced toxicity occurs predominantly in these organs. Pulmonary fibrosis is a well-known adverse effect of bleomycin, and bleomycin-induced lung injury in rodents is an established model for human pulmonary fibrosis. In 1983, Mountz et al. [4] reported that rats injected repeatedly with sublethal doses of bleomycin over a 58-week period developed severe dermal fibrosis similar to those found in human scleroderma with structural abnormalities of collagen fibers; however, histological features were not shown in their paper. On the other hand, we established bleomycin-induced murine scleroderma model by repeated local injections of bleomycin into the shaved back skins and published in a series of studies [5–10]. Thereafter, this model has been admitted worldwide as a representative scleroderma model, and making use of this model, a number of studies have been performed. Further, modified models have also been reported [11, 12].

Histopathological examination revealed definite dermal sclerosis characterized by thickened collagen bundles and deposition of homogenous materials in the thickened dermis with cellular infiltrates, which mimicked human scleroderma. Dermal thickness gradually increased with the onset of the sclerosis. Cellular infiltrates were composed of T cells, monocytes/macrophages, and mast cells, which are supposed to play an important role in the induction of dermal sclerosis. By contrast, dermal sclerosis can be compulsorily induced by bleomycin treatment, even in nude mice, severe combined immunodeficiency (SCID) mice, and mast cell-deficient mice [6, 8, 10]. A study shows that transfer of CD4+ T cells from bleomycin-treated mice induced the same pathological changes and antibody production in untreated Balb/c nude mice [12]. Mast cells increased in number in tandem with the induction of dermal sclerosis. Also, a marked degranulation was found in particular in the early phase, with elevated plasma histamine levels [5]. In some strains, epidermal thickness was also induced as well [6]. Further, lung fibrosis showing thickened alveolar walls with cellular infiltrates was also induced early on. Cutaneous changes were generally localized to the area surrounding the injected site, and sclerotic changes were not induced in the remote regions, such as fingers or abdominal skin. After the stoppage of bleomycin injections, sclerotic changes remained at least 6 weeks, suggesting that the induction of dermal sclerosis is not transient but persistent. Thickness of vascular wall in the deep dermis was also observed [13].

There was some variation among strains in the intensity of the symptoms and the period required to induce dermal sclerosis, C3H/He, DBA/2, B10.D2, and B10. A strain demonstrated intense dermal sclerosis by bleomycin treatment, suggestive of bleomycin "susceptibility" [7, 14]. Hydroxyproline contents in the bleomycin-treated skin were significantly increased in comparison with those of the PBS-treated skin. Increased production as well as upregulation of mRNA levels of type I collagen was found in the sclerotic skin [5, 7]. In the bleomycin-induced scleroderma, α-SMA-positive myofibroblasts were observed in the dermis and gradually increased in tandem with the induction of dermal sclerosis [9]. Interestingly, autoantibodies were detected in the serum after bleomycin treatment [5]. Bleomycin hydrolase inactivates bleomycin by hydrolyzing the amide bond in the β-aminoalanineamide moiety. Due to the lack or shortage of this enzyme in the lungs and the skin, bleomycin-induced fibrosis and sclerosis occur predominantly in these organs. A recent report shows that a one-time injection of bleomycin-poly (l-lactic acid) microspheres can induce dermal sclerosis in mice [11]; however, this technique is difficult and can be available in limited institutes. The induction of dermal sclerosis is considered to be, in part, mediated by inflammatory and fibrogenic cytokines, as well as by the direct effect of bleomycin on ECM synthesis in fibroblasts.

2 Materials

1. Mice weighing 20–25 g (*see* **Notes 1** and **2**).
2. 80 mg/kg ketamine + 10 mg/kg xylazine solution.
3. 1-ml syringes and 25 G needles for anesthesia.
4. Alcohol wipes.
5. Electric shaver.
6. 1-ml syringes and 27 G needles for intradermal injection.

3 Methods

1. Anesthetize the mouse by intraperitoneal injection of ketamine/xylazine using 25 G needles.
2. Shave the back of the mouse gently.
3. Wipe the injection site with alcohol swabs.
4. Inject 100 μl of bleomycin at a concentration of 100–1000 μg/ml intradermally (*see* **Note 3**).
5. Repeat the above steps 3–7 times per week (i.e., every other day, every weekday, or every day, depending on the desired degree of fibrosis) (*see* **Note 4**).

4 Notes

1. Mice at the age of 4–6 weeks are usually chosen. Although dermal sclerosis can be induced by bleomycin in various mice strains, C3H/He, A/J, DBA2, B10.D2, and B10.A, Balb/c mice develop intense dermal sclerosis, characterized by deposition of homogenous materials and thickened collagen bundles in the dermis. By contrast, Ruzehaji et al. [15] reported that male Balb/c mice developed the most severe fibrosis phenotype. Although dermal sclerosis was not very strongly induced in C57BL/6 J strain, a frequently used strain as a control wild type in studies using gene deficient mice, C57BL/6 J strain, can be used in those experiments.
2. Both males and females can be used, and there are no definite differences of the degrees in induced fibrosis.
3. Bleomycin administration is recommended to the superficial areas in the skin to avoid diffusion. Bleomycin at a concentration less than 1 mg/ml is commonly used, because mice are getting thin with weight loss and easily die if higher concentration than 1 mg/ml of bleomycin is frequently given. If mice lose too much weight, adjustment at 500 μg/ml is recommended. A modified method by continuous subcutaneous bleomycin injection from implanted osmotic minipumps also developed skin and pulmonary fibrosis [16].
4. Typical treatment is 4 weeks, but the length of treatment can be adjusted based on results.

Acknowledgment

This work was supported in part by a grant from project research on intractable diseases from the Japanese Ministry of Health, Labour and Welfare.

References

1. Yamamoto T (2009) Scleroderma–pathophysiology. Eur J Dermatol 19(1):14–24. doi:10.1684/ejd.2008.0570
2. Yamamoto T (2010) Animal model of systemic sclerosis. J Dermatol 37(1):26–41. doi:10.1111/j.1346-8138.2009.00764.x
3. Yamamoto T (2006) Bleomycin and the skin. Br J Dermatol 155(5):869–875. doi:10.1111/j.1365-2133.2006.07474.x
4. Mountz JD, Downs Minor MB, Turner R et al (1983) Bleomycin-induced cutaneous toxicity in the rat: analysis of histopathology and ultrastructure compared with progressive systemic sclerosis (scleroderma). Br J Dermatol 108(6):679–686. doi:10.1111/j.1365-2133.1983.tb01080.x
5. Yamamoto T, Takagawa S, Katayama I et al (1999) Animal model of sclerotic skin. I: local injections of bleomycin induce sclerotic skin mimicking scleroderma. J Invest Dermatol 112(4):456–462. doi:10.1046/j.1523-1747.1999.00528.x
6. Yamamoto T, Takahashi Y, Takagawa S et al (1999) Animal model of sclerotic skin. II. Bleomycin induced scleroderma in genetically mast cell deficient WBB6F1-W/W(V) mice. J Rheumatol 26(12):2628–2634
7. Yamamoto T, Kuroda M, Nishioka K (2000) Animal model of sclerotic skin. III: histopathological comparison of bleomycin-induced scleroderma in various mice strains. Arch Dermatol Res 292(11):535–541. doi:10.1007/s004030000183
8. Yamamoto T, Nishioka K (2001) Animal model of sclerotic skin. IV: induction of dermal sclerosis by bleomycin is T cell independent. J Invest Dermatol 117(4):999–1001. doi:10.1046/j.0022-202x.2001.01509.x
9. Yamamoto T, Nishioka K (2002) Animal model of sclerotic skin. V: increased expression of alpha-smooth muscle actin in fibroblastic cells in bleomycin-induced scleroderma. Clin Immunol 102(1):77–83. doi:10.1006/clim.2001.5138
10. Yamamoto T, Nishioka K (2004) Animal model of sclerotic skin. VI: evaluation of bleomycin-induced skin sclerosis in nude mice. Arch Dermatol Res 295(10):453–456. doi:10.1007/s00403-003-0439-y
11. Shibusawa Y, Negishi I, Tabata Y et al (2008) Mouse model of dermal fibrosis induced by one-time injection of bleomycin-poly(L-lactic acid) microspheres. Rheumatology (Oxford) 47(4):454–457. doi:10.1093/rheumatology/ken058
12. Ishikawa H, Takeda K, Okamoto A et al (2009) Induction of autoimmunity in a bleomycin-induced murine model of experimental systemic sclerosis: an important role for CD4+ T cells. J Invest Dermatol 129(7):1688–1695. doi:10.1038/jid.2008.431
13. Yamamoto T, Katayama I (2011) Vascular changes in bleomycin-induced scleroderma. Int J Rheumatol 2011:270938. doi:10.1155/2011/270938
14. Oi M, Yamamoto T, Nishioka K (2004) Increased expression of TGF-beta1 in the sclerotic skin in bleomycin-'susceptible' mouse strains. J Med Dent Sci 51(1):7–17
15. Ruzehaji N, Avouac J, Elhai M et al (2015) Combined effect of genetic background and gender in a mouse model of bleomycin-induced skin fibrosis. Arthritis Res Ther 17:145. doi:10.1186/s13075-015-0659-5
16. Liang M, Lv J, Zou L et al (2015) A modified murine model of systemic sclerosis: bleomycin given by pump infusion induced skin and pulmonary inflammation and fibrosis. Lab Invest 95(3):342–350. doi:10.1038/labinvest.2014.145

Chapter 4

Assessing the Effects of Fibrosis on Lung Function by Light Microscopy-Coupled Stereology

Bartosz Pilecki and Grith Lykke Sørensen

Abstract

Pulmonary diseases such as fibrosis are characterized by structural abnormalities that lead to impairment of proper lung function. Stereological analysis of serial tissue sections allows detection and quantitation of subtle changes in lung architecture. Here, we describe a stereology-based method of assessing pathology-induced changes in lung structure.

Key words Design-based stereology, Systematic uniform random sampling, Lung, Morphometry, Volume density, Point counting, Surface density, Intersection counting, Numerical density, Physical disector

1 Introduction

The three-dimensional (3D) structure of the lung is tightly linked to its primary function as the gas-exchanging organ. The mammalian lung is characterized by a large surface area with a thin diffusion barrier, thus providing means for very efficient gas exchange [1]. Alterations in lung architecture are common in pulmonary diseases and result in functional impairment, which underlines the importance of accurate quantitation of lung structure parameters when assessing pathology or treatment effects [2]. Such precise estimation of disease-induced structural changes requires the use of stereological methods, which have become a golden standard for lung morphometry in pulmonary research [3–5].

Stereology can be defined as science that provides sampling and measurement tools to obtain quantitative 3D data (volume, surface area, length, particle number) based on simple measurements on 2D microscopic sections (Table 1) [6]. Design-based stereology is unbiased to size, shape, spatial distribution, or spatial orientation of the investigated tissue [7]. The main steps in stereology are sampling and estimation/measurement. To ensure randomization for location (i.e., that each part of the lung has an

Laure Rittié (ed.), *Fibrosis: Methods and Protocols*, Methods in Molecular Biology, vol. 1627,
DOI 10.1007/978-1-4939-7113-8_4, © Springer Science+Business Media LLC 2017

Table 1
Basic parameters estimated by stereology

Parameter	Test probe	Method	Example
Volume (3D)	Test points (0D)	Point counting	Lung parenchyma Alveolar septa
Surface area (2D)	Test lines (1D)	Intersection counting	Alveolar epithelium
Length (1D)	Test planes (2D)	Transect counting	Fibers
Particle number (0D)	Disector (3D)	Top counting	Alveoli Type II epithelial cells

Overview of basic structural parameters possible to evaluate by stereological methods together with the appropriate geometric probes and methods to estimate them. Numbers in brackets indicate the dimension of the parameter or test probe. (Modified from Weibel et al. 2007 [9])

equal chance of being sampled), one of the unbiased sampling strategies needs to be used. The most common sampling method in small animal research is systematic uniform random sampling (SURS). In SURS, the first cut is made randomly after initial tissue processing, and the subsequent parallel slices are made with a constant thickness interval [7]. The microscopic fields of view (FOV) of the section are then themselves sampled with a predefined step length. The stereological measurements are most often simple counts of test points (specified tissue components) interacting with geometric probes, such as lines or point grids, superimposed on the FOV. The obtained parameters are first calculated as relative densities (volume density, surface density, etc.) and should be converted to absolute quantities through multiplication with a reference volume (total lung volume) [8].

Pulmonary fibrosis, characterized by excessive deposition of interstitial tissue within the septa, is a consequence of several interstitial lung diseases. Among them, idiopathic pulmonary fibrosis (IPF) represents the most prevalent and most fatal disorder [10]. The common pathophysiological features of IPF include the increase of septal thickness, alveolar collapse, tissue scarring, and alveolar epithelial type II cell hyperplasia as well as hypertrophy, all of which can be determined by stereology (Table 2) [11]. Indeed, two recent studies have used design-based stereology to investigate pulmonary changes in the rodent model of fibrosis as well as human IPF tissue and shown that structural alterations assessed by stereology are significantly correlated with severity of fibrosis and lung function parameters [12, 13].

Here, we show how to use stereology to assess the impact of fibrosis on lung structure at the light microscopy level, based on previously published material [14]. We describe in detail all the crucial steps related to tissue processing, proper sampling, measurement types, and calculation of results.

Table 2
Stereological parameters in fibrotic research accessible by light microscopy

Structure	Parameter	Method	Magn
Parenchymal damage	Volume of functional (ventilated) and destroyed (nonventilated) lung parenchyma	Point counting	5X
Alveolar disturbances	Volume of alveolar airspace and septal wall tissue within functional parenchyma	Point counting	20X
Functional gas exchange area	Surface area of alveolar epithelium within functional parenchyma	Intersection counting	20X
Septal thickening	Mean septal wall thickness within functional parenchyma	Septal wall volume-to-surface ratio	20X
Alveolar collapse	Number of ventilated alveoli	Physical disector	20X
Alveolar collapse	Number-weighed mean volume of alveoli	Ratio of alveolar airspace volume to alveolar number	20X
AEIIC hyperplasia	Number of AEIIC per lung	Physical disector	100X

AEIIC alveolar epithelial type II cells

2 Materials

2.1 Lung Isolation

1. Surgical instruments (clean and sterilized with 70% ethanol (v/v)).
2. Thin suture (size 5-0 or similar).
3. Catheter (*see* **Note 1**).

2.2 Sample Preparation

2.2.1 Reagents

1. 0.15 M HEPES buffer, pH 7.35.
2. Fixative (*see* **Note 2**): 1.5% paraformaldehyde and 1.5% glutaraldehyde in 0.15 M HEPES buffer, pH 7.35.
3. Agar or low-melt agarose (4% w/v, in distilled water).
4. 0.1 M sodium cacodylate buffer, pH 7.35.
5. 1% osmium tetroxide (OsO_4) in 0.1 M sodium cacodylate buffer (*see* **Note 3**).
6. Distilled water.
7. Half-saturated uranyl acetate (*see* **Note 4**).
8. Acetone solutions (70, 80, 90, 100% v/v, in distilled water).
9. Glycol such as Technovit 8100 (Heraeus Kulzer, Wehrheim, Germany) (*see* **Note 5**).

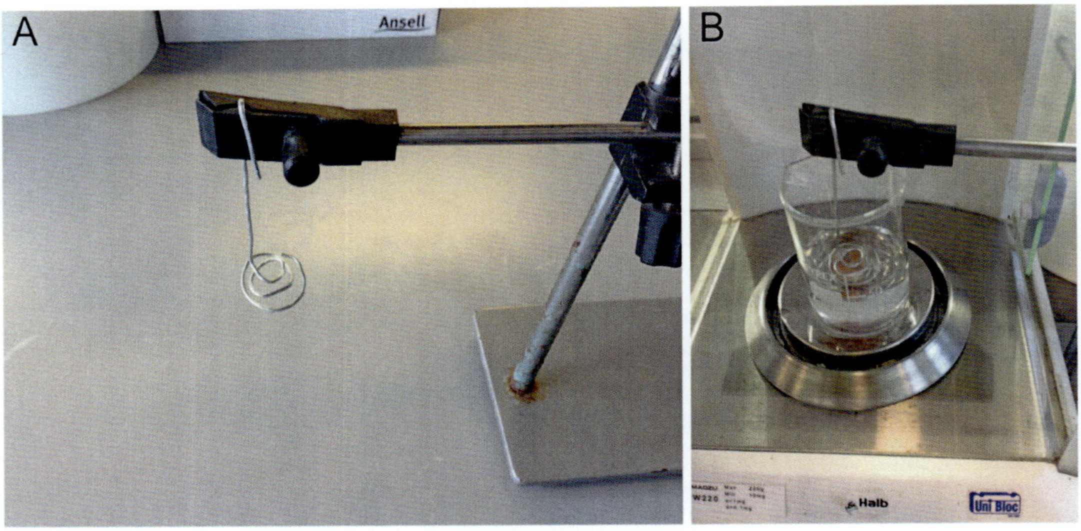

Fig. 1 A wire with a coiled end attached to the stand can be used as a lung diver (**a**). The lung diver keeps the lung from emerging to the surface (**b**) (Figure courtesy of Anne Trommelholt Holm)

10. Toluidine blue staining solution: 1 g toluidine blue and 2.5 g sodium hydrogen carbonate in 100 mL distilled water (1% stock solution). For staining, dilute to 0.1% (w/v).
11. 96% ethanol solution (v/v, in distilled water), from absolute ethanol.
12. Xylene.
13. Mounting medium.

2.2.2 Equipment

1. Beaker with water.
2. Scale.
3. "Lung diver" device (*see* **Note 6**) (Fig. 1).
4. Scalpel.
5. Tissue slicer (*see* **Note 7**).
6. Rectangular point grid or millimeter graph paper.
7. Embedding molds.
8. Microtome.
9. Glass slides positively charged.
10. Cover glasses.

2.3 Microscopes

1. Light microscope with a motorized stage, equipped with low-power and high-power objective lenses (1X, 5X, 20X).
2. Digital camera attached to the microscope.
3. Image analysis software (*see* **Note 8**).

3 Methods

3.1 Lung Fixation

1. Euthanize the animal.
2. Carefully expose the trachea. Using fine scissors, make a small hole in the trachea and insert the catheter. Fix the catheter in place by placing a ligature below the insertion site.
3. Open the abdomen and the thorax.
4. Fix the lungs by intratracheal instillation of a fixative solution through the catheter at the constant pressure of 25 cm H_2O (*see* **Note 9**).
5. Ligate the trachea below the catheter (*see* **Note 10**).
6. Carefully remove the lungs from the thorax and immerse in the fixative. Store at 4 °C until further processing (at least 24 h).

3.2 Measuring a Reference Volume

Total lung volume can be estimated by two methods.

3.2.1 Scherle's Method: Fluid Displacement

1. Carefully remove as much non-lung tissue (e.g., trachea, esophagus, etc.) from the lung as possible.
2. Place the beaker with water on the scale, submerge the lung diver, and zero the scale.
3. Lift the device, attach the lungs, and lower the device so that the lungs are fully submerged in water and the device is in the same initial position (*see* **Note 11**). The device or the lungs should not touch the walls or the bottom of the beaker (Fig. 1).
4. Record the weight change, and calculate the corresponding volume based on Archimedes' principle [15]: the buoyant force acting on a submerged body is equal to the weight of the displaced liquid. As the specific gravity of water is close to 1, the measured weight gain (in grams) corresponds to the volume of the immersed tissue in mL ($V \approx W$).

3.2.2 Cavalieri's Principle

Estimation of total lung volume by Cavalieri's method is based on point counting of the cut tissue surfaces after serial sectioning [16]. The total volume can then be calculated as multiplication of slab thickness by the sum of cut face areas. The procedure is to be performed after **step 4** of the sampling protocol described in Subheading 3.3.

1. Overlay the square point grid onto the cut slabs (*see* **Note 12**).
2. Count the total number of points hitting the cut face area (*see* **Note 13**). As the points are crossings of horizontal and vertical lines, only one of four corners of such crossings should be chosen for counting and kept throughout the whole counting process (Fig. 2).

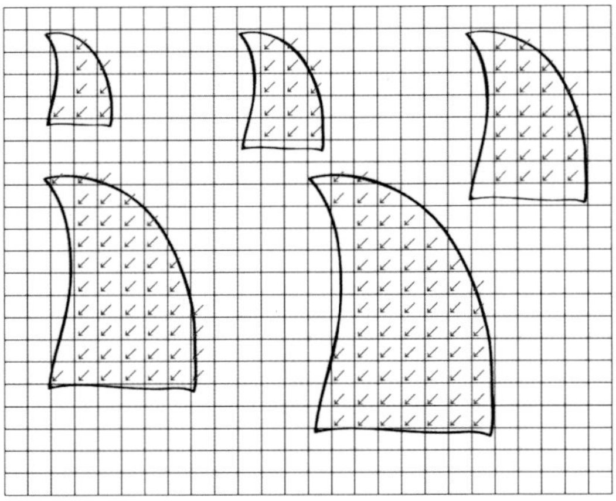

Fig. 2 Lung volume estimate by Cavalieri's principle. A square point grid is laid over the same cut faces of the lung slabs. The test points (here, upper right corner of the line crossings) hitting the cut area are counted (marked with *red arrows*). The lung volume is then estimated by multiplying the total number of counted points by the slab thickness *t* and known area per point *a*(*p*), corresponding to the area of a single square: $V_{lung} = a(p) \times t \times \sum P$. Assuming that $a(p) = 3\ mm^2$ and $t = 1$ mm, the lung volume in this particular example can be calculated as follows: $V_{lung} = 3\ mm^2 \times m\ 1\ mm \times (8 + 14 + 25 + 49 + 63) = 477\ mm^3$

3. Calculate the total lung volume by using the following formula, where t = slab thickness, P = total number of counted points, and $a(p)$ = area per point (*see* **Note 14**):

   $V_{lung} = a(p) \times t \times \sum P$

3.3 Systematic Uniform Random Sampling (SURS)

1. Carefully remove as much non-lung tissue (e.g., trachea, esophagus, etc.) as possible.
2. Embed the lungs in fluid agar and allow it to harden (*see* **Note 15**).
3. Cut the agar block into slabs of equal, defined thickness (t) using the tissue slicer (Fig. 3).
4. Orient the slabs so that the same cut side is facing upward.
5. If the lung volume is to be estimated by Cavalieri's principle, follow procedure detailed in Subheading 3.2.2.
6. Number the slides according to their natural order.
7. Beginning from a random slab, select every i-th slab for embedding and further analysis (*see* **Note 16**).

3.4 Embedding and Further Processing

1. Remove the surrounding agar from the chosen slabs.
2. Incubate the samples subsequently in:
   (a) 0.15 M HEPES buffer for 5 min (repeat twice).

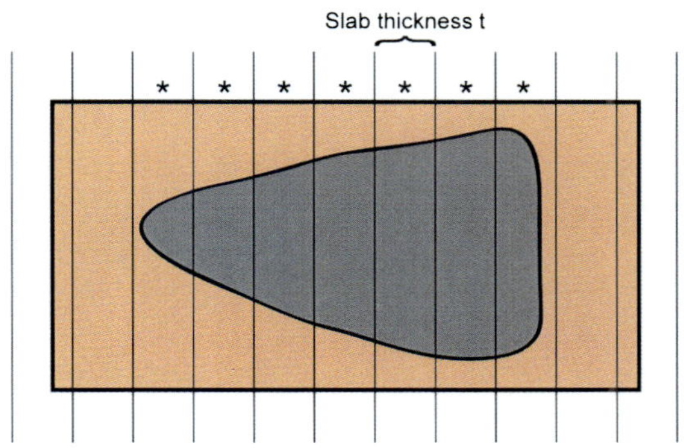

Fig. 3 Slab preparation by tissue slicer. The lung is placed into the tissue slicer and sectioned with a constant thickness *t*. Slabs containing tissue (marked with *asterisks*) are used for further sampling

(b) 0.1 M sodium cacodylate buffer for 5 min (repeat three times).

(c) 1% OsO_4 in 0.1 M sodium cacodylate buffer for 2 h.

(d) 0.1 M sodium cacodylate buffer for 5 min (repeat four times).

(e) Distilled water for 5 min (repeat twice).

(f) Uranyl acetate solution for 20 h, protected from light.

(g) Distilled water for 5 min (repeat five times).

(h) 70% acetone for 10 min (repeat twice).

(i) 80% acetone for 10 min (repeat twice).

(j) 90% acetone for 10 min (repeat twice).

(k) 100% acetone for 10 min (repeat three times).

(l) 1:1 mixture of 100% acetone/Technovit 8100 containing hardener I, overnight.

(m) Technovit 8100 containing hardener I for 48 h.

3. Embed the samples in Technovit 8100 containing hardener I and hardener II.
4. Cut thin (1.5 μm) sections from the glycol methacrylate-embedded samples onto glass slides.
5. Randomly sample the sections to be stained and analyzed (e.g., every first and third section from each block).
6. Stain the sections with toluidine blue (0.1% solution):

(a) Wash the sections in distilled water for 30 s.

(b) Stain with toluidine blue for 45 s.

(c) Rinse in distilled water.

(d) Incubate in 96% ethanol for 1 min.

(e) Incubate in absolute ethanol for 1 min (repeat twice).

(f) Incubate in xylene for 1 min (repeat twice).

(g) Mount in resinous medium and cover glass.

3.5 Morphometry of Lung Parenchyma

3.5.1 Volume Estimation by Point Counting

Point counting is used to estimate the volume of a structure of interest in relation to the reference space. All points hitting the structure of interest as well as all points hitting the reference space are counted on random FOV (*see* **Note 17**). The volume density can then be calculated by dividing the total number of points hitting the structure of interest by the total number of reference points:

$$V_V(\text{struct}/ref) = \sum P_{\text{struct}} / \sum P_{ref}$$

The multiplication of the volume density by the volume of the reference space gives the total volume of the structure of interest:

$$V(\text{struct}, ref) = V_V(\text{struct}/ref) \times V(ref)$$

As an example, the estimation of total parenchymal volume should proceed as follows (Fig. 4):

1. Mount the section on the microscope.
2. Select a low magnification (e.g., 5X objective).
3. Define the structure of interest and the reference space (e.g., for parenchymal volume density, the reference space would be the whole lung, and the structure of interest would be lung non-parenchyma—*see* **Note 18**).

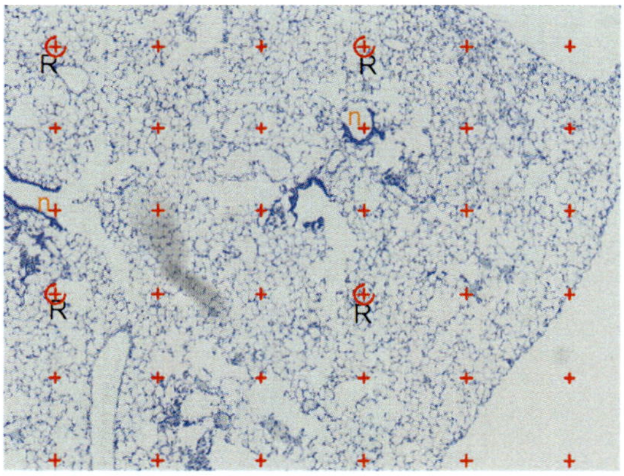

Fig. 4 Estimation of parenchymal volume density by point counting. A point grid with coarse (*encircled*) and fine points in a fixed relation (here, 1:9) is used for counting. Coarse points are counted if they hit a reference space (here, lung tissue). Fine points are counted if they hit non-parenchyma. In the analyzed FOV, there are four course points (marked "*R*") and two fine points (marked "*n*") counted. The picture was taken with a 5X objective. For example, assuming that the total number of counted course points was 130, and the total number of fine points was 145, the parenchymal volume density would be calculated as follows: V_V(par/lung) = 1 − (145/(9 × 130)) ≈ 0.88

4. Superimpose the grid consisting of coarse and fine points in a fixed relation for counting of reference points and non-parenchyma points, respectively. Using two grids of different densities in a fixed relation to each other ensures that the counting process is efficient.
5. Sample the random FOV according to the SURS principle (meander sampling) (*see* **Note 19**).
6. Count the number of points hitting non-parenchyma: airways, blood vessels, or pleura (P_{nonpar}).
7. Count the coarse points hitting the lung tissue (cP_{ref}). Multiply by the ratio between the grids (e.g., nine fine points for every coarse point) to calculate the total number of reference points (P_{ref}).
8. Calculate the parenchymal volume density:
   $V_V(\text{par/lung}) = 1 - \sum P_{\text{nonpar}} / \sum P_{\text{ref}}$
9. Calculate the total volume of lung parenchyma per lung by multiplying the parenchymal volume density by the total lung volume (obtained from fluid displacement or Cavalieri's method):

   $V_{\text{par, lung}} = V_V(\text{par/lung}) \times V_{\text{lung}}$

3.5.2 Surface Estimation by Intersection Counting

The surface density of a structure of interest within the reference space can be estimated by overlaying a grid containing both lines and points. The counting events are all intersections of test lines with the surface of a given structure (I_{struct}) and all points hitting the reference space (P_{ref}). When the length of a test line per point ($l(p)$) is known, the surface density can be estimated based on the following equation: $S_V(\text{struct/ref}) = 2 \times \sum I_{\text{struct}} / [l(p) \times \sum P_{\text{ref}}]$.

The total surface of the structure of interest can then be calculated by multiplying the surface density by the reference volume: $S_{\text{struct, ref}} = S_V(\text{struct/ref}) \times V_{\text{ref}}$.

As an example, the estimation of total alveolar surface should proceed as follows (Fig. 5):

1. Mount the section on the microscope.
2. Select a magnification (e.g., 20X objective) (*see* **Note 20**).
3. Define the structure of interest and the reference space. For alveolar surface density, the reference space would be lung parenchyma, and the structure of interest would be alveolar epithelium.
4. Superimpose a test system consisting of test lines associated with points at their ends.
5. Sample the FOV.
6. Count the points hitting the lung parenchyma (P_{par}).
7. Count the intersections of test lines with alveolar surface (I_{alv}). Keep in mind that a line crossing one alveolar septum results in two intersections, not one.

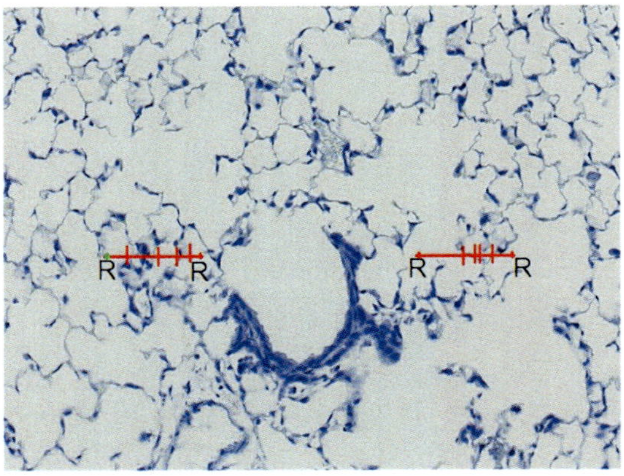

Fig. 5 Estimation of alveolar surface density by intersection counting. A test system consisting of lines of known length associated with points (both ends of each line) is used for counting. Line ends are counted if they hit a reference space (here, lung parenchyma). In addition, all intersections of the test lines with alveolar septa are counted. In the analyzed FOV, there are four reference points (marked "*R*") and eight intersections (marked with *vertical red lines*) counted. The picture was taken with a 20X objective. For example, assuming that the total number of counted intersections was 193, the total number of counted line ends was 98, and $l(p) = 50\ \mu m$, the alveolar surface density would be calculated as follows: $S_V(\text{alv/par}) = 2 \times 193/(50 \times 98) \approx 0.08$

8. Calculate the alveolar surface density related to lung parenchyma:

   $$S_V\,(\text{alv/par}) = 2 \times \sum I_{\text{alv}}/[l(p) \times \sum P_{\text{par}}]$$

9. Calculate the total alveolar surface area inside the lung by multiplying the alveolar surface density by the parenchymal volume density and the total lung volume:

   $$S_{\text{alv, lung}} = S_V\,(\text{alv/par}) \times V_V\,(\text{par/lung}) \times V_{\text{lung}}$$

3.5.3 Particle Number Estimation

Simple point counting of particles on single near-2D sections is not a correct method for estimating particle number and may lead to erroneous results. Therefore, particle number estimation should be carried out using the disector method [17]. The physical disector can be described as a small volume probe composed of two paired sections of the same specimen within a known distance from each other and the unbiased counting frame of a known area (*see* **Note 21**). One of the sections, the so-called sampling section, is used for counting, while the other one, called the look-up section, is used for comparison. The particle is counted only when it falls within the counting frame in the sampling section but is absent in the look-up section (*see* **Note 22**). The counting frame on the reference section can be associated with a point, and the volume of the disector can be estimated by counting all points hitting the reference space using the following equation, where V_{dis} = total

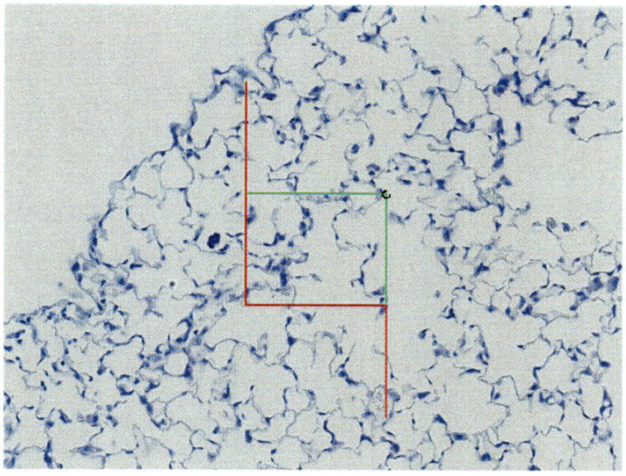

Fig. 6 For particle number estimation, a counting frame consisting of two inclusion lines (upper and right, *green*) and two exclusion lines (lower and left, *red*) together with an associated point (upper right corner, marked with a *black circle*) is used. The frame should be superimposed on corresponding FOV of two adjacent sections. The particle is counted only when it is present within the counting frame in the sampling section but absent in the look-up section

disector volume, A_{cf} = area of a counting frame, h = disector height (distance between the sections), and P_{ref} = number of counted reference points (*see* **Note 23**): $V_{dis} = A_{cf} \times h \times \sum P_{ref}$.

The numerical density of particles related to the reference space can then be estimated by dividing the total number of counted particles (Q) by the total disector volume: N_V (particle/ref) = $\sum Q/V_{dis}$

$$N_V\left(\text{particle}/ref\right)=\sum Q/\left(A_{cf}\times h\times\sum P_{ref}\right)$$

Finally, the total particle number inside the reference space can be calculated by multiplying the particle's numerical density by the total reference volume: $N_{\text{part, ref}} = N_V$ (particle/ref) $\times V_{ref}$.

As an example, the estimation of total number of alveoli should proceed as follows (Fig. 6):

1. From a stack of consecutive sections of known thickness, mount the first and the fourth together on the microscope. Note the disector height (here, corresponding to tripled section thickness). Align the sections as well as possible, and make sure that you are able to meander through both sections simultaneously, so that the sections stay aligned throughout sampling.
2. Select a magnification (e.g., 20X objective).
3. Define the structure of interest and the reference space. For alveolar numerical density, the reference space would be the lung parenchyma, and the structure of interest would be bridges connecting the free edges of alveolar septa, creating a closed alveolus [18, 19].

4. Superimpose an unbiased counting frame associated with one point.
5. Sample the FOV from both sections simultaneously.
6. Define the reference section and the look-up section.
7. Compare the sections and count all bridges (n) visible within the counting frame on the reference section but missing from the look-up section.
8. Count all frame-associated points hitting lung parenchyma (P_{par}).
9. Calculate the numerical density of alveoli related to the lung parenchyma:

   $N_V\,(\text{alv/par}) = \sum n / (A_{cf} \times h \times \sum P_{par})$
10. Calculate the total number of alveoli per lung by multiplying the alveolar numerical density by the parenchymal volume density and the total lung volume:

    $N_{alv,\,par} = N_V\,(\text{alv/par}) \times V_V\,(\text{par/lung}) \times V_{lung}$

4 Notes

1. We use 18 G cannulas (Angiocath, Becton Dickinson) shortened to approximately 1 cm of length.
2. Different fixatives can be used, and the choice depends on the purpose. Formaldehyde alone should not be used, as it does not adequately stabilize tissue structure. Glutaraldehyde rapidly stabilizes tissue structure, but high concentrations of glutaraldehyde compromises protein immunogenicity. To adequately preserve both lung structure and immunogenicity, a fixative containing 4% paraformaldehyde and 0.1% glutaraldehyde in 0.2 M HEPES buffer is recommended. The final fixative needs to be prepared freshly or aliquoted and stored frozen at −20 °C.
3. Post-fixation with OsO_4 and uranyl acetate, routinely used for electron microscopy, is also recommended for light microscopy-based morphometry in order to avoid differential tissue deformation (i.e., nonuniform deformation of certain structures) [20].
4. Uranyl acetate has a solubility of approximately 77 g/l at room temperature. To make a half-saturated solution, mix equal volumes of saturated uranyl acetate with distilled water. Saturated uranyl acetate should be prepared a day before and stirred thoroughly.
5. Paraffin is not a preferred embedding medium for stereology due to significant tissue shrinkage that occurs during embedding. The degree of shrinkage after paraffin embedding might

differ between experimental groups (control vs. fibrotic), making the reliable analysis impossible [21].

6. Lung diver is a device that helps submerge lungs in water so that they don't emerge during the measurement. We have used a piece of wire with a coiled end attached to a stand (Fig. 1).
7. Tissue slicer is made of several spacers of equal thickness with cavities in between them that allow preparation of slabs of constant shape and thickness. Tissue slicers are commercially available but can also be custom-made, and the size and spacer distance of the slicer can be customized to match specific experimental requirements.
8. Several commercial stereology software systems are available. In our description of computer-based stereology, we refer to the newCAST system (Visiopharm, Hørsholm, Denmark), which we have personal experience with.
9. A relatively high pressure and rapid flow ensures homogeneous fixation. To prevent erythrocytes from stacking up behind fixed capillary segments, the pulmonary artery can be clamped just before instillation [22].
10. Ligating the airways prevents the fixative from escaping the lungs. If fluid displacement method is to be used, the ligature should be placed as close to the hilum as possible.
11. The lungs should be dried before being submerged as any carry-over liquid would influence the measurement. If the tissue is not dry enough, swab it gently with a paper towel.
12. The denser the point grid is, the more precise the volume estimate will be. Counting of 100–200 points is enough to reach sufficient precision. This is true not only for a Cavalieri's estimate but also for other analyses.
13. As the first slab most probably has no visible tissue cut face (only embedding agar is visible), it is important to exclude it from the Cavalieri's estimate.
14. Area per point can be calculated by measuring the side lengths of the rectangular grid and dividing their product by the number of points within the rectangular grid.
15. Pre-embedding in agar/agarose facilitates tissue sectioning. However, if immunohistochemistry is to be used, agar should be cooled below 50 °C before embedding to avoid potential loss of antigenicity.
16. In most studies, five appropriately sampled tissue blocks per animal (from at least five animals per experimental group) should give sufficient precision [23].
17. A pilot study is usually necessary to customize the sampling so that the selected number of analyzed sections and FOV gives

rise to the desired 100–200 counting events. If the counting events need to be increased, the result will be more precise if sampling is modified on a higher level (i.e., it's better to increase a number of analyzed sections per lung than increase a number of analyzed FOV per section, and it's better to increase a number of analyzed FOV than to increase a number of counting events per FOV) [24].

18. It is more efficient to count non-parenchyma as structure of interest because the fraction of non-parenchyma is much lower (and thus easier to count) than the fraction of parenchyma, and together they add up to 1. In this indirect approach, the parenchymal volume density can then be calculated by subtracting the volume density of non-parenchyma to 1:

    $V_V\,(\text{par/lung}) = 1 - V_V\,(\text{nonpar/lung})$

    $V_V\,(\text{par/lung}) = 1 - \sum P_{\text{nonpar}} / \sum P_{\text{ref}}$

19. When using the newCAST software and a motorized microscope, FOV sampling is semiautomatic. After selecting the region of interest and defining the fraction of the area to be sampled, the software automatically selects randomly sampled FOV. It is crucial that the magnification and sampling scheme is kept constant between the samples of the same specimen (same lung).
20. The results obtained from surface estimation depend on magnification. When the higher magnification is used, more surface irregularities become visible, leading to higher values.
21. The unbiased counting frame has two inclusion lines and two exclusion lines. If a structure of interest lies within the frame but touches the exclusion line, it should not be counted.
22. To increase efficiency, the counting can be repeated in the other direction—with the "old" reference section used as the "new" look-up section and vice versa.
23. The appropriate disector height depends on the size of objects to be counted. For alveoli, disector heights of 3 μm for mice, 4.5 μm for rats, and 9 μm for humans are recommended [14].

References

1. Weibel ER (2013) It takes more than cells to make a good lung. Am J Respir Crit Care Med 187(4):342–346. doi:10.1164/rccm.201212-2260OE
2. Hsia CC, Hyde DM, Ochs M et al (2010) An official research policy statement of the American Thoracic Society/European Respiratory Society: standards for quantitative assessment of lung structure. Am J Respir Crit Care Med 181(4):394–418. doi:10.1164/rccm.200809-1522ST
3. Ferrando RE, Nyengaard JR, Hays SR et al (2003) Applying stereology to measure thickness of the basement membrane zone in bronchial biopsy specimens. J Allergy Clin Immunol 112(6):1243–1245
4. Tschanz SA, Salm LA, Roth-Kleiner M et al (2014) Rat lungs show a biphasic formation of

new alveoli during postnatal development. J Appl Physiol (1985) 117(1):89–95. doi:10.1152/japplphysiol.01355.2013

5. Holm AT, Wulf-Johansson H, Hvidsten S et al (2015) Characterization of spontaneous air space enlargement in mice lacking microfibrillar-associated protein 4. Am J Physiol Lung Cell Mol Physiol 308(11):L1114–L1124. doi:10.1152/ajplung.00351.2014
6. Schneider JP, Ochs M (2013) Stereology of the lung. Methods Cell Biol 113:257–294. doi:10.1016/B978-0-12-407239-8.00012-4
7. Ochs M, Muhlfeld C (2013) Quantitative microscopy of the lung: a problem-based approach. Part 1: basic principles of lung stereology. Am J Physiol Lung Cell Mol Physiol 305(1):L15–L22. doi:10.1152/ajplung.00429.2012
8. Hyde DM, Tyler NK, Plopper CG (2007) Morphometry of the respiratory tract: avoiding the sampling, size, orientation, and reference traps. Toxicol Pathol 35(1):41–48. doi:10.1080/01926230601059977
9. Weibel ER, Hsia CC, Ochs M (2007) How much is there really? Why stereology is essential in lung morphometry. J Appl Physiol (1985) 102(1):459–467. doi:10.1152/japplphysiol.00808.2006
10. Datta A, Scotton CJ, Chambers RC (2011) Novel therapeutic approaches for pulmonary fibrosis. Br J Pharmacol 163(1):141–172. doi:10.1111/j.1476-5381.2011.01247.x
11. Muhlfeld C, Ochs M (2013) Quantitative microscopy of the lung: a problem-based approach. Part 2: stereological parameters and study designs in various diseases of the respiratory tract. Am J Physiol Lung Cell Mol Physiol 305(3):L205–L221. doi:10.1152/ajplung.00427.2012
12. Lutz D, Gazdhar A, Lopez-Rodriguez E et al (2015) Alveolar derecruitment and collapse induration as crucial mechanisms in lung injury and fibrosis. Am J Respir Cell Mol Biol 52(2):232–243. doi:10.1165/rcmb.2014-0078OC
13. Birkelbach B, Lutz D, Ruppert C et al (2015) Linking progression of fibrotic lung remodeling and ultrastructural alterations of alveolar epithelial type II cells in the amiodarone mouse model. Am J Physiol Lung Cell Mol Physiol 309(1):L63–L75. doi:10.1152/ajplung.00279.2014
14. Muhlfeld C, Knudsen L, Ochs M (2013) Stereology and morphometry of lung tissue. Methods Mol Biol 931:367–390. doi:10.1007/978-1-62703-056-4_18
15. Scherle W (1970) A simple method for volumetry of organs in quantitative stereology. Mikroskopie 26(1):57–60
16. Michel RP, Cruz-Orive LM (1988) Application of the Cavalieri principle and vertical sections method to lung: estimation of volume and pleural surface area. J Microsc 150(Pt 2):117–136
17. Sterio DC (1984) The unbiased estimation of number and sizes of arbitrary particles using the disector. J Microsc 134(Pt 2):127–136
18. Ochs M, Nyengaard JR, Jung A et al (2004) The number of alveoli in the human lung. Am J Respir Crit Care Med 169(1):120–124. doi:10.1164/rccm.200308-1107OC
19. Hyde DM, Tyler NK, Putney LF et al (2004) Total number and mean size of alveoli in mammalian lung estimated using fractionator sampling and unbiased estimates of the Euler characteristic of alveolar openings. Anat Rec A Discov Mol Cell Evol Biol 277(1):216–226. doi:10.1002/ar.a.20012
20. Schneider JP, Ochs M (2014) Alterations of mouse lung tissue dimensions during processing for morphometry: a comparison of methods. Am J Physiol Lung Cell Mol Physiol 306(4):L341–L350. doi:10.1152/ajplung.00329.2013
21. Dorph-Petersen KA, Nyengaard JR, Gundersen HJ (2001) Tissue shrinkage and unbiased stereological estimation of particle number and size. J Microsc 204(Pt 3):232–246
22. Vock R, Weibel ER (1993) Massive hemorrhage causes changes in morphometric parameters of lung capillaries and concentration of leukocytes in microvasculature. Exp Lung Res 19(5):559–577
23. Cruz-Orive LM, Weibel ER (1990) Recent stereological methods for cell biology: a brief survey. Am J Phys 258(4 Pt 1):L148–L156
24. Gundersen HJ, Osterby R (1981) Optimizing sampling efficiency of stereological studies in biology: or 'do more less well!'. J Microsc 121(Pt 1):65–73

Chapter 5

Transplanting Human Skin Grafts onto Nude Mice to Model Skin Scars

Jie Ding and Edward E. Tredget

Abstract

Hypertrophic scar (HTS) is a common outcome of deep dermal wound healing mainly followed mechanical, chemical, and thermal injuries in the skin. Because of the lack of the most effective prevention and treatment, it is particularly important to establish an ideal dermal animal model for improving the understanding of the pathogenesis and exploring therapeutic approaches of HTS. Compared to other dermal fibrotic animal models in rabbits, red Duroc pigs, guinea pigs, rats, and mice, the approach that uses normal human split-thickness skin grafted onto nude or other immunodeficient mice which develop scars that resemble human HTS offers the advantages of lower cost, easier manipulation, and shorter research period. In this chapter, we will introduce the detailed procedures to create the ideal dermal fibrotic mouse model.

Key words Hypertrophic scar, Dermal fibrotic mouse model, Immunodeficient mice

1 Introduction

The skin is the largest organ of human bodies with three layers. The epidermis is the outer layer of the skin. It provides vital barrier function and regulates the amount of water released from the body into the atmosphere. The dermis layer is beneath the epidermis. It provides tensile strength and elasticity to the skin because of the existence of extracellular matrix (ECM), which is mainly produced by resident cells such as fibroblasts and composed of fibrous proteins like collagen and glycosaminoglycans. The hypodermis contains loose connective tissue and considerable adipose tissue. It connects the skin to underlying bone and muscle, supplies it with blood vessels and nerves, and contributes to thermoregulation of the body in furred animals.

Wound healing is an intricate process, in which the skin repairs itself after injury. A normal process of wound healing has four phases. Hemostasis phase is from initial injury to 3 h. In this phase, blood vessels constrict, clot forms, and cytokines release from platelet cells. Inflammatory phase is from injury to 3 days in

Laure Rittié (ed.), *Fibrosis: Methods and Protocols*, Methods in Molecular Biology, vol. 1627,
DOI 10.1007/978-1-4939-7113-8_5, © Springer Science+Business Media LLC 2017

uncomplicated normal wound healing. During this time, leukocytes and macrophages infiltrate to wound site, clean the wound, and destroy the bacterial and cell debris. The proliferation phase is from 3 days to 3 weeks during which new blood vessels and granulation tissue start to form and fill the wound cavity. The remodeling phase is from 3 weeks to a year, during which the disorganized collagen fibers are rearranged, cross-linked, and aligned under the direction of remodeling enzymes. Wound healing is a mixture of regeneration and replacement. Regeneration means that wound heals with creation of the same cell types as original ones, whereas replacement is the substitution of new cell types for preexisting native cell types after healing of the wound. Regeneration-based wound healing in a normal wound restores the normal skin. However, replacement-based wound healing is the common expected form of wound repair, creating either mature scars or abnormal scars such as hypertrophic scars (HTS) and keloids. The abnormal scars are the dermal form of profibrotic disorders defined by overgrowth, hardening, and scarring of various tissues and can be responsible for the deaths of millions of people where it is often progressive, irreversible, and fatal (*see* [1] and Chap. 1). Dermal scars can result in critical physical and psychological problems such as loss of skin function, limited movement of joints, and changes in appearance for patients even if they have survived serious trauma and skin injuries [2].

HTS and keloids have critical epidemiological, clinical, and histological differences [3]. Morphologically, HTS are red, raised, uncomfortable scars confined to the boundaries of original wounds, which can result in functional limitations due to the development of contracture and disfigurement and especially lead to cosmetic problems for burn survivors (Fig. 1). Histologically, HTS are thicker in both the epidermis and dermis; have ultrastructural nodules or whorls, hypervascularity, and hypercellularity in the dermis; lack rete ridges structure in the epidermis; and have excessive ECM where abnormal morphology of collagen fibril structure occurs as compared to normal skin (Fig. 2). Biochemically, HTS were found to have higher proportions of types III and V collagens; increased expression of transforming growth factor beta 1 (TGF-β1), connective tissue growth factor (CTGF/CCN2), vascular endothelial growth factor (VEGF), and platelet-derived growth factor (PDGF); and decreased decorin compared to normal skin [5–8].

There are several hypotheses regarding the cellular and molecular mechanisms of hypertrophic scarring. Although inflammation is not the only critical step in the development of HTS, the secretion and activation of pro-inflammatory cytokines and immunoregulators during the inflammatory phase of wound healing are prerequisites for fibrogenic response, such as TGF-β action and its downstream mediators comprising the SMAD signal-transduction pathway [3], type 2 helper T-cell-derived cytokines [9, 10], and

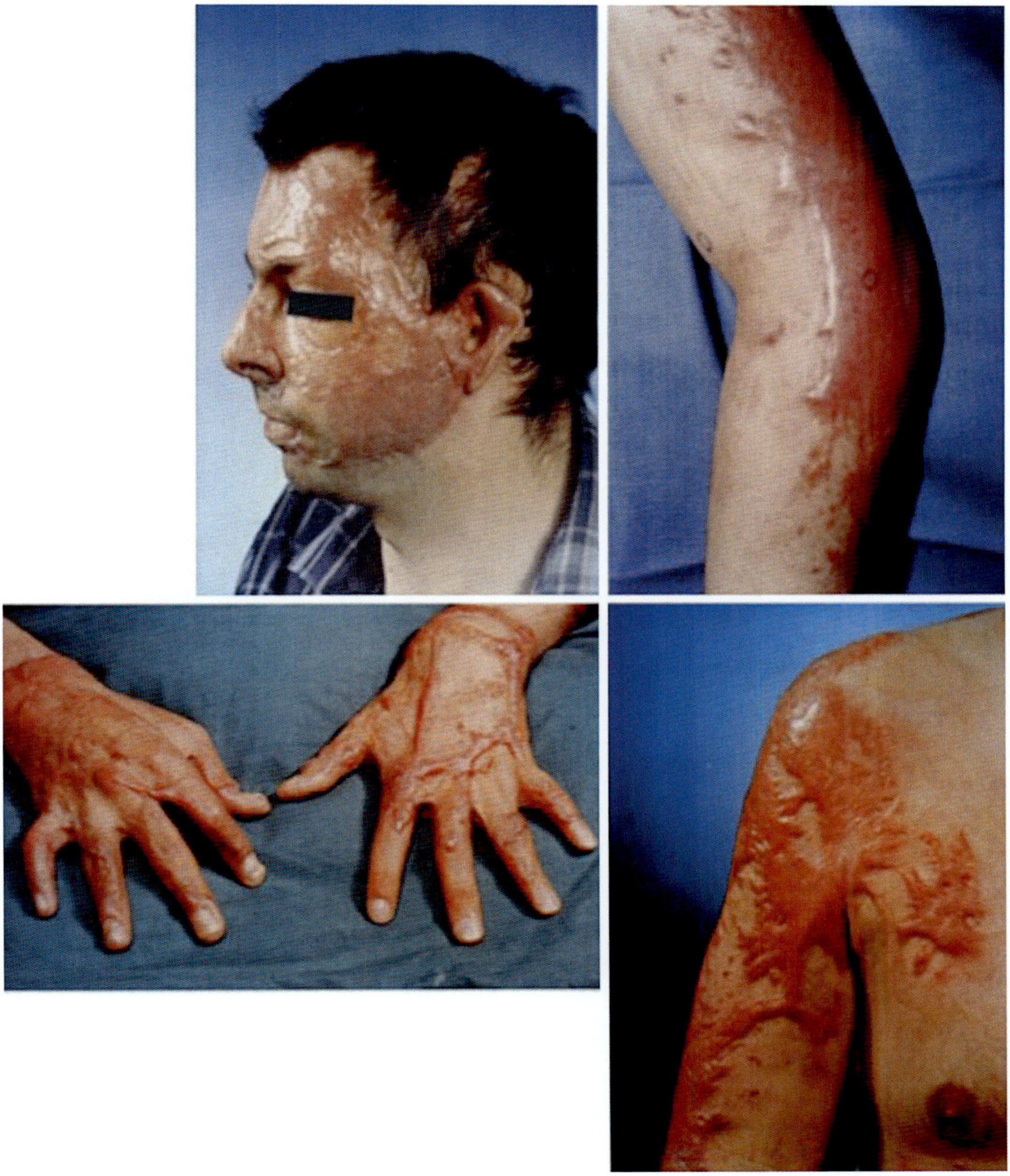

Fig. 1 Hypertrophic scarring in a 34-year-old man, 8 months after 60% total-body-surface-area burn of the face, upper extremities, and hands (from ref. [4])

toll-like receptor signaling [11]. The recruitment of blood-borne cells such as mast cells, macrophages, and fibrocytes has been thought to be an important source to fibrotic regulation of local dermal cells and to promote myofibroblast formation [12–15]. Studies demonstrate that recruitment of blood-borne cells into wound sites is tightly regulated by chemokines contributing to

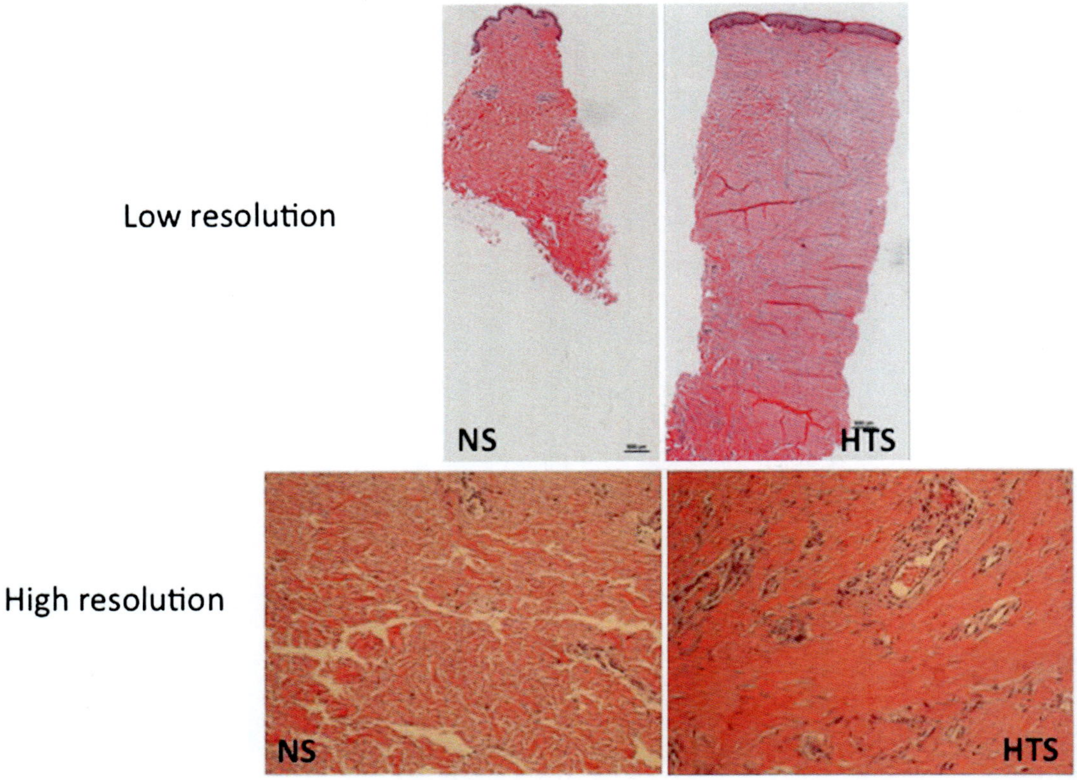

Fig. 2 Histological characteristics of human hypertrophic scar (HTS) and site-matched normal skin (NS) stained by H&E (from ref. [2])

reepithelialization, tissue remodeling, and angiogenesis during wound healing and fibrotic induction during scar formation as well. Many studies have emphasized the pathogenic role of chemokine pathways (CCL2/CCR2 [16] and CXCL12/CXCR4 [17, 18]). As major effectors of ECM degradation and remodeling, matrix metalloproteinase 1 (MMP1) has been found reduced in postburn HTS fibroblasts [19], which might explain collagen accumulation in hypertrophic scarring.

Decorin is a small cellular or pericellular matrix proteoglycan. It plays a role in collagen fibrillogenesis and inactivates fibrotic factors such as TGF-β and CTGF. It is significantly downregulated in HTS [7, 20], and microRNA 181b (miR181b) has been found responsible for low expression of decorin in HTS fibroblasts, suggesting a possible molecular mechanism for scarring. HTS displays excessive signaling via the Wnt pathway. The regional variation in the activation of this pathway would be a reasonable contributor to the pathogenesis of HTS occurring in certain susceptible body areas [5]. One of the histological characteristics of HTS is hypercellularity. In the remodeling phase of wound healing, the cell number is reduced gradually due to cell apoptosis. In HTS tissue, the induction of apoptosis in myofibroblasts was found delayed and correlated with the size of original burns [21]. Clinically, deep dermal injury is one of the risk factors for HTS development and supports the concept of fibroblast heterogeneity linked to profibrotic microenvironment after deep injury: Studies have reported that, compared to superficial dermal fibroblasts, deep dermal fibroblasts have more fibrotic features by expressing low MMP-1 mRNA, producing more TGF-β, CTGF, type I collagen, alpha smooth muscle actin (α-SMA), and versican and less decorin and decorin-induced apoptosis in deep dermal fibroblasts [22, 23]. Thus, dermal injury beyond a critical depth appears to select for the profibrotic fibroblast within the heterogeneity of fibroblast populations at different levels in the skin [24].

Some forms of treatment have been used for HTS patients, including surgical, nonsurgical, immunological, and biomolecular treatments. Traditional methods of nonsurgical management focus on attenuation of ongoing fibrotic response and improvement of existing scar tissues, whereas preventative strategies intend to inhibit profibrotic responses before hypertrophic scarring. However, no method can prevent and replace the pathological scars completely. Therefore, improved understanding of HTS development may lead to exciting therapy for dermal scars and other fibrotic disorders.

Extensive studies on dermal scar pathogenesis and therapeutic strategies have been done in a wide variety of animal models in pigs, rabbits, rats, guinea pigs, and mice [25]. Red Duroc pigs were used to induce HTS formation successfully early in 1972 by Silverstein et al., in which repeated deep dermal injuries were sustained on the backs of red Duroc pigs [26, 27]. Thirty years later, Zhu studied deep tangential wounds using electric Padgett dermatome and suggested that a further study was needed so that it could be accepted or rejected as a model of human HTS [28, 29]. Using this pig model, Duroc dermal fibroblasts were reported to have inherent myofibroblastdifferentiation that may account for the pathological scarring [30]. Beta-2 adrenergic receptor agonist reduced both scar area and hyperpigmentation by almost 50% and significantly improved scar quality in this Duroc dermal scar model [31]. In contrary, Gallant-Behm reported that the healing of full-thickness excisional skin wounds in Yorkshire pigs closely resembles normal healing in humans, but not the identical wounds in red Duroc pigs, which form hypercontracted, hyperpigmented scars [32]. However, the structure differences in the epidermis, sweat glands, and hair follicles, costs, and difficulty to maintain and evaluate burns or other deep dermal injuries in this species limit its widespread usage [25]. In 1997, promoted by previous report on scar formation after healing of dermal ulcers created in the rabbit ears [33], Morris et al. quantified the excessive scars for a rabbit dermal scar model, in which full-thickness excisional wounds to the cartilage surface in New Zealand white rabbit ears healed with irregular elevated scars [34]. Due to perichondrial hypertrophy and cartilage thickening, the scar tissues are not completely same as human HTS [34]. Even so, it has been used for studying molecular mechanism and new therapeutic approaches of HTS (*see* [35–38] and Chapter 6). Since 1999 when Yamamoto et al. established a dermal sclerosis model in BALB/C mouse [39], murine dermal fibrosis models were induced by bleomycin also in C3H/HeJ, C57BL/6, DBA/2 and nude mice (*see* [40–42] and Chapter 3). The Balb/C mice are reported more susceptible to bleomycin-induced fibrosis [42]. By using these models, IL-13 was suggested to promote the progression of cutaneous fibrosis/sclerosis [40], and lysophosphatidic acid-3 antagonist was found to improve dermal and lung fibrosis [43]. In 2002, Aksoy et al. created a new, practical, and economical experimental dermal scar model in guinea pig. They produced a circular skin excision wound on the dorsal skin of the torso followed by panniculectomy on both sides. HTS developed after healing when the wounds were treated with coal tar [44]. Unfortunately, the toxic, carcinogenic effects of coal tar also limit its usage in the lab. Because the human skin has a unique wounding response and scarring behavior [45], implantation of human abnormal scar tissues such as HTS to athymic mice or nude rats [46, 47] or hamster [48] is an interesting approach to establish dermal fibrotic models. These models are based on animals that are either immune deficient or have an immune-privileged site, which allows transplanted human tissue to survive without rejection. In 2007, Xia's group established a HTS model by transplanting full-thickness human skin grafts onto backs of nude mice, which had morphologic and histologic properties similar to human HTS [49]. Our group modified this model later by transplanting split-thickness human skin grafts onto full-thickness excisional wounds on the dorsum of nude mice and found the human skin grafts developed more scar tissues in a shorter period of time (Fig. 3) [13].

Similar models of human skin transplantation have been performed in RAG-1, RAG-2, and T-cell receptor (TCR) knockout mice, in which functional T, B, and NK cells are deficient [50]. We further modified the nude mouse model by grafting full-thickness human skin with a deep wound created by using a jig before or after grafting. It has proved to be a more promising dermal fibrotic mouse model (Fig. 4) [51]. In this chapter, we will introduce materials and method to establish dermal fibrotic mouse models; dermal fibrotic RAG-1$^{-/-}$, RAG-2$^{-/-}\gamma$ c$^{-/-}$, and TCR $\beta^{-/-}$ $\delta^{-/-}$ mouse models; and dermal fibrotic nude mouse model with a deep wound.

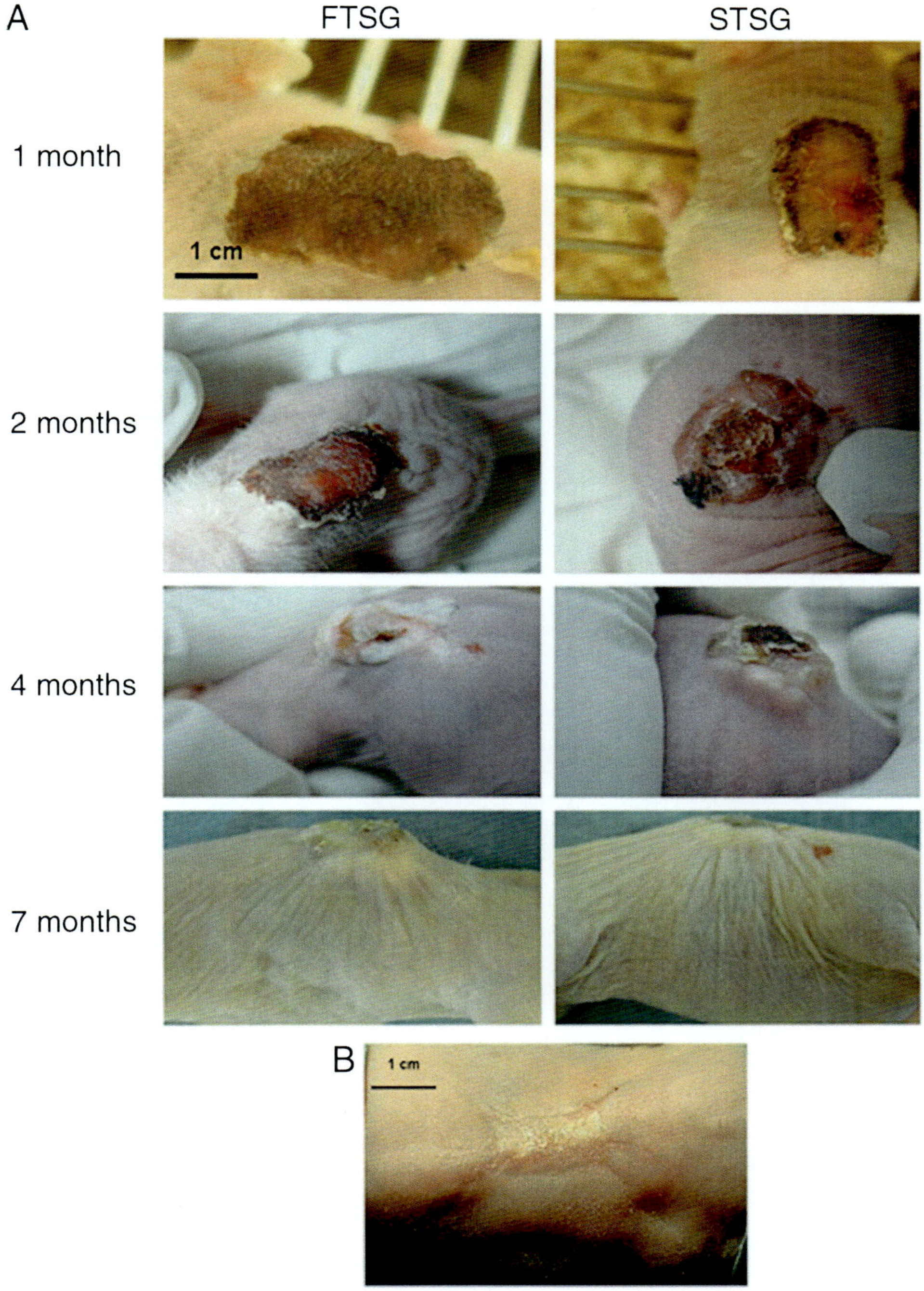

Fig. 3 Photographs of scar after full-thickness and split-thickness skin graft. (**a**) Macroscopic observation of scar development in full-thickness skin and split-thickness skin graft. Scars were photographed using the same exposure and lighting settings, at the indicated time after transplantation. Representative results for the three animals in each group are shown. (**b**) Macroscopic observation of rat skin transplantation (scale bar = 1 cm). FTSG, full-thickness skin graft; STSG, split-thickness skin graft (from ref. [13])

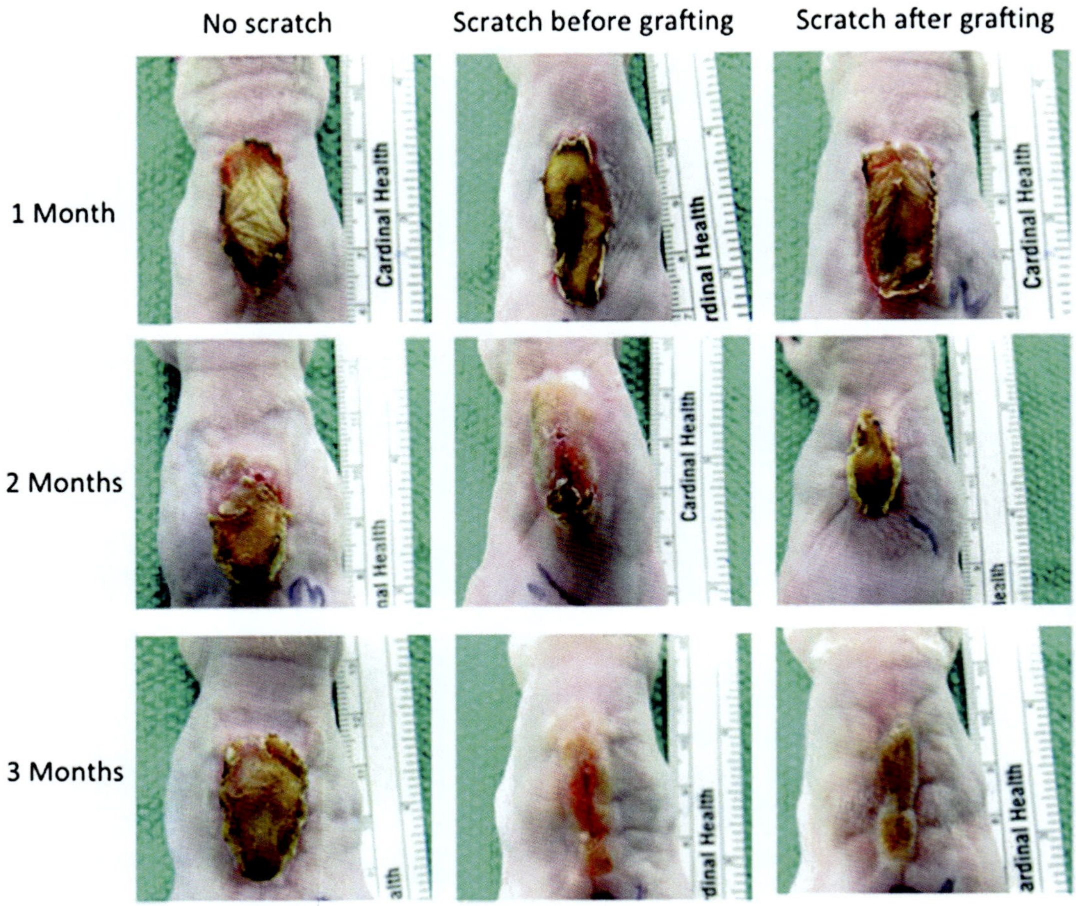

Fig. 4 Morphological observation of the graft development over time showing the red elevated grafts compared to the mouse skin. The scratch in the grafts made wound contract more than the ones without scratch (from ref. [51])

2 Materials

1. Human skin (*see* **Notes 1** and **2**).
2. Dermatome and sterile blades.
3. Sterile skin graft carriers.
4. 0.9% NaCl (w/v) (thereafter referred to "normal saline").
5. Nude mice, RAG-1^{-}/$^{-}$, RAG-2^{-}/$^{-}$ γ c^{-}/$^{-}$, and TCR β^{-}/$^{-}$ δ^{-}/$^{-}$. Male mice (18–22 g) should be conditioned in individual cages (*see* **Notes 3** and **4**) in viral antibody-free biocontainment facility for 1–2 weeks before surgery to allow for an acclimatizing period.
6. Induction chamber with isoflurane inhalant and nosecone.
7. Ocular ointment.

8. Electric heating pads (circulating water pad).
9. Skin marker.
10. Betadine.
11. 70% ethanol (v/v in sterile water).
12. Surgical instruments: sterile paper sheet, gloves, scissors, forceps, needle holder, scalpel, and blades.
13. Sterile cotton tipped applicators.
14. Sterile Topper*8 cotton gauze.
15. 4-0 silk suture.
16. Mesh gauze impregnated with a blend of petrolatum and 3% Bismuth Tribromophenate (w/v) for wound dressing (we use Xeroform®, Covidien, Mansfield, MA).
17. Analgesic and fever reducer: we use 1 mg/ml Meloxicam (Sandoz, Boucherville, QC) in normal saline.
18. 0.5 ml insulin syringes.
19. 80 mg/100 ml sulfamethoxazole and 16 mg/100 ml trimethoprim solution in autoclaved deionized/UV filtered water (we use Teva-Sulfamethoxazole Trimethoprim oral suspension from TEVA Pharmaceutical Industries Ltd., Petach Tikva, Israel).
20. Digital camera.
21. Anesthetic machine.
22. Garbage bags.
23. Sharp container.
24. Jigsaw (lab made) and blade.
25. Hair removal cream.

3 Methods

3.1 Dermal Fibrotic Nude Mouse Model

3.1.1 Preoperative Procedures

1. Generate human split-thickness skin grafts using a dermatome set at 0.03 cm.
2. Cut grafts with a scalpel using a 2.0 × 1.5 cm plastic template made of skin graft carrier, and store in sterile normal saline at room temperature until grafting.
3. Anesthetize acclimated animals using an anesthetic machine with isoflurane inhalant 4~5% and maintained by 1~2% with a nosecone under a fume hood during the surgical procedure (*see* **Note 5**).
4. Check mouse for an acceptable surgical plane of anesthesia by pinching the back of the skin.
5. Apply ocular ointment and place the mouse on a circulating water pad.

3.1.2 Surgical Procedures

Surgical procedures are summarized in Fig. 5.

1. Use aseptic technique throughout the surgical procedure.
2. Disinfect the surgical area of the dorsum with Betadine, wash with 70% ethanol using sterile cotton tipped applicators, and finally dry with sterile cotton gauze.
3. Mark a 2.0 × 1.5 cm surgical area with sterile plastic template made of skin graft carrier.
4. Create a full-thickness excision skin wound 2.0 × 1.5 cm in size on the dorsum using fine forceps and scissors (*see* **Note 6**).
5. Graft split-thickness human skin on the mouse wound by suturing in place with 4-0 silk sutures, one stitch at each of four corners, one stitch on each of two short sides (1.5 cm), and three stitches on each of two long sides (2 cm).
6. Place a piece of Xeroform slightly larger than the defect on top of the wound.
7. Cover the wound with a piece of cotton gauze on the top of Xeroform. Fix the dressing into place over the wound using a tie over bolus technique (*see* **Note 7**).

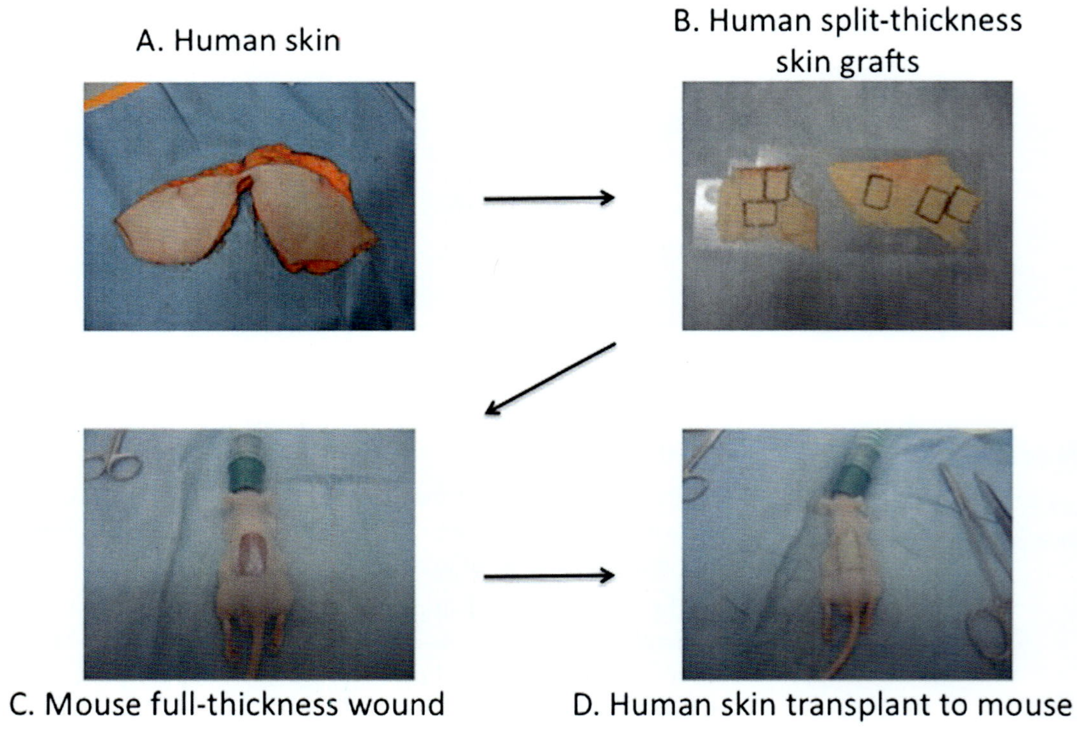

Fig. 5 Surgical procedures to establish fibrotic nude mouse model. (**a**) Collection of the human skin from patients who underwent abdominoplasty. (**b**) Preparation of split-thickness skin grafts from it. (**c**) Preparation of full-thickness excision wound on the back of nude mouse. (**d**) Transplantation of human skin graft onto the wound of mouse

8. Administer preventative pain reliever immediately following surgery by injecting 4 mg/kg Meloxicam subcutaneously (*see* **Notes 8** and **9**).
9. Stop the anesthesia and maintain mouse on the heating pad until the mouse starts to move.
10. Return the mouse back to its cage.
11. Discard all garbage into garbage bag or appropriate containers and clean the work area.
12. House the mouse individually until the end of the experiment.

3.1.3 Postoperative Procedures

1. Administer sulfamethoxazole/trimethoprim suspension orally (the drug is in the drinking water) during the first week after surgery to prevent infections.
2. Observe the mouse cage environment including food and water consumption; cage contamination by blood, pus, diarrhea, or other exudate; and mouse bedding.
3. Monitor the health status of mice based on postoperative monitoring sheet daily until removing the dressing for signs of responsiveness, posture, and respiration rate and effort (*see* **Note 10**).
4. Remove the dressing and stitches on day 7 under anesthesia machine with isoflurane inhalation (as in Subheading 3.1.1, **step 3**).
5. Document healing and scar formation by digital photography weekly after removing stitches (*see* **Note 11**).
6. Collect scar tissue from the mice for further histological analysis at the end of experiment under anesthesia machine with isoflurane inhalation.
7. Euthanatize the mice using CO_2 chamber or other acceptable euthanasia methods (check with local Animal Care and Use Committee).

Dermal Fibrotic RAG-1$^{-/-}$, RAG-2$^{-/-}\gamma c^{-/-}$, and TCR $\beta^{-/-}\delta^{-/-}$ Mouse Models

Procedures are the same as those we make the nude mouse model besides the following:

1. After **step 2** of Subheading 3.1.2, remove the hair from the mouse dorsal surface with hair remover cream.
2. Proceed to **step 3** of Subheading 3.1.2 onward.

3.2 Dermal Fibrotic Nude Mouse Model with a Deep Wound

The procedures are the same as in Subheading 3.1 except for the followings mentioned specifically:

1. As the first step in Subheading 3.1.1, perform a deep wound in the full-thickness human skin grafts:
   (a) Remove excessive subcutaneous fat manually from the skin sample with curved scissors.

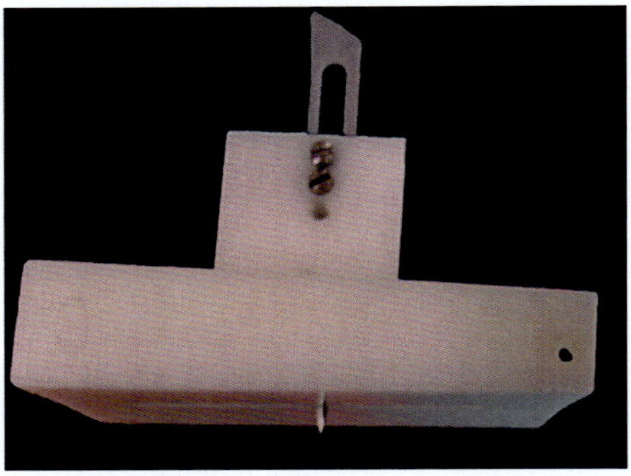

Fig. 6 The jigsaw used to make scratch wound on human skin grafts (from ref. [51])

(b) Cut full-thickness human skin into 3.0 × 1.5 cm grafts with a scalpel and blade.

(c) Make a 0.6 mm deep and 2 cm long incision wound in the center of each graft using a jigsaw with #11 blade in a specially designed modification of a jig originally described by Dunkin et al. [52] and illustrated in Fig. 6.

(d) Proceed to **step 3** of Subheading 3.1.1 onward.

2. After **step 3** of Subheading 3.1.2

   (a) Mark a 3.0 × 1.5 cm surgical area with sterile plastic template made of skin graft carrier.

   (b) Create a 3.0 × 1.5 cm full-thickness excision skin wound on the dorsum of mouse using fine forceps and scissors.

   (c) Graft full-thickness human skin graft containing a deep wound on the mouse wound following **step 6** of Subheading 3.1.2 onward.

3. After remove dressing and stitches as described in **step 4** of Subheading 3.1.3., make a 0.6 mm deep and 2 cm long incision wound in the center of each grafted tissue using a jigsaw with a blade.

4. Let the wound heal by itself (the wound causes more reaction, which causes more scarring).

4 Notes

1. Full-thickness human skin obtained as surgical remnants from patients undergoing abdominoplasty. Carefully follow local regulations regarding requirements for written informed consent, handling human tissue, and any protection-related features.

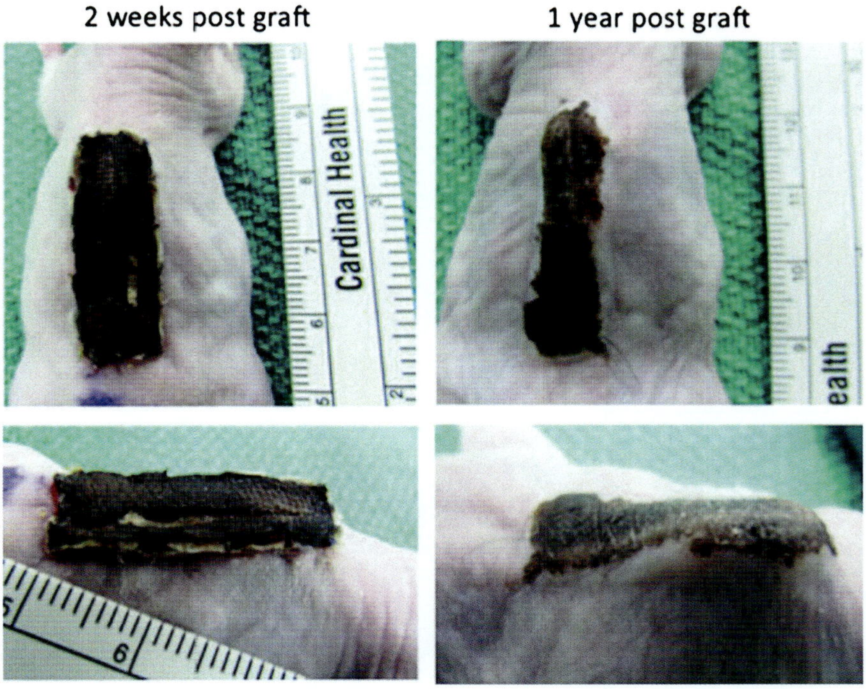

Fig. 7 The graft survived, and the scratch in it healed preserving the color of the human skin for 1 year after grafting (from ref. [51])

2. Skin samples from African-American patient undergoing abdominoplasty can be used to specifically study human skin survival and migration of the dark melanin-containing keratinocytes in this mouse model. A deep wound (as the ones described in Subheading 3.3) is typically made before grafting onto the back of nude mice. Scratched grafts may be followed for 1 year after transplantation (Fig. 7) [51].
3. Prevent skin wound caused by mouse fighting, and protect the wound after surgery.
4. Animal protocol should be approved by local Animal Care and Use Committee and in accordance with the standards of the local Council on Animal Care prior to starting experimentation.
5. It takes 15~20 min to complete a mouse model. The maximum we did was 24 models in a day.
6. Ensure the panniculus carnosus is intact.
7. Tie over bolus dressing to ensure adherence of the graft to the wound bed. Make sure the dressing is not too tight, or it will prevent the animals from breathing or moving. Utmost care must be taken to avoid animal mortality from this step onward.
8. We typically administer pain reliever at a dose based on an average weight of 20 g.

9. Start with a single dose of the meloxicam once after surgery. If the mice are not active or if there is evidence that their nests are not well built, this should be indications that mice are struggling with pain. In this case, give an additional dose on each of the following 2 postoperative days.
10. Any mouse that appears to be becoming moribund should be euthanized immediately.
11. Including a ruler always positioned similarly relative to the mouse (as in Fig. 4) helps assessing wound and scar sizes overtime.

Acknowledgment

This work was supported by Firefighter's Burn Trust Fund, Edmonton Civic Employees Research Awards, and University of Alberta Hospital Foundation.

References

1. Ding J, Tredget EE (2015) Cellular and molecular mechanism of dermal fibrosis following burn injury, and exploration of therapeutic approaches. J Aesthet Reconstr Surg 1(1):6. doi:10.4172/2472-1905.10003
2. Ding J, Tredget EE (2015) The role of chemokines in fibrotic wound healing. Adv Wound Care (New Rochelle) 4(11):673–686. doi:10.1089/wound.2014.0550
3. Gauglitz GG, Korting HC, Pavicic T et al (2011) Hypertrophic scarring and keloids: pathomechanisms and current and emerging treatment strategies. Mol Med 17(1–2):113–125. doi:10.2119/molmed.2009.00153
4. Tredget EE, Ding J (2009) Wound healing: from embryos to adults and back again. Lancet 373(9671):1226–1228. doi:10.1016/S0140-6736(09)60705-4
5. Tziotzios C, Profyris C, Sterling J (2012) Cutaneous scarring: pathophysiology, molecular mechanisms, and scar reduction therapeutics part II. Strategies to reduce scar formation after dermatologic procedures. J Am Acad Dermatol 66(1):13–24. doi:10.1016/j.jaad.2011.08.035
6. Stewart TL, Ball B, Schembri PJ et al (2012) The use of laser Doppler imaging as a predictor of burn depth and hypertrophic scar Postburn injury. J Burn Care Res 33(6):764–771. doi:10.1097/BCR.0b013e318257db36
7. Kwan P, Ding J, Tredget EE (2015) MicroRNA 181b regulates Decorin production by dermal fibroblasts and may be a potential therapy for hypertrophic scar. PLoS One 10(4). doi:10.1371/journal.pone.0123054
8. Qing C, Wang ZY, Song F et al (2016) Dynamic biological changes in fibroblasts during hypertrophic scar formation and regression. Int Wound J 13(2):257–262. doi:10.1111/iwj.12283
9. Tredget EE, Yang L, Delehanty M et al (2006) Polarized Th2 cytokine production in patients with hypertrophic scar following thermal injury. J Interf Cytokine Res 26(3):179–189. doi:10.1089/jir.2006.26.179
10. Wong VW, Paterno J, Sorkin M et al (2011) Mechanical force prolongs acute inflammation via T-cell-dependent pathways during scar formation. FASEB J 25(12):4498–4510. doi:10.1096/fj.10-178087
11. Wang J, Hori K, Ding J et al (2011) Toll-like receptors expressed by dermal fibroblasts contribute to hypertrophic scarring. J Cell Physiol 226(5):1265–1273. doi:10.1002/jcp.22454
12. Wynn TA (2008) Cellular and molecular mechanisms of fibrosis. J Pathol 214(2):199–210. doi:10.1002/path.2277
13. Wang J, Ding J, Jiao H et al (2011) Human hypertrophic scar-like nude mouse model: characterization of the molecular and cellular biology of the scar process. Wound Repair Regen 19(2):274–285. doi:10.1111/j.1524-475X.2011.00672.x

14. Liu HB, Ding J, Ma ZS et al (2015) A novel subpopulation of peripheral blood mononuclear cells presents in major burn patients. Burns 41(5):998–1007. doi:10.1016/j.burns.2014.12.005
15. Zhu Z, Ding J, Ma Z et al (2016) Systemic depletion of macrophages in the subacute phase of wound healing reduces hypertrophic scar formation. Wound Repair Regen 24(4):644–656. doi:10.1111/wrr.12442
16. Wong VW, Rustad KC, Akaishi S et al (2012) Focal adhesion kinase links mechanical force to skin fibrosis via inflammatory signaling. Nat Med 18(1):148–152. doi:10.1038/nm.2574
17. Ding J, Hori K, Zhang R et al (2011) Stromal cell-derived factor 1 (SDF-1) and its receptor CXCR4 in the formation of postburn hypertrophic scar (HTS). Wound Repair Regen 19(5):568–578. doi:10.1111/j.1524-475X.2011.00724.x
18. Ding J, Ma Z, Liu H et al (2014) The therapeutic potential of a C-X-C chemokine receptor type 4 (CXCR-4) antagonist on hypertrophic scarring in vivo. Wound Repair Regen 22(5):622–630. doi:10.1111/wrr.12208
19. Ghahary A, Shen YJ, Nedelec B et al (1996) Collagenase production is lower in post-burn hypertrophic scar fibroblasts than in normal fibroblasts and is reduced by insulin-like growth factor-1. J Invest Dermatol 106(3):476–481. doi:10.1111/1523-1747.ep12343658
20. Scott PG, Dodd CM, Tredget EE et al (1996) Chemical characterization and quantification of proteoglycans in human post-burn hypertrophic and mature scars. Clin Sci (Lond) 90(5):417–425. doi:10.1042/cs0900417
21. Nedelec B, Shankowsky H, Scott PG et al (2001) Myofibroblasts and apoptosis in human hypertrophic scars: the effect of interferon-alpha2b. Surgery 130(5):798–808. doi:10.1067/msy.2001.116453
22. Wang J, Dodd C, Shankowsky HA et al (2008) Deep dermal fibroblasts contribute to hypertrophic scarring. Lab Investig 88(12):1278–1290. doi:10.1038/labinvest.2008.101
23. Honardoust D, Ding J, Varkey M et al (2012) Deep dermal fibroblasts refractory to migration and decorin-induced apoptosis contribute to hypertrophic scarring. J Burn Care Res 33(5):668–677. doi:10.1097/BCR.0b013e31824088e3
24. Kwan P, Hori K, Ding J et al (2009) Scar and contracture: biological principles. Hand Clin 25(4):511–528. doi:10.1016/j.hcl.2009.06.007
25. Seo BF, Lee JY, Jung SN (2013) Models of abnormal scarring. Biomed Res Int 2013:423147. doi:10.1155/2013/423147
26. Silverstein P, Goodwin M Jr, Raulston G (1972) Hypertrophic scarring, etiology and control of a disabling complication in burned soldiers. Ann Res Prog Rep US Army Instit Surg Res Sec 37:1–5
27. Silverstein P, Goodwin MN, Raulston GL et al (1976) Hypertrophic scar in the experimental animal. In: Longacre JJ (ed) The ultrastructure of collagen; its relation to the healing of wounds and to the management of hypertrophic scar. Thomas, Springfield, IL, pp 213–236
28. Zhu KQ, Engrav LH, Gibran NS et al (2003) The female, red Duroc pig as an animal model of hypertrophic scarring and the potential role of the cones of skin. Burns 29(7):649–664. doi:10.1016/S0305-4179(03)00205-5
29. Zhu KQ, Engrav LH, Tamura RN et al (2004) Further similarities between cutaneous scarring in the female, red Duroc pig and human hypertrophic scarring. Burns 30(6):518–530. doi:10.1016/j.burns.2004.02.005
30. Sood RF, Muffley LA, Seaton ME et al (2015) Dermal fibroblasts from the red Duroc pig have an inherently Fibrogenic phenotype: an in vitro model of Fibroproliferative scarring. Plast Reconstr Surg 136(5):990–1000. doi:10.1097/prs.0000000000001704
31. Le Provost GS, Pullar CE (2015) beta2-adrenoceptor activation modulates skin wound healing processes to reduce scarring. J Invest Dermatol 135(1):279–288. doi:10.1038/jid.2014.312
32. Gallant CL, Olson ME, Hart DA (2004) Molecular, histologic, and gross phenotype of skin wound healing in red Duroc pigs reveals an abnormal healing phenotype of hypercontracted, hyperpigmented scarring. Wound Repair Regen 12(3):305–319. doi:10.1111/j.1067-1927.2004.012311.x
33. Mustoe TA, Pierce GF, Morishima C et al (1991) Growth factor-induced acceleration of tissue repair through direct and inductive activities in a rabbit dermal ulcer model. J Clin Invest 87(2):694–703. doi:10.1172/jci115048
34. Morris DE, Wu L, Zhao LL et al (1997) Acute and chronic animal models for excessive dermal scarring: quantitative studies. Plast Reconstr Surg 100(3):674–681
35. Li Y, Kilani RT, Rahmani-Neishaboor E et al (2014) Kynurenine increases matrix metalloproteinase-1 and -3 expression in cultured dermal fibroblasts and improves scarring in vivo.

J Invest Dermatol 134(3):643–650. doi:10.1038/jid.2013.303

36. Zhang Q, Liu LN, Yong Q et al (2015) Intralesional injection of adipose-derived stem cells reduces hypertrophic scarring in a rabbit ear model. Stem Cell Res Ther 6:145. doi:10.1186/s13287-015-0133-y
37. Çaliskan E, Gamsizkan M, Açikgoz G et al (2016) Intralesional treatments for hypertrophic scars: comparison among corticosteroid, 5-fluorouracil and botulinum toxin in rabbit ear hypertrophic scar model. Eur Rev Med Pharmacol Sci 20(8):1603–1608
38. Rha EY, Kim YH, Kim TJ et al (2016) Topical application of a silicone gel sheet with verapamil microparticles in a rabbit model of hypertrophic scar. Plast Reconstr Surg 137(1):144–151. doi:10.1097/prs.0000000000001889
39. Yamamoto T, Takagawa S, Katayama I et al (1999) Animal model of sclerotic skin. I: local injections of bleomycin induce sclerotic skin mimicking scleroderma. J Invest Dermatol 112(4):456–462. doi:10.1046/j.1523-1747.1999.00528.x
40. Matsushita M, Yamamoto T, Nishioka K (2004) Upregulation of interleukin-13 and its receptor in a murine model of bleomycin-induced scleroderma. Int Arch Allergy Immunol 135(4):348–356. doi:10.1159/000082331
41. Serratrice N, Bruzzese L, Magalon J et al (2014) New fat-derived products for treating skin-induced lesions of scleroderma in nude mice. Stem Cell Res Ther 5(6):138. doi:10.1186/scrt528
42. Ruzehaji N, Avouac J, Elhai M et al (2015) Combined effect of genetic background and gender in a mouse model of bleomycin-induced skin fibrosis. Arthritis Res Ther 17:145. doi:10.1186/s13075-015-0659-5
43. Ohashi T, Yamamoto T (2015) Antifibrotic effect of lysophosphatidic acid receptors LPA1 and LPA3 antagonist on experimental murine scleroderma induced by bleomycin. Exp Dermatol 24(9):698–702. doi:10.1111/exd.12752
44. Aksoy MH, Vargel I, Canter IH et al (2002) A new experimental hypertrophic scar model in guinea pigs. Aesthet Plast Surg 26(5):388–396. doi:10.1007/s00266-002-1121-z
45. Rittié L (2016) Cellular mechanisms of skin repair in humans and other mammals. J Cell Commun Signal 10(2):103–120. doi:10.1007/s12079-016-0330-1
46. Polo M, Kim YJ, Kucukcelebi A et al (1998) An in vivo model of human proliferative scar. J Surg Res 74(2):187–195. doi:10.1006/jsre.1997.5251
47. Wang X, Smith P, Pu LL et al (1999) Exogenous transforming growth factor beta(2) modulates collagen I and collagen III synthesis in proliferative scar xenografts in nude rats. J Surg Res 87(2):194–200. doi:10.1006/jsre.1999.5757
48. Hochman B, Vilas Boas FC, Mariano M et al (2005) Keloid heterograft in the hamster (*Mesocricetus auratus*) cheek pouch, Brazil. Acta Cir Bras 20(3):200–212. doi:S0102-86502005000300003
49. Yang DY, Li SR, Wu JL et al (2007) Establishment of a hypertrophic scar model by transplanting full-thickness human skin grafts onto the backs of nude mice. Plast Reconstr Surg 119(1):104–109. doi:10.1097/01.prs.0000244828.80490.62. discussion 110-101
50. Momtazi M, Ding J, Kwan P et al (2015) Morphologic and histologic comparison of hypertrophic scar in nude mice, T-cell receptor, and recombination activating gene knockout mice. Plast Reconstr Surg 136(6):1192–1204. doi:10.1097/PRS.0000000000001782
51. Alrobaie S, Ding J, Ma Z et al (2015) A novel nude mouse model of hypertrophic scarring using scratched full-thickness human skin grafts. Wound Repair Regen 23(4):A2–A2. doi:10.1089/wound.2015.0670
52. Dunkin CSJ, Pleat JM, Gillespie PH et al (2007) Scarring occurs at a critical depth of skin injury: precise measurement in a graduated dermal scratch in human volunteers. Plast Reconstr Surg 119(6):1722–1732. doi:10.1097/01.prs.0000258829.07399.f0

Chapter 6

Hypertrophic Scarring in the Rabbit Ear: A Practical Model for Studying Dermal Fibrosis

Layla Nabai and Aziz Ghahary

Abstract

Excessive fibrous tissue deposition after injury in the form of hypertrophic scar remains a major clinical challenge. The development of an animal model for such scarring has been extremely difficult because of a major difference between the healing process in laboratory animals and humans. Here, we describe the rabbit ear model for excessive dermal scarring which has some clinical and histological resemblance to human hypertrophic scar. Since its development, this model has been widely used to study the cellular and molecular biology of hypertrophic scarring and evaluate the efficacy of new therapeutic agents.

Key words Hypertrophic scar, Animal model, Rabbit ear, Dermal fibrosis

1 Introduction

Hypertrophic scar (HSc) can occur as a consequence of healing process in humans. This fibro-proliferative disorder has characteristic clinical and histological features. It begins to develop weeks after deep trauma, severe burn injury, and surgical incision as red, thick, and irritable scar over the site of injury [1]. HSc continues to enlarge for 3–6 months, remains static for several months, and gradually regresses over approximately 1 year after injury [2]. Histologically, HSc is characterized by an excessive deposition of extracellular matrix components, especially type I collagen. Despite decades of research, the underlying mechanism(s) of this abnormal scarring is still obscured, so an effective preventive or therapeutic option remains as an unachieved ideal.

The dynamic nature of skin scarring and the ethical limitations for human studies encourages the development of scar models. Over the past decades, different animal models, in vitro cell culture, and tissue-engineered models have been developed to investigate the pathophysiology of HSc and test the new therapeutic modalities [3]. While cell/tissue cultures are suitable for studying the pathophysiological mechanisms, the animal models are usually

Laure Rittié (ed.), *Fibrosis: Methods and Protocols*, Methods in Molecular Biology, vol. 1627,
DOI 10.1007/978-1-4939-7113-8_6, © Springer Science+Business Media LLC 2017

needed to assess the efficacy and safety of a new therapy. An ideal animal model should resemble human hypertrophic scarring in clinical characteristics and histological, immunological, and biochemical aspects [4]. One of the obstacles to the development of a suitable animal model is the presence of the panniculus carnosus, the striated muscle found in superficial fascia beneath the skin in laboratory animals. This fibro-muscular layer is responsible for rapid contraction and faster healing of the wounds in those animals. Among a wide variety of animal models which have been generated, the red Duroc pigs have the most similar skin architecture to humans and may develop scars resembling human hypertrophic scars. However they are costly and difficult to maintain [5].

The rabbit ear model was first established by Morris et al. in 1997 following observations made by the authors that some surgical wounds in the rabbit ear remain raised for months after healing [2]. In this model a full-thickness excisional wound to the cartilage surface was created over the ventral side of rabbit ear. Depending on the size of the original wound, this technique was used to develop an acute or chronic scarring model. Clinically, the large wounds (1.5 × 4.5–7.0 cm) healed with visibly raised and palpable scars which remained elevated up to 90 days or more post wounding. The healed small wounds (6 mm in diameter) also remained elevated until they were harvested at 22 days post wounding. Histologically, the chronic scars showed increased collagen fibers, irregularly arranged with circular or whorled pattern in elevated area, which resembled the characteristic collagen nodules of human hypertrophic scar. Horizontally oriented collagen fibers were located in deeper layers. In addition, increased vascularity and mild chronic inflammatory infiltrate were observed [2, 6]. The thickening of the subdermal cartilaginous layer and focal areas of cartilage proliferation was apparent in the scar area as well [2]. In order to quantify the newly deposited scar connective tissue, the authors introduced a formula to derive the hypertrophy index (HI) (also called as scar elevation index) from the measurement of total area of new scar and the thickness of adjacent unwounded dermis [2]. Since its development, many laboratories including ours have used the rabbit ear model to further elucidate the factors involved in pathogenesis of dermal scarring [7–9] or investigate the antifibrogenic effect of prospective treatment options [1, 10–22].

The rabbit ear model of hypertrophic scarring has several advantages over other models of fibro-proliferative disorders. First of all as it is evident in Fig. 1, the rabbit ear has no panniculus carnosus; as a result, significant wound contraction is excluded, and healing occurs primarily by granulation tissue formation and re-epithelialization, which mimics the wound healing process in humans. Second, the histology of the HSc in rabbit ear shows increases in the deposition of collagen fibers, the number of cells, and the density of blood vessels similar to the HSc in human. The presence of irregularly arranged collagen fibers with circular or whorled pattern in elevated

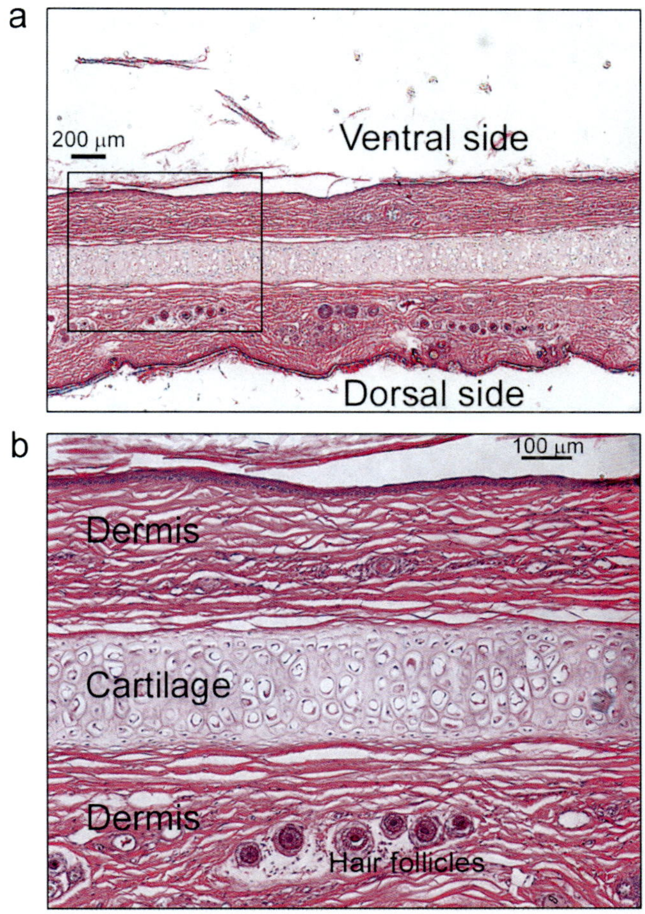

Fig. 1 Histology of the normal rabbit ear. (**a**, **b**) Hematoxylin- and eosin-stained section at 20- and 100-fold magnification, respectively. No hair follicle is observed in the dermis of the ventral side compared with the dorsal side

area is also common between rabbit ear model and human HSc (Fig. 2) [23, 24]. In addition, the relatively simple procedures needed to generate hypertrophic scar in rabbit ear and its reproducibility make it a useful model to evaluate the efficacy of the newly developed anti-fibrotic agents in preclinical studies.

Although the rabbit ear model is widely used as a model of hypertrophic scarring, there are some limitations. Like any other animal model, the physiology of rabbit skin and its immune system is very different from humans, so the identification of essential factors responsible for differences between normotrophic and hypertrophic scar formation is not possible. In addition, genetic predisposition plays an important role in hypertrophic scarring in humans, influencing the entire process of healing from the inflammatory phase to the tissue remodeling and scar formation. This predisposition is not considered in rabbit ear model [3]. Other major limitation of the ear model is the fact that ear skin is

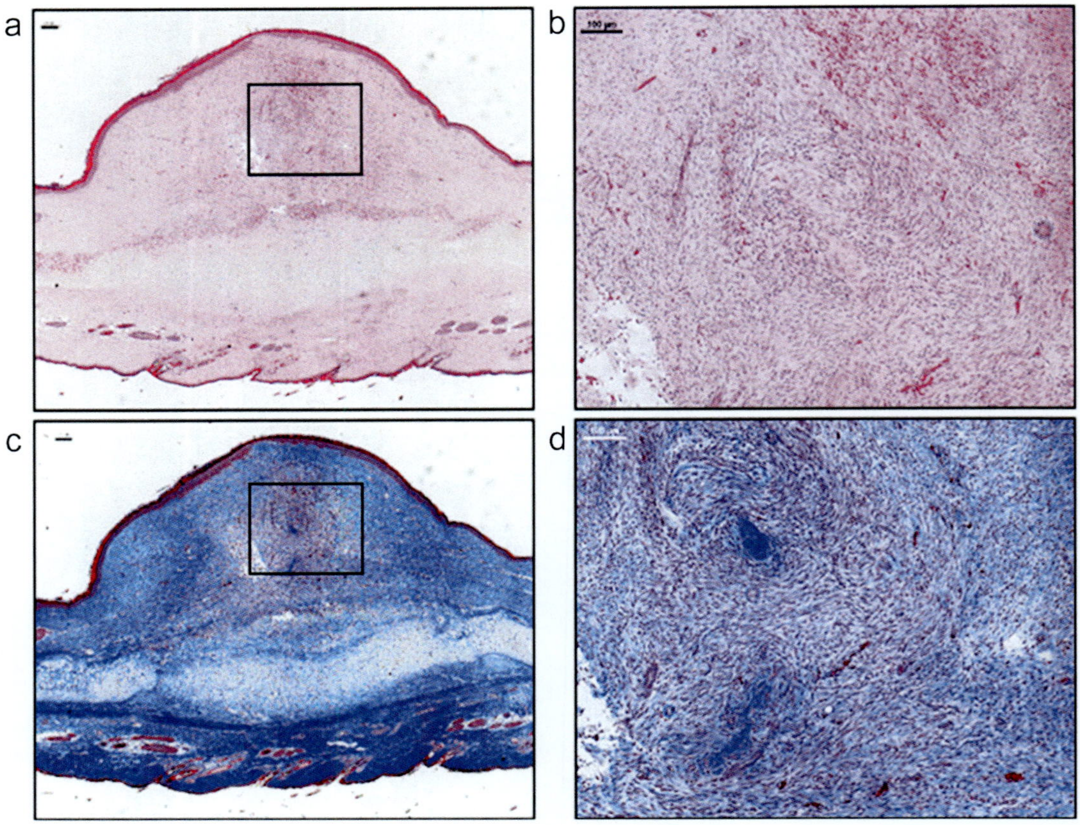

Fig. 2 Histology of HSc in rabbit ear. (**a**, **b**) Hematoxylin- and eosin-stained section at 20- and 100-fold magnification, respectively, shows increased cellularity and vascular density in the scar area. (**c**, **d**) Masson's Trichrome staining of the same sample shows irregularly arranged collagen fibers with circular or whorled pattern in the same area. 20- and 100-fold magnification, respectively. Scale bars = 200 μm in (**a**) and (**c**), 100 μm in (**b**) and (**d**)

histologically simpler than trunk skin and both the inner and outer skin are firmly attached to the underlying auricular cartilage with no intervening muscle or adipose tissue. Therefore, the healing process occurs over an avascular cartilage base [25].

2 Materials

2.1 Generation of Skin Wounds

1. New Zealand White rabbits (*see* **Notes 1** and **2**).
2. Depilatory cream (such as Nair®).
3. Betadine (10% povidone-iodine).
4. 70% alcohol (isopropyl or ethanol) in distilled water.
5. Dressing materials: plain gauze roll, gauze squares, paraffin gauze, antibiotic ointments, Mepitel, semiocclusive dressing (such as Tegaderm® (3M, St. Paul, MN)).

6. Sterile basic surgical tools (fine forceps, surgical blades #10 and #11, scissors, needle holder, tweezers).
7. Sutures (nylon 5–0 or 6–0).
8. Gown, gloves.
9. Punch biopsy tool (6 mm or larger).
10. Electrical heating pad (or other heat source that will not burn).
11. Gas anesthesia machine and isoflurane gas.
12. Endotracheal tube (size 2–3.5 mm).
13. Beck Airway Airflow Monitor (BAAM) (optional).
14. Laryngoscope (optional).
15. Meloxicam 5 mg/mL diluted with sterile water 1:10 or buprenorphine.
16. Ketamine.
17. Xylazine.
18. 1 mL syringes.
19. 27 G ½ needle.
20. Sterile eye lubricant.

2.2 Rabbit Sacrifice and Sample Harvest

1. Pentobarbital.
2. Sterile syringe.
3. 25–27 G needle.
4. Formalin 10%.
5. Ethanol 70%.
6. Tissue cassettes, cryotubes, and eppendorfs.
7. Tissue forceps.
8. Scissors.
9. Punch biopsy tool.
10. Paper towel.
11. RNAlater.

3 Methods

3.1 Generation of Skin Wounds

1. Restrain the animal manually (another operator or a towel).
2. Administer pain killer meloxicam 0.1–0.2 mg/kg or buprenorphine 0.01–0.05 mg/kg by subcutaneous injection.
3. Administer 35–50 mg/kg ketamine mixed with 5–10 mg/kg xylazine through subcutaneous or intramuscular injection for induction of anesthesia (*see* **Note 3**).
4. Monitor animal's breathing and circulation (*see* **Note 4**).

5. Once sedated, place the animal in supine position on electrical heating pad covered with towel.
6. Intubate the animal (*see* **Note 5**).
7. Begin administering isoflurane gas 1–3% in oxygen using precision vaporizer for maintaining general anesthesia.
8. Verify level of anesthesia (negative response to toe pinch).
9. Apply small amount of eye lubricant to both eyes.
10. Depilate the ventral surface of the ear using a quick application and removal of Nair (*see* **Note 6**).
11. Disinfect with betadine, followed by 70% alcohol.
12. By using aseptic techniques, cut a circular skin wound with a 6.0 mm or larger punch biopsy tool without compromise of ear cartilage or puncturing the back of the ear.
13. Dissect the perichondrial membrane off the cartilage using forceps and scissors.
14. Cover the wound with dressing paraffin gauze or similar.
15. Cover with Tegaderm (or similar) and suture in place one piece of gauze over top.
16. Bandages should remain in place for 1–2 days until hemostasis and a firm clot has formed (*see* **Note 7**).

3.2 Rabbit Sacrifice

Rabbit sacrifice by overdose of pentobarbital: It is preferable to sedate the animal before this procedure. Manual restraint (another technician or a towel) can be used with EMLA cream applied to the ear 45 min prior to injection.

1. Restrain the animal manually (another operator or a towel).
2. Administer 35–50 mg/kg ketamine mixed with 5–10 mg/kg xylazine through subcutaneous or intramuscular injection.
3. Once sedated, inject 120 mg/kg of pentobarbital (2–3 mL/4.5 kg of euthanyl-pentobarbital 240 mg/mL) intravenously into the marginal ear vein. Additional euthanyl may be used as required.
4. Alternatively, 2–3 mL/4.5 kg euthanyl may be injected intracardiac while the animal is anesthetized.

3.3 Sample Harvest

1. Harvest each scar separately with a 0.5 cm margin of surrounding unwounded tissue.
2. Bisect through the maximum point of scar hypertrophy on visualization and palpation.
3. One half of each scar is fixed in 10% neutral buffered formaldehyde for 24 h and after dehydration in ethanol will be embedded in paraffin and used for histology and immunohistochemistry. The other half is stored in RNAlater at −80 °C for RNA extraction (*see* **Note 8**).

4 Notes

1. The age of the rabbit is an important factor when you are looking for more prominent fibrotic response. It has been shown that young rabbits (3–6 months old) demonstrate significantly greater scar elevation/area compared with aged ones (44–62 months old) [7].
2. Males and females can be used with this model, and no differences in wound healing processes can be found between young male and young female rabbits [2].
3. Drugs may be delivered separately. In this case xylazine should be delivered 10–20 min in advance.
4. Significant respiratory depression, reduced respiratory rate, and reduction in heart rate are often observed (with exception to ketamine alone). Many protective reflexes are not abolished, and so monitoring the depth of anesthesia is not similar to other general anesthetics.
5. Following sedation by injecting ketamine/xylazine, open the mouth and pull the tongue forward into the diastema and insert the endotracheal tube into the trachea using a laryngoscope (you can insert it blindly). To confirm correct placement, use a BAAM (Beck Airway Airflow Monitor) or listen by stethoscope while pushing air through a 5 mL syringe attached to the tube. Then inflate the cuff, tie a roll gauze around the tube, and secure it behind the neck of the animal.
6. It is better to perform all surgical procedures on the ventral surface of the ear, where there is minimal hair, and create full-thickness wounds so the possibility of hair cycle influences on wound healing and scar formation is minimized [2] (Fig. 1).
7. After removal of the bandages, for topical preparations of the anti-fibrogenic factors, Elizabethan neck collar should be used upon application for 2 h.
8. Dermal fibrosis can be measured in a number of ways in this model. Scar elevation index (SEI) or hypertrophy index (HI), cellularity, and collagen content are validated outcome measures usually used [1, 21]. The SEI measures the ratio of total scar area to the area of normal underlying dermis as described previously by Morris et al. [2]. As shown in Fig. 3, the height of the normal underlying dermis is determined based on the thickness of the normal adjacent unwounded dermis. The epithelial height is not considered in SEI calculations. Total tissue cellularity and infiltrated immune cells are quantified in 5 μm-thick paraffin-embedded tissue sections under 400-fold magnification (high-power field [hpf]). Infiltrated T-cells are immunostained using rabbit anti-T cell CD3 peptide (1:50;

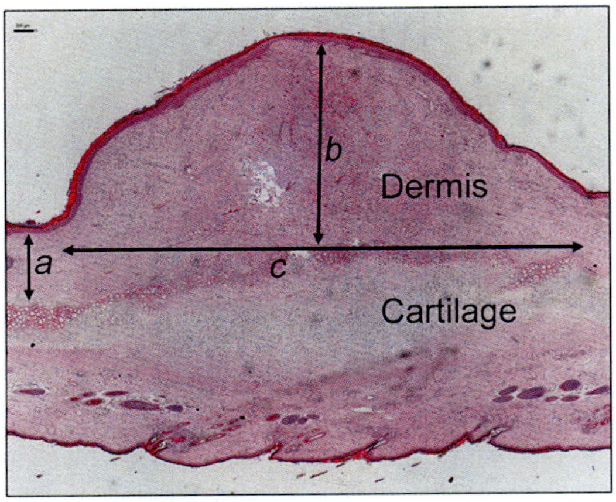

Fig. 3 Measurement of Scar Elevation Index (SEI). (**a**) Height of the normal underlying dermis. (**b**) Height of the new scar area. (**c**) Width of scar portion to be quantified. SEI is the ratio of total scar area to the area of normal underlying dermis (SEI = [b × c]/a). SEI = 1 indicates no newly formed hypertrophied dermis, whereas an SEI > 1 denotes HSc formation. Scale bar = 200 μm

Abcam, Cambridge, MA) as primary and Alexa Fluor® 488 goat anti-rabbit IgG (1:1000; Invitrogen) as secondary antibody. Infiltrated macrophages are stained using rabbit anti-F4/80 (1:50; Abcam) as primary and rhodamine-conjugated goat anti-rabbit antibody (1:1000; Invitrogen) as secondary antibody. The total tissue cellularity is measured by counterstaining the sections with 4′,6-diamidino-2-phenylindole (DAPI) [16]. The collagen content in scar area can be quantified by the Masson's Trichrome staining of the 4–5 μm-thick paraffin-embedded tissue sections and further determination of collagen density using Image Pro Plus 4.5 software [1]. Alternatively, it can be estimated by the measurement of hydroxyproline in samples obtained from scar area [19].

References

1. Rahmani-Neishaboor E, Yau FM, Jalili R et al (2010) Improvement of hypertrophic scarring by using topical anti-fibrogenic/anti-inflammatory factors in a rabbit ear model. Wound Repair Regen 18(4):401–408. doi:10.1111/j.1524-475X.2010.00598.x
2. Morris DE, Wu L, Zhao LL et al (1997) Acute and chronic animal models for excessive dermal scarring: quantitative studies. Plast Reconstr Surg 100(3):674–681
3. van den Broek LJ, Limandjaja GC, Niessen FB et al (2014) Human hypertrophic and keloid scar models: principles, limitations and future challenges from a tissue engineering perspective. Exp Dermatol 23(6):382–386. doi:10.1111/exd.12419
4. Ramos ML, Gragnani A, Ferreira LM (2008) Is there an ideal animal model to study hypertrophic scarring? J Burn Care Res 29(2):363–368. doi:10.1097/BCR.0b013e3181667557
5. Seo BF, Lee JY, Jung SN (2013) Models of abnormal scarring. Biomed Res Int 2013:423147. doi:10.1155/2013/423147
6. Harunari N, Zhu KQ, Armendariz RT et al (2006) Histology of the thick scar on the female, red Duroc pig: final similarities to

human hypertrophic scar. Burns 32(6):669–677. doi:10.1016/j.burns.2006.03.015

7. Marcus JR, Tyrone JW, Bonomo S et al (2000) Cellular mechanisms for diminished scarring with aging. Plast Reconstr Surg 105(5):1591–1599
8. Lu L, Saulis AS, Liu WR et al (2005) The temporal effects of anti-TGF-beta1, 2, and 3 monoclonal antibody on wound healing and hypertrophic scar formation. J Am Coll Surg 201(3):391–397. doi:10.1016/j.jamcollsurg.2005.03.032
9. Kryger ZB, Sisco M, Roy NK et al (2007) Temporal expression of the transforming growth factor-Beta pathway in the rabbit ear model of wound healing and scarring. J Am Coll Surg 205(1):78–88. doi:10.1016/j.jamcollsurg.2007.03.001
10. Saulis AS, Mogford JH, Mustoe TA (2002) Effect of mederma on hypertrophic scarring in the rabbit ear model. Plast Reconstr Surg 110(1):177–183. discussion 184-176
11. Saulis AS, Chao JD, Telser A et al (2002) Silicone occlusive treatment of hypertrophic scar in the rabbit model. Aesthet Surg J 22(2):147–153. doi:10.1067/maj.2002.123023
12. Kim I, Mogford JE, Witschi C et al (2003) Inhibition of prolyl 4-hydroxylase reduces scar hypertrophy in a rabbit model of cutaneous scarring. Wound Repair Regen 11(5):368–372
13. Brown RJ, Lee MJ, Sisco M et al (2008) High-dose ultraviolet light exposure reduces scar hypertrophy in a rabbit ear model. Plast Reconstr Surg 121(4):1165–1172. doi:10.1097/01.prs.0000302512.17904.2a
14. Jia S, Zhao Y, Mustoe TA (2011) The effects of topically applied silicone gel and its silver derivative on the prevention of hypertrophic scarring in two rabbit ear-scarring models. J Plast Reconstr Aesthet Surg 64(12):e332–e334. doi:10.1016/j.bjps.2011.05.008
15. Chavez-Munoz C, Hartwell R, Jalili RB et al (2012) Application of an indoleamine 2,3-dioxygenase-expressing skin substitute improves scar formation in a fibrotic animal model. J Invest Dermatol 132(5):1501–1505. doi:10.1038/jid.2011.467
16. Rahmani-Neishaboor E, Jallili R, Hartwell R et al (2013) Topical application of a film-forming emulgel dressing that controls the release of stratifin and acetylsalicylic acid and improves/prevents hypertrophic scarring. Wound Repair Regen 21(1):55–65. doi:10.1111/j.1524-475X.2012.00857.x
17. Poormasjedi-Meibod MS, Hartwell R, Kilani RT et al (2014) Anti-scarring properties of different tryptophan derivatives. PLoS One 9(3):e91955. doi:10.1371/journal.pone.0091955
18. Wo Y, Zhang Z, Zhang Y et al (2014) Enhanced in vivo delivery of 5-fluorouracil by ethosomal gels in rabbit ear hypertrophic scar model. Int J Mol Sci 15(12):22786–22800. doi:10.3390/ijms151222786
19. Li Y, Kilani RT, Rahmani-Neishaboor E et al (2014) Kynurenine increases matrix metalloproteinase-1 and -3 expression in cultured dermal fibroblasts and improves scarring in vivo. J Invest Dermatol 134(3):643–650. doi:10.1038/jid.2013.303
20. Liu YL, Liu WH, Sun J et al (2014) Mesenchymal stem cell-mediated suppression of hypertrophic scarring is p53 dependent in a rabbit ear model. Stem Cell Res Ther 5(6):136. doi:10.1186/scrt526
21. Hartwell R, Poormasjedi-Meibod MS, Chavez-Munoz C et al (2015) An in-situ forming skin substitute improves healing outcome in a hypertrophic scar model. Tissue Eng Part A 21(5–6):1085–1094. doi:10.1089/ten.TEA.2014.0271
22. Zhang Q, Liu LN, Yong Q et al (2015) Intralesional injection of adipose-derived stem cells reduces hypertrophic scarring in a rabbit ear model. Stem Cell Res Ther 6:145. doi:10.1186/s13287-015-0133-y
23. Ehrlich HP, Desmouliere A, Diegelmann RF et al (1994) Morphological and immunochemical differences between keloid and hypertrophic scar. Am J Pathol 145(1):105–113
24. Lee JY, Yang CC, Chao SC et al (2004) Histopathological differential diagnosis of keloid and hypertrophic scar. Am J Dermatopathol 26(5):379–384
25. Davidson JM, Yu F, Opalenik SR (2013) Splinting strategies to overcome confounding wound contraction in experimental animal models. Adv Wound Care (New Rochelle) 2(4):142–148. doi:10.1089/wound.2012.0424

Chapter 7

Mouse and Rat Models of Induction of Hepatic Fibrosis and Assessment of Portal Hypertension

Sabine Klein, Robert Schierwagen, Frank Erhard Uschner, and Jonel Trebicka

Abstract

Portal hypertension either develops due to progressive liver fibrosis or is the consequence of vascular liver diseases such as portal vein thrombosis or non-cirrhotic portal hypertension. This chapter focuses on different rodent models of liver fibrosis with portal hypertension and also in few non-cirrhotic portal hypertension models. Importantly, after the development of portal hypertension, the proper assessment of drug effects in the portal and systemic circulation should be discussed. The last part of the chapter is dedicated in these techniques to assess the in vivo hemodynamics and the ex vivo techniques of the isolated liver perfusion and vascular contractility.

Key words Portal hypertension, Bile duct ligation, Carbon tetrachloride, Methionine-choline-deficient diet, High-fat diet, Partial portal vein ligation, Colored microsphere technique, Isolated in situ liver perfusion, Aortic ring contraction

1 Introduction

Portal hypertension is the consequence of progressive fibrosis together with vasoconstriction in the hepatic vascular bed. The increase in portal pressure is associated with vascular dysfunction in terms of hypo-contractility in extrahepatic vessels together with an increase in cardiac output. Both intra- and extrahepatic changes characterize full picture of portal hypertension during liver fibrosis and lead to major complications occurring in human liver disease.

To mimic the development of portal hypertension, animal models of liver fibrosis are important. In order to have a balance between the feasibility in the lab and the representativeness of the disease, we will present in the following different animal models which have been used in our lab for different purposes. While bile duct ligation in rats and mice is an aggressive but fast model of severe liver fibrosis with portal hypertension, carbon tetrachloride (CCl_4) intoxication via inhalation is slow but mimics more

Laure Rittié (ed.), *Fibrosis: Methods and Protocols*, Methods in Molecular Biology, vol. 1627,
DOI 10.1007/978-1-4939-7113-8_7, © Springer Science+Business Media LLC 2017

adequate the toxic genesis of liver disease especially alcoholic liver disease [1–6]. An emerging need is the development of good models of nonalcoholic liver disease. During this condition the portal hypertension is slightly different and the underlying mechanisms of diseases and complications also. Therefore, we offer a novel model, recently published, to analyze this condition, which is very similar to the human disease [7]. In addition methionine-choline-deficient (MCD) diet might be another complementary model, which might be useful to specifically analyze nonalcoholic fatty liver disease in lean individuals [7].

Portal hypertension defined as the gradient between the portal pressure and hepatic venous (or central venous) pressure above 5 mmHg is clinically relevant only if it exceeds 10 mmHg and leads to complications in human disease. Besides the portal hypertension developing due to liver injury, also non-cirrhotic idiopathic portal hypertension might occur in patients, and this is important to dissect the differences between the cirrhotic and non-cirrhotic portal hypertension. Therefore, besides the typical liver injury such as bile duct ligation and CCl_4 intoxication, partial portal vein ligation and recently published embolization model might also be useful as comparison to cirrhotic portal hypertension and to investigate drugs in the non-cirrhotic portal hypertension [8, 9].

To date the treatment of portal hypertension and complications is still challenging, and new treatments are needed. To develop new treatment strategies, understanding the pathophysiology is pivotal; therefore, animal models are indispensable, especially the hemodynamic characterization of these animals. The necessary techniques to characterize portal hypertension are on the one hand in vivo hemodynamic assessment using pressure measurements and assessment of regional blood flows, as well as in situ liver perfusion assessing the responsiveness of the hepatic vascular bed and in vitro extrahepatic vessel contractility. All these techniques are useful to characterize the conditions and drug effects before starting the testing in humans [1, 2, 10–14].

In this chapter, we detail the state-of-the-art protocols used in the investigation of liver fibrosis and portal hypertension. The models and techniques highlighted were previously successfully used and reproducible in different laboratories and by different researchers. Importantly, the effects of any drugs should be investigated by different techniques and in different models in order to avoid model-specific effects and bias. Moreover, in the hemodynamic situation, one should always investigate first the in vivo situation before going into more detail, meaning that if a drug has a portal pressure-lowering effect through splanchnic vasoconstriction and/or decreased mesenteric blood inflow, then isolated liver perfusion would probably not reveal much insight, but the contraction of mesenteric arteries or aorta would give the answer regarding the real effect underlying the beneficial portal pressure-lowering effect. Vice versa an effect on the portal hypertension in vivo associated with a decrease in hepatic vascular resistance, liver perfusion using agonist and antagonist of the respective pathway might demonstrate the real mechanism of action. For these reasons, we present here different techniques to model liver cirrhosis and portal hypertension, including bile duct ligation, CCl_4 intoxication, various diets, partial portal vein ligation, and a model of non-cirrhotic idiopathic portal hypertension.

In liver cirrhosis and portal hypertension, the portal vein is contracted, and thus less blood enters the liver with a higher pressure. The cirrhotic intrahepatic changes lead to a changed blood distribution intra- and extrahepatic. Angiogenesis occurs due to the portal hypertension and the nodular changes of the liver, leading to shunts to bypass the liver. To treat liver cirrhosis and portal hypertension, it is indispensable to determinate blood flow of organs in the cirrhotic rat and also the intrahepatic resistance. We thus present a method for hemodynamic assessment of portal hypertension. This method utilizes colored microspheres to assess blood flow in organs and organ resistances. Colored microspheres are commercially available and are not harmful to health, like radioactive microspheres used in former times. This method enables researchers to investigate the effects of new developed drugs on lowering resistances and portal hypertension, which is the main lethal complication of liver cirrhosis. Careful assessments of hepatic and extrahepatic effects are needed before any treatment might be used in humans, and this chapter might contribute to the safety of experimental testing in that regard.

2 Materials

2.1 Anesthesia

All solutions should be prepared with deionized water, sterilized, and stored at room temperature.

1. Eye lubrication ointment.
2. 0.9% (w/v) NaCl solution.
3. Antiseptic solution and skin and wound disinfectant.
4. Carprofen.
5. Perform anesthesia according to your local animal care-approved protocol. Commonly used anesthetics include ketamine/xylazine and isoflurane:
   (a) Ketamine/xylazine cocktail: mix a dose of 80–100 mg/kg ketamine with 5–10 mg/kg xylazine in 0.9% (w/v) sodium chloride. Inject cocktail intraperitoneally.
   (b) Isoflurane is administered by inhalation: 4% (v/v) isoflurane in pure oxygen at a flow rate of 4 L/min.

2.2 Surgical Material

Surgical materials are typically similar for all procedures, except that scissors, forceps, ligation, and sutures need to be smaller when used in mice *vs.* rats. As a general recommendation, work should be performed in conditions as sterile as possible (e.g., using sterile gloves, skin and wound disinfectant, sterilized surgical cutlery and dressing):

1. Scalpel.
2. Curved very fine precision tip forceps.
3. High precision 45° angle broad point forceps.
4. Forceps with straight tip.
5. Tissue forceps.
6. Surgical terminal.
7. Needle holder.
8. Cuticle scissors.
9. Small scissors.
10. Sterile dressings.
11. For ligations: silk (3-0) and (5-0), needle holder, and 20G needles (i.e., 0.889 mm diameter).
12. For sutures: 3-0 or 5-0 prolene and 5-0 monocryl monofilament absorbable.
13. Heating mat.
14. Adhesive tape.
15. Electric clippers.
16. Razor for rats and mice.
17. Heated, filter-topped recovery cage.
18. Subcutaneous injection material: 27-G needles and 1 ml syringes.

2.3 Materials Specific for CCl_4 Intoxication

1. Liquid carbon tetrachloride (CCl_4) (*see* **Note 1**).
2. Drinking water with 300 mg/L phenobarbital to increase liver-associated enzymes.
3. Fume hood.
4. Individually ventilated cages.
5. Compressed air.
6. Glass flask with gas bubbler/washing attachment.
7. Gas flowmeter.
8. Rubber tubes.

2.4 Materials Specific for Special Diets

1. Mice, with an initial body weight between 20 g and 25 g:
   - (a) Western diets are supplied to Apoetm1Unc mice on a C57BL/6J background.
   - (b) Methionine-choline-deficient diet is supplied to mice (we use mice with C57BL/6J background).

2. Special diets:
   (a) Western diet containing 20.9% crude fat and 1.25% cholesterol (we use diet # S0279-S011, from Ssniff Spezialdiäten GmbH, Germany).
   (b) Methionine-choline-deficient diet (we use diet # E15653-94 from Ssniff Spezialdiäten GmbH, Germany).
3. Precision scale.
4. Blood glucose meter.

2.5 Materials Specific for Colored Microsphere Techniques

1. Glass tubes with lids (10 per rat).
2. Basic Tween solution: 20% (w/v) Tween-80 in 4 M KOH; prepare nine glass tubes per rat, each tube filled with 7 ml of solution.
3. 5.26 M KOH: prepare one glass tube per rat filled with 3.8 ml of solution.
4. 0.5% Tween solution: mix 0.5% (w/v) Tween-80 in 0.9% NaCl.
5. Dimethylformamide.
6. PE-50 catheters (3 per rat).
7. 1 ml plastic syringes filled with 0.9% NaCl with 10,000 U heparin (3 per rat).
8. Two 500 ml glass tubes with lids (one for the liver, one for the gastrointestinal tract).
9. Colored microspheres (we recommend white and blue microspheres, 15 μm diameter; we use the ones from Triton Technologies).
10. 2 ml gas-tight glass syringe (we use the ones from Hamilton).
11. Two 1 ml gas-tight glass syringe (we use the ones from Hamilton).
12. Vortex.
13. Water bath heated at 60 °C.
14. Withdrawal pump with a 2 ml syringe mount (ours is from Hugo-Sachs Electronics).
15. Compressed air pump connected to a closed glass vessel and glass vessel connected to a metal filter.
16. Polycarbonate membranes 13 mm diameter with 0.8 μm pore size (we use Whatman® Nuclepore™ track-etched types).
17. Plastic paraffin film such as Parafilm M®.
18. Microplate reader for absorbances between 300 and 800 nm.
19. 96-well glass microplate.
20. Pressure transducers (ours are from ADInstruments).
21. Data acquisition hardware for pressure measurement (ours is from ADInstruments).

2.6 Materials Specific for Isolated Liver Perfusions in Rats

1. Water bath at 37 °C.
2. Oxygen bottle (95% oxygen, 5% carbon dioxide).
3. Tubes (connecting tubes, semipermeable tube adapters for connection).
4. Drip chamber.
5. Flask with two necks.
6. Pressure transducers (ours are from ADInstruments).
7. Bio/Bridge Amplifier and data acquisition hardware (ours are from ADInstruments).
8. Glass spiral hose.
9. Peristaltic pump.
10. Thermometer.
11. Hot plate with integrated stirrer.
12. pH meter.
13. Peripheral venous catheter (22G).
14. Krebs-Henseleit (KH) buffer made in diH_2O: for 1 L, mix 9.55 g of Krebs-Henseleit buffer modified (we get ours from Sigma), 9.55 g $NaHCO_3$, 2.1 g $CaCl_2{\bullet}H_2O$ (MW = 147.02), and 2000 IU of heparin to reduce risk of thrombosis; adjust pH to 7.4 using 1 M HCl or 5 M NaOH (*see* **Notes 2** and **3**).

2.7 Materials Specific for Aortic Contraction in Rats

1. Tissue and organ bath system (we use the one from Hugo-Sachs).
2. Water bath with included water pump.
3. Four force transducers (up to 20 g) (ours are from ADInstruments).
4. Bio/Bridge Amplifier and data acquisition hardware (ours are from ADInstruments).
5. Oxygen bottle (95% oxygen, 5% carbon dioxide).
6. Thermometer.
7. Hot plate with integrated stirrer.
8. pH meter.
9. Crushed ice.
10. KH buffer (**item 14** in Subheading 2.6).

3 Methods

3.1 Anesthesia

We recommend a mixture of ketamine and xylazine for injection anesthesia in rats. Although ketamine/xylazine can be injected as an intraperitoneal, subcutaneous, or intramuscular route, we highly recommend intraperitoneal injection because it leads to a fast increase in serum anesthesia levels and thereby is better controllable with fewer side effects (*see* **Notes 4** and **5**).

3.2 Median Laparotomy

1. Prepare a heated surgical field by positioning sterile drapes and fixing them with adhesive tapes.
2. Shave the rat in area corresponding to the operation field, including the whole abdomen and the lower end of the sternum using electric clippers.
3. Place the animal on an individual sterile field for aseptic preparation: Prepare the rat's surgical site with alternating applications of chlorhexidine scrub solution and alcohol. Repeat this process twice. Reapply eye lubrication ointment if necessary.
4. Place the shaved and disinfected rat on the heated surgical field. Immobilize the rat in supine position and make sure to reevaluate the anesthesia depth by pain stimulation with a surgical forceps (e.g., in the soft tissue between the toes).
5. Disinfect the operation area with skin disinfectant.
6. Use a sterile dressing moistened with wound disinfectant and cut a hole in its center (big enough for the incision) to cover the operation area from dirt and hair.
7. Perform a median laparotomy using the scalpel: first incise the cutis at the lower abdomen (Fig. 1) and then bluntly dissect the cutis from the peritoneum, using an anatomical forceps.
8. Cut the cutis from the lower abdomen up to the lower end of the sternum (Fig. 1).
9. When incising the peritoneum, lift it tightly up, using a surgical forceps (*see* **Note 6**) and make sure to cut on the linea alba (*see* **Note 7**).

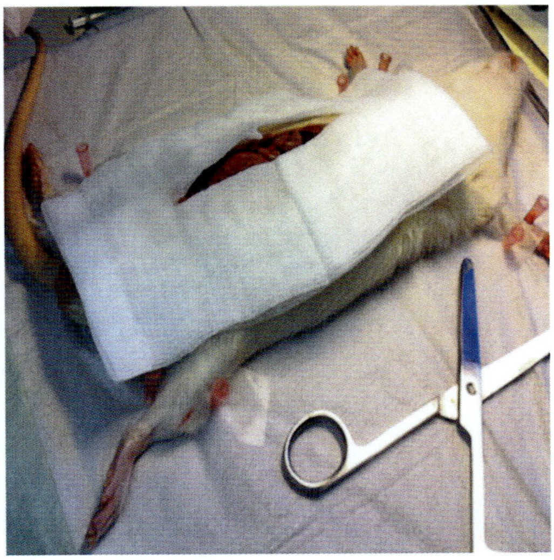

Fig. 1 Rat after median laparotomy to perform bile duct ligation

3.3 Induction of Liver Fibrosis in Rodents

3.3.1 Bile Duct Ligation Model in Rats

The bile duct ligation is an obstructive jaundice model resulting in cholestasis. For preclinical or research studies involving jaundice or liver fibrosis due to extrahepatic cholestasis, the rat is the most common animal model. Moreover, the effects of biliary drainage on hepatic blood flow and portal hypertension can be investigated with this model.

Male and female rats of any stain can be used for bile duct ligation. They should weigh at least 200 g, but no special diet is required. Rats can be group-housed after the bile duct ligation:

1. Prepare and anesthetize the rat, fix, disinfect, and perform a median laparotomy as described in Subheadings 3.1 and 3.2.
2. Lift the liver slightly with straight tip forceps to visualize the duodenum.
3. Take out the duodenum carefully with the thumb and finger, to avoid squeezing the duodenum.
4. Separate the bile duct from the portal vein and hepatic artery with very fine curved precision tip forceps.
5. Place the 3-0 silk around the bile duct and ligate it with two surgical knots.
6. Fix the ends of the 3-0 silk to the surgical terminal, placing it cranially to ensure that the knot is as close to the liver as possible.
7. Tie a second 3-0 silk with two surgical knots, placing it ventrally, around the bile duct.
8. Dissect the bile duct in between the knots with small scissors and cut the loose ends of the 3-0 silks.
9. Clean the peritoneal cavity: rinse it with 0.9% NaCl solution and place the abdominal organs back into their physiological locations.
10. Sew the abdominal peritoneum with 3-0 prolene, followed by the cutis with running sutures.
11. Cut the loose ends of the sutures and sterilize the rat's surgical area with antiseptic solution.
12. To avoid pain, inject rats with 5 mg/kg/day carprofen subcutaneously and once a day for the next 5 days.
13. Following surgery, place the rat on a cellulose sheet inside a heated, filter-topped recovery cage. Rats need to be regularly observed until they recover from anesthesia.
14. Observe postoperative rats daily and record observations in score sheets until rats develop ascites, a definitive sign for liver cirrhosis with portal hypertension. Liver cirrhosis is present after approximately 4–6 weeks, when ascites developed and rats can be further investigated.

3.3.2 Bile Duct Ligation Model in Mice

Another common animal model for bile duct ligation is the mouse. Beneficial effects in mice are that they develop faster liver fibrosis with portal hypertension than rats and, of course, they are much more space-saving than rats. Just like in rats, male and female mice of any stain can be used for bile duct ligation, and they should be at least 21 days old. The conditions of feeding and housing of mice after bile duct ligation are the same as of rats:

1. Anesthetize the mouse as described in Subheading 3.1.
2. Shave the abdominal fur of the mouse and check the adequacy of anesthesia (e.g., regular spontaneous breathing, no reflex after setting of pain stimuli between toes, and no response to pain).
3. Apply eye and nose ointment to protect eyes from drying.
4. Place the mouse on an individual sterile field for aseptic preparation.
5. Clean the surgical site twice with disinfection solution and alcohol.
6. Reapply eye lubrication ointment if necessary.
7. Place the shaved and disinfected mouse on a heated surgical field, fixed with adhesive tapes on a sterile operation table.
8. Perform a median laparotomy as described in Subheading 3.2, **steps 6–9**.
9. Follow **steps 2–7** of Subheading 3.3.1 using 5-0 silk in mice (instead of 3-0 for rats) to isolate the bile duct.
10. Also ligate the mouse gallbladder with 5-0 silk and carefully remove it to avoid contamination of the liver with bile.
11. Dissect the bile duct in between the knots with a small scissor.
12. Cut off the loose ends of the 5-0 silks.
13. Rinse the peritoneal cavity with 0.9% NaCl solution and place the abdominal organs back into their physiological locations.
14. Sew the abdominal peritoneum and cutis with 5-0 prolene with running sutures.
15. Cut the loose ends of the sutures and sterilize the operation area of the mouse with antiseptic solution.
16. Following surgery, place the mouse on a cellulose sheet inside a heated, filter-topped recovery cage. Mice need to be regularly observed until they recover from anesthesia.
17. Liver fibrosis and portal hypertension are present in mice after 14 days.

3.3.3 CCl_4 Intoxication in Mice and Rats

1. Switch the fume hood on and wait until the flow is sufficient.
2. Connect the compressed air valve with a rubber tube to the intake valve of the gas bubbler.

Table 1
Treatment pattern of CCl_4 intoxication in rats

Treatment time	Time with CCl_4 aerosol flow	Time in CCl_4 aerosol atmosphere
Week 1	30 s	30 s
Week 2	60 s	60 s
Week 3	120 s	120 s
Week 4	180 s	180 s
Week 5	240 s	240 s
Weeks 6–16	300 s	300 s

3. Connect the exhaust valve of the gas bubbler with the intake valve of the flowmeter and plug a rubber tube to the exhaust valve of the flowmeter.
4. Carefully fill the CCl_4 into the glass flask until the nozzle of the gas bubbler is fully covered.
5. Insert the rubber tube coming from the flowmeter into the ventilation orifice of the cage.
6. Turn up the compressed air to a final flow of 1 L/min. The compressed air should bubble the CCl_4 and carry the air/CCl_4 aerosol to the cage (*see* **Note 8**).
7. Keep animals in the cage with closed lid in CCl_4-enriched atmosphere for the required time, which is as long as the flow was switched on.
8. Treatment regimens for rats and mice differ:
   (a) Rats should have an initial body weight of 100 g at treatment initiation. Intoxication of rats is performed twice weekly (typically, Mondays and Fridays) for 16 weeks. In the first week of treatment, rats are intoxicated for 30 s, and in the second week they are intoxicated for 1 min. Increase intoxication from week 3 to week 6 by 1 min weekly. From week 6 to week 16, rats are intoxicated for 5 min. The treatment pattern for rats is summarized in Table 1.
   (b) Mice should have an initial body weight of 20–25 g at treatment initiation. Intoxication of mice is performed three times a week (typically, Mondays, Wednesdays, and Fridays) for 4 weeks. From week 1 to week 4, intoxication time increases by 30 s weekly, starting with 30 s at week 1. The treatment pattern for mice is summarized in Table 2.
9. At the end of the required intoxication time, open the lid to let remaining CCl_4 evaporate for at least 10 min.

Table 2
Treatment pattern of CCl_4 intoxication in mice

Treatment time	Time with CCl_4 aerosol flow	Time in CCl_4 aerosol atmosphere
Week 1	30 s	30 s
Week 2	60 s	60 s
Week 3	90 s	90 s
Week 4	120 s	120 s

10. Close the lid and return the cage to the ventilation unit (*see* **Notes 9** and **10**).
11. Pour the CCl_4 back into the storage container.

3.3.4 Western Diet in ApoE$^{-/-}$

1. Record mouse weight prior to the initiation of the diet.
2. Feed mice for 7 weeks continuously with Western diet.
3. Record body weight weekly.
4. After the last day of diet, keep mice fasting overnight and measure the fasting glucose levels the next morning.
5. Record mice weight before organ withdrawal and liver weight after withdrawal (*see* **Notes 11** and **12**).

3.3.5 Methionine-Choline-Deficient Diet

1. Use mice with an initial body weight between 20 and 25 g and weigh mice prior to the initiation of the diet.
2. Feed mice for 7 weeks continuously with MCD diet.
3. Record body weight weekly.
4. After the last day of diet, keep mice fasting overnight and measure the fasting glucose levels the next morning.
5. Record body weight before organ withdrawal and liver weight after withdrawal (*see* **Note 13**).

3.4 Other Models of Portal Hypertension

3.4.1 Partial Portal Vein Ligation

1. Prepare and anesthetize the rat, fix, disinfect, and perform a median laparotomy as described in Subheadings 3.1 and 3.2.
2. Tightly grab the cecum with an anatomical forceps, mobilize it together with the small intestine, and put it on the left side of your sterile dressing (*see* **Notes 14** and **15**).
3. After mobilizing, you will identify the portal vein located right next to the caval vein embedded in the mesenterial tissue collecting blood from the small intestine (Fig. 2).
4. Use a small anatomical forceps to bluntly uncover the portal vein from the mesenterial tissue (*see* **Note 16**).

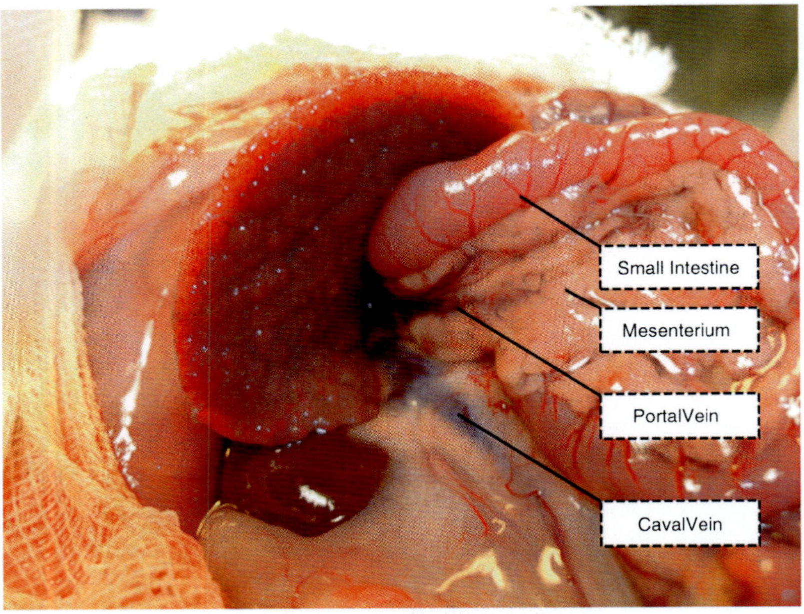

Fig. 2 Illustration of upper abdominal topography. View on the caval vein and the portal vein embedded in the mesenterial tissue

5. Use silk (3-0) to make a loop around the portal vein close to the liver.
6. Position a 20G needle in the longitudinal direction, on top of the portal vein.
7. Ligate the portal vein together with the needle (*see* **Note 17**).
8. When successfully ligated, you will see hyperemia (the intestine turns dark blue/violet) of the small intestine as well as stagnant mesenterial veins.
9. Slowly remove the needle, which will lead to partly reopening of the portal vein blood flow (*see* **Note 18**).
10. After the removal, the original intestine color should return. Still, the vessels will remain more stagnant then before the ligation.
11. Close the peritoneum with an ongoing suture (5-0 monocryl) (*see* **Note 19**).

Close the skin separately with single-knot sutures (5-0 monocryl) (*see* **Note 20**).

3.4.2 Non-cirrhotic Idiopathic Portal Hypertension

Non-cirrhotic idiopathic portal hypertension occurs in the absence of chronic liver injury and splanchnic venous thrombosis. This disease is poorly understood and is benign (5 year survival of almost 100%). Non-cirrhotic idiopathic portal hypertension arises from various conditions, including chronic infectious diseases, toxins or drug exposures, and genetic and immunologic disorders. The

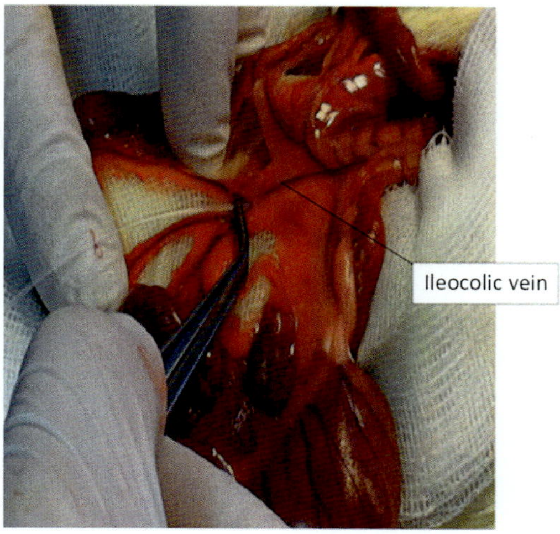

Fig. 3 PE-50 catheter placing. Injection of a sharpened PE-50 catheter into an ileocecal vein pushed to the portal vein is shown, as a mean to measure the portal pressure and for injection of blue microspheres

symptoms are splenomegaly and pancytopenia. The major burden of non-cirrhotic idiopathic portal hypertension in patients is the development of gastroesophageal varices, bleeding, and complications. The initial causes of non-cirrhotic idiopathic portal hypertension are micro-thrombotic lesions in small portal venules. Therefore, we developed a rat model of non-cirrhotic idiopathic portal hypertension by repetitive injections of colored microspheres to induce micro-thrombotic lesions in small portal venules:

1. Prepare and anesthetize the rat, fix, disinfect, and perform a median laparotomy as described in Subheadings 3.1 and 3.2.
2. Take out the cecum with a straight forceps and expose the jejunum to visualize the ileocecal veins.
3. Slightly insert a sharpened PE-50 catheter into the ileocecal vein and advance to the portal vein for the measurement of portal pressure (Fig. 3).
4. Aspirate the blood and fix the catheter with two surgical knots of a 5-0 silk.
5. After measuring the portal pressure in the rat, weekly embolized rats receive every week 100 μl of colored microspheres diluted in 200 μl sodium chloride with 0.5% Tween.
6. After application of the colored microspheres, ligate the ileocecal vein with surgical knots of 3-0 silk.
7. Rinse the peritoneal cavity with 0.9% NaCl and place the abdominal organs back into the physiological positions.
8. Sew the abdominal peritoneum and cutis with 5-0 prolene with running sutures.

9. Cut the ends of the sutures and sterilize the operation area of the rat with antiseptic solution.
10. Following surgery, place the rat on a cellulose sheet inside a heated, filter-topped recovery cage.
11. Inject 5 mg/kg/day carprofen subcutaneously in the rat for 5 days to prevent pain.
12. Repeat surgical steps three times (every 7 days), except for the two control groups:
    (a) The "single embolization" group receives microspheres only one time, at the beginning, and will undergo the microsphere technique after 3 weeks (*see* below).
    (b) The "no embolization" group receives no microspheres, but fake surgery is performed and their portal pressure is measured every 7 days (*see* below).
13. After the third repetition of embolization with microspheres, perform the method of the colored microsphere technique (Subheading 3.5.1) to investigate the blood flow and resistances of organs.

3.5 Hemodynamic Assessment of Portal Hypertension

3.5.1 Systemic and Portal Hemodynamics In Vivo (Microsphere Technique)

1. Prepare and anesthetize the rat, fix, disinfect, and perform a median laparotomy as described in Subheadings 3.1 and 3.2.
2. Insert a PE-50 catheter into the ileocecal vein and advance to the portal vein as described in **steps 2–4** in the methods of noncirrhotic idiopathic portal hypertension (Subheading 3.4.2).
3. Sew the peritoneum and the cutis with 3-0 prolene. Make sure that the catheter is not moved and still pervasive to blood.
4. Expose the femoral artery using tissue forceps: First, cut the cutis and dissect the tissue. Then carefully isolate the femoral artery using curved high precision 45° angle broad point forceps.
5. Cut a little hole in the femoral artery using a scalpel.
6. Lift up the hole in the femoral artery using curved very fine precision tip forceps and insert a second PE-50 catheter for measurement of mean arterial pressure (MAP) and blood withdrawal.
7. After aspirating the blood from the femoral artery, fix the catheter with two surgical knots of 3-0 silk (Fig. 4).
8. Cut the cutis of the throat, mobilize the thyroids with curved and straight broad point forceps, and insert the last catheter in the carotid artery (it will be used for microsphere injection).
9. Repeat the procedure (**steps 4–8**) for the femoral vein.
10. Expose the tissue close to the trachea to visualize the carotid.
11. Isolate the carotid from surrounding tissue, and place two 3-0 silks around the carotid. Fix the cranial 3-0 silk with two surgical knots and tie the second 3-0 silk with a surgical terminal.

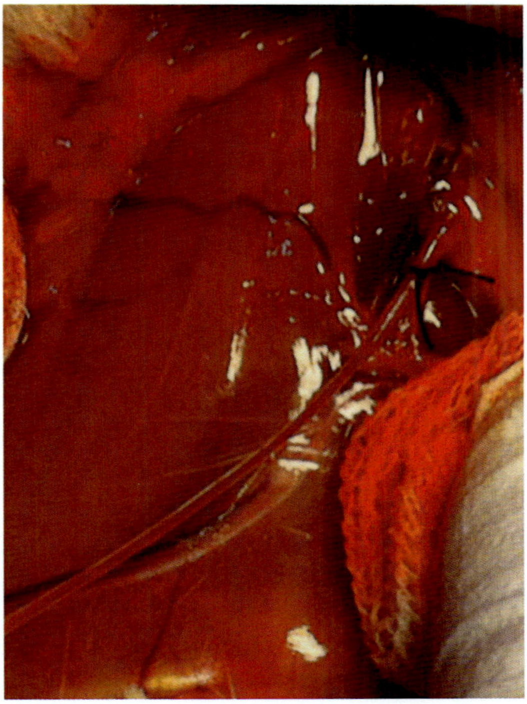

Fig. 4 The cannulated femoral vein and artery for mean arterial pressure measurement and blood withdrawal

12. Cut a hole in the carotid using a scalpel.
13. Insert the third PE-50 catheter in the hole using curved very fine precision tip forceps and push the catheter forward until it reaches the left atrium (Fig. 5).
14. Loosen the second 3-0 silk from the surgical terminal and aspirate blood.
15. Fix the 3-0 silk with two surgical knots. This catheter is ready for microsphere injection.
16. Connect the first two catheters (in the femoral artery and the portal vein) to a pressure transducer for blood pressure measurement.
17. Fill a 2 ml gas-tight glass syringe with 250 μl of 0.5% Tween-80 solution. Fix the syringe in the mount of the withdrawal pump and connect the femoral catheter to the syringe.
18. Fill a 1 ml gas-tight glass syringe with 100 μl of 0.5% Tween-80 solution and 200 μl white microspheres (*see* **Note 21**). Connect the syringe to the carotid catheter.
19. Set the withdrawal pump at 0.65 ml/min and start the pump.
20. 10 s after soaking blood from the femoral vein in the 2 ml glass syringe, slowly inject the white microspheres in the carotid for exactly 20 s.

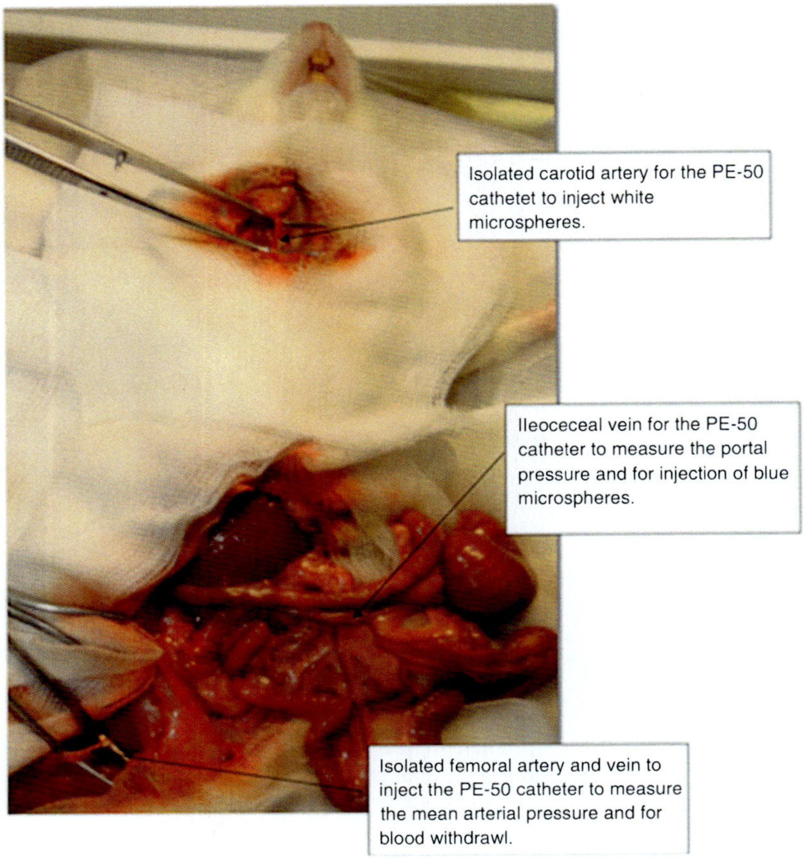

Fig. 5 Illustration of the carotid artery, the ileocecal vein, and the femoral artery to perform the colored microsphere technique

21. After an additional 30 s, stop the withdrawal pump and inject the content of the 2 ml glass syringe into the glass tube with 3.8 ml of 5.26 M KOH and 0.5 ml of 20% Tween-80.
22. Rinse the 2 ml glass syringe with 2 ml of 0.5% Tween solution and add the rinsing solution to the same glass tube.
23. Rinse the 1 ml glass syringe with 1 ml of 0.5% Tween-80 solution and add the rinsing solution to a glass tube with 7 ml of Basic Tween solution to get the rest of the white microspheres.
24. Prepare the second 1 ml gas-tight glass syringe by filling it with 200 μl of 0.5% Tween solution and 100 μl of blue microspheres (*see* **Note 21**). Connect the syringe to the portal vein catheter and slowly inject the blue microsphere solution.
25. After 15 min, sacrifice the rat by injecting 1 ml of 10X ketamine solution in the carotid catheter or other appropriate method (*see* **Note 22**).
26. Remove the spleen, the right kidney, and the left kidney, cut them into two pieces, and record their weight.

27. Put every piece into another glass tube filled with Basic Tween solution.
28. Remove the right lung and the left lung, record their weight, and put them also into separate glass tubes filled with Basic Tween solution.
29. Remove the whole liver, record the liver's weight, and transfer it in a 500 ml glass tube.
30. Multiply the weight of the liver (g) by 14. The result is the Basic Tween solution volume (in ml) that has to be added to the liver-containing glass tube.
31. Remove the whole gastrointestinal tract, clean it by flushing it with water, record the weight, and transfer it into the second 500 ml glass tube. Add 14 times (in ml) the weight of the gastrointestinal tract (g) in ml of Basic Tween solution to the glass tube.
32. Close all glass tubes with lids and boil the organs for 2 h at 60 °C.
33. Prepare the compressed air pump by connecting it to a closed glass vessel, itself connected to a metal holder with a metal filter.
34. The metal filter is covered with a standard thick filter paper. Place a polycarbonate membrane on top of the filter paper.
35. Fix the metal filter, the paper filter, and the polycarbonate membrane very tightly with a metal funnel to ensure the absence of leaks during filtration.
36. Filter all the organs dissolved in **step 32**, each through a separate polycarbonate membrane. After filtration, transfer each polycarbonate membrane to a separate glass test tube using forceps, and close the glass tube with plastic paraffin film. The boiled liver and gastrointestinal tract should be filtered three times through separate polycarbonate membranes, and each membrane should be transferred into a separate tube.
37. Add 200 μl of dimethylformamide to each test tube with a membrane (*see* **Note 23**).
38. Vortex the membrane with dimethylformamide thoroughly and centrifuge at 2,000 *g* for 5 min.
39. Transfer 100 μl of each supernatant to separate wells of a 96-well glass plate using pipette and filtered tips.
40. Add microsphere controls to the glass plate. The controls are prepared by dissolving 50 μl of white and blue microspheres (one control per color) in 1 ml DMF. After centrifugation at 2,000 *g* for 5 min, transfer 100 μl of supernatant into a well of the glass plate.
41. Place the glass plate into a plate reader and measure the 300–800 nm absorption spectrum for each well.

42. Calculate the cardiac output and organ blood flow using Excel spreadsheet macros (obtained online from Triton Technologies), expressed per 100 g body weight. Splanchnic perfusion pressures are defined as "mean arterial pressure" minus "portal pressure." Splanchnic vascular resistances are the ratios between splanchnic perfusion pressures and measured splanchnic blood flows, without including hepatic arterial flows. Mesenteric portal-systemic shunt flows are measured as the fraction of white/blue microspheres in the lung from total white/blue microspheres injected in an ileocecal vein. Hepatic portal-vascular resistances are "portal pressure" divided by sum of gastrointestinal and splenic perfusions minus mesenteric portal-systemic shunt flow. "Systemic vascular resistance" is the ratio between "mean arterial pressure" and cardiac output. Arterial vascular resistances of specific organs (kidney, spleen, liver, stomach-gut) are the ratios between "mean arterial pressure" and organ blood flows.

3.5.2 Isolated Liver Perfusions in Rats

1. Arrange your experimental setup according to Fig. 6 and corresponding legend (*see* **Note 24**).
2. Fill up the system with KH buffer so that at least 150 ml remain in the buffer bowl (perform all calculations concerning the test specimen on this amount). Refill during the experiment if necessary (*see* **Note 3**).
3. Turn on the oxygen, the water bath, and the peristaltic pump.
4. Prepare and anesthetize the rat, fix, disinfect, and perform a median laparotomy as described in Subheadings 3.1 and 3.2.
5. Identify the caval and the portal vein as described in Subheading 3.4.1, **steps 2–4**.
6. Using silk (3-0), prepare the following loops:
   (a) Around the portal vein (similarly to the partial portal vein method described in Subheading 3.4.1, **steps 5–10**)
   (b) Around the caval vein right above both renal veins (Fig. 7)
7. Identify and ligate the ligamentum *teres hepatis*, which is connecting the liver and peritoneum (Fig. 8) (*see* **Note 25**).
8. Take a peripheral venous catheter (22 G) and puncture the portal vein (*see* **Note 26**).
9. Slightly push the catheter forward until you reach the portal vein bifurcation (*see* **Note 27**) (Fig. 7).
10. Attach the catheter with a silk (3-0) ligation and immediately connect the catheter with the KH buffer tube (*see* **Note 28**).
11. Perfuse the liver with the KH buffer (30 ml/min) (*see* **Note 29**).

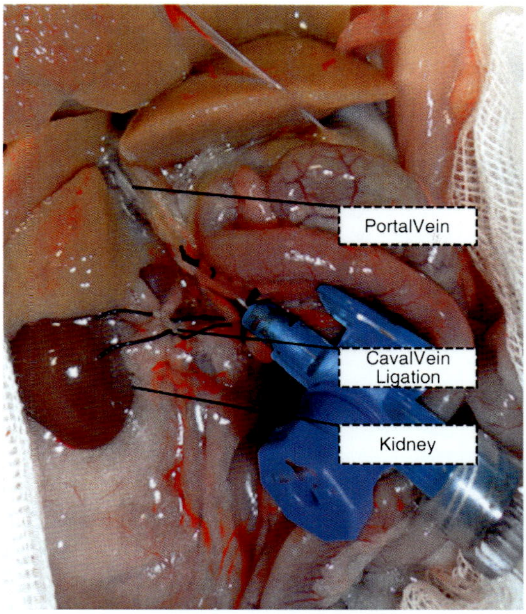

Fig. 6 Experimental setup for isolated liver perfusion in rats. The experimental setup should provide physiological conditions for the liver tissue to stay vital. The Krebs-Henseleit (KH) buffer is formulated to maintain liver tissue stability and is maintained warm and oxygenated during the entire experiment. A peristaltic pump circulates the buffer solution at 30 ml/min through the isolated liver. To guarantee oxygenation of the KH buffer, a semipermeable tube of 1–2 meters in length should be interposed. This tube is coiled and filled in a two-neck flask, closed by plugs. A mixture of 95% oxygen/5% carbon dioxide is pumped into the flask. Increasing pressure transfers oxygen through the semipermeable tube and thereby oxygenates the buffer solution. Surplus of air is released from the flask by a second tube to prevent overpressure (this tube might be connected to the buffer bowl for additional oxygenation). Downstream of the oxygenator, a glass spiral hose immersed in a water bath keeps the buffer solution at 37 °C. It is very important that the KH buffer remains free of air bubbles, since it may lead to venous embolism and thereby destroy the hepatic tissue. This is the role of the drip chamber, which is installed between the water bath and the liver. Lastly, a pressure transducer, connected with an amplifier and data acquisition hardware, is installed right before the portal vein catheter for invasive pressure measurements and analysis

12. Liver color should turn bright since the blood is replaced by KH buffer (*see* **Note 30**).
13. The next steps should be performed as fast as possible, since the KH buffer is already flooding the vascularity of the rat (*see* **Note 31**).
14. Open the thorax and mobilize the sternum by detaching it from the rips. You may use a needle holder or clamp to fix the sternum.
15. Grab the right heart ear with an anatomical forceps.

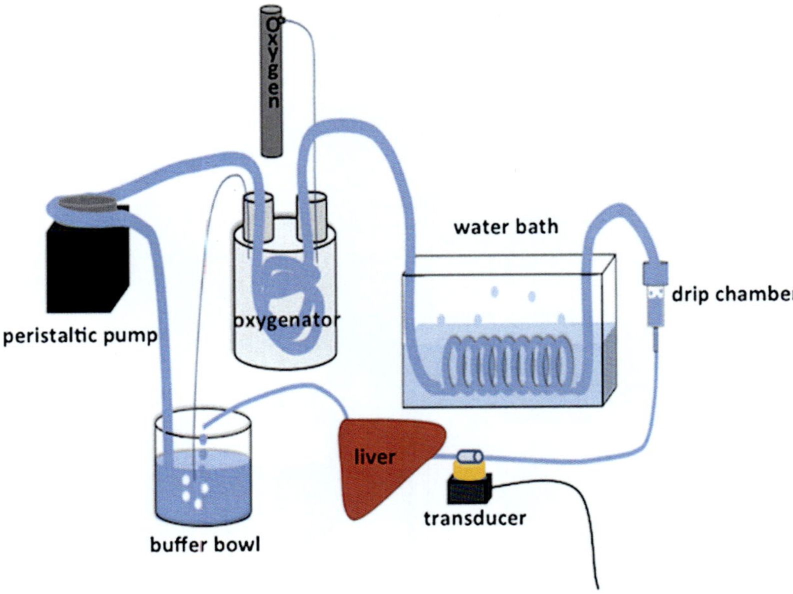

Fig. 7 Abdominal ligations for liver perfusion. Illustration of the placed peripheral venous catheter and the caval vein ligation

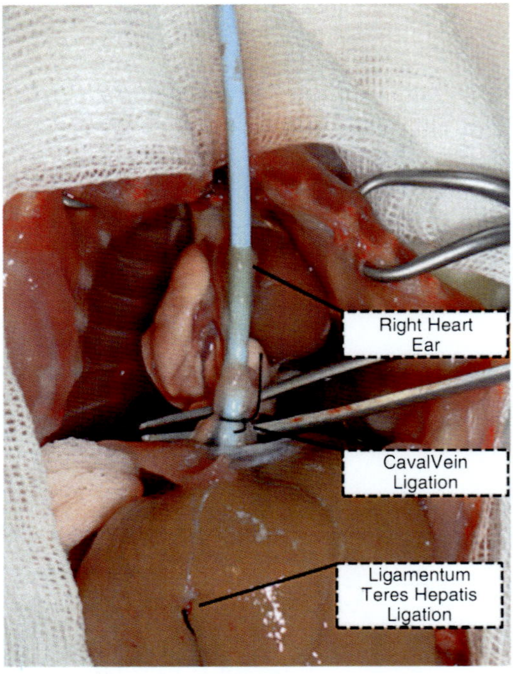

Fig. 8 Upper abdominal and thoracic ligations. Illustration of the ligamentum *teres hepatis* ligation as well as the catheterization of the right heart ear and upper caval ligation

16. Incise the heart ear and introduce a long catheter, which should stay with its end inside the inferior caval vein (at diaphragm level) (Fig. 8).
17. Attach the catheter at diaphragm level with a silk (3-0) ligation (*see* **Note 32**).
18. To prevent a loss of KH buffer, close/ligate the loops you previously prepared at the caval vein.
19. At this point, the KH buffer should circulate through the liver in a closed system (*see* **Note 33**).
20. Wait until the measured pressure stabilizes to start with contraction/relaxation experiments.

3.5.3 Aortic Contraction in Rats

1. Arrange your experimental setup according to the following tips:
   (a) The aorta preparation should be performed in a deep bowl. There are two options to maintain aorta vitality during dissection: either by cooling down the KH buffer to 4 °C while maintaining the bowl on crushed ice or by using a heated bowl to maintain the KH buffer at 37 °C. Be aware that the 37 °C temperature needs to stay stable during the entire preparation. Without continuous warming, the temperature will drop rapidly.
   (b) Always use a small tube to oxygenate the KH buffer in the bowl (warm or cold) during the entire preparation.
   (c) Maintaining the vitality of the aorta is the most challenging part of the contraction experiments. The aorta should be immersed in KH buffer all time (*see* **Note 24**).
   (d) The organ bath consists of four chambers, each containing a movable holder to attach an aortic ring. Included in each holder is an opening for oxygen so that the KH buffer can be oxygenated during the whole experiment.
   (e) Since the KH buffer should stay warmed at 37 °C, the frame of the chambers should be connected to a water bath with a pump that circulates warm water.
   (f) The upper attachment for the aortic rings is the force transducer, which directly measures the tension and tension changes in grams. The transducer should be connected to a data acquisition hardware and calibrated prior to the experiment.
   (g) The transducer itself is installed on a height regulator. By turning a button, the height of the transducer can be changed, leading to higher tension on the aortic rings.
2. Fill in preheated (*see* **Note 34**), oxygenated, and pH-normalized KH inside the chambers (20 ml per chamber).

3. Prepare and anesthetize the rat, fix, disinfect, and perform a median laparotomy as described in Subheadings 3.1 and 3.2.
4. The abdominal aorta is the best section to use for aortic ring contraction and is usually located directly behind the caval vein.
5. Use a small anatomical forceps to bluntly uncover the aorta. Start at the mesenterial artery and dissect the aorta till the femoral artery bifurcation (*see* **Note 35**).
6. Take two small clamps and occlude the aorta close to the mesenterial artery as well as close to the bifurcation.
7. Cut off the aorta so that it is still attached to the two clamps, and place the aorta in the dissecting bowl with chilled or heated KH buffer.
8. Start cleaning the aorta and removing surrounding adipose and connective tissues until the aorta is completely white (*see* **Note 36**).
9. Cut the aorta in small, about 2 mm (max.4–5 mm) long rings (*see* **Note 37**).
10. Push two silk (3-0) strings through the aortic rings and make two sized loops with a 3–5 mm distance from the aortic tissue (*see* **Note 38**). The first loop should be small, since it will later be connected to the holder inside the organ bath chamber. The second loop should be longer, since it will be attached to the force transducer when the ring is inside the organ bath (*see* **Note 39**).
11. Place the aortic ring inside the organ bath chamber, connect it to the transducer, and adjust a passive tension of 0.5 g by changing the height of the transducer (*see* **Note 36**).
12. Wait until tension stabilizes.
13. Perform the following washing steps three times:
    (a) Remove the KH buffer from the chamber and immediately fill it up with 20 ml of fresh pre-warmed KH buffer.
    (b) Readjust the pretension to 0.5 g.
14. After the third wash, wait until the tension stabilizes at 0.5 g to start contraction experiments (*see* **Note 40**).
15. It may be useful to test the aorta vitality by using increasing doses of phenylephrine (10^{-8} to 10^{-5} M). If viable, the aortas should have a dose-dependent contraction. The effect of pre-contraction can be washed out by repeating the three washing steps. Alternatively, pre-contraction may be used for relaxation experiments.
16. Repeat washing steps at the end of each experiment.

4 Notes

1. CCl_4 is very toxic and harmful to the ozone layer. Therefore, it is important to perform every step with CCl_4 under the fume hood.
2. The KH buffer should be pre-warmed at 37 °C prior to the experiment and oxygenated during the whole experiment, as the diluted ingredients precipitate in the absence of oxygen. When not directly used, you should stabilize the KH buffer on a hot plate with magnetic stirrer and oxygenation.
3. You should always have extra KH buffer on hands, ready to use.
4. When injected subcutaneously, slower drug uptake in adipose tissue may lead to delayed anesthesia effects and thereby entails the risk of overdosing.
5. If applied intramuscularly, a maximum of 300 mg ketamine/30 mg xylazine in a single injection should not be exceeded, since it may cause severe tissue necrosis.
6. It is important to lift up the peritoneum while cutting, since fragile structures, such as the intestine or other abdominal organs, are located right beneath the peritoneum and might be injured by deep incisions.
7. *Linea alba* is avascular. More laterally incisions might cause bleeding.
8. A higher flow of the CCl_4 aerosol than 1 L/min could cause severe side effects, leading to the death of the animals.
9. In rats development of ascites is a sign of severe liver fibrosis.
10. Animals should be three days without CCl_4 intoxication prior to proceed with experiments to avoid measuring effects of the acute intoxication, rather than the effects of the chronic intoxication.
11. Make sure that Western diet supply in the cage is always sufficient.
12. Due to the high fat content, Western diet needs to be stored at 4 °C. In case of storage at room temperature for a longer time period, the diet turns rancid and crumbly. Therefore, it is advised to give smaller portion more often, rather than bigger portions only once per week.
13. Special attention has to be paid to the weight development of the mice during the time they are fed MCD diet. Severe weight loss might be life-threatening for some animals. If severe weight loss occurs, the diet needs to be stopped before the end of the experiment.
14. Be careful handling the intestine. If the traction is high, it might lead to vascular or intestinal lacerations.

15. Make sure to secure the intestine on disinfected dressings to prevent infections.
16. Make sure to conserve surrounding and suppling vessels and do not put pressure directly on the portal vein.
17. Make sure the needle does not slip while ligating.
18. Since the needle may have sharp edges, make sure to remove the needle slowly without destroying the portal vein.
19. Before closing the peritoneum, check for bleeding inside the abdomen. If so, try to stop the bleeding by ligation.
20. It is important to close the skin with single knots. Otherwise, when stitched ongoing, the rats may bite the suture and open up their whole skin. Single knots provide more safety.
21. Vortex microspheres just prior to aspirate with the syringe to ensure that the suspension is homogeneous.
22. Animal euthanasia should be performed according to methods (e.g., overdose of 10% ketamine solution, cervical dislocation, carbon dioxide inhalation) approved by your local animal regulatory committee.
23. Dimethylformamide is toxic by inhalation and should be handled under a fume hood.
24. It is important to know that the live tissue constantly consumes the glucose within the KH buffer. Therefore, it is highly recommended to change KH buffer every 30–45 min during the experiment (this also applies to the KH buffer inside the organ bath chamber in the case of aortic contraction experiments).
25. Inside the ligamentum *teres hepatis* is a small vein. If not ligated, it may lead to a loss of KH buffer.
26. Be careful not to destroy the portal vein when puncturing. Once snatched, it will be almost impossible to bring the catheter in the correct position. When punctured successfully, blood will flow back in the catheter.
27. Make sure that you are not entering one of these two veins; otherwise, only a part of the whole liver will be perfused by the KH buffer.
28. KH buffer should already be inside the tubes and circulate. It is very important that you remove all trapped air bubbles in the tubes before connecting with the catheter.
29. The faster you perfuse the liver, the better you can reduce the risk of liver tissue ischemia.
30. It is necessary that the liver changes color homogeneously. If not, this may indicate that you are not perfusing all areas of the liver and thus distort your results.
31. As pressure rises, it will end up causing severe tissue damage.

32. You should check for the absence of caval kinking (it may be caused by the catheter and lead to blockage of the perfusion).
33. If KH buffer volume decreases in the buffer bowl, you will have to find the causal leak and close it. Possible reasons for leakage include incomplete ligations and vessel destruction during preparation.
34. The KH buffer should be heated on a hot plate with stirrer.
35. Be careful not to destroy smaller vessels that are leaving the aorta, since this might lead to bleeding.
36. Don't apply too much pressure or tension on the aorta while cleaning and later while attaching it to the organ bath. This might lead to irreversible tissue damage.
37. This way you will get more than four aortic rings. You can store the remaining rings in 4 °C in KH buffer and use them later. If so, make sure to change the KH buffer every 30 min.
38. The knots should not be made directly at the aortic ring, since it may lead to tissue damage.
39. After preparing the loops, make sure that you have no loose ends or free silk parts, till they may vibrate or swing inside the organ bath. This may lead to wrong results.
40. Don't change the passive tension after this point, or this would lead to altered results. When viable, the aortic rings should relax and reach 0.5 g passive tension.

Acknowledgment

The Laboratory is supported by grants from the Deutsche Forschungsgemeinschaft (SFB TRR57 to P18), the H. J. & W. Hector Stiftung, Ernst-Bertha-Grimmke-Stiftung (6/15) and European Union's Horizon 2020 research and innovation programme (No 668031).

References

1. Trebicka J, Hennenberg M, Laleman W et al (2007) Atorvastatin lowers portal pressure in cirrhotic rats by inhibition of RhoA/Rho-kinase and activation of endothelial nitric oxide synthase. Hepatology 46(1):242–253. doi:10.1002/hep.21673
2. Trebicka J, Leifeld L, Hennenberg M et al (2008) Hemodynamic effects of urotensin II and its specific receptor antagonist palosuran in cirrhotic rats. Hepatology 47(4):1264–1276. doi:10.1002/hep.22170
3. Trebicka J, Hennenberg M, Odenthal M et al (2010) Atorvastatin attenuates hepatic fibrosis in rats after bile duct ligation via decreased turnover of hepatic stellate cells. J Hepatol 53(4):702–712. doi:10.1016/j.jhep.2010.04.025
4. Granzow M, Schierwagen R, Klein S et al (2014) Angiotensin-II type 1 receptor-mediated Janus kinase 2 activation induces liver fibrosis. Hepatology 60(1):334–348. doi:10.1002/hep.27117

5. Klein S, Herath CB, Schierwagen R et al (2015) Hemodynamic effects of the non-peptidic angiotensin-(1-7) agonist AVE0991 in liver cirrhosis. PLoS One 10(9):e0138732. doi:10.1371/journal.pone.0138732
6. Klein S, Rick J, Lehmann J et al (2015) Janus-kinase-2 relates directly to portal hypertension and to complications in rodent and human cirrhosis. Gut. doi:10.1136/gutjnl-2015-309600
7. Schierwagen R, Maybuchen L, Zimmer S et al (2015) Seven weeks of Western diet in apolipoprotein-E-deficient mice induce metabolic syndrome and non-alcoholic steatohepatitis with liver fibrosis. Sci Rep 5:12931. doi:10.1038/srep12931
8. Uschner FE, Ranabhat G, Choi SS et al (2015) Statins activate the canonical hedgehog-signaling and aggravate non-cirrhotic portal hypertension, but inhibit the non-canonical hedgehog signaling and cirrhotic portal hypertension. Sci Rep 5:14573. doi:10.1038/srep14573
9. Klein S, Hinuber C, Hittatiya K et al (2016) Novel rat model of repetitive portal venous embolization mimicking human non-cirrhotic idiopathic portal hypertension. PLoS One 11(9):e0162144. doi:10.1371/journal.pone.0162144
10. Heller J, Trebicka J, Shiozawa T et al (2005) Vascular, hemodynamic and renal effects of low-dose losartan in rats with secondary biliary cirrhosis. Liver Int 25(3):657–666. doi:10.1111/j.1478-3231.2005.01053.x
11. Hennenberg M, Biecker E, Trebicka J et al (2006) Defective RhoA/Rho-kinase signaling contributes to vascular hypocontractility and vasodilation in cirrhotic rats. Gastroenterology 130(3):838–854. doi:10.1053/j.gastro.2005.11.029
12. Zhou Q, Hennenberg M, Trebicka J et al (2006) Intrahepatic upregulation of RhoA and Rho-kinase signalling contributes to increased hepatic vascular resistance in rats with secondary biliary cirrhosis. Gut 55(9):1296–1305. doi:10.1136/gut.2005.081059
13. Hennenberg M, Trebicka J, Biecker E et al (2007) Vascular dysfunction in human and rat cirrhosis: role of receptor-desensitizing and calcium-sensitizing proteins. Hepatology 45(2):495–506. doi:10.1002/hep.21502
14. Trebicka J, Hennenberg M, Schulze Probsting A et al (2009) Role of beta3-adrenoceptors for intrahepatic resistance and portal hypertension in liver cirrhosis. Hepatology 50(6):1924–1935. doi:10.1002/hep.23222

Chapter 8

Mouse Models of Corneal Scarring

Laure Rittié, Audrey E.K. Hutcheon, and James D. Zieske

Abstract

Corneal scarring is an obligatory consequence of stroma corneal injury and is a major cause of decreased visual quality and vision loss worldwide. There are currently no satisfactory intervention therapies for corneal fibrosis. In this chapter, we describe well-established in vivo corneal wound models to allow researchers to investigate epithelial and stromal responses to corneal injury.

Key words Cornea, Epithelial debridement, Incision, Keratectomy, Mouse

1 Introduction

The cornea is an excellent model system for the analysis of the wound repair response because it is of relatively simple anatomy, is readily accessible, and lacks vascularization. Corneal injuries may involve only the superficial epithelial layer or may penetrate deeper into the stromal layer. While the reepithelialization of the corneal epithelium is an important process for restoring the imaging properties of the eye after injury, stromal repair should be regarded as equally important, as corneal scarring is a major cause of decreased visual quality and vision loss worldwide [1, 2]. Causes of corneal scaring include all insults that disrupt the corneal stroma, including ocular trauma (chemical, physical, or surgical) or corneal dystrophies. There is currently no means to control or cure corneal fibrosis during wound repair or once established. To positively influence research efforts, it is important to develop and validate animal models to test drugs that potentially mitigate corneal fibrosis. Here we describe well-established in vivo corneal wound models to allow researchers to investigate epithelial and stromal responses to injury.

Laure Rittié (ed.), *Fibrosis: Methods and Protocols*, Methods in Molecular Biology, vol. 1627, DOI 10.1007/978-1-4939-7113-8_8,

2 Materials

2.1 Anesthesia

1. 27 G, 1/2″ sterile needles and 1 ml sterile syringes for intraperitoneal (IP) injections.
2. Ketamine/xylazine is used at 100–200 mg/kg ketamine with 20 mg/kg xylazine to provide approximately 20–40 min of anesthesia (*see* **Notes 1–3**). Prepare a ketamine/xylazine mix based on a 0.1 ml/10 g body weight dose rate. To prepare ~50 doses, mix 0.6 ml of 100 mg/ml ketamine hydrochloride (60 mg) with 0.5 ml of20 mg/ml xylazine (10 mg) and 3.9 ml of water for injection (WFI). Ketamine/xylazine in this mixture will be at 120/20 mg/kg when injected at 100 μl/10 g body weight.
3. Scale.
4. Proparacaine hydrochloride ophthalmic solution, 0.5% (w/v), sterile.
5. Sterile gauze.
6. Atropine solution, 1% (w/v), sterile.
7. Heated pad.

2.2 Corneal Surgery

1. 25 G, 1/2″ needles and 1 ml syringes for subcutaneous (SC) injections.
2. Meloxicam, used at 5–10 mg/kg in SC injections (*see* **Notes 2** and **4**).
3. Trephine (surgical instrument with a cylindrical blade): 1.0–2.0 mm diameter for epithelial debridement or 1.5–2.5 mm diameter for superficial keratectomy.
4. Surgical blades.
5. Forceps and other needed surgical instruments.
6. Triple antibiotic ointment.

2.3 Postoperative Examination

One or several of the following, according to needs:

2.3.1 Slit Lamp or Fluorescent Microscopy

1. 0.5% fluorescein eye drops.
2. Sterile PBS.
3. Gauze.
4. Slit lamp (we use one from Topcon Medical Systems) or fluorescent microscope.
5. Image processing software (we use ImageJ).

2.3.2 In Vivo Scanning Confocal Microscopy

1. In vivo scanning confocal microscope: we use the Heidelberg Retina Tomograph (HRT) from Heidelberg Engineering. This

is a confocal laser scanning system for imaging of the anterior and posterior segments of the eye.

2. Eye lubricant (we use GenTeal Liquid Gel Drops from Novartis).

3 Methods

3.1 Anesthesia and Preparation for Surgery

1. Prepare surgical field with heated pads and reagents.
2. Anesthetize adult mice of either sex by performing an IP injection of ketamine/xylazine using 27 G sterile needles and according to mouse weight (*see* **Note 5**).
3. Apply proparacaine eye drops to topically anesthetize the cornea.
4. Blot the excess proparacaine from the corner of the eye with gauze.
5. Apply one drop of atropine solution (for penetrating wounds only) (*see* **Note 6**).
6. Evaluate the depth of systemic anesthesia by performing a toe pinch (i.e., pinching the mouse toes with your fingers should not trigger any reaction from the animal). Proceed to surgical procedure only when the animal no longer responds to toe pinch stimulation, indicating adequate anesthesia levels.
7. Transfer the animal to a heated pad and proceed with experimentation.

3.2 Corneal Surgery

1. Administer preemptive pain relieving medication by performing a SC injection of meloxicam using a 25 G sterile needle.
2. Perform a wound on the center of the cornea, according to the desired following method:
   (a) *Epithelial debridement*: Perform a 1.0–2.0 mm diameter epithelial wound by demarcating an area on the center of the cornea with a trephine and removing the epithelium within the circle with a small scalpel (Fig. 1b) (*see* **Note 7**).
   (b) *Superficial keratectomy*: Place a 1.5–2.5 mm diameter trephine on the center of the cornea, and gently rotate two times to cut into the stroma. Use forceps to pull and separate the epithelial layer, the basement membrane, and a thin segment of the anterior stroma from the remaining stroma (Fig. 1c).
   (c) *Penetrating incision*: Place a 1.0–1.5 mm surgical blade on the center of the cornea and cut through the entire epithelium, stroma, and endothelium.
3. Wound only one eye per animal and keep the other eye as contralateral control.

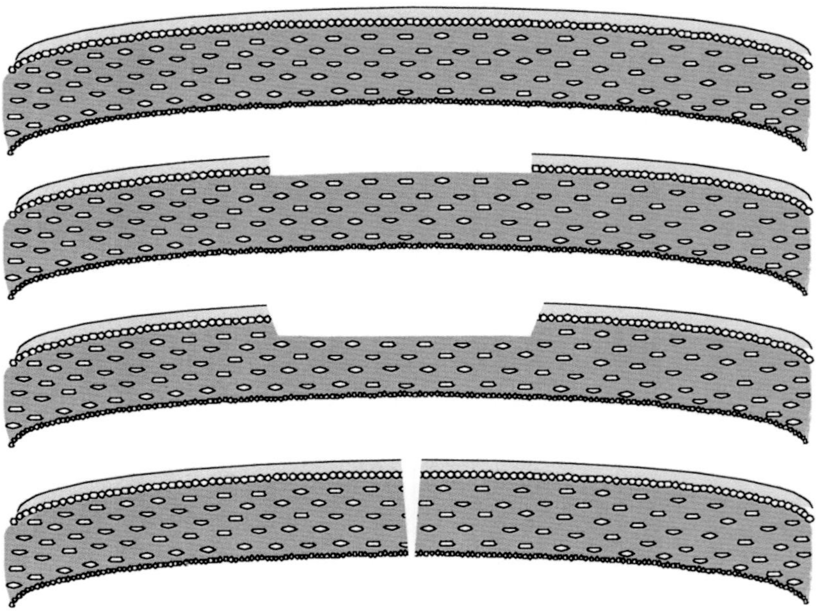

Fig. 1 Corneal wound diagram. (**a**) In the unwounded eye, the cornea is in *light green* and the stroma is in *gray*. (**b**) A debridement wound removes the corneal epithelium and leaves the basement membrane intact. (**c**) A keratectomy wound removes the epithelial layer, the basement membrane, and a thin segment of the anterior stroma. (**d**) A penetrating incision cuts through the entire epithelium, stroma, and endothelium

4. Apply triple antibiotic ointment immediately after wounding.
5. The day following surgery, administer pain relieving medication as described in **step 1**, and apply triple antibiotic ointment as described in **step 4**.
6. Allow the corneas to heal from 4 h to 12 weeks, at which time the animals will be euthanized for postoperative examination (*see* Subheading 3.3) (*see* **Notes 8** and **9**).

3.3 Postoperative Examination

3.3.1 General Considerations

Corneas are typically observed in vivo by slit lamp, in vivo scanning confocal microscope, and/or fluorescent microscopy on days 1, 2, 4, 7, and 14. After day 14, the eyes are typically examined once every other week. The animals are generally not anesthetized for the slit lamp examination if they can be restrained by hand with minimal stress. If this is not possible, or if the slit lamp examination occurs on the same days as other examination, anesthetize the animals as described in Subheading 3.1 (*see* **Note 10**).

3.3.2 Slit Lamp or Fluorescent Microscopy

During these examinations, we typically stain the corneas with fluorescein to highlight any defects in the epithelium.

1. Apply a drop of fluorescein dye to both eyes.
2. After 2 min, rinse the eyes three times with sterile PBS. Blot excess liquid from the inside corner of the eye.

3. Apply a drop of eye lubricant to both eyes to prevent drying of the corneal surface.
4. Examine the eyes by slit lamp and/or fluorescent microscopy for any epithelial defects: Place the animal on a pad or cushion on the microscope stand, and examine the eye under fluorescent light with green filters.
5. Evaluate the rate of epithelial healing by measuring the wound size overtime with image processing software (such as ImageJ).

3.3.3 Scanning In Vivo Confocal Microscope

We typically use HRT to observe morphological changes in the cornea. Mice will be prepared for direct observation under a microscope, without prior eye dissection.

1. Anesthetize the animals and place them on a heated pad as described in Subheading 3.1.
2. Apply a drop of eye lubricant on the tip of the objective lens and another drop on the animal's eye to maintain immersion contact between the objective lens and the eye.
3. Take HRT images of each layer of the cornea for both eyes. This will take 5–10 min per eye.
4. Save all images prior to analysis.

3.4 Tissue Processing for Analysis

Biochemical assays or immunoassays can be performed on ocular tissue as well. These techniques require prior enucleation (i.e., surgical removal of the eyeball). A video-based enucleation protocol was described in detail by Mahajan et al. [3]. Following enucleation, the eye can be prepared for histology of biochemical analysis by several methods:

1. For whole mounts, dissect the corneas, fix them in prechilled methanol/dimethyl sulfoxide (4:1, v/v) for 2 h at −20 °C, and store in methanol at −20 °C until use.
2. For frozen sections, embed the whole globes with the epithelial side down in an optimal cutting temperature (OCT) medium-filled mold. Place the mold on dry ice to allow the OCT with globe to freeze. Make sure that there is OCT on all sides of the globe and no part of the globe is touching the sides of the mold. Store at −80 °C until use.
3. For paraffin sections, fix the eyes in 10% buffered formalin or in 4% paraformaldehyde for 24–48 h, dehydrate, and embed in paraffin block.
4. For transmission electron microscopy, fix the eyes in 1/2 strength Karnovsky's.
5. For Western blot analysis, scrape the epithelium from limbus to limbus immediately after euthanizing the mice. Flash freeze the epithelium in liquid nitrogen, and solubilize protein in lysis buffer. Proceed to standard Western blot analysis.

4 Notes

1. Ketamine and xylazine are regulated substances in many countries. Handle injectable drugs according to the local Drug Enforcement Administration, and store under double lock and key where required. Maintain appropriate use and disposal records at all times.
2. Sterile technique must be used in the preparation and administration of injectable drugs. All needles, syringes, and containers used to deliver or store drugs must be sterile. The use of nonsterile equipment can result in animal infections and/or illness.
3. Isoflurane (2–4%) inhalation can also be used, unless otherwise specified.
4. Meloxicam is a nonsteroidal anti-inflammatory drug with analgesic and fever reducer effects.
5. The amount of drug administered to each animal is based on its body weight. Each animal needs to be weighed on the day of anesthesia. Mice and rats, especially young, growing animals, can change weight rapidly. A body weight recorded last week may not be accurate today.
6. Atropine is used to dilate the iris. We have found that, in some of our wound-healing studies, the iris adheres to the endothelium during the wound-healing process.
7. Ensure you leave an intact basement membrane. This will appear as a smooth shiny surface. If basement membrane is removed or damaged, a rough dull surface will be observed.
8. Methods for mice euthanasia should be chosen in accordance to local regulations and should be consistent with recommendations of local authorities. All protocols should be approved prior to the experiment.
9. Animals should always be examined to ensure that death has occurred.
10. We do not recommend using isoflurane due to the length of time that the animals will need to be restrained for HRT and/or the fluorescent microscope exam (~5–10 min).

References

1. Friedlander M (2007) Fibrosis and diseases of the eye. J Clin Invest 117(3):576–586. doi:10.1172/JCI31030
2. Dawson DG (2010) Corneal scars A2 - Dartt, Darlene A. In: Encyclopedia of the eye. Academic Press, Oxford, pp 499–514. doi:10.1016/B978-0-12-374203-2.00073-7
3. Mahajan VB, Skeie JM, Assefnia AH et al (2011) Mouse eye enucleation for remote high-throughput phenotyping. J Vis Exp 57. doi:10.3791/3184

Chapter 9

Modeling Cardiac Fibrosis in Mice: (Myo)Fibroblast Phenotype After Ischemia

Daniela Fraccarollo, Paolo Galuppo, and Johann Bauersachs

Abstract

Cardiac (myo)fibroblasts play a key role in the regulation of wound healing and pathogenic remodeling after myocardial infarction. Impaired scar formation and alterations of the extracellular matrix network precipitate cardiac dysfunction leading to increased morbidity and mortality. Therapeutic approaches addressing (myo)fibroblast phenotype appear to be useful in preventing progressive structural, electrical, and functional impairment and heart failure.

Permanent ligation of the left anterior descending coronary artery has proven to be a valuable experimental model to investigate the arrays of pathways/mechanisms involved in cardiac repair and extracellular matrix remodeling in ischemic heart failure. Here we describe the surgical procedure to occlude the left coronary artery in mice. Moreover, we present an accurate method to isolate (myo)fibroblasts from ischemic myocardium, with maintenance of the functional phenotype, using the specific marker for mouse cardiac fibroblasts mEF-SK4. The protocol can be completed within a few hours, and the isolated fibroblasts/myofibroblasts are suitable for downstream molecular biology applications, like gene expression profiling and cell culture.

Key words Myocardial infarction, Fibrosis, Cardiac fibroblasts, mEF-SK4, Fluorescence-activated cell sorting

1 Introduction

Ischemic cell death and the consequent loss of contractile myocardium trigger a cascade of cellular activities that promote infarct wound healing and dynamic time-dependent structural changes of the infarcted region and the residual viable myocardium [1]. The pivotal role of (myo)fibroblasts as regulators and effectors of infarct wound healing and fibrotic remodeling has been recognized, indicating a potential therapeutic target for preventing progressive functional deterioration and heart failure [1, 2].

Cardiac fibroblasts, as a heterogeneous population of mechanosensitive/sentinel cells, modulate several biochemical/biophysical interactions among immune cells, cardiomyocytes, and vascular and endothelial cells, under the coordination of matricellular

Laure Rittié (ed.), *Fibrosis: Methods and Protocols*, Methods in Molecular Biology, vol. 1627,
DOI 10.1007/978-1-4939-7113-8_9,

macromolecules, growth factor, and cytokine-mediated pathways [3, 4]. After ischemic injury, cardiac fibroblasts sense the loss of extracellular matrix structural integrity as well as microenvironmental signals and phenotypically differentiate into myofibroblasts, which secrete large quantities of extracellular matrix molecules [5–7]. Formation of a well-organized scar tissue (reparative fibrosis) is a crucial stage of infarct repair. Weak and poorly structured collagen matrix renders the scar less resistant to distension during overload, leading to infarct thinning and adverse chamber dilation. In contrast, excessive myofibroblast differentiation, particularly in the remote non-infarcted myocardium, results in deposition of extracellular matrix proteins (reactive fibrosis) and significant increase in myocardial stiffness, leading to relaxation abnormalities, arrhythmogenicity, and ultimately progressive cardiac hypertrophy and systolic dysfunction [1, 8–10].

Ligation of the left anterior descending coronary artery permanently (myocardial infarction) or temporarily (ischemia/reperfusion) is the standard surgical technique to induce myocardial ischemic injury in rodents in preclinical research [11]. Especially, application of this experimental model to genetically modified mice allowed identifying gene targets and pathways involved in the remodeling processes and concomitantly to explore potential therapeutic strategies. Given the variable anatomy of the mouse left coronary artery, permanent ligation generates infarcts of variable size and a broad spectrum of cardiac dysfunction, ranging from minor impairment to overt heart failure, in relation to the technique and the exact location [11, 12]. Targeted ligation of the left anterior descending artery just below the left auricular level ensures reproducible and large infarcts (more than 40% of the left ventricular myocardium). The non-reperfused myocardial infarction model is particularly useful to investigate cellular/molecular mechanisms regulating cardiac infarct scar formation as well as to explore the pathophysiology of chronic heart failure and fibrotic remodeling. In contrast, the ischemia/reperfusion model is more clinically relevant to mimic the pathological course of acute myocardial infarction in patients undergoing coronary intervention and is particularly suitable to study reperfusion injury and the early inflammatory response to ischemia. Other methods to generate myocardial ischemic injury include cryocoagulation of the free left ventricular wall with a cryoprobe. Similar to the model of reperfused infarction, cryoinjury produces infarcts of smaller size and no overt heart failure and fibrotic remodeling. The cryoinfarction model is suitable for cell engraftment studies [11–13].

Here we describe the surgical procedure to occlude the left coronary artery in mice (Subheading 3.1). Moreover, a protocol for efficient isolation of cardiac fibroblasts/myofibroblasts, with preservation of the functional phenotype, is also provided (Subheading 3.2).

Several methods have been described for the isolation of mouse cardiac fibroblasts. Standard procedure involves steps of mincing, repetitive enzymatic digestion, plating of cardiac cell suspension in tissue culture dishes, washing away of nonadherent cells, culturing in DMEM supplemented with fetal bovine serum, and finally, passaging using Accutase or trypsin. However, adult cardiac fibroblasts cultured on rigid plastic surfaces and/or in serum-containing media undergo phenotypic and functional changes, which is an often overlooked or perhaps deliberately disregarded feature [14–16].

Current knowledge regarding (myo)fibroblasts biology were hampered by the lack of specific and reliable cardiac fibroblast markers [3, 17, 18]. Markers such as vimentin, CD90, and DDR2 are not specific for fibroblasts. In an elegant study, Pinto et al. [18] recently showed that the antibody mEF-SK4 labeled cardiac fibroblasts with high sensitivity and specificity.

Here, we present a fluorescence-activated cell-sorting strategy to isolate cardiac fibroblasts/myofibroblasts, using the mEF-SK4 antibody. Our approach allows to preserve cell surface antigens along with cell viability, permitting to obtain highly purified fibroblasts from the normal and ischemic mouse myocardium, with maintenance of the phenotype. The protocol can be completed within a few hours, and the isolated fibroblasts are suitable for downstream molecular biology applications, like gene expression profiling and cell culture.

2 Materials

2.1 Coronary Artery Ligation

1. Glass bead sterilizer or autoclave.
2. Surgical instruments (Fig. 1A).
3. Surgical tape.
4. Rubber band.
5. Intubation tube (22G intravenous catheter, 22 mm long) fitted with a 22G blunt needle as support (Fig. 1C).
6. Animal clipper.
7. Dental mirror.
8. Anesthesia equipment (Fig. 1B, a–d).
9. Mouse ventilator (Fig. 1B, e).
10. 5% (v/v) isoflurane.
11. Buprenorphine.
12. Surgical heating plate.
13. *Light source* (bright enough to allow transillumination of the larynx).
14. 70% (v/v) ethanol in water.

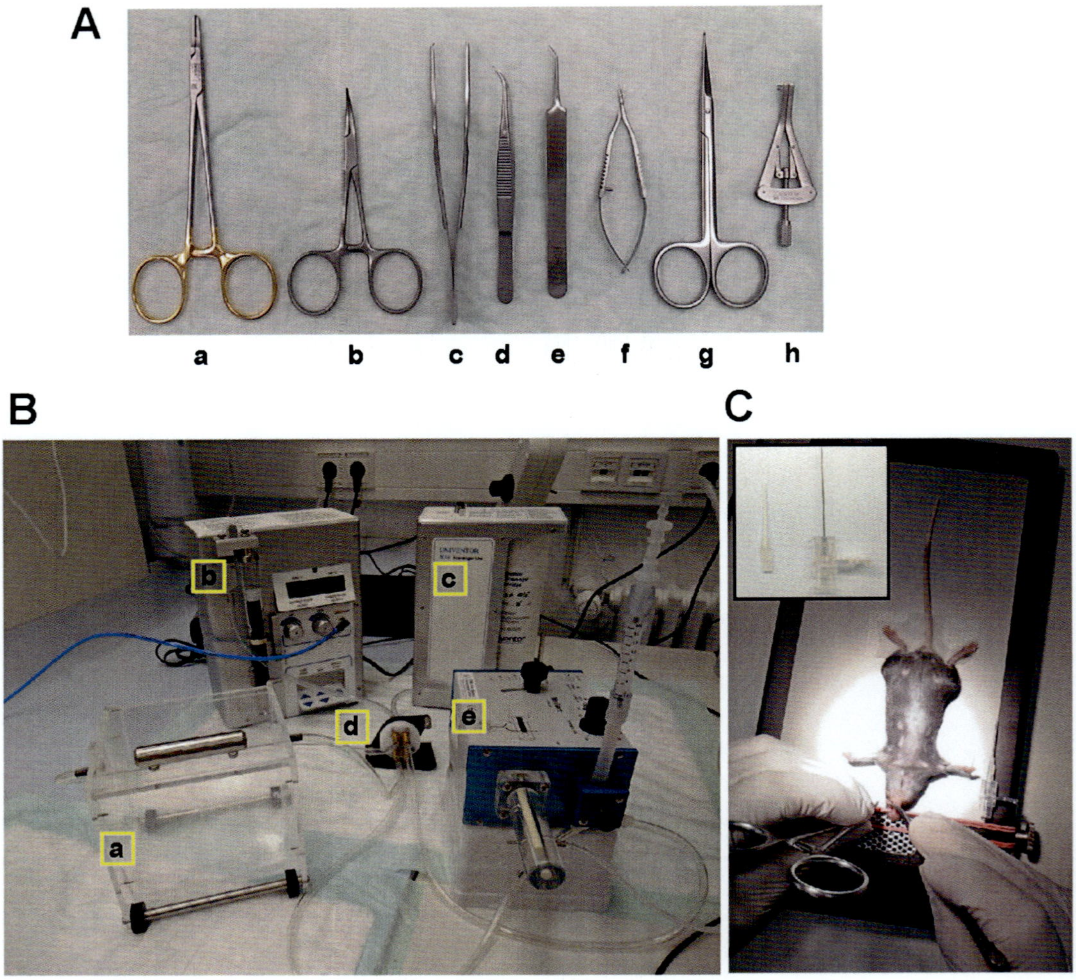

Fig. 1 Surgical instruments and settings. (**A**) Surgical instruments: **a**, Durogrip needle holder; **b**, artery forceps; **c**, appling forceps; **d**, splinter forceps; **e**, micro forceps; **f**, eye scissors; **g**, vessel scissors; **h**, self-retaining retractor. (**B**) anesthesia/ventilation equipment: **a**, induction chamber; **b**, anesthesia unit; **c**, scavenger unit; **d**, gas scavenger routing switch; **e**, ventilator. (**C**) orotracheal intubation; inset: intubation tube, 22G blunt needle

15. Silk suture 5-0, FS-2 needle, 45 cm black.
16. Silk suture 6-0, FS-33 needle, 45 cm black.
17. Surgical clips.
18. Sterile gauze sponges.
19. Sterile cotton sticks.
20. Animal weighing balance.

2.2 Isolation of Adult Mouse Cardiac Fibroblasts/Myofibroblasts

1. Bottle-top sterile filter units, pore size 0.2 μm.
2. 15 ml and 50 ml conical tubes.
3. 100 μm cell strainer.

4. 60 mm and 100 mm petri dishes.
5. 5 ml and 10 ml serological pipettes.
6. Heat-inactivated fetal bovine serum (HI-FCS).
7. Phosphate-buffered saline (PBS).
8. Water for injection.
9. Perfusion buffer (*see* **Note 1**): 113 mM sodium chloride (NaCl), 4.7 mM potassium chloride (KCl), 0.6 mM potassium phosphate monobasic (KH_2PO_4), 0.6 mM sodium phosphate dibasic (Na_2HPO_4), 1.2 mM magnesium sulfate heptahydrate ($MgSO_4{\bullet}7H_2O$), 12 mM sodium bicarbonate ($NaHCO_3$), 10 mM potassium bicarbonate ($KHCO_3$), 10 mM HEPES, 30 mM taurine, 5.5 mM glucose, 10 mM 2,3-butanedione monoxime, pH = 7.46.
10. Prepare the solution on the day of isolation (~50 ml per heart) with ultrapure water, sterilize by filtering with a 0.2 μm filter, and keep refrigerated until use.
11. Digestion buffer: 0.20 mg/ml Liberase (we use Liberase from Roche Diagnostics) and 400 μM calcium chloride in perfusion buffer. Prepare the solution on the day of isolation (~25 ml per heart) with ultrapure water, sterilize by filtering with a 0.2 μm filter, and keep refrigerated until use.
12. Stop buffer: perfusion buffer supplemented with 10% (v/v) HI-FCS.
13. Low waste syringe (we use 1 ml Injekt®-F from B. Brown).
14. Aortic cannula OD 1.0 mm.

2.3 Fluorescence-Activated Cell Sorting

1. 70 μm cell strainer.
2. 5 ml polypropylene round-bottom tubes.
3. FACS buffer: PBS, pH 7.2, supplemented with 0.5% (m/v) bovine serum albumin and 2 mM EDTA. Filter through a 0.22 μm filter and store at 4 °C.
4. Polystyrene microparticles for fluorescence compensation (we use the BD™ CompBeads Compensation Particles Anti-Rat Ig, κ Set from BD Biosciences).
5. Fc Block (we use Mouse BD Fc Block™ from BD Biosciences).
6. Fluorochrome-conjugated antibodies (we use the ones summarized in Table 1).
7. Sorting medium: Dulbecco's Modified Eagle Medium (DMEM), supplemented with 5% (v/v) HI-FCS.
8. Flow cytometer/cell sorter (*see* **Note 2**).

Table 1
Antibodies used for fluorescence-activated cell sorting

Antibody	Fluorochrome	Clone	Concentration	Supplier
anti-CD31	Alexa Fluor® 488	390	5 μg/ml	BioLegend
anti-TER-119	FITC	TER-119	5 μg/ml	BioLegend
anti-CD45	PerCP/Cy5.5	104	2 μg/ml	BioLegend
anti-CD11b	eVolve 605	M1/70	dil. 1:40	eBioscience
anti-NG2	PE	1E6.4	5 μg/ml	Miltenyi Biotec
anti-PDGFRβ	PE	APB5	2 μg/ml	BioLegend
anti-mEF-SK4	APC	mEF-SK4	2.5 μg/ml	Miltenyi Biotec

3 Methods

3.1 Coronary Artery Ligation

1. Sterilize surgical instruments (Fig. 1A) using a glass bead sterilizer (10–15 s) or autoclave at 121 °C (15 min).
2. Anesthetize mouse (*see* **Note 3**) with a mixture of isoflurane (5%) and oxygen, using an induction chamber (Fig. 1B, a).
3. Weigh the animal.
4. Place the anesthetized mouse on his back to a surgical heating plate at 37 °C and tape forelimbs and hind limbs (Fig. 1C).
5. Proceed with orotracheal intubation: illuminate the tracheal area with strong external light source that penetrates the skin for transillumination of the larynx, hold the upper jaw in place using a surgical thread or thin rubber band placed horizontally under the top teeth, lift laterally the tongue with splinter forceps, and insert the intubation tube (Fig. 1C). Remove the blunt needle; confirm successful endotracheal placement by observing condensation on a dental mirror held in close proximity of the tracheal tube.
6. Connect the intubation tube to the ventilator and the anesthesia unit; fix the tubing connection with a tape. Maintain anesthesia with a constant mixture of isoflurane (1.5–2%) and oxygen (ventilation rate 120 breaths/min). The tidal volume is adjusted based on the body weight (BW) (10 μl/g BW).
7. Check anesthesia: the mouse should be unresponsive to tail and/or toe pinch.
8. Administer buprenorphine (0.1 mg/kg BW) intraperitoneally for postoperative pain relief.
9. Slightly shave the chest and disinfect the skin using 70% ethanol.

10. Pull the skin up, away from the chest using splinter forceps and make a 0.5–1.0 cm incision along the midaxillary line using sterile scissors. Widen with the artery forceps.
11. Dissect and retract precordial muscle and make a small hole (~3 mm) between the third and fourth rib using the eye scissors.
12. Widen the intercostal space with the self-retaining retractor (Fig. 2A). Care has to be taken to avoid contact with the lungs during the surgery.
13. Pull the pericardium away from the heart and tear it open using splinter forceps. This procedure provides a good visualization and easier access to the left anterior descending the coronary artery.
14. Perform a ligature of the left anterior descending coronary artery: Using the Durogrip needle holder, place a 6-0 silk suture beneath the artery along the log axis of the heart and perpendicular to it, just below the left auricular level (Fig. 2B). Tie the ends of the suture with a double knot, using micro forceps in order to achieve a successful occlusion (Fig. 2C) (*see* **Note 4**).
15. Remove the retractor and close the thoracic cavity with 1–2 mattress sutures using a 5-0 silk suture.
16. Close the skin with two to three surgical clips.
17. Turn off isoflurane and administer 100% oxygen until recovery.
18. Extubate as soon as the mouse begins to breathe autonomously.
19. Remove the mouse from the isothermal plate and place the mouse in a cage on a warming pad. Mice resume their normal patterns of mobility within 1 h after recovering from the anesthesia. Perioperative death is less than 10%.

3.2 Isolation of Adult Mouse Cardiac Fibroblasts/Myofibroblasts

1. Prepare perfusion buffer (~50 ml per heart) and digestion buffer (~25 ml per heart) as described in Subheading 2.2, **items 9** and **10**.
2. Prepare the perfusion system (*see* **Note 5**):
   (a) *Set flow rate of the perfusion pump to 3 ml/min and adjust the temperature of circulating water so the outflow from the tip of the cannula is 37 °C* (Fig. 3A).
   (b) *Run 30 ml of water for injection through the perfusion system to eliminate air bubbles. Prime the perfusion system with perfusion buffer* (Fig. 3A, a) *and with digestion buffer* (Fig. 3A, b).
   (c) *Allow the system to reach the working temperature of 37 °C.*

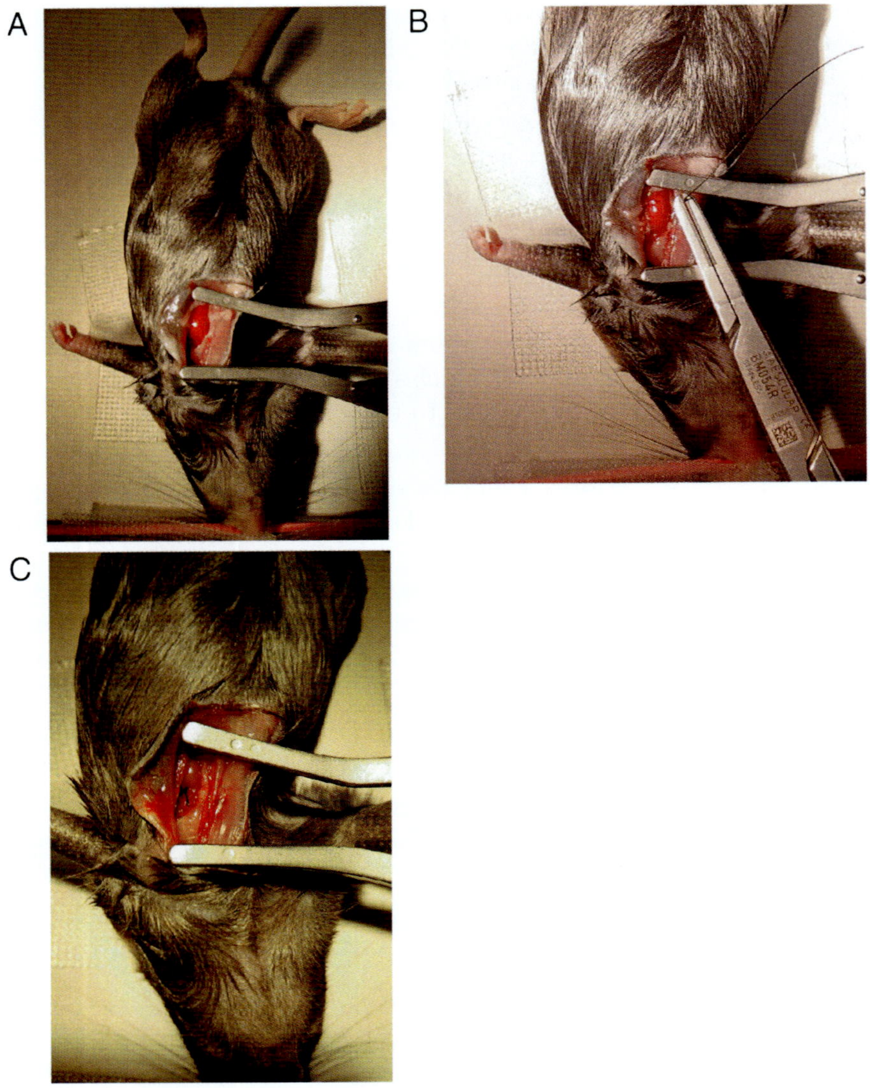

Fig. 2 Coronary artery ligation. (**a**) Chest opening. (**b**) Ligation of the left anterior descending the coronary artery just below the left auricular level. (**c**) A double knot is made to occlude the coronary artery permanently

3. Attach the aortic cannula to a perfusion buffer-filled syringe, with the tip close to the surface of a 60 mm petri dish, and prepare a loose knot with a piece of silk thread (~10 cm), necessary to secure the aorta to the cannula (Fig. 3B).

4. As for coronary artery ligation (Subheading 3.1, **steps 2–5**), anesthetize the mouse with a mixture of isoflurane (5%) and oxygen, transfer the unconscious mouse to the surgical isothermal plate, tape the mouse's limbs, perform orotracheal intubation, and connect the intubation tube to the ventilator and anesthesia unit adjusted to deliver an isoflurane (1.5–2%) and oxygen mix.

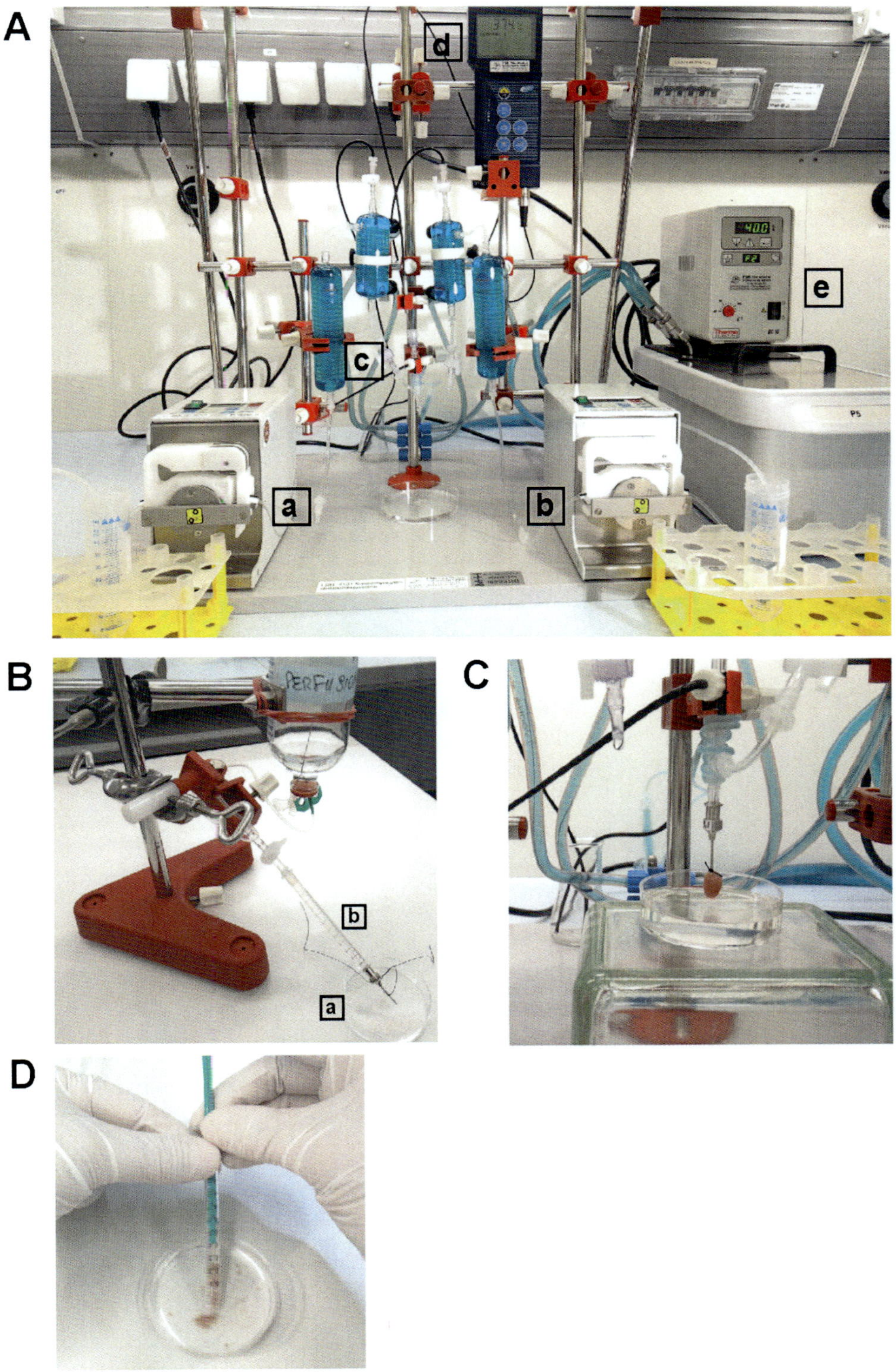

Fig. 3 Heart perfusion system. (**A**) Modified Langendorff unit for perfusion of mouse heart: (*a*) peristaltic pump for perfusion buffer; (*b*) peristaltic pump for digestion buffer; (*c*) water-jacked heat exchange coil; (*d*) digital thermometer; (*e*) circulating water bath. (**B**) System for cannulation: (*a*) aortic cannula; (*b*) syringe filled with perfusion buffer. (**C**) Perfusion of the heart. (**D**) Gentle pipetting with a sterile low waste syringe in order to obtain a cell suspension

5. Check with a toe pinch to ensure that the mouse is fully anesthetized.
6. Wipe the chest with 70% ethanol.
7. Cut open the chest cavity and carefully expose the heart (as described in Subheading 3.1, **steps 9–11**).
8. Cut the aorta, letting enough stem length for correct cannulation (i.e., 2–3 mm).
9. Discard foreign tissue and immediately transfer the excised beating heart to a 60 mm petri dish containing perfusion buffer.
10. Move the heart to the system for cannulation (Fig. 3B). Cannulate the aorta using fine forceps and a dissecting microscope and secure the aorta on the cannula with the silk suture (*see* **Note 6**). To ensure reproducibility, aortic cannulation should not exceed 2 min.
11. Connect the aortic cannula to the perfusion system (Fig. 3C) and start immediately to perfuse the heart (*see* **Note 7**).
12. Perfuse the heart with perfusion buffer for 5 min (3 ml/min) in order to flush blood from the vasculatures and left ventricle.
13. Switch to digestion buffer and perfuse for 8 min (3 ml/min). A swollen and slightly pale ventricle is indicative of a good perfusion during the enzyme digestion (Fig. 3C).
14. Collect the last 5 ml of the digestion buffer running through the heart in a 60 mm petri dish and transfer the heart in this solution afterwards.
15. Separate atria, right ventricle, and subsequently ischemic area und surviving myocardium, using a dissecting microscope.
16. Pipette smoothly the heart tissue several times through a sterile low waste syringe (Fig. 3D) in order to obtain a cell suspension.
17. Add 5 ml of stop buffer to inhibit enzyme activity and disperse again the cells by further gentle pipetting with a sterile low waste syringe (Fig. 3D).
18. Carefully filter the cell suspension through a 100 μm cell strainer in a 50 ml conical tube.
19. Wash the cell strainer with 30 ml of perfusion buffer.
20. Centrifuge the content of the tube at 10 *g*, 4 min at 4 °C.
21. Collect the supernatant in a fresh 50 ml tube (discard the pellet) and centrifuge the supernatant at 400 *g*, 20 min at 4 °C.
22. Discard all of the supernatant and gently resuspend the cells in 1 ml FACS buffer.

23. Once cells are in homogeneous suspension, add FACS buffer to a final volume of 40 ml.
24. Centrifuge at 400 *g*, 20 min at 4 °C.
25. Discard supernatant and resuspend cells in 15 ml FACS buffer.
26. Perform a cell count and viability analysis.
27. Centrifuge cells before FACS at 400 *g*, 20 min at 4 °C.

3.3 Fluorescence-Activated Cell Sorting

1. Resuspend cells in FACS buffer and filter through a 70 μm cell strainer in a 5 ml polypropylene tube on ice (*see* **Note 8**).
2. Prepare an unstained sample as autofluorescence control: add 50 μl of cell suspension to a flow cytometer tube and add FACS buffer to a final volume of 400 μl.
3. Prepare fluorescence-minus-one controls, i.e., a cell sample containing all but one of the fluorochrome-conjugated antibodies, for every fluorochrome being used (*see* **Note 9**).
4. Preincubate the cells with Fc Block for 10 min.
5. Add fluorochrome-conjugated antibodies at concentrations indicated in Table 1. Mix well and incubate for 30 min on ice.
6. Wash cells by adding 4 ml of ice cold FACS buffer and centrifuge at 400 *g*, 10 min at 4 °C.
7. Discard all of the supernatant and gently resuspend the cells in 1 ml FACS buffer.
8. Once cells are in a homogeneous suspension, add FACS buffer to a final volume of 5 ml.
9. Centrifuge at 400 *g*, 10 min at 4 °C.
10. Resuspend the cells in FACS buffer and perform a live/dead staining (*see* **Note 10**).
11. Filter the suspensions through a 70 μm cell strainer and perform fluorescence-activated cell sorting (Figs. 4 and 5) (*see* **Note 11**).

4 Notes

1. From *A*lliance *f*or Cellular *S*ignaling (AfCS, Solution Protocol PS00000452 [19]).
2. FACS data were acquired on a Gallios™ flow cytometer and analyzed with Gallios™ software (Beckman Coulter). Cell sorting was performed using a FACSAria Fusion cell sorter (BD Biosciences), at the **Research Facility Cell Sorting of the Hannover Medical School**.
3. C57BL/6 mice aged 8–12 weeks.

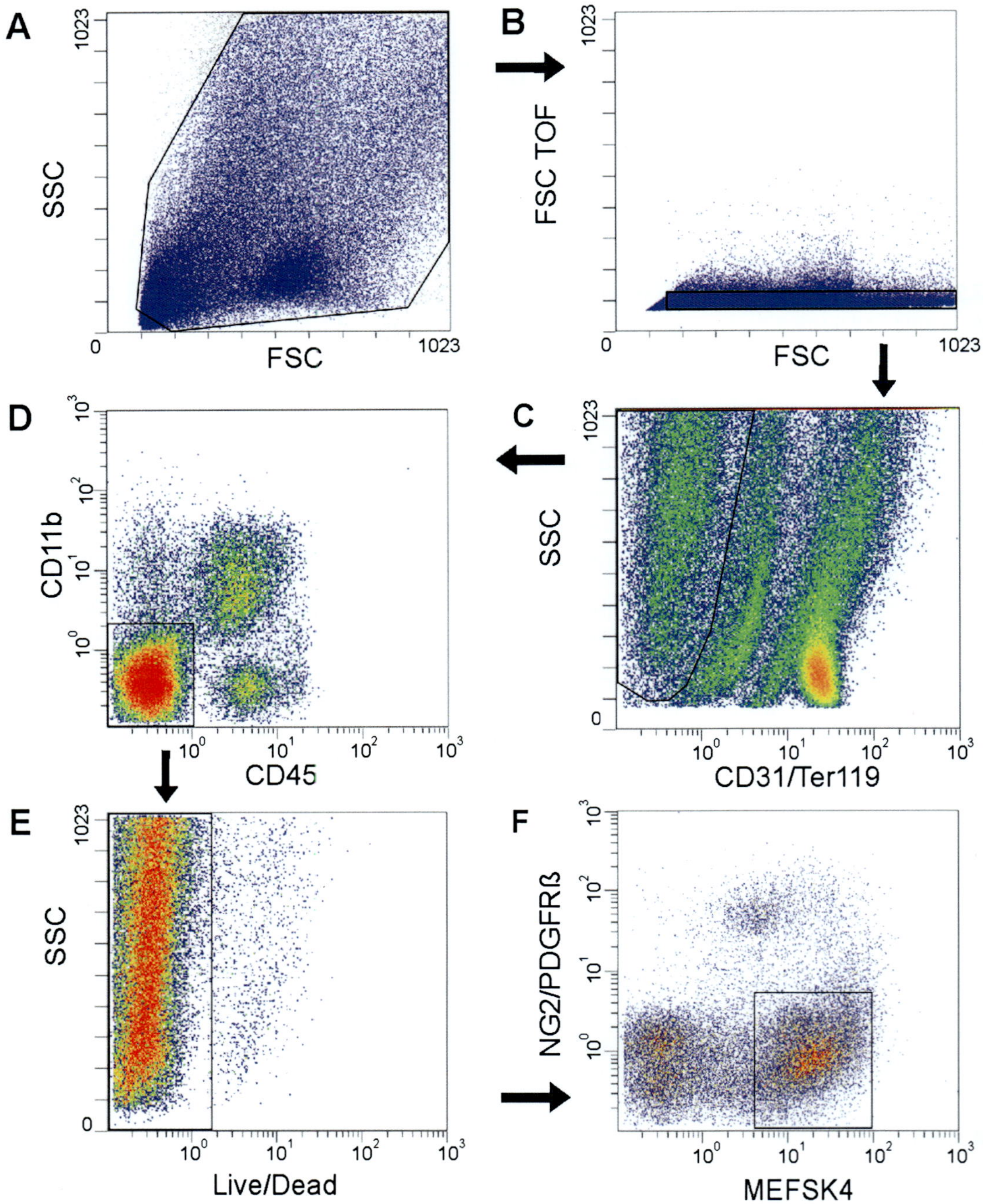

Fig. 4 Gating strategy for fluorescence-activated cell sorting. (**A**) In the forward scatter (FSC) versus side scatter (SSC) dot plot, draw a polygonal region to exclude debris. (**B**) Perform doublet discrimination by gating single cells in the FSC versus FSC-time-of-flight (ToF) dot plot as indicated. (**C**, **D**) Exclude endothelial and hematopoietic cells by selecting cells that are CD31⁻/TER-119⁻ and CD45⁻/CD11b⁻. (**E**) Live/Dead Violet was used to discriminate between live and dead cells. (**F**) Select the mEF-SK4⁺/NG2⁻/PDGFRβ⁻ population for sorting. Cells were isolated from ischemic myocardium 7 days after coronary artery ligation. FACS data were acquired on a Gallios™ flow cytometer

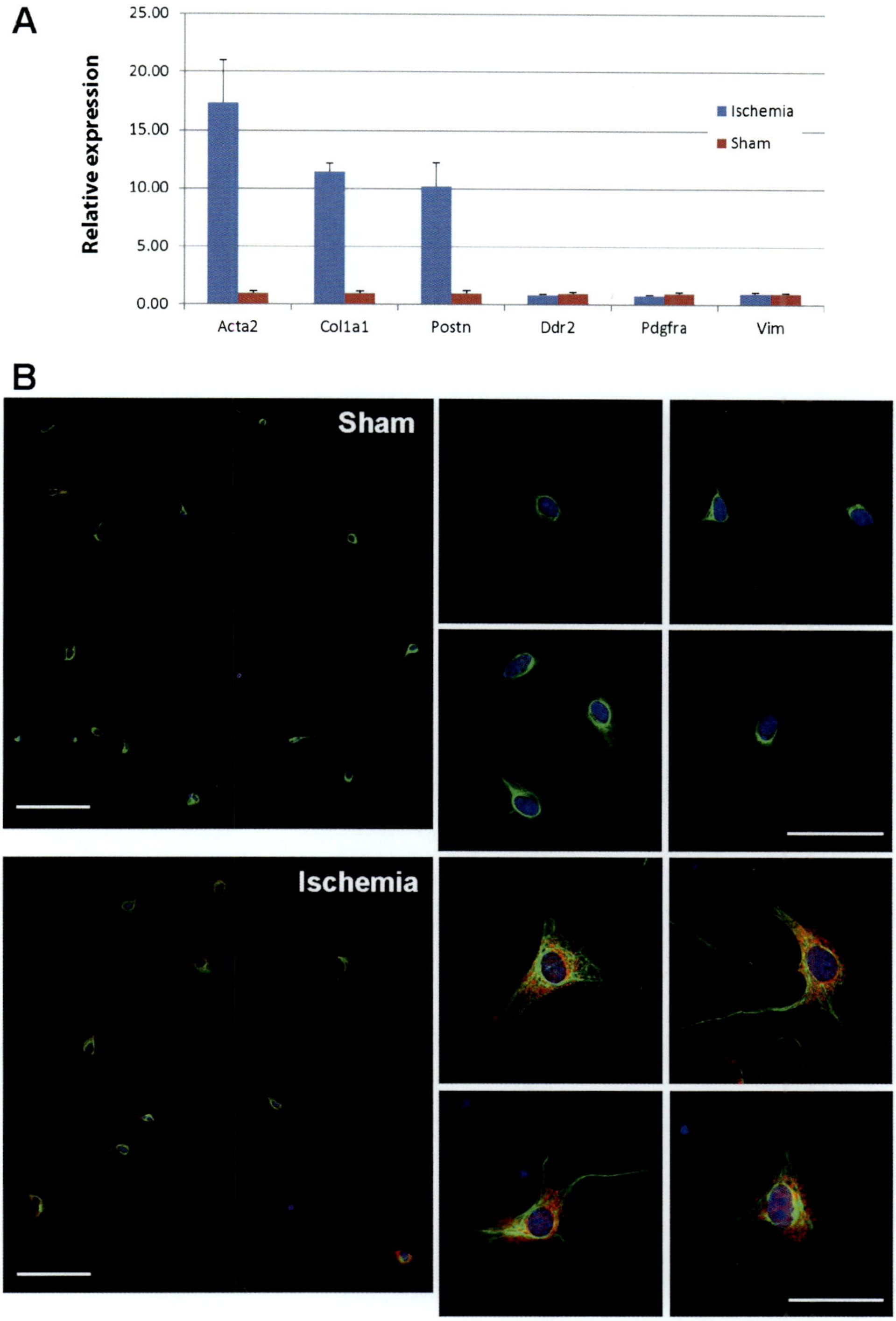

Fig. 5 Characterization of sorted fibroblasts/myofibroblasts. $CD31^-$/$TER\text{-}119^-$/$CD45^-$/$CD11b^-$/$NG2^-$/$PDGFR\beta^-$ and $mEF\text{-}SK4^+$ cells were isolated from sham-operated left ventricular myocardium or from ischemic myocardium 4 days after coronary artery ligation. (**A**) RT-PCR was employed to detect the relative gene expression of smooth muscle α-actin (Acta2), collagen I α1 (Col1a1), periostin (Postn), discoidin domain-containing receptor 2 (Ddr2), platelet-derived growth factor receptor α (Pdgfra) and vimentin (Vim); Data analysis was performed using the delta-delta Ct method with efficiency correction and GAPDH as reference. Sorted cells were directly collected in lysis buffer, and total RNA was immediately isolated using PrepEase RNA Spin Kit (PN78766, USB). (**B**) Immunocytochemical staining showing vimentin (*green*) and smooth muscle α-actin (*red*). Sorted cells were cultured in a sorting medium for 12 h. *Scale bar*: *left*, 100 μm, *right*, 50 μm

4. In sham-operated mice, the suture passing around the left anterior descending coronary artery was not tied.
5. This procedure is derived from AfCS Procedure Protocol PS00000125 [19].
6. To ensure reproducibility, aortic cannulation should not exceed 2 min.
7. Ensure the temperature is maintained at 37 °C during perfusion/digestion.
8. To prevent capping of antibodies on the cell surface and nonspecific cell labeling, perform all steps on ice and protected from light. Work fast and use precooled solutions. Cell concentration should be 1×10^6 to 1×10^7 cells per ml.
9. Fluorescence minus one (FMO) controls should be included during acquisition for gating analyses to distinguish positively from negatively staining cell populations.
10. We use Live/Dead® Fixable Violet Stain Kit from Thermo Fisher Scientific.
11. Cells are sorted in a sterile sorting medium or lysis buffer (PrepEase RNA Spin Kit, Affymetrix).

References

1. Fraccarollo D, Galuppo P, Bauersachs J (2012) Novel therapeutic approaches to post-infarction remodelling. Cardiovasc Res 94(2):293–303. doi:10.1093/cvr/cvs109
2. Prabhu SD, Frangogiannis NG (2016) The biological basis for cardiac repair after myocardial infarction: from inflammation to fibrosis. Circ Res 119(1):91–112. doi:10.1161/CIRCRESAHA.116.303577
3. Travers JG, Kamal FA, Robbins J et al (2016) Cardiac fibrosis: the fibroblast awakens. Circ Res 118(6):1021–1040. doi:10.1161/CIRCRESAHA.115.306565
4. Howard CM, Baudino TA (2014) Dynamic cell-cell and cell-ECM interactions in the heart. J Mol Cell Cardiol 70:19–26. doi:10.1016/j.yjmcc.2013.10.006
5. Ma Y, de Castro Bras LE, Toba H et al (2014) Myofibroblasts and the extracellular matrix network in post-myocardial infarction cardiac remodeling. Pflugers Arch 466(6):1113–1127. doi:10.1007/s00424-014-1463-9
6. Turner NA, Porter KE (2013) Function and fate of myofibroblasts after myocardial infarction. Fibrogenesis Tissue Repair 6(1):5. doi:10.1186/1755-1536-6-5
7. Tillmanns J, Hoffmann D, Habbaba Y et al (2015) Fibroblast activation protein alpha expression identifies activated fibroblasts after myocardial infarction. J Mol Cell Cardiol 87: 194–203. doi:10.1016/j.yjmcc.2015.08.016
8. Burchfield JS, Xie M, Hill JA (2013) Pathological ventricular remodeling: mechanisms: part 1 of 2. Circulation 128(4): 388–400. doi:10.1161/CIRCULATIONAHA.113.001878
9. Fraccarollo D, Berger S, Galuppo P et al (2011) Deletion of cardiomyocyte mineralocorticoid receptor ameliorates adverse remodeling after myocardial infarction. Circulation 123(4): 400–408. doi:10.1161/CIRCULATIONAHA.110.983023
10. Fraccarollo D, Galuppo P, Motschenbacher S et al (2014) Soluble guanylyl cyclase activation improves progressive cardiac remodeling and failure after myocardial infarction. Cardioprotection over ACE inhibition. Basic Res Cardiol 109(4): 421. doi:10.1007/s00395-014-0421-1
11. Patten RD, Hall-Porter MR (2009) Small animal models of heart failure: development of novel therapies, past and present. Circ Heart Fail 2(2):138–144. doi:10.1161/CIRCHEARTFAILURE.108.839761
12. Houser SR, Margulies KB, Murphy AM et al (2012) Animal models of heart failure: a scientific statement from the American Heart Association. Circ Res 111(1):131–150. doi:10.1161/RES.0b013e3182582523

13. Lara-Pezzi E, Menasche P, Trouvin JH et al (2015) Guidelines for translational research in heart failure. J Cardiovasc Transl Res 8(1):3–22. doi:10.1007/s12265-015-9606-8
14. Yong KW, Li Y, Huang G et al (2015) Mechanoregulation of cardiac myofibroblast differentiation: implications for cardiac fibrosis and therapy. Am J Physiol Heart Circ Physiol 309(4):H532–H542. doi:10.1152/ajpheart.00299.2015
15. van Putten S, Shafieyan Y, Hinz B (2016) Mechanical control of cardiac myofibroblasts. J Mol Cell Cardiol 93:133–142. doi:10.1016/j.yjmcc.2015.11.025
16. Rohr S (2011) Cardiac fibroblasts in cell culture systems: myofibroblasts all along? J Cardiovasc Pharmacol 57(4):389–399. doi:10.1097/FJC.0b013e3182137e17
17. Zhou P, WT P (2016) Recounting cardiac cellular composition. Circ Res 118(3):368–370. doi:10.1161/CIRCRESAHA.116.308139
18. Pinto AR, Ilinykh A, Ivey MJ et al (2016) Revisiting cardiac cellular composition. Circ Res 118(3):400–409. doi:10.1161/CIRCRESAHA.115.307778
19. O'Connell TD, Rodrigo MC, Simpson PC (2007) Isolation and culture of adult mouse cardiac myocytes. Methods Mol Biol 357:271–296. doi:10.1385/1-59745-214-9:271

Chapter 10

Characterization of Mesenchymal-Fibroblast Cells Using the *Col1a2* Promoter/Enhancer

Ian M.H. Li, Amy L. Horwell, Grace Chu, Benoit de Crombrugghe, and George Bou-Gharios

Abstract

Excessive deposition of extracellular matrix (ECM) is a common hallmark of fibrotic diseases in various organs. Chiefly among this ECM are collagen types I and III, secreted by local fibroblasts, and other mesenchymal cells recruited for repair purposes. In the last two decades, the search for a fibroblast-specific promoter/enhancer has intensified in order to control the regulation of ECM in these cells and limit the scarring of the fibrotic process In our previous work, we characterized an enhancer region 17 kb upstream of the *Col1a2* gene transcription start site. This enhancer in transgenic mice is expressed mainly in mesenchymal cells during development and in adults upon injury. When driving transgenes such as beta-galactosidase or luciferase, this construct acts as an informative reporter of collagen transcription and is predictive of collagen type I deposition. In this chapter, we provide detailed protocols for identifying similar enhancers and using the sequence to generate a construct for transfection and producing transgenic animals. We also provided information on the use of luminescence in transgenic mice, tissue processing, as well as using cre/lox system to obtain conditional gain and loss of function in mice.

Key words Collagen type I, Mesenchymal cells, Transfection, Enhancer, Transgenic mice, Transgene

1 Introduction

The origin of scar-producing cell(s) in tissues appears to be different depending on the tissue involved and the experimental injury model. In general, myofibroblasts are thought to be the cell type that generates and deposits collagen I- and collagen III-rich pathological extracellular matrix (ECM), leading to irreversible fibrosis and causing organ dysfunction [1]. Antibodies against the intermediate filament alpha-smooth muscle actin (α-SMA) have been widely used as a marker for collagen-producing myofibroblasts, and other less widely accepted markers such as the transcription factor S100A4 or fibroblast-specific protein (FSP) as it was termed, specifically in the kidney [2] and vimentin [3], have been reported to label myofibroblasts. However, none of these

Laure Rittié (ed.), *Fibrosis: Methods and Protocols*, Methods in Molecular Biology, vol. 1627,
DOI 10.1007/978-1-4939-7113-8_10

markers are unique to fibroblasts or myofibroblasts as they are expressed on many other cell types [4]. Furthermore, α-SMA is not necessary for myofibroblast formation and function and for wound closure as other filaments such as γ-actin and skeletal muscle α-actin may be able to functionally compensate for the lack of α-SMA in myofibroblasts [5].

One unique characteristic of fibroblasts is that they synthesize and secrete a number of ECM molecules including collagen type I, a fibril-forming collagen. Collagen type I is a heterotrimer formed from two α1-chains and one α2-chain. These chains are synthesized as precursor molecules termed pro-α1(I) and pro-α2(I). The genetic sequences coding for these precursors have been found to be located on separate chromosomes for a number of species. Our approach was to look for a fibroblast-specific element within the collagen type I gene regulatory elements since collagen is the terminal differentiating marker of fibroblasts. However, collagen type I is expressed in many other cell types such as osteoblasts [6, 7], smooth muscle cells [8], odontoblasts [9], tenocytes [10], etc.

Starting with a DNaseI hypersensitivity assay, we showed that separate *cis*-acting elements in the murine *Col1a1* gene drive expression in different cell lineages [9]. Similarly, we identified hypersensitive sites (HSs) in the mouse *Col1a2* gene as a cluster of three hypersensitive sites some 17 kb upstream of the transcription start site. These sites are found to be associated with an enhancer that expresses mainly in mesenchymal cells during development [11] (Fig. 1a). This region was later found to be similar in humans but was shifted further toward the 5′ end at −21 kb [12]. Other HSs were found in *Col1a1* [13] (shown as HS4 and HS5 in Fig. 1b). Transgenic mice carrying a GFP transgene were used to show that these elements control the expression pattern including hepatic stellate cells [14] and kidney fibroblasts [15].

The *Col1a2* 17 kb enhancer driving beta-galactosidase and luciferase [11] was shown to be an informative reporter of collagen transcription and predictive of collagen deposition in development. More importantly, when collagen type I is normally downregulated in adult fibroblasts, it is reactivated by this enhancer in adult tissue following injury [16]. We have used this mouse as a readout for collagen transcription and therefore fibrosis to understand the pathways involved [17, 18]. Furthermore, we used transgenes to track bone marrow cells in vivo after transplantation into recipient mice to show the extent of their participation in repair or fibrosis in injury models [19–21]. Similarly, we tracked fetal cells during gestation and postpregnancy to document the cell types actively transcribing collagen type I genes in fibrotic models or in response to injury [22–25] (Fig. 2).

In order to identify the shortest element capable of driving this enhancer, we deleted some sequences under HS5 and found that a 1.5 kb sequence between −17.0 and −15.5 kb in the mouse [26] is

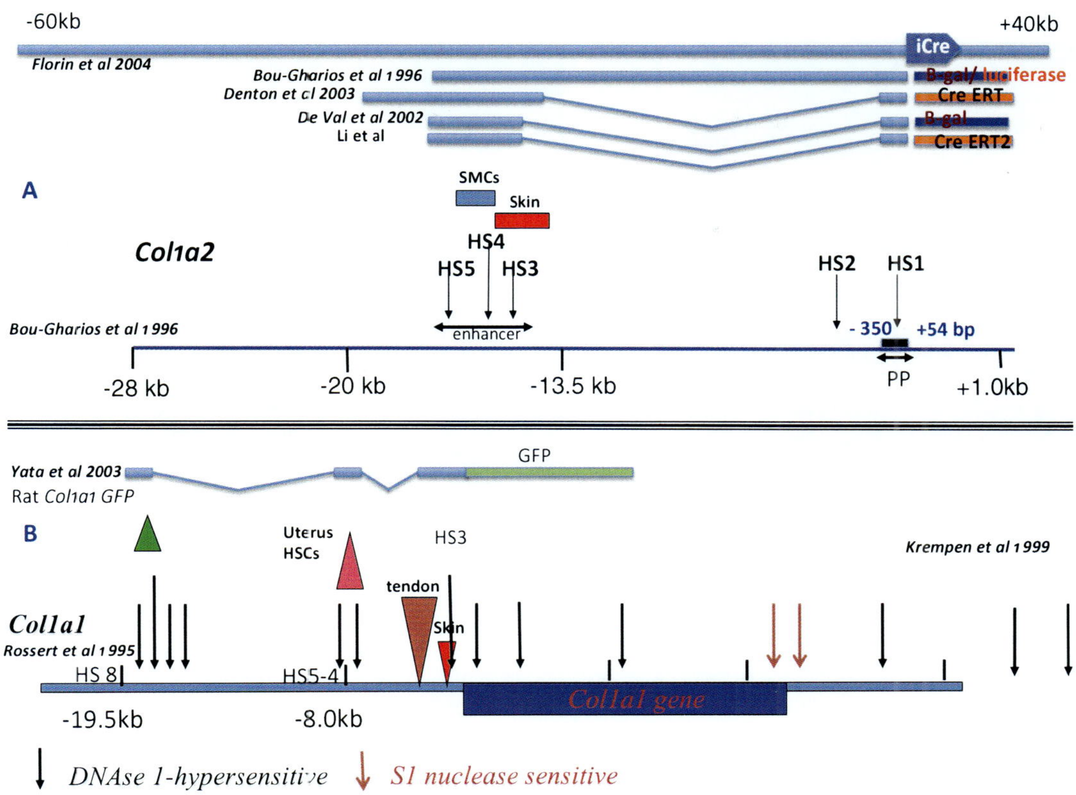

Fig. 1 Schematic diagram of the collagen alpha 2 gene with location of hypersensitive sites (HSs) and proximal promoter (pp). Illustration of where the elements are expressed in vivo. (**a**) Constructs used to generate mice expressing either transgene or cre recombinase are depicted with references at the *top*. (**b**) Transcriptional elements in the *Col1* genes are illustrated with HSs (*black arrows*) and S1 nuclease sensitive sites (*orange arrows*) depicted on the linear map with specific expression in mesenchymal cells. Reference to the GFP mouse generated using rat promoter

the shortest sequence that is functional. The expression of a reporter in transgenic mice starts at E10.5, in the aorta and pericardium, heart valve, and near the otic region in the head. As organogenesis expands, the transgene is seen in many tissues, including the developing dermis, while the epidermis is always devoid of expression. By E15.5, the meninges surrounding the brain and along the spinal cord are positive; the developing soft tissues such as the lung, kidney, spleen, and most but not all skeletal muscle interstitial cells expressed the transgene. In addition, the bladder wall and muscular layers of the stomach and intestines show expression of the transgene. The hard tissues, including long bones, do not express; the only osteoblasts that show expression belong to the intramembranous type, including the calvaria, mandible, and clavicles. Some chondrocytes in developing ribs show staining but to a lesser extent than other mesenchymal cells. Importantly, we have shown that in all of the data outlined above, the transgene expression mirrors the in situ hybridization results of the *col1a2* gene [16].

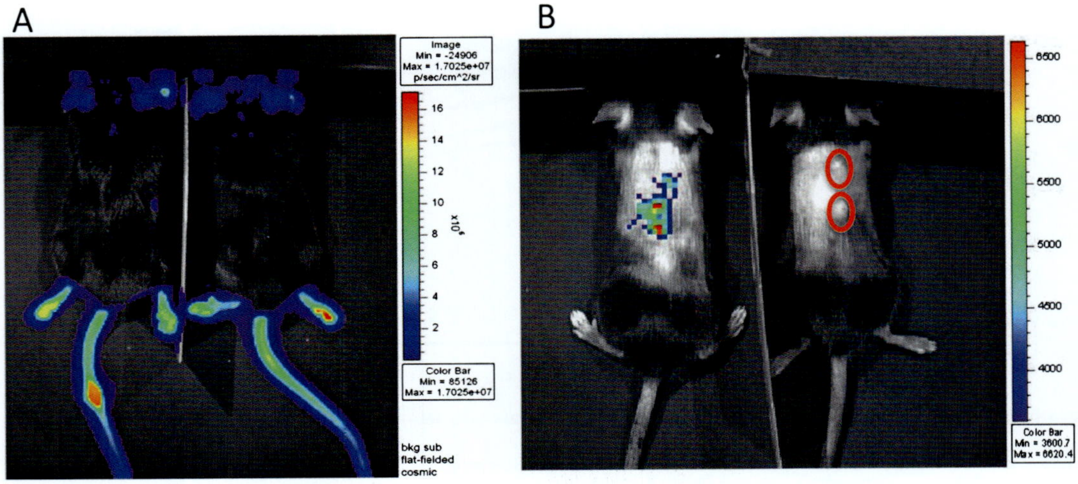

Fig. 2 Bioluminescence of 17 kb fibroblast enhancer in C57bl6 mice. (**A**) Bioluminescence expression in the tail, paws, and ears. Note the increase in collagen transcription in the tail injection site of the mouse on the left that was carried out 3 days earlier. In this example, we used bioluminescence as a genotyping method. (**B**) C57bl6 WT mice were injected with bone marrow from *Col1a2 luc* (*left*) and wild type (*WT*, *right*). Mice were then subjected to full skin thickness excisional wound (*red circle*). This example shows that bone marrow from *col1a2 luc* is transcribing the *col1a2* gene and participated in wound repair of the recipient mouse

In adult mice, the expression is significantly diminished but is reactivated during injury [16]. In particular, several kidney injury models have shown by in situ hybridization that the epithelial cells of the tubular network transcribe collagen type I genes *in situ* early on after injury. This was confirmed by transgene expression [16], by in situ hybridization of the transgene compared with the endogenous gene [19], and further by mRNA levels of cells using laser capture technique [27] suggesting that these cells contribute in situ to deposition of collagen in fibrosis.

In addition, the enhancer was used to drive expression of other genes to produce models of fibrosis. For example, overexpression of CCN2 using this enhancer showed clear fibrosis in the skin, lung, and kidney, but this was concentration dependent as only homozygote mice showed a phenotype [28]. Similarly, this enhancer was used to overexpress transforming growth factor (TGF)-β receptors to generate other fibrotic models [29–32] and also to generate a skin model for dystrophic epidermolysis bullosa [33].

We originally generated an inducible cre fused to a modified estrogen receptor that responds to tamoxifen and not estrogen (Cre ERT), using the larger 6 kb enhancer −19.5 to −13.5 kb [34]. Another non-inducible Cre mouse was created using a large (100 kb) *Col1a2* gene [35]. Having established the minimal sequence that drives mesenchymal cells, we generated a 1.5 kb enhancer driving tamoxifen-inducible cre recombinase (Cre ER^{T2}). Lineage tracing experiments can be accomplished using this *Col1a2 creER*^{T2} mouse mated with mice harboring a reporter gene preceded by a stop signal flanked by LOXP sites. Figure 3 shows soft tissues from a dual-fluorescent protein reporters B6.129(Cg)-Gt(ROSA)26Sortm4(ACTB-tdTomato,-EGFP) Luo/J (Jax Stock No: 007676) [36]. The mice were given tamoxifen at 6 weeks of age and sacrificed at 12 weeks, and we looked at the cells expressing collagen type I. As we have seen before during development, the floxed cells express EGFP in fibroblasts of the interstitium, around blood vessels of many soft tissues and in the eye. We describe below our current established protocols for vector cloning, transfection, generation of transgenic animals, and tissue processing and analysis.

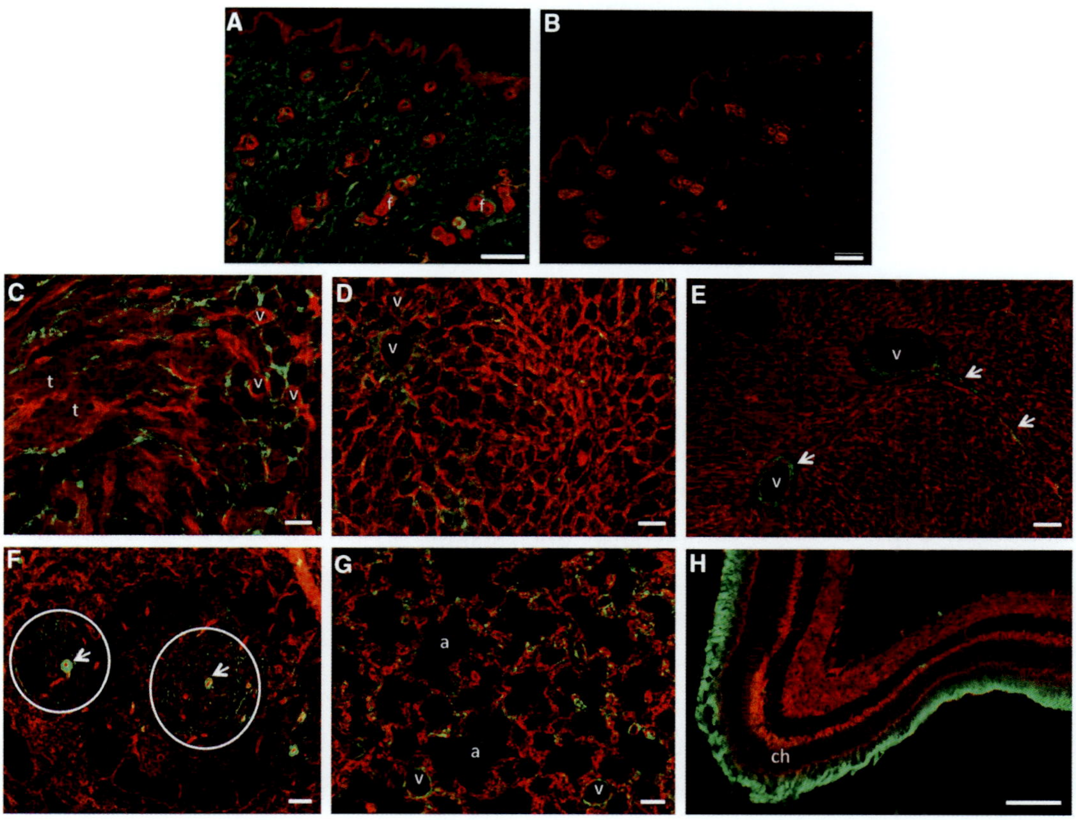

Fig. 3 Col1a2 fibroblasts enhancer driving CreER^{T2} mated with dual-fluorescent protein reporter [36] with tamoxifen given at 6 weeks of age and tissue collected at 12 weeks showing fibroblasts expressing GFP in tissues that are expressing *Col1a2.* Scale bar = 32 μm. (**A**) In the skin, GFP is detected in the dermis but not epidermis, nor in hair follicles (*f*) compared with no tamoxifen (**B**). (**C**) In the kidney, interstitial fibroblasts are green around tubules (*t*) and vessels (*v*). (**D**) In the liver, most of the diffuse staining is seen around the central vein (v). (**E**) In the heart, there are small cells outside some of the fascicles, but most of the staining is seen in vessels (*v, arrows*). In the spleen (**F**) GFP is found in splenic nodules (*round circles*) and blood vessels (*arrows*). (**G**) In the lungs, GFP is expressed in fibroblasts surrounding vessels (*v*) and alveoli (*a*). (**H**, f) In the eye, GFP is detected in the choroid (*ch*)

2 Materials

2.1 Cloning

1. High-purity genomic DNA as template.
2. Nuclease-free water.
3. Tris-EDTA (TE) buffer.
4. pβgal-Basic vector (Clontech).
5. HSP68-LacZ-Gateway™ vector (Addgene plasmid #37843).
6. Luciferase-based vector (we use the pGl4.10[*luc*] vector from Promega).
7. Taq polymerase.
8. Platinum™ Pfx DNA polymerase.
9. Thermal cycler.
10. Monarch®PCR & DNA Cleanup Kit (NEB) or similar kit.
11. QIAquick gel extraction kit (Qiagen) or similar.
12. pCR™8/GW/TOPO® TA cloning kit (Invitrogen, K2500–20).
13. 50 μg/ml streptomycin-containing LB-agar plates.
14. 100 μg/ml ampicillin-containing LB-agar plates.
15. Gateway™ LR Clonase II enzyme mix (Life Technologies, 11791-020).
16. rSAP or Antarctic phosphatase.
17. Lambda DNA-HindIII ladder.
18. UV transilluminator with a wavelength of 312 nm.
19. T4 DNA ligase.
20. T4 polynucleotide kinase.
21. TOP10 chemically competent E.coli (we use the One Shot® format from Invitrogen).
22. JM109 competent cells.
23. Ultrapure water for embryo transfer.
24. PVDF 0.22 μm centrifuge filters.
25. Inducible Cre plasmid pCreER^{T2} [37].
26. Restriction enzymes.
27. Bacterial shaking incubator.

2.2 In Vitro Analysis of Enhancer Regions

1. High-glucose (4.5 g/l) DMEM.
2. Complete DMEM: high-glucose DMEM supplemented with L-glutamine, 10% fetal bovine serum (FBS), 100 IU/penicillin, and 100 μg/ml streptomycin. Alternatively use complete media for the specific cell type of interest.

3. Opti-MEM® medium (Gibco).
4. Lipofectamine 2000 (Invitrogen).
5. Renilla luciferase control vector (we use pRL-TK from Promega).
6. Dual-Luciferase®Reporter Assay System (Promega).
7. 48-well clear bottom tissue culture-treated plates.
8. Cell culture material (biosafety cabinet, cell culture incubator, sterile pipettes, etc.).
9. White 96-well plate that can be used in luminometers.
10. Luminometer that accommodates 96-well plates (we use the Promega GloMax®-Multi Detection System).

2.3 ß-Galactosidase Staining

1. 1 M sodium phosphate (NaPi) buffer pH 7.4:
   (a) Dissolve 138 g of sodium dihydrogen phosphate (NaH_2PO4 –H_2O) in 1 l of ddH_2O and adjust pH to 7.4.
   (b) Dissolve 142 g sodium phosphate dibasic (Na2HPO4) in 1 l of ddH_2O, and adjust pH to 7.4.
   (c) Mix 423 ml of NaH_2PO4 –H_2O and 577 ml of Na2HPO4 to make 1 l of 1 M NaPi buffer.
2. X-gal fixative (FIX solution): 0.2% (v/v) glutaraldehyde, 0.1 M sodium phosphate buffer (pH 7.3), 5 mM ethylene glycol-*bis*(2-aminoethylether)-*N*, *N*, *N′*, *N′*- tetraacetic acid (pH 8.0), 2 mM $MgCl_2$, and 2% (v/v) formalin.
3. Rinse solution: 0.1 M sodium phosphate buffer, 2 mM $MgCl_2$, 0.1% (w/v) sodium deoxycholate, and 0.2% (w/v) NP40 (or substitute).
4. STAIN solution: 1 mg/ml 5-bromo-4-chloro-3-indolyl-β-D-galactosidase (X-gal), 5 mM potassium ferrocyanide, 5 mM potassium ferricyanide, 0.1% sodium deoxycholate, 0.2% (w/v) Nonidet P-40, 2 mM $MgCl_2$, and 0.1 M NaPi buffer. Add the X-gal fresh before use (stored in the dark).
5. 10% (v/v) neutral-buffered formalin: 100 ml 37–40% (v/v) formaldehyde, 4 g sodium phosphate monobasic, and 6.5 g sodium phosphate dibasic anhydrous in 1 l of water.
6. 1% (w/v) potassium hydroxide (KOH) in water.
7. 100% (w/v) glycerol.
8. Tube rotator that can hold 15 and 50 ml centrifuge tubes.

2.4 In Vitro ß-Galactosidase Staining

1. 1X phosphate-buffered saline.
2. 4% paraformaldehyde.
3. STAIN solution with X-gal substrate at 1 mg/ml (from **step 4** of Subheading 2.3).

4. Foil.
5. Laboratory rocker or 37 °C incubator.

2.5 Processing of Stained Tissue

1. Ethanol.
2. Xylene.
3. Paraffin wax for histology.
4. Tissue processor (such as from TP1020 Leica Biosystems).

2.6 In Vivo Bioluminescent Imaging

1. 150 mg/kg D-luciferin in PBS.
2. 30 G × 8 mm needle and syringes.
3. 2.5% isoflurane.
4. In vivo imager (we use the IVIS Spectrum in vivo imager system from PerkinElmer).

3 Methods

3.1 Identification of a Specific Enhancer in a Given Gene

In the 1990s when we first investigated enhancers in *Col1a2*, we knew that enhancers are able to act independently of distance and orientation in relation to their target gene and are generally highly conserved in evolution. DNaseI hypersensitive sites were one of the few indicative experiments for possible enhancer sites, since areas of active enhancers are generally void of nucleosomes allowing these DNA regions to be accessible to DNaseI. Such sites therefore coincide with DNaseI hypersensitivity which can be used as a part of a criterion to identify possible enhancers [38]. Today, we know that enhancers are marked by certain histone modifications to show a permissive chromatin such as acetylation of the third histone at the 27th lysine (H3K27ac) and methylation of the 4th lysine (H3K4me1) [39, 40]. Most importantly, if you are starting fresh, we would recommend that you start with the Encyclopedia of DNA Elements (ENCODE) project, which provides publically available data sets on functional elements of the genome:

1. Open the University of California at Santa Cruz genome browser webpage (https://genome.ucsc.edu/) [41].
2. Under "Genomes" in the upper left part of the page, select the mouse assembly July 2007 mm9 (NCBI37/mm9) and search for *Col1a2* as target gene in the box that reads "enter position, gene symbol or search terms."
3. In the tab "Expression and Regulation" which is the seventh tab down the page, click on the link "LICR Histone" (i.e., ChIP-seq from the ENCODE Ludwig Institute for Cancer Research (ENCODE/LICR) project track data) and select the

epigenetic signatures H3K4me1, H3K27ac, and H3K4me3 in E14.5 mouse limb and in mouse embryonic fibroblasts (MEFs) (Fig. 4). Click on "Submit."

4. In the tab "Expression and Regulation" which is the seventh tab down the page, click on the link "UW DNaseI HS" (i.e., DNaseI hypersensitivity by Digital DNaseI from ENCODE project at the University of Washington) and select the E11.5 mouse fibroblasts and the immortalized mouse fibroblast cell line (NIH3T3) (Fig. 4). Click on "Submit."
5. Ensure the conservation throughout vertebrate genomes is selected (i.e., "full"); this can be found in the eighth tab of the genome browser under "Comparative Genomics" (you can pick the genomes of particular interest by clicking on the tabs).
6. Look for regions that have high conservation and good histone peaks and DNaseI peaks; you can use other tracks as exclusion criteria's, but, generally, these marks are good indicators for enhancers without needing to conduct ChIP-seq or DNaseI hypersensitivity experiments (Fig. 5).
7. Identify these sequences with a 100 bp extra nucleotides from both side, and clone them out in an expression vector for in vitro and in vivo analysis as described in Subheading 3.2.

3.2 Cloning for In Vivo and In Vitro Analysis and Inducible Systems

3.2.1 Producing the Insert by PCR

1. Design primers for PCR that are ±100 bp from the regions identified in the ENCODE, ChIP, or DNaseI analysis (*see* **Note 1**).
2. Resuspend primers in nuclease-free water or TE buffer to a concentration of 100 pmol/μl to create a stock and then use in a 1 in 10 dilution in nuclease-free water.
3. Amplify DNA fragments by PCR from high-purity genomic DNA (for mouse Promega, G3091), cosmids, or genomic clones. There are two methods used in this lab to generate plasmids for examining enhancer function in vivo: cloning the minimal promoter and enhancer directly in the pβgal-Basic or just the enhancer into the HSP68-*LacZ*-Gateway [42]. For in vitro analysis, enhancers and minimal promoters are cloned into the pGl4.10-*luc* (but other luciferase-based vectors can be used). The pβgal-Basic and luciferase vectors are cloned using standard cloning methods (*see* **Notes 2**), while the HSP68 vector is cloned using Gateway™ (*see* **Notes 3** and **4**).
4. All PCR reactions should be verified by electrophoresis, run 5 μl on 1% agarose gel.
5. After verification, clean up the remaining PCR reaction using the Monarch® PCR & DNA Cleanup Kit (*see* **Note 5**).

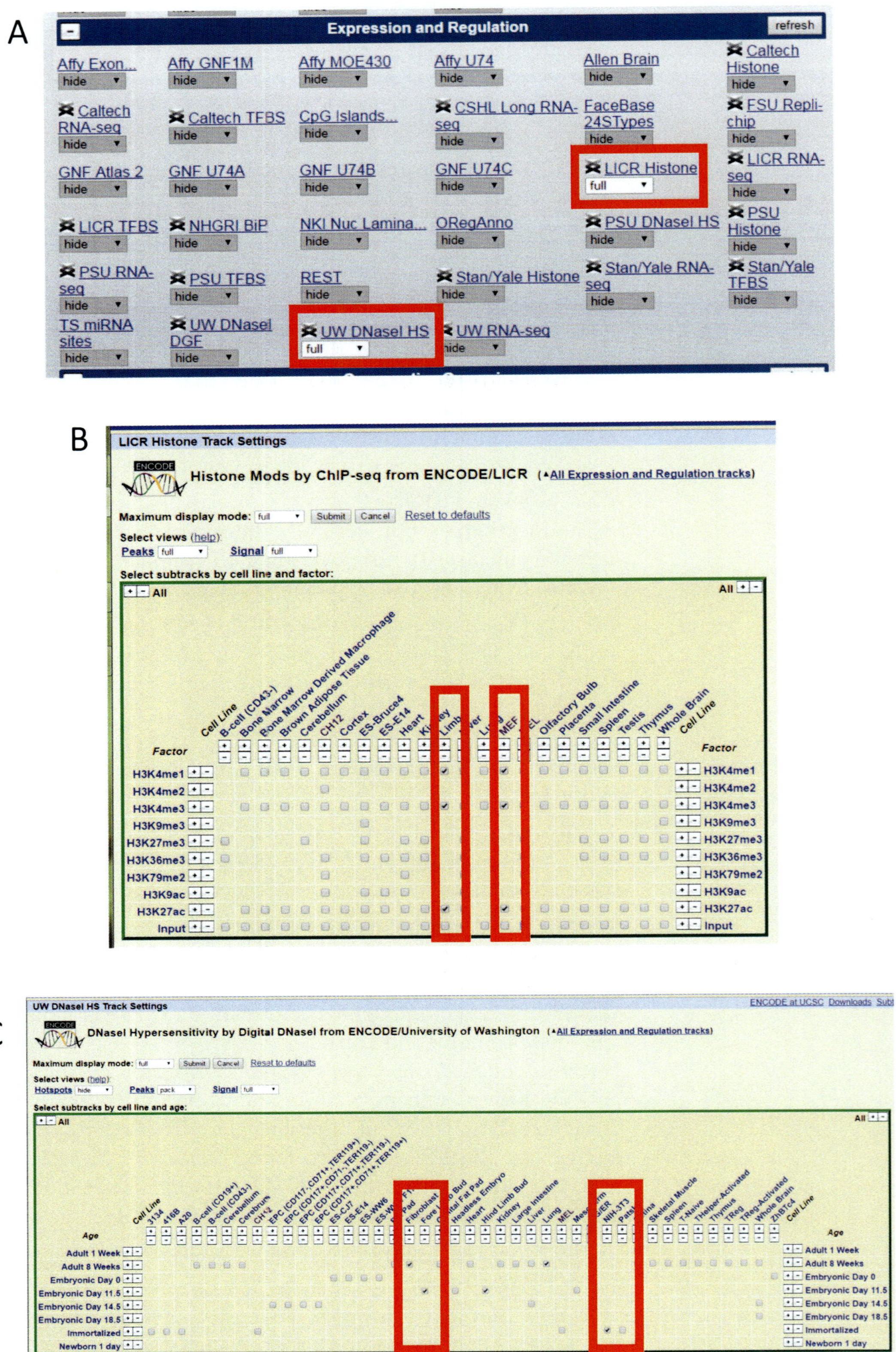

Fig. 4 UCSC window for selection of enhancer criteria. (**A**) Browser window showing "Expression and Regulation" tracks after scrolling down to the seventh tab of the mouse/mm9. (**B**) Display window after clicking on the "LICR Histone." From this window, you can select the cell type and the different histone modifications

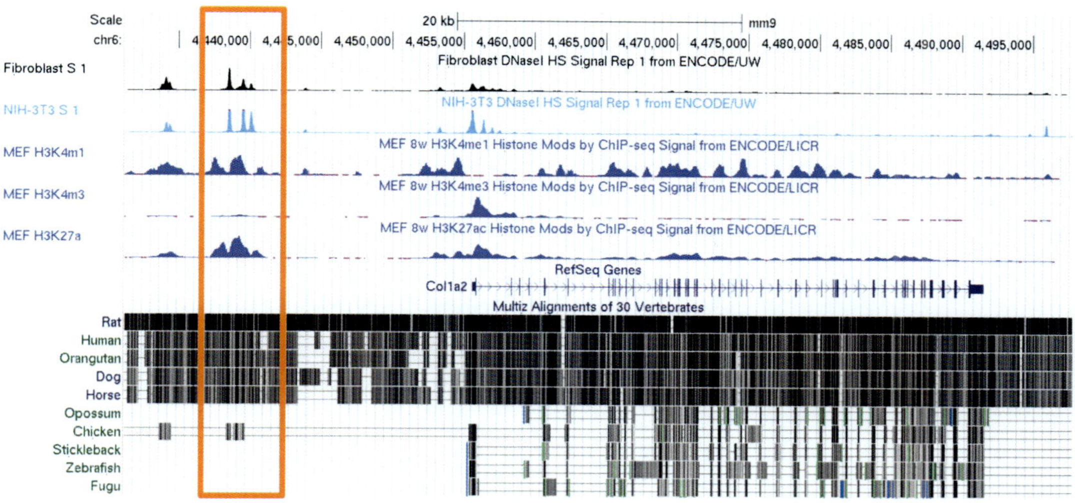

Fig. 5 ENCODE readout showing histone methylation and acetylation in two types of fibroblasts and MEF cells showing peaks of activity in acetylation and methylation of H3K4m1 that represent enhancers (*orange box*) in the 5′ sequences of the *Col1a2* mouse gene. The *peaks* correspond to high homology of sequence from humans to chicken

6. Clone PCR fragment into vector as described in Subheading 3.2.3 "Gateway Cloning" or Subheading 3.2.2 "Standard Cloning."
7. Once cloned into the vector, it is advised to perform sequencing to verify the inserted regions.

3.2.2 Standard Cloning

1. Digest the vectors and inserts (containing restriction enzyme recognition sites on the 5′ and 3′ ends) with the desired restriction enzyme overnight at the recommended temperature.
2. Dephosphorylate the vector using rSAP or Antarctic phosphatase (*see* **Note 6**). Add the phosphatase to the reaction at 1–5 units per pmol of DNA ends based on the following calculation:

$$\mu g\ DNA \times \frac{\text{pmol}}{600\,pg} \times \frac{10^6\,pg}{1\,\mu g} \times \frac{1}{N} \times 2 \times \frac{kb}{1000bp} = \text{pmol}\ DNA\ ends$$

N is the nucleotides in kilobases, 660 pg/mol is the average molecular weight of a nucleotide pair, 2 is the number of ends, and Kb/1000 bp is the conversion factor.

Fig. 4 (continued) that mark enhancers and other regulatory elements (for the *Col1a2* gene, we selected MEFs and limb-specific modifications (*red boxes*)). Once submitted, they will appear as tracks in the browser. (**C**) The window is presented to the user once "UW DNaseI HS" is selected. You can select different cell types that may be of interest, but for the *Col1a2* fibroblast and the cell line, NIH3T3 was used. For the purpose of searching for enhancers, the ENCODE Ludwig Institute for Cancer Research (ENCODE/LICR) tracks for histone modifications and ENCODE project University of Washington (UW DNaseI HS), highlighted in *red boxes*, can be selected

3. Incubate the reaction for another hour at 37 °C for rSAP and 30 min for Antarctic phosphatase.
4. Heat inactivate at 65 °C for 5 min for rSAP or 80 °C for 2 min for Antarctic phosphatase. If possible this will denature the restriction enzyme too; if the enzyme cannot be heat inactivated, perform gel electrophoresis and gel purification or column-based purification.
5. Run 2 μl of the insert and vector on 1% agarose gel alongside 0.5 μg and 1 μg of lambda DNA-HindIII digest ladder.
6. Estimate the concentration based on the HindIII ladder or use programs to estimate the concentration such as the BioRad Image Lab™ software. Additional verification by UV spectroscopy is also possible.
7. Carry out ligations at a 4:1 molar ratio of insert to vector (*see* **Note 7**):

   (a) Determine the amount of insert in a 10 μl ligation mix based on the calculation:

$$\text{mass of insert } (g) = \text{desired } \frac{\text{insert}}{\text{vector}} \text{ molar ratio} \times \text{mass of vector } (g) \times \text{ratio of insert to vector lengths}$$

   (b) Carry out the ligation in the following reaction: 1 μl 10X T4 ligase buffer, 1 μl vector, x μl insert, 1 μl T4 DNA ligase (NEB), and complete to 10 μl with ddH_2O (*see* **Notes 8–10**).

   (c) Incubate at 37 °C for 1 h.

   (d) Heat inactivate at 65 °C for 20 min in a thermal cycler.
8. Incubate ligations at 16 °C overnight.
9. Heat inactivate at 65 °C for 10 min.
10. Use 5 μl of ligation mix to transform competent bacteria (we use JM109 from Promega) and plate onto ampicillin selective plates.
11. After growing selected clones into ~5 ml LB broth with ampicillin, extract DNA with miniprep kit following manufacturer's instructions.
12. Check vectors for correct insertion using restriction enzyme digestion and Sanger sequencing.

3.2.3 Gateway Cloning

Fragments are first inserted into the pCR™8/GW/TOPO® vector using the pCR™8/GW/TOPO® TA cloning kit according to manufacturer's instructions as follows:

1. Place 2 μl of freshly extracted DNA product, 1 μl salt solution, and 0.5 μl TOPO® vector with 2.5 μl dH_2O in a 1.5 ml centrifuge tube, touch down centrifuge to ensure all reagents are

together, and then incubate at room temperature for 30 min for short fragments of up to 1.5 kb and 1 h for fragments longer than 1.5 kb.

2. Transform 4 μl of the TOPO® reaction into TOP10 *E. coli* bacteria and incubate overnight at 37 °C on streptomycin LB-agar plates. Include a negative control and the pCR™8/GW/TOPO positive control that is provided in the kit.
3. The following day, select colonies and perform colony PCR. Colonies that contain the insert can then be used to inoculate starter cultures for minipreps. Cloning success and correct orientation of insertion should be checked and verified by restriction enzyme digestion and Sanger sequencing.

   The enhancer sequences are transferred from the pCR8/GW/enhancer entry vector to the HSP68/LacZ/Gateway® destination vector using Gateway LR Clonase II enzyme mix.
4. Set up a reaction of 1 μl of HSP68/LacZ/Gateway® (37 ng/μl) with 1 μl of the TOPO entry vector (37 ng/μl) in a 1.5 ml centrifuge tube.
5. Thaw the LR Clonase II enzyme for 2 min on ice then vortex for 2 s twice.
6. Add 0.5 μl of LR Clonase II to the reaction mix, mix, and then incubate at room temperature for 1 h or up to 16 h for larger fragments.
7. Stop the reaction by the addition of 0.25 μl of 2 μg/μl Proteinase K solution and incubate at 37 °C in a water bath for 15 min.
8. Transform the entire reaction into TOP10 chemically competent *E. coli* bacteria and plate onto ampicillin selection plates. Incubate at 37 °C overnight.
9. The following day, perform colony PCR and create starter cultures for minipreps; verify constructs using restriction enzyme digestion and Sanger sequencing.

3.3 In Vitro Transfection

We use a fibroblast cell line to determine the activation of the enhancer, but different cell types can be used based on the expression pattern or predicted expression of the enhancer. We use the murine embryonic fibroblast, NIH3T3, maintained in complete DMEM:

1. Seed the NIH3T3 at a density of 1.75×10^4 cells/well in a 48-well tissue culture-treated plate and incubate overnight (around 12 h) in a cell culture incubator. Only conduct transfection when cells are ~80% confluent.
2. Co-transfect the cells in triplicates with the enhancer constructs and any Renilla luciferase control vector to allow normalization of transfection efficacy. Blanks, luciferase vector with no

insert, and pRL-TK alone are included in each experiment as controls.

3. For each well set up the following two reaction tubes:
   (a) Tube 1: 80 μl Opti-MEM®, 2 μg DNA, and 120 ng pRL-TK vector
   (b) Tube 2: 80 μl Opti-MEM® and 3 μl Lipofectamine® 2000
4. Incubate 5 min at room temperature.
5. Add 80 μl from tube 2 to tube 1 and mix by flicking.
6. Incubate at room temperature for 25 min.
7. Add 40 μl of the mix to each well (so the final concentration of DNA is 500 ng with 0.75 μl of Lipofectamine and 30 ng of TK vector).
8. Assay the cells after 24–48 h.

3.4 Luciferase Assays

We conduct luciferase assays using the Dual-Luciferase®Reporter Assay System. Reagents are prepared fresh for each experiment, with the exception of the Luciferase Assay Reagent II (LARII):

1. Prepare the passive lysis buffer by adding one volume of 5X concentrate into four volumes of distilled water and invert to mix.
2. Prepare the LARII by adding 10 ml of luciferase assay buffer II to the lyophilized luciferase assay substrate and store in aliquots of 1 ml at −80 °C.
3. Add 1 volume of Stop & Glo® substrate to 50 volumes of Stop & Glo® buffer and invert to mix (*see* **Note 11**). Wrap in foil to protect from light.
4. Equilibrate cells to room temperature for 10 min.
5. Add 65 μl of passive lysis buffer to each well and incubate at room temperature for 15 min while rocking.
6. Add 50 μl of LARII to each well of a white 96-well plate and perform a background reading in a luminometer.
7. Transfer 10 μl of cell lysate into the plate and mix by pipetting six times.
8. Read the plate within 10 min of mixing.
9. Add 50 μl of Stop & Glo® Reagent mix by pipetting four times and read the Renilla luminescence.
10. Normalize the luminescence to the control vector and calculate the relative response ratio (RRR) using the following formula:

$$RRR = \frac{(\text{experimental sample ratio}) - (\text{negative control ratio})}{(\text{positive control ratio}) - (\text{negative control ratio})}$$

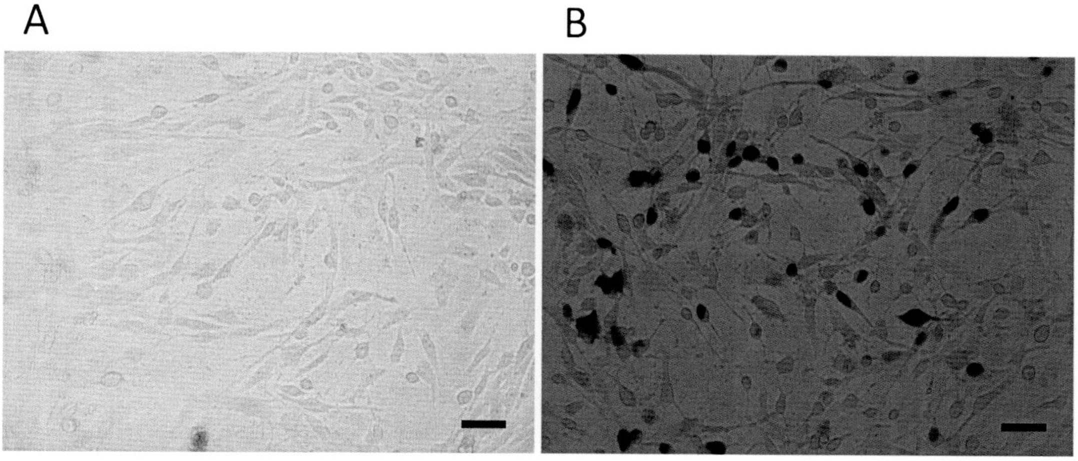

Fig. 6 X-gal staining in fibroblasts after transfection with control vector (**A**) and Col1a2 transgene (**B**) showing positive *blue* staining. Scale bar = 10 μm

3.5 X-gal Staining in Cells

Cells that are transfected with a β-gal-based vector or primary cells taken from mice harboring a β-gal transgene can be stained for β-galactosidase (Fig. 6):

1. Remove cells from cell culture incubator and allow time to equilibrate to room temperature.
2. Remove growth medium and wash with ice-cold 1X PBS twice.
3. Fix cells in 4% paraformaldehyde on ice for 2–5 min.
4. Wash cells twice with ice-cold 1X PBS.
5. Add enough stain solution with X-gal to cover the cells and incubate in the dark at 37 °C for 8 h (longer incubations can be done). Alternatively, cover in foil and incubate at room temperature with agitation or on a laboratory rocker for 16 h (or overnight).
6. Wash in PBS and image cells (Fig. 6).

3.6 In Vivo Bioluminescence Imaging

In vivo imaging of transgenic mice that harbor a luciferase gene can be used as a noninvasive longitudinal monitoring of the gene expression. To visualize the expression in vivo, we use the following method:

1. Inject D-luciferin intraperitoneally into the mice using 30 G needle (*see* **Note 12**).
2. Anesthetize mice using 2.5% isoflurane. If looking at specific tissues, cull the animal and dissect the tissue of interest.
3. Place mouse or tissue into an in vivo imager.
4. Collect data depending on study parameters. Adjust camera settings to obtain a signal level of 600–60,000 counts/easy

Table 1
Embryo fixation time relative to gestation stage

Gestation state	Fixation time
E7.5–8.5	10 min
E8.5–9.0	20 min
E9.5	30 min
E10–11.5	45 min
E12.5	1 h
E13.5	2.5–2 h
E14.5	2.5 h
E15.5	3 h
E16.5–17.5	4 h

with autoexposure setting. Make sure to determine plateau of constant luciferase activity rather than peak of activity (*see* **Notes 13**). You may need to shade high-expressing areas to see other low levels (*see* **Notes 14** and **15**).

3.7 X-gal Staining in Embryos and Adult Tissues

3.7.1 X-gal Staining of Mouse Embryos

1. Transgenic mouse embryos can be collected at different time points during gestation. Embryos taken after E15.5 will require de-skinning or opening up along the vertical axis from head to tail to allow penetration of the fix/stain solution. After dissection, keep the yolk sac and placenta for genotyping.
2. Rinsed samples in ice-cold 1X PBS and fix embryos in FIX solution at 4 °C. Recommended fixation times relative to gestation stages are shown in Table 1.
3. Rinse embryos twice in PBS (*see* **Note 16**).
4. Place embryos into 50 ml tubes with 25–40 ml of STAIN solution; cover the tubes with foil paper and incubate overnight in the dark at room temperature.
5. Rinse in PBS.
6. At this stage you can photograph the embryos then fix overnight in 4% PFA at 4 °C (if >E15.5 fix for 1–2 h) for further histology (*see* Subheading 3.7.3).

3.7.2 X-gal Staining of Adult Tissues Collected from Mice

1. Incubate tissues in six times their volume of FIX solution for 2 h at room temperature while rotating.
2. Continue from **step 3** of Subheading 3.7.1.

Table 2
Dehydration and paraffin-embedding protocol for β-gal-stained embryos less than E14.5

Reagent	Immersion period (min) under vacuum
70% ethanol	30
90% ethanol	30
100% ethanol	10
100% ethanol	10
100% ethanol	10
100% ethanol	10
Xylene	10
Xylene	10
Wax	100
Wax	100

3.7.3 Paraffin Embedding for Histology of X-gal-Stained Samples

After overnight fixation samples can be processed to allow histological interrogation. The LacZ staining may be reduced significantly with xylene. We have adopted a processing procedure of LacZ-stained embryos to minimize exposure to xylene in the processing (*see* **Note 17**). Alternatively, samples can be cryopreserved and then cryo-sectioned.

For embryos up to E14.5, dehydrate and paraffin-embed fixed samples by successively immersing them in ethanol, xylene, and wax (strictly follow reagents and times indicated in Table 2).

For larger LacZ-stained embryos (E14.5–E18.5) and soft tissue, open the embryos down the center to allow better infiltration and follow reagents and times indicated in Table 3.

3.8 Generation of a Fibroblast-Specific Cre-Inducible Strain

For inducible systems, we use the plasmid pCreER^{T2}, which contains the cDNA for the protein Cre recombinase (causes recombination of two *LoxP* sequences) with a modified estrogen receptor (ER^{T2}) [37]. The pCreER^{T2} is digested with the enzymes *SfiI* and *PvuII*, blunted with T4 DNA polymerase, and dephosphorylated with Antarctic phosphatase. Cloning into the vector of interest is performed following the cloning procedures detailed in Subheadings 3.2.3 or 3.2.2. The 1.9 kb fragment of the *Col1a2* enhancer (−17.0/−15.45 kb) and the mouse minimal proximal promoter (SDV150) [26] are prepared by *BamHI* excision and gel extraction using the QIAquick gel extraction kit. The insert is ligated to the linear pCreER^{T2} by T4 DNA ligase and verified by

Table 3
Dehydration and paraffin-embedding protocol for β-gal-stained large embryos (E14.5 to E18.5) and adult tissues

Reagent	Immersion period (min) under vacuum
70% ethanol	30
90% ethanol	30
100% ethanol	10
100% ethanol	10
100% ethanol	10
100% ethanol	10
Xylene	30
Xylene	30
Wax	120 (2 h)
Wax	Overnight

restriction enzyme digest and Sanger sequencing. For oocyte injection, the vector is digested with *FspI* and the 6181 bp fragment is gel purified. This mouse model can be used in different strategies to target fibroblasts in gain and loss of function experiments as illustrated in Fig. 7.

4 Notes

1. Primers can be generated using a web-based program primer blast (http://www.ncbi.nlm.nih.gov/tools/primer-blast/). Generally, primers should be 18–30 nt with an annealing temperature of 60 °C with a difference of ±2 °C (for anything greater, a touchdown PCR may be required). Standard desalt or high-purity salt-free purification can be used with no deleterious effects to cloning; the GC content of the primers should be about 40–60% with no more than three similar nucleotides between primer pairs (inter-homology) to reduce primer dimers and no more than four repeats. For sticky end cloning, it is generally advisable to leave or add 3-4 bases between restriction enzyme cleavage site and the end of the primer for successful digestion.
2. For standard cloning, we use proofreading Platinum™ *PfX* DNA polymerase. If PCR fails or the temperature between primer pairs is greater than 5 °C, a touchdown PCR can be

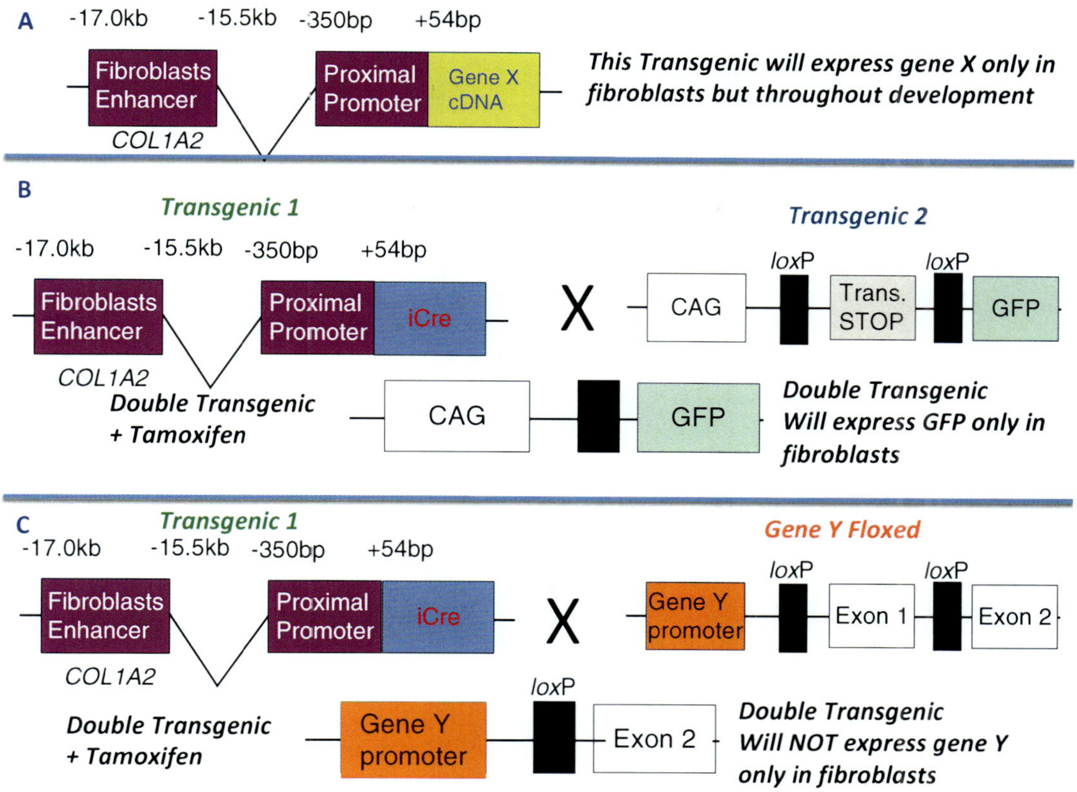

Fig. 7 Transgenic strategies for Col1a2 CreER[T2]. (**A**) Strategy for using fibroblast-specific enhancers to overexpress a specific gene in mesenchymal cells. (**B**) Gain of function experiment where two transgenic mice are generated. One mouse expresses cre recombinase, the other expresses a gene of interest (in this case GFP) with a transcriptional STOP, flanked by LoxP sites (floxed). In the presence of tamoxifen (or in non-inducible cre lines), the recombinase enzyme will flox out the transcriptional stop to express GFP only in mesenchymal cells. (**C**) In loss of function experiments, a mouse harbouring a floxed exon on a specific gene is mated with a mouse expressing cre recombinase in mesenchymal cells. The floxed exon will be deleted in the mesenchymal cells when tamoxifen is added

conducted starting at 5 °C higher than the lowest temperature of the primer pairs can be. The standard three-step cycling is carried out by an initial denaturing step at 94 °C for 5 min, then 35–40 cycles of 94 °C for 15 s, 55 °C for 30 s, and an extension step of 68 °C at 1 kb/min; the reaction can then be maintained at 4 °C or frozen and stored at −20 °C for future use. Alternatively, a two-step PCR can be performed, of 94 °C for 5 min, then 30 cycles of 94 °C for 15 s, the extension is carried out at 68 °C, at 1 kb/min. The *PfX* taq polymerase produces a blunt-ended product that can be used in blunt-ended cloning if no restriction enzymes are suitable.

3. For Gateway™-based cloning, a non-high-fidelity DNA*taq* polymerase, in our case REDExtract™-N-Amp ReadyMix™ (Sigma, E3004), is used to utilize the ability of the *taq* poly-

merase to perform A-tailing to allow for TA cloning. Reaction parameters of 94 °C for 3 min to denature the DNA, 30 s at the specific primer annealing temperature (58–62 °C), extension of 2 min at 72 °C for 30 cycles, a prolonged final extension time of 10 min is then carried out (to allow A-tailing), and a soak step at 4 °C to end.

4. The advantage of the gateway cloning is that once you generate a recipient vector, many more enhancers can be directly cloned in. The disadvantage is the use of proprietary LR Clonase II and specific bacteria. To propagate a new destination vector that has not been used in a LR reaction or has no insert, a bacteria that is able to withstand the *ccdB* gene product such as the *ccd*B Survival™ 2 T1^R chemically competent cells from Invitrogen should be used.
5. If the PCR yields multiple bands, but a band of the correct size is seen, the correct band can be extracted from the gel using kits such as the QIAquick gel extraction kit.
6. rSAP can be added directly to the restriction mix, whereas Antarctic phosphatase buffer should supplement the restriction mix and the volume brought up to 30 μl.
7. You can use different ratios of 1:1, 2:1, 5:1, 10:1, or even 1:10 if there are problems with ligation.
8. If using blunt-ended cloning, treat the purified PCR product using T4 polynucleotide kinase (T4 PNK) in the following reaction in 0.2 ml PCR reaction tube; if using a different buffer than the T4 ligase, add 10 mM ATP to the mix to allow the T4 PNK to work. Set up the reaction as follows: up to 1 μg PCR product, 2 μl 10X T4 ligase buffer, 1 μl T4 PNK, and dH_2O up to 20 μl.
9. Phosphatased inserts can be used in blunt-end cloning in blunted vector (i.e., that has been digested with a restriction enzyme that blunts) or sticky ends that have been filled in by DNA polymerase I large (Klenow) fragment or by T4 DNA polymerase.
10. Blunt-end ligations can be carried out in the presence of the blunt-end enzyme to prevent vector religation and increase efficiency of the ligation.
11. The yellow color should be uniform throughout the solution.
12. Luciferin has to be distributed evenly inside the animal before measuring luciferase activity (in our experience 10 min).
13. In our 17 kb black mouse, tail, periodontal ligaments, and ears are seen as baseline expression without shaving (Fig. 2a) or with shaving to obtain low activity as in bone marrow contribution to repair (Fig. 2b).

14. Calibrated units are photons per second, representing the flux radiating omnidirectionally from a user-defined region of interest (ROI).
15. Factors that will affect imaging of luciferase include relative placement of animal versus camera, fur color and presence (may need to shave), imaging time point, luciferin dose per mouse (keep weight record of mice and inject constant dose), and biological factors (e.g., circadian rhythm, surgery, implantation).
16. The larger the embryos, the more rinse they require.
17. The xylene steps have been reduced to minimize the leeching of the X-gal staining.

References

1. Leask A, Denton CP, Abraham DJ (2004) Insights into the molecular mechanism of chronic fibrosis: the role of connective tissue growth factor in scleroderma. J Invest Dermatol 122(1):1–6. doi:10.1046/j.0022-202X.2003.22133.x
2. Strutz F, Okada H, Lo CW et al (1995) Identification and characterization of a fibroblast marker: FSP1. J Cell Biol 130(2):393–405. doi:10.1083/jcb.130.2.393
3. Goodpaster T, Legesse-Miller A, Hameed MR et al (2008) An immunohistochemical method for identifying fibroblasts in formalin-fixed, paraffin-embedded tissue. J Histochem Cytochem 56(4):347–358. doi:10.1369/jhc.7A7287.2007
4. Sugimoto H, Mundel TM, Kieran MW et al (2006) Identification of fibroblast heterogeneity in the tumor microenvironment. Cancer Biol Ther 5(12):1640–1646. doi:10.4161/cbt.5.12.3354
5. Tomasek JJ, Haaksma CJ, Schwartz RJ et al (2013) Whole animal knockout of smooth muscle alpha-actin does not alter excisional wound healing or the fibroblast-to-myofibroblast transition. Wound Repair Regen 21(1):166–176. doi:10.1111/wrr.12001
6. Rossert J, Eberspeacher H, De Crombrugghe B et al (1996) Identification of a minimal sequence of the mouse pro-a1(1) collagen promoter that confers high level osteoblast expression in transgenic mice, and that binds a protein selectively present in osteoblasts. Proc Natl Acad Sci U S A 93:1027–1031
7. Kalajzic Z, Liu P, Kalajzic I et al (2002) Directing the expression of a green fluorescent protein transgene in differentiated osteoblasts: comparison between rat type I collagen and rat osteocalcin promoters. Bone 31(6):654–660. doi:10.1016/S8756-3282(02)00912-2
8. Ponticos M, Partridge T, Black CM et al (2004) Regulation of collagen type I in vascular smooth muscle cells by competition between Nkx2.5 and deltaEF1/ZEB1. Mol Cell Biol 24(14):6151–6161. doi:10.1128/MCB.24.14.6151-6161.2004
9. Rossert J, Eberspaecher H, de Crombrugghe B (1995) Separate cis-acting DNA elements of the mouse pro-alpha 1(I) collagen promoter direct expression of reporter genes to different type I collagen-producing cells in transgenic mice. J Cell Biol 129(5):1421–1432. doi:10.1083/jcb.129.5.1421
10. Terraz C, Brideau G, Ronco P et al (2002) A combination of cis-acting elements is required to activate the pro- alpha 1(I) collagen promoter in tendon fibroblasts of transgenic mice. J Biol Chem 277(21):19019–19026. doi:10.1074/jbc.M200125200
11. Bou-Gharios G, Garrett LA, Rossert J et al (1996) A potent far-upstream enhancer in the mouse pro alpha 2(I) collagen gene regulates expression of reporter genes in transgenic mice. J Cell Biol 134(5):1333–1344. doi:10.1083/jcb.134.5.1333
12. Antoniv TT, De Val S, Wells D et al (2001) Characterization of an evolutionarily conserved far-upstream enhancer in the human alpha 2(I) collagen (COL1A2) gene. J Biol Chem 276(24):21754–21764. doi:10.1074/jbc.M101397200
13. Krempen K, Grotkopp D, Hall K et al (1999) Far upstream regulatory elements enhance position-independent and uterus-specific expression of the murine a1 (I) collagen promoter in transgenic mice. Gene Expr 8:151–163

14. Yata Y, Scanga A, Gillan A et al (2003) DNase I-hypersensitive sites enhance alpha1(I) collagen gene expression in hepatic stellate cells. Hepatology 37(2):267–276. doi:10.1053/jhep.2003.50067
15. Lin SL, Kisseleva T, Brenner DA et al (2008) Pericytes and perivascular fibroblasts are the primary source of collagen-producing cells in obstructive fibrosis of the kidney. Am J Pathol 173(6):1617–1627. doi:10.2353/ajpath.2008.080433
16. Ponticos M, Abraham D, Alexakis C et al (2004) Col1a2 enhancer regulates collagen activity during development and in adult tissue repair. Matrix Biol 22(8):619–628. doi:10.1016/j.matbio.2003.12.002
17. Ponticos M, Harvey C, Ikeda T et al (2009) JunB mediates enhancer/promoter activity of COL1A2 following TGF-beta induction. Nucleic Acids Res 37(16):5378–5389. doi:10.1093/nar/gkp544
18. Ponticos M, Papaioannou I, Xu S et al (2015) Failed degradation of JunB contributes to overproduction of type I collagen and development of dermal fibrosis in patients with systemic sclerosis. Arthritis Rheumatol 67(1):243–253. doi:10.1002/art.38897
19. Roufosse C, Bou-Gharios G, Prodromidi E et al (2006) Bone marrow-derived cells do not contribute significantly to collagen I synthesis in a murine model of renal fibrosis. J Am Soc Nephrol 17(3):775–782. doi:10.1681/ASN.2005080795
20. Higashiyama R, Moro T, Nakao S et al (2009) Negligible contribution of bone marrow-derived cells to collagen production during hepatic fibrogenesis in mice. Gastroenterology 137(4):1459–1466. doi:10.1053/j.gastro.2009.07.006e1451
21. Higashiyama R, Nakao S, Shibusawa Y et al (2011) Differential contribution of dermal resident and bone marrow-derived cells to collagen production during wound healing and fibrogenesis in mice. J Invest Dermatol 131(2):529–536. doi:10.1038/jid.2010.314
22. Lee ES, Bou-Gharios G, Seppanen E et al (2010) Fetal stem cell microchimerism: natural-born healers or killers? Mol Hum Reprod 16(11):869–878. doi:10.1093/molehr/gaq067
23. Bou-Gharios G, Amin F, Hill P et al (2011) Microchimeric fetal cells are recruited to maternal kidney following injury and activate collagen type I transcription. Cells Tissues Organs 193(6):379–392. doi:10.1159/000321172
24. Seppanen EJ, Hodgson SS, Khosrotehrani K et al (2012) Fetal microchimeric cells in a fetus-treats-its-mother paradigm do not contribute to dystrophin production in serially parous mdx females. Stem Cells Dev 21(15):2809–2816. doi:10.1089/scd.2012.0047
25. Seppanen E, Roy E, Ellis R et al (2013) Distant mesenchymal progenitors contribute to skin wound healing and produce collagen: evidence from a murine fetal microchimerism model. PLoS One 8(5):e62662. doi:10.1371/journal.pone.0062662
26. De Val S, Ponticos M, Antoniv TT et al (2002) Identification of the key regions within the mouse pro-alpha 2(I) collagen gene far-upstream enhancer. J Biol Chem 277(11):9286–9292. doi:10.1074/jbc.M111040200
27. Fragiadaki M, Witherden AS, Kaneko T et al (2011) Interstitial fibrosis is associated with increased COL1A2 transcription in AA-injured renal tubular epithelial cells in vivo. Matrix Biol 30(7–8):396–403. doi:10.1016/j.matbio.2011.07.004
28. Sonnylal S, Shi-Wen X, Leoni P et al (2010) Selective expression of connective tissue growth factor in fibroblasts in vivo promotes systemic tissue fibrosis. Arthritis Rheum 62(5):1523–1532. doi:10.1002/art.27382
29. Denton CP, Zheng B, Shiwen X et al (2001) Activation of a fibroblast-specific enhancer of the proalpha2(I) collagen gene in tight-skin mice. Arthritis Rheum 44(3):712–722. doi:10.1002/1529-0131(200103)44:3<712::AID-ANR121>3.0.CO;2-1
30. Denton CP, Zheng B, Evans LA et al (2003) Fibroblast-specific expression of a kinase-deficient type II transforming growth factor beta (TGFbeta) receptor leads to paradoxical activation of TGFbeta signaling pathways with fibrosis in transgenic mice. J Biol Chem 278(27):25109–25119. doi:10.1074/jbc.M300636200
31. Denton CP, Lindahl GE, Khan K et al (2005) Activation of key profibrotic mechanisms in transgenic fibroblasts expressing kinase-deficient type II transforming growth factor-{beta} receptor (T{beta}RII{delta}k). J Biol Chem 280(16):16053–16065. doi:10.1074/jbc.M413134200
32. Beyer C, Schramm A, Akhmetshina A et al (2012) Beta-catenin is a central mediator of pro-fibrotic Wnt signaling in systemic sclerosis. Ann Rheum Dis 71(5):761–767. doi:10.1136/annrheumdis-2011-200568

33. Ito K, Sawamura D, Goto M et al (2009) Keratinocyte−/fibroblast-targeted rescue of Col7a1-disrupted mice and generation of an exact dystrophic epidermolysis bullosa model using a human COL7A1 mutation. Am J Pathol 175(6):2508–2517. doi:10.2353/ajpath.2009.090347
34. Zheng B, Zhang Z, Black CM et al (2002) Ligand-dependent genetic recombination in fibroblasts: a potentially powerful technique for investigating gene function in fibrosis. Am J Pathol 160(5):1609–1617. doi:10.1016/S0002-9440(10)61108-X
35. Florin L, Alter H, Grone HJ et al (2004) Cre recombinase-mediated gene targeting of mesenchymal cells. Genesis 38(3):139–144. doi:10.1002/gene.20004
36. Muzumdar MD, Tasic B, Miyamichi K et al (2007) A global double-fluorescent Cre reporter mouse. Genesis 45(9):593–605. doi:10.1002/dvg.20335
37. Indra AK, Warot X, Brocard J et al (1999) Temporally-controlled site-specific mutagenesis in the basal layer of the epidermis: comparison of the recombinase activity of the tamoxifen-inducible Cre-ER(T) and Cre-ER(T2) recombinases. Nucleic Acids Res 27(22):4324–4327. doi:10.1093/nar/27.22.4324
38. Lelli KM, Slattery M, Mann RS (2012) Disentangling the many layers of eukaryotic transcriptional regulation. Annu Rev Genet 46:43–68. doi:10.1146/annurev-genet-110711-155437
39. Heintzman ND, Stuart RK, Hon G et al (2007) Distinct and predictive chromatin signatures of transcriptional promoters and enhancers in the human genome. Nat Genet 39(3):311–318. doi:10.1038/ng1966
40. Heintzman ND, Hon GC, Hawkins RD et al (2009) Histone modifications at human enhancers reflect global cell-type-specific gene expression. Nature 459(7243):108–112. doi:10.1038/nature07829
41. Consortium EP (2012) An integrated encyclopedia of DNA elements in the human genome. Nature 489(7414):57–74. doi:10.1038/nature11247
42. Pennacchio LA, Ahituv N, Moses AM et al (2006) In vivo enhancer analysis of human conserved non-coding sequences. Nature 444(7118):499–502. doi:10.1038/nature05295

Part II

Cell Culture Models

Chapter 11

Isolation and Culture of Primary Murine Hepatic Stellate Cells

Sabine Weiskirchen, Carmen G. Tag, Sibille Sauer-Lehnen, Frank Tacke, and Ralf Weiskirchen

Abstract

Hepatic stellate cells (HSCs) are found in the perisinusoidal space of the liver (i.e., the space of Dissé). They represent 5–8% of the total number of liver cells. In normal liver, these cells have a quiescent phenotype and are characterized by numerous fat vacuoles that store vitamin A in a form of retinyl ester. In injured liver, these cells transdifferentiate into a myofibroblast phenotype, become highly proliferative and are responsible for excess collagen synthesis and deposition during fibrosis. Due to their exceptional pathophysiological relevance, several isolation and purification protocols of primary HSCs have been established that provide the basis for studying HSC biology in vitro. We here describe a method for high-purity isolation of HSCs from mice. This protocol includes the enzymatic digestion of the liver tissue by pronase and collagenase, cellular enrichment by centrifugation of the crude cell suspension through a Nycodenz density gradient, and a final (optional) flow cytometric enrichment that allows generating ultrapure HSC fractions.

Key words Hepatic stellate cells, Myofibroblasts, Nycodenz, FACS, Density gradient, Desmin, Phalloidin

1 Introduction

Based on their central role in the pathogenesis of chronic liver disease, HSCs have been the focus of many studies during the last decades [1]. They are the primary cell type in the liver responsible for scar tissue formation during fibrosis. Understanding HSC biology is therefore considered a promising basis to identify novel therapeutic options designed to attenuate or even reverse extracellular matrix production. First protocols for the isolation of HSCs were established in 1982 [2]. In the respective protocol, HSCs were released from rat liver by digesting the liver with pronase E and collagenase and enriched by metrizamide density centrifugation and centrifugal elutriation resulting in a final cell fraction that contained more than 70% of HSCs [2]. Subsequently, protocols

Laure Rittié (ed.), *Fibrosis: Methods and Protocols*, Methods in Molecular Biology, vol. 1627, DOI 10.1007/978-1-4939-7113-8_11,

were established that introduced a few other compounds for preparing continuous or discontinuous density gradients. These were made of arabinogalactan (Stractan) [3, 4], metrizamide (Amipaque) [5], iohexol (Nycodenz) [6–8], iodixanol (OptiPrep) [9, 10], or colloidal silica particles that are coated with polyvinylpyrrolidone (Percoll) [11]. All these protocols take advantage of the fact that the average volume of parenchymal cells (i.e., hepatocytes) is an order of magnitude higher than that of HSCs and that the retinoid content of HSCs results in a significant lower cell density, allowing HSCs to float on the diverse gradient materials. This is the reason why most of these pioneering protocols used livers from old, fatty rats as cell donors that are particularly suitable when choosing density centrifugation for enrichment.

In the past, all these "conventional" HSC isolation procedures have long been considered the "gold standard" methodology to purify fairly large numbers of HSCs with a morphologically acceptable purity and a typical "HSC phenotype." When these cells are kept in primary culture on uncoated ordinary culture dishes, the cells characteristically become activated and undergo the typical gradual phenotypic transition from a quiescent, retinoid-containing cell type to an activated, highly proliferative, fat- and retinoid-losing phenotype. This transdifferentiation process mimics the hallmarks of this cell type that also occur during hepatic fibrosis. However, although these "purified HSCs" had significantly contributed to the knowledge in HSC biology for many years, the contamination with other cell types may lead to falsification or misinterpretation of some experimental in vitro data. Particularly, such experimental hindrances may become visible when highly sensitive techniques are applied (e.g., qRT-PCR) or findings at the single cell level (e.g., single cell sequencing) are interpreted. Moreover, different methods for HSC isolation, which leverage distinct properties of HSCs, showed that the HSC population in a healthy, uninjured liver is heterogeneous with regard to its capacity for retinoid and lipid storage and expression of HSC activation markers [12]. Therefore, nearly two decades ago, first attempts were made to isolate HSCs from rats by use of side scatter-activated cell sorting that allowed to sort on average $1.4 \pm 0.4 \times 10^6$ cells with practically feasible sorting runs for up to 4 h resulting in more than 5.0×10^6 highly purified viable cells [13].

However, there is today an urgent need to isolate highly pure HSCs from a wide range of transgenic mouse models. Therefore, we and others have developed novel fluorescence-activated cell sorting (FACS) or magnetic cell sorting (MACS) protocols that are suitable for isolating ultrapure HSCs from mouse livers [14–16]. In principle, these FACS-based purification strategies take advantage of the endogenous retinoid fluorescence of HSCs that can be used for separation in FACS machines that are equipped with a UV laser, allowing to distinguish these cells by their vitamin A-specific autofluorescence from other cell subpopulations.

In the following, we provide a standard operation protocol for the isolation of primary mouse HSCs that includes the classical enzymatic digestion of the liver tissue, cellular enrichment by centrifugation through a discontinuous Nycodenz density gradient, and an optional UV light flow cytometric sorting step allowing the optimal purification of HSCs.

2 Materials

2.1 Animals

The mice that we used in the outlined experiments were from a C57BL/6 genetic background and generated by in-house crossings. However, this protocol is also suitable for mice from other genetic backgrounds (e.g., Balb/c). The optimal weight of animals that we use for HSC isolation is 20–25 g, which is typically reached at the age of 20–50 weeks. The animals were housed at four to five mice per cage in a room maintained at constant 20 °C with a relative humidity of 50% and a 12 h on/off light cycle. The animals had free access to a regular standard mouse chow and trap water. In our animal facility, the animals are housed under specific-pathogen-free conditions, according to the guidelines of the Federation for Laboratory Animal Science Associations (FELASA).

2.2 Instruments

1. Standard laboratory equipment.
1. Heated water bath.
2. Magnetic stirrer.
3. Peristaltic pump with sterile hoses.
4. Precooled centrifuges.
5. Perfusion system.
6. Sterile surgical instruments and preparation tools (scissors, forceps, bulldog clamp).
7. Electric shaver.
8. Adhesive tapes for mouse fixation.
9. Sterile 50 ml plastic tubes.
10. Pasteur pipettes.
11. Standard cell culture room equipped with a sterile hood and a humidified incubator with 5% CO_2 fumigation.
12. Cell culture plates (Petri dishes, 12-well plates).
13. 70 μm cell strainer.
14. Cannula (Luer Lock, 1.5 × 120 mm, chromed brass neck, stainless beveled steel tip) for preparing Nycodenz gradient.
15. 10 ml Luer Lock syringes.
16. Venous cannula G16 (Luer Lock, 2.0 × 70 mm).

17. Sterile Erlenmeyer flask.
18. Cell sorter.
19. FACS collection tubes.
20. Cell counting chamber.
21. Glass slides (poly-L-lysine coated).
22. Tissue culture plates.
23. Light/fluorescence microscope.

2.3 Reagents

All materials must be sterile filtered with a 0.20 μm filter or autoclaved at 121 °C for 20 min and kept at 4 °C until use. The formulation of Perfusion buffer 1 and Perfusion buffer 2 was slightly modified from an established protocol for isolation of rat HSC. In the respective protocol, these buffers were named SC-1 and SC-2 [17].

1. Perfusion buffer 1 (SC-1): 8 g/l NaCl, 400 mg/l KCl, 78 mg/l $NaH_2PO_4 \cdot H_2O$, 151 mg/l $Na_2HPO_4 \cdot 2\ H_2O$, 2.38 g/l HEPES, 350 mg/l $NaHCO_3$, 190 mg/l EGTA, 900 mg/l glucose, and 6 mg/l phenol red. Adjust pH to 7.3–7.4 with 10 M NaOH.
2. Perfusion buffer 2 (SC-2): 8 g/l NaCl, 400 mg/l KCl, 78 mg/l $NaH_2PO_4 \cdot H_2O$, 151 mg/l $Na_2HPO_4 \cdot 2\ H_2O$, 2.38 g/l HEPES, 350 mg/l $NaHCO_3$, 560 mg/l $CaCl_2$ 2 H_2O, and 6 mg/l phenol red. Adjust pH to 7.3–7.4 using 10 M NaOH.
3. Gey's balanced salt solution (GBSS): 370 mg/l KCl, 210 mg/l $MgCl_2 \cdot 6\ H_2O$, 70 mg/l $MgSO_4 \cdot 7\ H_2O$, 75 mg/l $Na_2HPO_4 \cdot 2\ H_2O$, 30 mg/l KH_2PO_4, 991 mg/l glucose, 227 mg/l $NaHCO_3$, 225 mg/l $CaCl_2 \times 2\ H_2O$, 8 g/l NaCl, and 6 mg/l phenol red. Adjust pH to 7.3–7.4 with 10 M NaOH.
4. GBSS for Nycodenz solution: GBSS without 8 g/l NaCl.
5. Xylazine hydrochloride.
6. Ketamine hydrochloride.
7. 70% ethanol (v/v, in water) or approved polyalcohol antiseptic for the skin (we use a colorless one that contains 70% (v/v) 2-propanol, water, butane-1,3-diol, perfume oil, and traces of quinoline yellow).
8. Hank's balanced salt solution (HBSS) (without Ca^{2+}/Mg^{2+}): 0.4 g KCl, 0.06 g KH_2PO_4, 8 g NaCl, 0.35 g $NaHCO_3$, 0.048 g Na_2HPO_4, and 1 g D-glucose per liter of water.
9. Phosphate-buffered saline (PBS): 8 g NaCl, 0.2 g KCl, 1.44 g Na_2HPO_4, and 0.24 g KH_2PO_4 are dissolved in water, adjusted with 1 M HCl to pH 7.4, and filled to 1 liter.
10. Sheath fluid: 1X HBSS supplemented with 4.7 ml/l of 7.5% sodium bicarbonate solution.

11. FACS sort buffer: HBSS supplemented with 10 mM 4-(2-hydroxyethyl)-1-piperazineethanesulfonic acid (HEPES), 0.06% (w/v) bovine serum albumin (BSA), and 0.3 mM EDTA and adjusted to pH 7.3–7.4 with 10 M NaOH.
12. FACS collection buffer: HBSS supplemented with 10 mM HEPES and 20% (v/v) fetal bovine serum (FBS).
13. 0.5 mg/ml pronase E (EC 3.4.24.4, 4.000.000 PU/g) from *Streptomyces griseus*, in Perfusion buffer 2. The solution should be freshly prepared and sterilized by filtration (0.20 μm) (*see* **Note 1**).
14. 0.75 U/ml collagenase P (EC 3.4.24.3) from *Clostridium histolyticum* in Perfusion buffer 2. The solution should be freshly prepared and sterilized by filtration (0.20 μm) (*see* **Note 1**).
15. 0.4 mg/ml pronase E, 1.5 U/ml collagenase P in Perfusion buffer 2. The solution should be freshly prepared and sterilized by filtration (0.20 μm) (*see* **Note 1**).
16. 2 mg/ml DNase I, grade II, from bovine pancreas (EC 3.1.21.1) in GBSS. Sterilize by filtration (0.20 μm) and store in 1 ml aliquots at −20 °C.
17. 28.6% (w/v) Nycodenz in GBSS without NaCl. Sterilize by filtration (0.20 μm) and store at 4 °C. The final concentration during the density gradient centrifugation prepared from this stock solution is 8% (w/v). Please note that other compounds for preparation of density gradients suitable for HSC preparation are available (*see* **Note 2**). If you choose another compound, you have to adapt the concentration to form optimal gradients for HSC isolation.
18. Triton X-100.
19. Monoclonal rabbit anti-mouse desmin antibody. We use clone Y66 (Cat#NB110-56931, Novus Biologicals LLC, R&D Systems, Abingdon, UK), which was generated using a synthetic peptide corresponding to the C-terminus of human desmin and is reactive against desmin of human, mouse, rat, and guinea pig. Prepared aliquots and stored at −20 °C.
20. Labeled anti-rabbit IgGs. We use the freeze-dried powder of the Cy3 AffiniPure Fab fragment donkey anti-rabbit IgG (H + L) (Cat#711-167-003, Jackson ImmunoResearch Laboratories Inc., Suffolk, UK). Rehydrate to 1.0 mg/ml with distilled water, and store aliquots at −80 °C.
21. 0.4% trypan blue solution (w/v): The ready-to-use, sterile filtered solution is stored at room temperature.
22. Rhodamine phalloidin. We use the one from Molecular Probe (Cat#R415, Thermo Fisher Scientific GmbH) to label F-actin. Reconstitute in methanol to a final concentration of 200 U/l

(~6.6 μM). This stock solution is stable for at least 1 year when stored frozen at −20 °C.

23. 4% paraformaldehyde (w/v) in PBS. Mix 4 g of extra pure paraformaldehyde with 60 ml sterile water and heat to 60 °C while stirring on a heated magnetic stirrer. Slowly add two or three drops of 2 M NaOH until the solution becomes almost clear. Turn the heater off, and add 33.3 ml of 3 × PBS (0.411 M NaCl, 8.1 mM KCl, 30 mM Na_2HPO_4, 5.4 mM KH_2PO_4). Adjust pH to 7.2 with 1 M HCl and store in aliquots at −20 °C until use.
24. 5 mg/ml 4′,6-diamidino-2-phenylindole (DAPI): stains preferentially double-stranded DNA and is used for nuclear counterstain. Dissolve 10 mg DAPI (the entire vial) in 2 ml deionized, sterile water. This stock solution is stable for at least 6 months when stored protected from light at −20 °C.
25. Dulbecco's Modified Eagle medium (DMEM) with 4.5 g/l glucose without L-glutamine.
26. 200 mM L-glutamine: This solution contains 29.23 mg/ml L-glutamine in 0.85% (w/v) NaCl solution and should be "tissue culture grade."
27. Penicillin-streptomycin solution: This bacteriostatic and bactericidal solution contains 10.000 IU potassium penicillin and 10 mg streptomycin sulfate per ml.
28. FBS, tissue culture grade.
29. HSC culture medium: 10% FBS, 4 mM L-glutamine, 1% penicillin-streptomycin solution in DMEM.
30. Trypsin/EDTA solution for dissociation of cell monolayers.

3 Methods

The outlined protocol allows purifying approximately 0.5–2 × 10^6 HSCs from one mouse. In our laboratory, we successively prepare three to five mice in a batch to obtain sufficient amounts of cells for subsequent in vitro experiments. The optimal workflow when preparing more than one mouse requires two well-trained persons working in parallel. One person performs the in situ perfusion of the liver and the in vitro digestion; the other person takes care of the FACS sorter setup, FACS, and seeding of the cells. The different steps take about 4 h for preparation of single cell suspension, 1 h for separating HSCs from parenchymal cells by gradient centrifugation, and 1–2 h for FACS. Additional times may be necessary for setup and calibration of FACS machine.

All experiments depicted here were approved by the official state animal care and use committee (LANUV, Recklinghausen, Germany). The implementation of this protocol at other locations may require approval by authorities that are responsible for respective localities. All experiments were conducted in accordance with the German federal law regarding the protection of animals and *Guide for the Care and Use of Laboratory Animals* (National Institutes of Health publication 8th Edition, 2011).

All surgical procedures are carried out under clean conditions. Therefore, all surgical forceps and scissors that are needed during the procedure are sterilized prior usage according to the guidelines necessary to perform surgeries in animals. The method described here is optimized for the isolation of HSC from the livers of five mice, while other hepatic cell fractions are discarded during the purification (*see* **Note 3**).

In the described protocol, the liver is first perfused with solutions containing pronase and collagenase. Thereafter, the liver cells are dispersed from the digested liver and further purified by centrifugation on a discontinuous Nycodenz density gradient. The individual steps are schematically summarized in Fig. 1.

3.1 Surgical Procedures and Liver Perfusion

1. Anesthetize the mouse by intraperitoneal injection with 6–8 mg/kg body weight xylazine and 90–120 mg/kg body weight of ketamine. Anesthesia is sufficient when the following vital criteria are reached: regular spontaneous breathing, no reflex after setting of pain stimuli between toes, and no response to pain.
2. Shave the operation area with an electric fur shaver.
3. Sterilize the shaved abdominal skin with 70% ethanol (or an approved polyalcohol antiseptic for the skin).
4. Place the mouse on the working surface and fix the limbs with tapes so that the animal stays as straight as possible. Optional: cover the operational area with a fluid-impermeable, self-adhesive drape (Fig. 2a).
5. Open the abdomen with a midline laparotomy up to the sternum by cutting the cutis plus fascia at the same time with an 11.5 cm surgical scissor (Fig. 2b).
6. Cut the peritoneum along the *linea alba* to open the peritoneal cavity (Fig. 2c, d). Expose the abdominal cavity as wide as possible.
7. Place the intestine sideways and lift the liver with a cotton swab so that the ventral side sticks to the diaphragm and the *hilum* is clearly visible. The portal vein is now exposed (Fig. 2e).
8. Setup and actuate the liver perfusion system by equilibrating it with sterile, prewarmed Perfusion buffer 1. Important: To avoid contaminations, it is essential that the hoses of the perfusion system are autoclaved. Allow the water bath to reach the correct temperature (37 °C), place a Microlance hypodermic needle (26 G cannula) at the end of the hose system, and

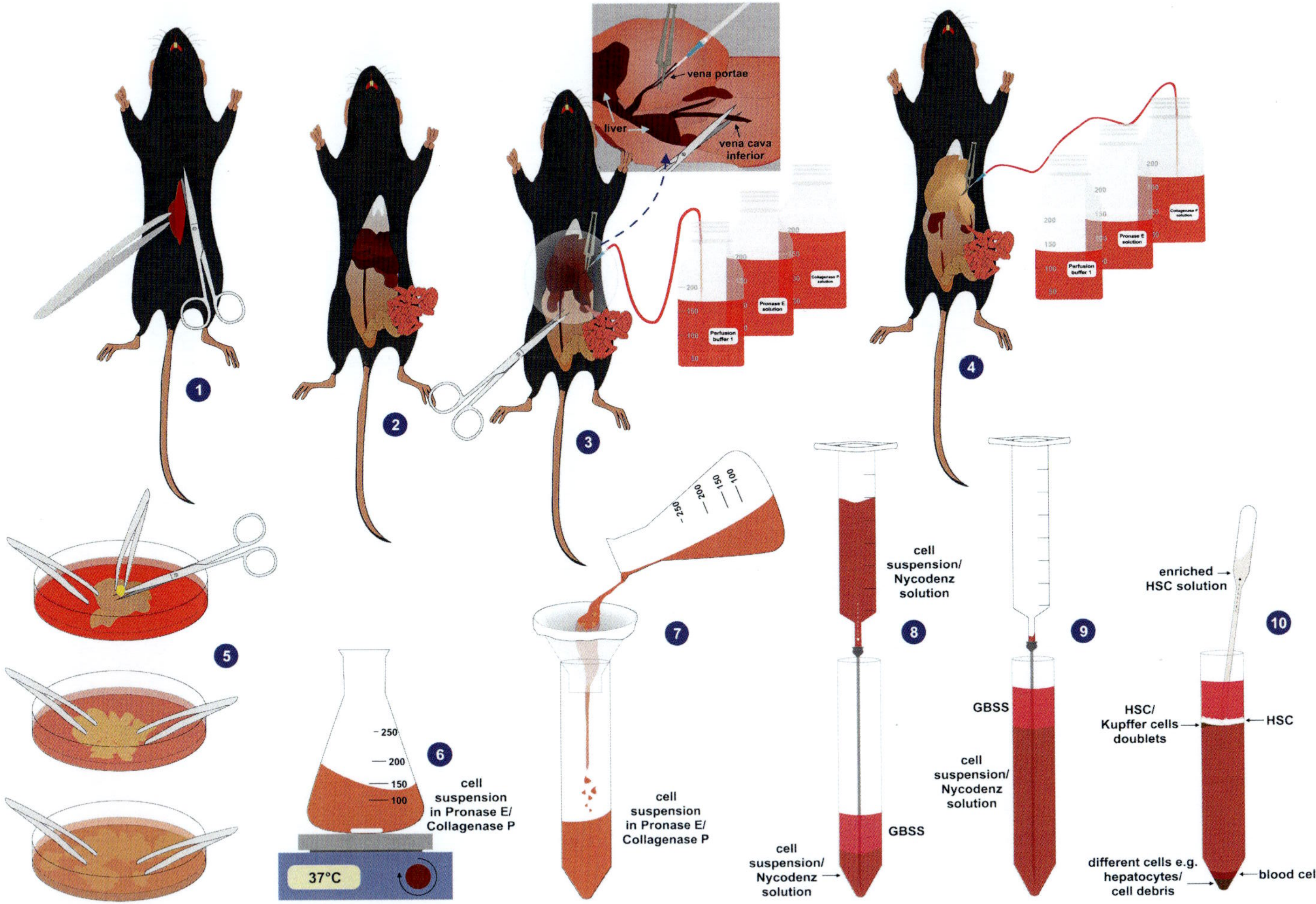

Fig. 1 Schematic overview of the protocol for isolation of murine HSC. In a first step, the mouse is anesthetized and the abdominal cavity is opened (*1*). The liver is exposed by placing the intestine to the side (*2*). Then the liver is perfused through the portal vein (*3*) with different enzymatic perfusion solutions (*4*). The liver cells are dispersed in a sterile plastic culture dish (*5*). Remaining cell clumps are dissolved by stirring at 37 °C on a magnetic stirrer (*6*). Thereafter, the solution is filtered through a mesh (*7*) and prepared for density centrifugation. Therefore, the cell suspension is supplemented with Nycodenz solution and layered under GBSS (*8, 9*). After centrifugation, HSCs are enriched in the white shining interphase, while hepatocytes and blood cells are found at the bottom of the gradient (*10*). For details of each step, refer to the text

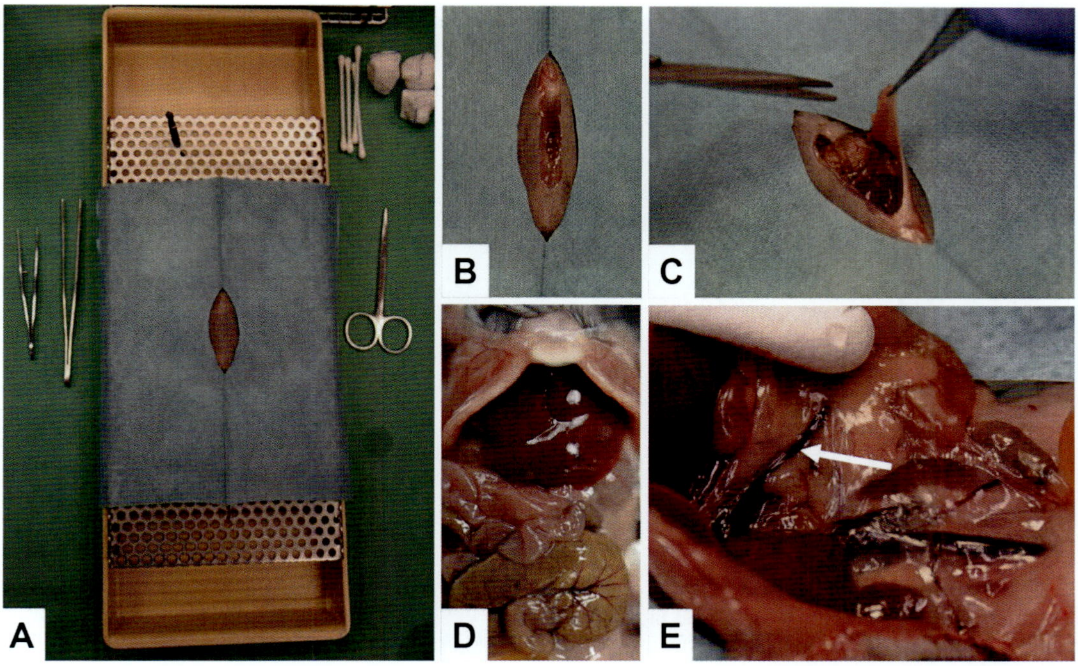

Fig. 2 Experimental setup for isolation of murine HSC. (**a**) Prior to starting, the work space is prepared and the sterilized instrumentation is arranged. The anesthetized and shaved mouse is placed onto the working area and prepared for surgery. (**b**, **c**) The abdomen is opened. (**d**) The liver is uncovered, and (**e**) the ventral side of the liver is lifted with a cotton swab so that the portal vein is freely exposed (marked with a *white arrow*)

remove all air bubbles within the system. Set the flow rate of the perfusion pump to 6.5 ml/min.

9. Stop the perfusion pump and insert the cannula of the perfusion set in the portal vein (parallel to the orientation of the vein, close to where the splenic vein is entering the portal vein) in the direction to the liver (Fig. 3a).

10. Fix the cannula at the portal vein with a bulldog clamp in the middle of the injection site and the cannula tip (Fig. 3b). Ensure that you simultaneously clamp the silvery bile duct to guarantee that the perfusion buffers flows through the liver. Make sure that the bulldog clamp does not squeeze the *vena cava inferior*.

11. Start the perfusion pump and immediately cut the *vena cava inferior* with sharp scissors (Fig. 3c) to reduce the pressure within the liver. Perfusion buffer 1 now flows through the liver.

12. Perfuse the liver for 4 h and 30 min with a flow rate of 6.5 ml/min (Fig. 3d).

13. Stop the perfusion pump and carefully change Perfusion buffer 1 to prewarmed pronase E solution (prewarmed at 37 °C). Take care not to introduce bubbles into the perfusion system.

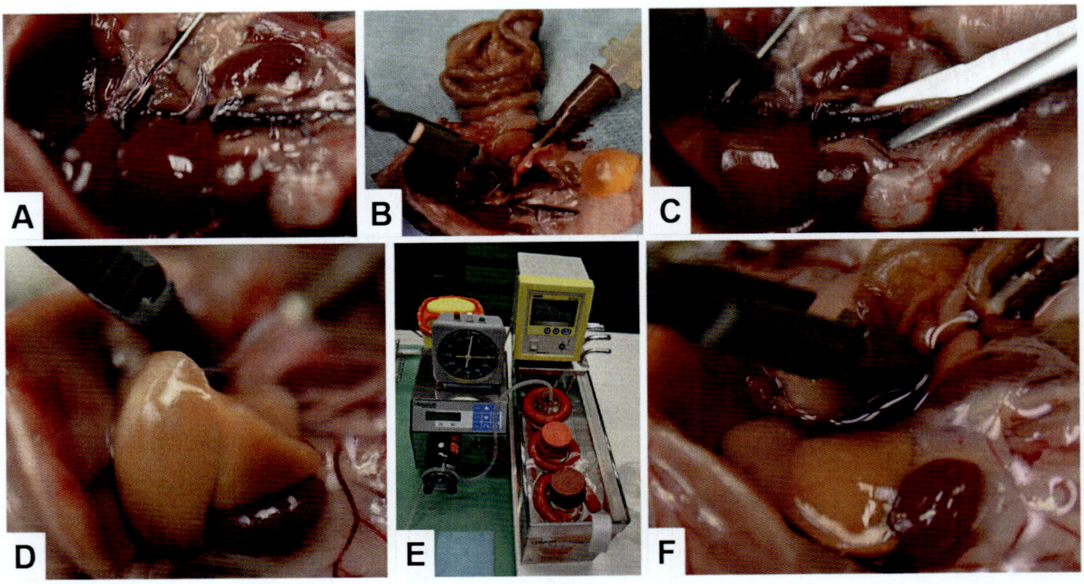

Fig. 3 Liver perfusion. (**a**) A cannula is carefully plugged into the portal vein without rupturing the vessel wall and (**b**) positioned into a stable position by fixing it with a bulldog clamp. (**c**) The *vena cava inferior* is cut with scissors and (**d**) the peristaltic pump started allowing the perfusion buffer to flow freely through the liver. (**e**) During the complete liver perfusion, the perfusion buffers are prewarmed to 37 °C by storing them in a heated water bath. (**f**) The perfusion is successively continued with different perfusion solutions. During this process, the liver is cleaned from blood (visible by a change from *dark red* to *brown*), and the ongoing enzymatic digestion is associated with a swelling of the liver lobules and a loss of the typical liver shape

In our laboratory, we prewarm all buffers during the perfusion process in a water bath. To change buffers, we only shift the hose of the perfusion apparatus into the next flasks, while the other flasks that are not in use are closed with a cover (Fig. 3e).

14. Perfuse the liver for 4 h and 30 min with a flow rate of 6.5 ml/min.
15. Again, stop the perfusion pump and change buffer to collagenase P solution. Start the pump and perfuse the liver for 4 h and 30 min with a flow rate of 6.5 ml/min. Ongoing enzymatic digestion is reflected by swelling of the liver lobules and loss of typical liver shape (Fig. 3f). When the liver is digested (Fig. 4a, b), immediately cut the thoracic part of the *vena cava inferior* and stop the inflow before air enters the liver.
16. Separate the liver from the gastric band and cut the *arteria hepatica* with small scissors.
17. Gently remove the liver (take care not to damage the liver capsule) from the body cavity with sterile forceps (Fig. 4c). To do so, grab the liver carefully with large tweezers to avoid leakage.

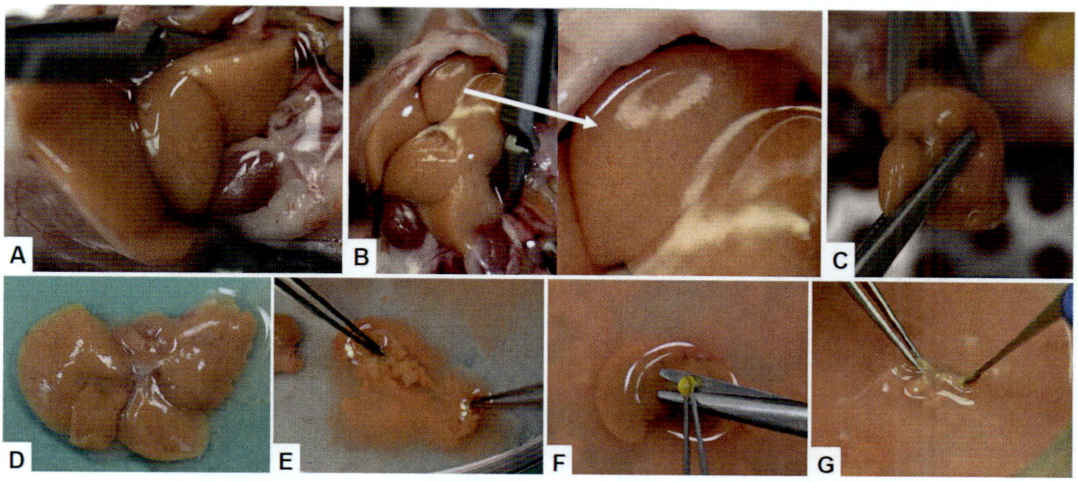

Fig. 4 Removal of digested liver and releasing of dispersed cells. (**a**, **b**) After successful digestion, the liver architecture is amorphous and has a very light color. (**c**) The liver is grabbed with anatomic tweezers and removed from the abdominal cavity. (**d**) The typical appearance of a digested liver is shown. (**e**) The Glisson's capsule removed to release the dispersed cells. (**f**) The gallbladder is carefully removed, and (**g**) the digested liver is grabbed with forceps and intensively shaken to release the dispersed cells

3.2 In Vitro Liver Digestion

1. Place the liver into a 50 ml plastic tube on ice with 20 ml pronase E/collagenase P solution and start to prepare the next mice following the advice given above. Collect all livers in this tube. The following steps are optimized for a total amount of five livers. In case of different numbers of livers, the protocol can be adapted accordingly.
2. Transfer all digested livers into a sterile Petri dish. The typical appearance of the liver is depicted in Fig. 4d.
3. Add 1 ml DNase I solution.
4. Remove the Glisson's capsule of each liver and disperse the liver cells with the help of tweezers (Fig. 4e–g). Remove the gallbladder (that is normally colored yellow) using scissors and tweezers. At the end of this process, the liver tissue is completely disbanded, and only a few cell clumps remain.
5. Transfer this cell suspension into a sterile Erlenmeyer flask, in which a magnetic stir bar is placed. Fill up to a volume of 120 ml with prewarmed, sterile pronase E/collagenase P solution (Fig. 5a).
6. Remove the remaining cell clumps by carefully stirring the cell suspension at 37 °C for 20 min (Fig. 5b). During the digestion, adjust the pH with 1 M NaOH: the Perfusion buffer 2 should keep its red color (phenol red) indicating pH 7.4. Typically, one drop of 1 M NaOH is required every other minute.

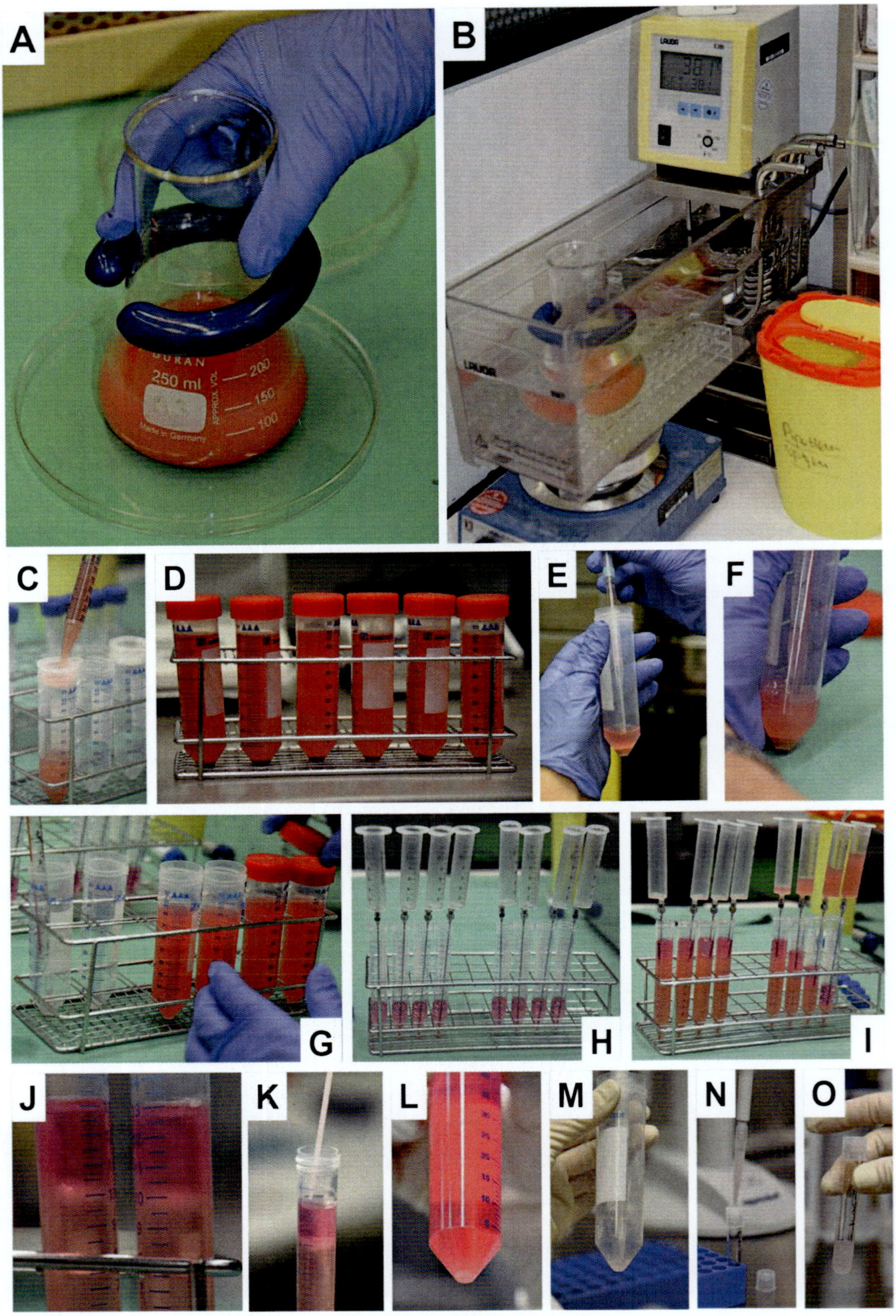

Fig. 5 Enrichment of hepatic stellate cells by Nycodenz gradient centrifugation. (**a**) The tissue cell suspension is transferred into a sterile 250 ml glass Erlenmeyer flask, in which a magnetic stir bar is placed. (**b**) Remaining cell clumps in the cell suspension are removed by stirring at low speed at 37 °C. (**c**) The cell suspension is filtered into six 50 ml plastic tubes. (**d**, **e**) After centrifugation, the supernatant is removed. (**f**, **g**) The cell pellets are then resuspended in GBSS, DNase I is added, and the suspension is combined into four 50 ml plastic tubes and centrifuged. (**h**, **i**) Preparation of 15 ml tubes for Nycodenz density centrifugation (~two tubes for each animal).

7. Filter the dispersed cell suspensions through a 70 μm cell strainer (Fig. 5c) into six 50 ml plastic tubes (~20 ml per tube). Thereafter, fill each tube up to 50 ml with cold Perfusion buffer 2 (Fig. 5d) and centrifuge them for 10 min at 4 °C and 600 *g*.
8. Remove the supernatants with a sterile Pasteur pipette (Fig. 5e) and resuspend each pellet in 10 ml cold GBSS.
9. Add 150 μL DNase I solution to the cell suspensions (Fig. 5f). Combine all suspensions into four 50 ml plastic tubes (Fig. 5g). Fill up the tubes with cold GBSS and centrifuge again for 10 min at 4 °C and 600 *g*.
10. After centrifugation, aspirate the supernatants completely with a sterile Pasteur pipette. Resuspend each pellet in 10 ml cold GBBS, add 150 μL DNase I, and pool pellets into two 50 ml plastic tubes.

3.3 Nycodenz Density Gradient Centrifugation

1. Fill up each tube to 36.0 ml with cold GBSS and add 14.0 ml Nycodenz solution to each tube to reach a final Nycodenz concentration of 8% (w/v) and mix the solution by carefully inverting the tubes several times.
2. Arrange ten 15 ml plastic tubes into a rack and pre-fill each tube with 1.5 ml cold GBSS (~two tubes/animal). Place a sterile barrel with a special Luer Lock cannula (120 mm, autoclaved) into each tube (Fig. 5h).
3. Fill 10 ml of the cell/Nycodenz solution into each syringe. The solution flows through the cannula under the pre-filled GBSS (Fig. 5i).
4. Centrifuge the tubes for 22 min at 4 °C and 1500 *g* (without break).
5. After centrifugation, a pellet containing hepatocytes (brown) and blood cells (red) is visible in each tube. HSCs are found in the interphase of both solutions. They appear as a white condensed band (Fig. 5j). Collect the respective cell fractions that accumulate from the different gradients (Fig. 5k) and combine them in a 50 ml plastic tube. For this step, we recommend to use a blunt cannula made out of plastic and a smooth operating syringe, in which the plunger is equipped with a manual rubber stopper.

Fig. 5 (continued) (**j**) After density centrifugation, HSCs can be identified as a white cell layer that is floating at the surface of the gradient. (**k**) The HSC-containing layers are collected and combined, filled with GBSS, and centrifuged again. (**l**) After centrifugation, a white pellet is visible. (**m**) The supernatant is removed, resuspended in FACS sort buffer, and (**n**) filtered through a 40 μm filter. (**o**) The solution is now ready for FACS

6. Fill the cell suspension to 50 ml with cold GBSS (or FACS sort buffer) and centrifuge for 10 min at 4 °C and 600 *g*, if the cells are intended to be further sorted by FACS. After centrifugation, a clear white pellet containing the enriched fraction of HSCs should be visible at the bottom of the tube (Fig. 5l). For FACS, proceed to Subheading 3.4. If the cells are intended to be cultured without subsequent FACS, resuspend the cell pellet in culture medium as detailed in Subheading 3.7. Surplus of cells may potentially be cryopreserved at this stage (*see* **Note 4**).

3.4 Fluorescence-Activated Cell Sorting (FACS)

Although flow cytometry and FACS have become standard methods for separating individual subsets of cells from heterogeneous populations, there are several potential pitfalls when using these techniques. A good introduction to this technique, its principles, sample preparation, FACS sorter setup, sort strategies, and a troubleshooting guide is given elsewhere [18]. In addition, it should be noticed that all sorters will produce biological/chemical hazards and aerosols that might have potential (bio)safety implications.

In our laboratory, we use the BD FACSAria II SORP Cell sorter that is equipped with a 355 nm UV laser and a 488 nm blue laser. For sorting of HSCs, we use a gating strategy, in which the cells are first gated based on their forward and sideward scattering where smaller and granulated cells are framed. In the gating hierarchy, we perform a doublet discrimination gating, which is recommended by the manufacturer. From the generated single cells, we select the HSCs by their emission of autofluorescence after excitation of vitamin A with a UV laser, which is measured in the "Indo-1" channel of the corresponding detector, passing 505 nm long-pass (505LP) and a 530 ± 30 nm (530/30) band-pass filter. A short overview of the FACS workflow is given in Fig. 6.

1. Setup and activate the FACS machine. For sorting of HSCs, we use the following parameters: sample loading port to 4 °C at 300 rpm, 100 μm nozzle, pressure 20 psi, threshold rate ~ 5000 events/sec, threshold 5000, precision mode purity (yield mask 32, purity mask 32, phase mask 0), and collection device set to 4 °C.
2. Verify that the suitable cytometer configuration for HSC sorting is chosen and perform the calibration steps recommended by the manufacturer. Verify that the side stream formation and the drop break-off are properly adjusted (Fig. 7a–d).
3. Fill the collection tubes with 1 ml FACS collection buffer and set one into the collection device at the position of the left side stream (Fig. 7e).
4. Discard the supernatant from **step 6**, Subheading 3.3 (Fig. 5m), resuspend the cells in FACS buffer, and filter them through a 40 μm filter for FACS (Fig. 5n). After this step the solution should have a white opaque appearance (Fig. 5o).

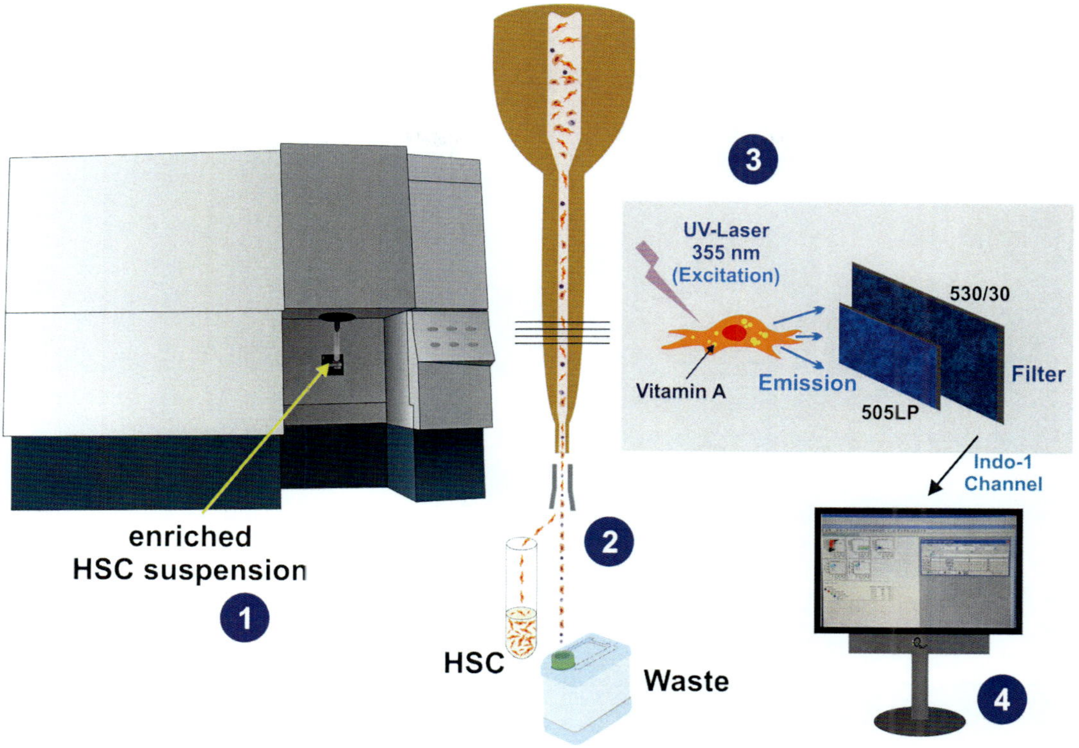

Fig. 6 Schematic overview of the protocol for FACS of murine HSCs. The enriched HSC suspension is placed into the FACS machine (*1*). Sorting of HSCs is done by excitation with UV light from a 355 nm laser (*2*) and measuring the emission resulting from the cellular retinol content in the "Indo-1" channel that uses a 505 nm long-pass and a 530 ± 30 nm band-pass filter (*3*). The sorting is monitored and documented using appropriate hard- and software (*4*). For details of each step, refer to the text

5. Insert the enriched HSC suspension into the sample injection chamber of the FACS sorter and acquire a representative amount of cells (Fig. 7f).
6. Dilute the enriched HSC suspension with FACS sort buffer so that the intended threshold rate during the measurement will not be exceeded and start sorting. During the process you can follow the correct sorting into the HSC vs. waste fractions by inspecting the different streams (Fig. 7g).
7. Based on the chosen gating strategy, sorting of HSCs is done by exciting the cell suspension with a UV laser and measuring the emission in the "Indo-1" channel. The emission measured in the "DAPI" channel (450/50) serves as a control (Fig. 7h). The "Indo-1"-positive population with higher size contains an amount of contaminating cell doublets which should be excluded by adjusting the gate [16, 19].
8. During the cell sorting, the collection tube located in the collection device will fill up with sorted HSCs and buffer. Make sure to change the tubes in time to prevent overload (Fig. 8a–c).

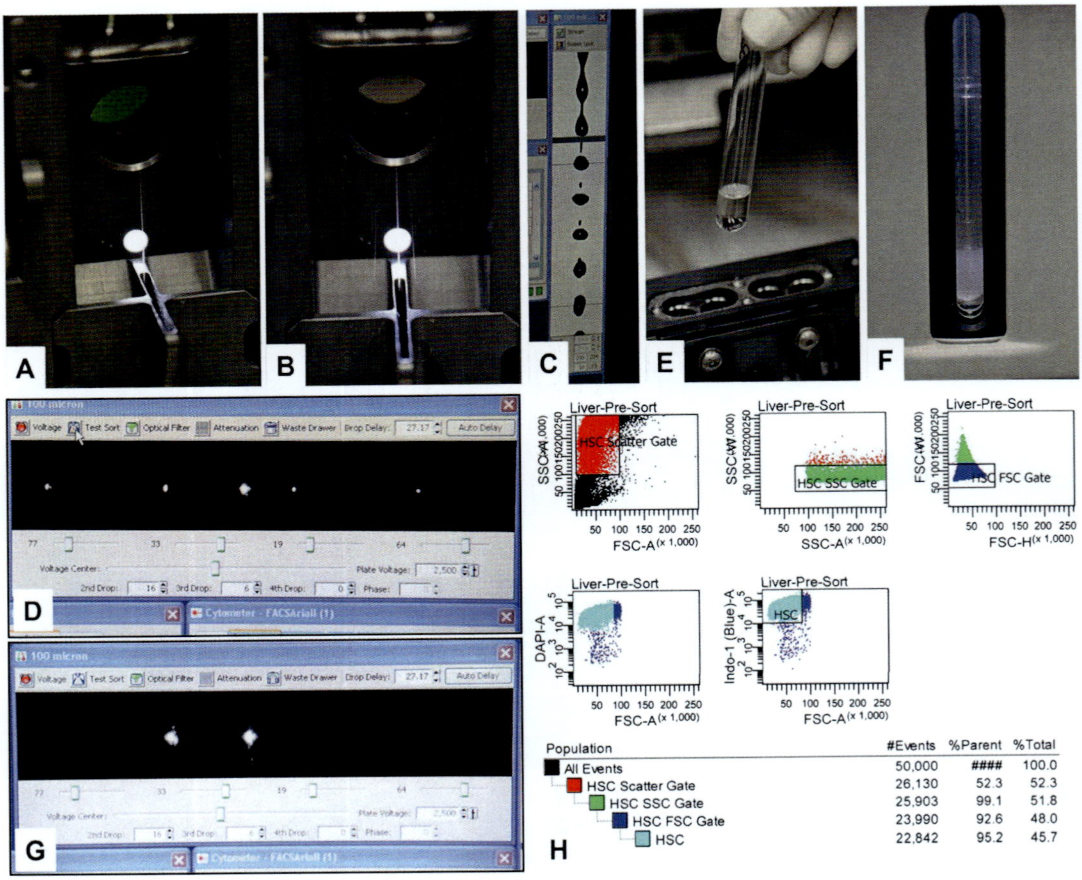

Fig. 7 FACS setup and FACS. The sorting conditions, drop formation, and deflection are crucial in FACS. (**a**–**d**) The side stream formation and the drop break-off are shown as a live image of the corresponding cameras. (**e**) The cells are sorted in the collection device (**f**) after acquiring in the collection chamber. (**g**) Representative results of sorting and cell separation into HSC fraction and waste are depicted. (**h**) Sorting of the cell suspension is conducted using the granularity and autofluorescence of HSC as sorting criteria

9. To confirm successful cell sorting and to determine the purity of the sorted HSC preparation, an aliquot of the sorted suspension is analyzed by FACS. Modify the given gating strategy to include all cells in the forward and sideward scatter ignoring the doublet discrimination and remark the resulting purity in the hierarchy (% parent) (Fig. 8d–f).
10. Centrifuge the collecting tubes at 4 °C for 10 min at 750 *g* without break and discard the supernatants. Resuspend the pellets and pool them into one tube in a total of 1 ml HSC culture medium (Fig. 9a–c). The resulting pellet of ultrapure HSCs harbors a white color with diffuse shape and is very delicate.

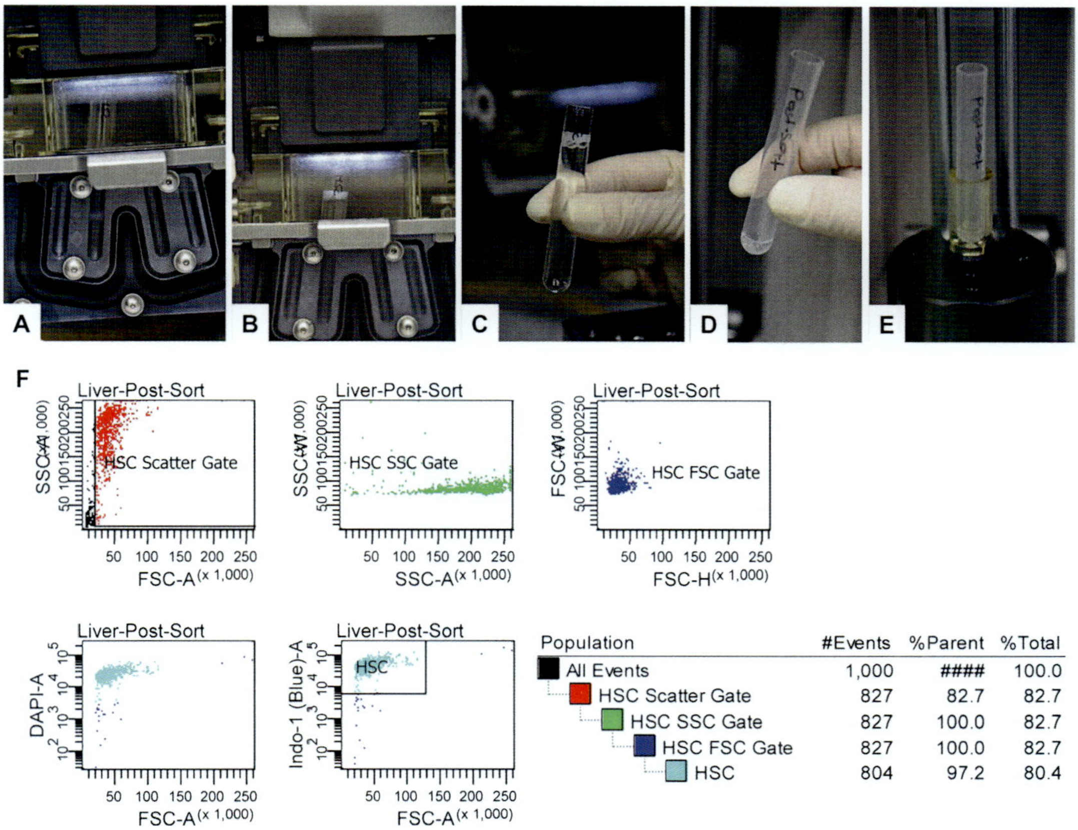

Fig. 8 HSC FACS. (**a**–**e**) For the determination of the purity of sorted HSCs, an aliquot of cells (at least 1000 events) is once analyzed under the same conditions as during the initial sorting. (**f**) The results of a typical "post-sort" purity control run are depicted

3.5 Determination of Cell Yield and Viability

The final yield of the cell isolation will be determined by counting, using an automated cell counter or a hemocytometer. In our laboratory, we determine the number of purified cells in a Neubauer bright-line chamber with a depth of 0.1 mm and a counting area of 0.0025 mm^2 (*see* **Note 5**).

1. Dilute an aliquot of the resuspended cell suspension, e.g., 20 μL with 80 μL of FACS sort buffer, and mix 20 μL of this dilution with 20 μL of trypan blue solution (Fig. 9d–e).
2. Place the cover glass on the top of the Neubauer chamber so that it covers the central counting area. In this step, it is important to achieve the correct depth between the cover glass and the central counting area. To guarantee this we moisten the outer sections with breath and carefully position the slip onto the counting chamber. The formation of multicolor Newton's rings confirms the proper attachment.

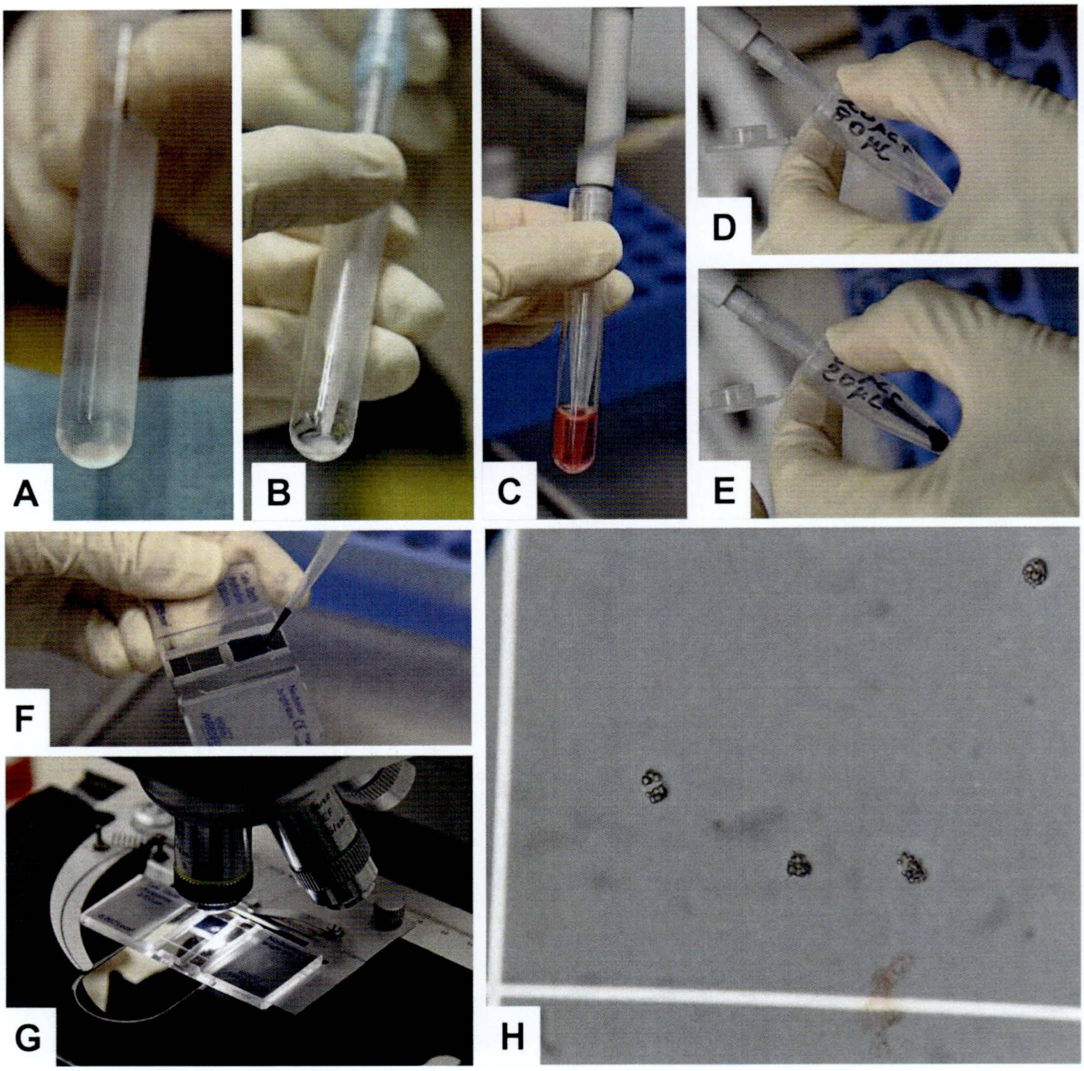

Fig. 9 Cell counting and plating. (**a**, **b**) The FACS-separated HSCs are concentrated by centrifugation and (**c**) resuspended in cell culture medium. (**d–f**) An aliquot of the cell fraction is mixed with trypan blue solution. (**g**, **h**) Viable and dead cells are counted in a counting chamber

3. Load the hemocytometer with 10 μL from the solution prepared in **step 2** (Fig. 9f). Avoid introducing air bubbles into the counting chamber.
4. Place the Neubauer chamber on the microscope stage (Fig. 9g) and count the unstained and stained cells in four big squares in the corners of the central counting area (which is equal to 16 small squares). The staining with trypan blue is a dye exclusion method used to selectively mark dead cells. Vital cells with intact cell membranes do not incorporate the dye, while dead cells appear in blue color. The typical appearance (i.e., high content of fat droplets with their specific bright shine and

rounded cell phenotype) of four cells in a small square of the counting chamber is shown in Fig. 9h.

5. Calculate the total cell number of the cell suspension using the following formula: Total cell number in the cell suspension = (number of counted cells/4) × dilution factor × ml suspension × 10,000.
6. Calculate the viability (%) in the cell suspension using the following formula: Viability (%) = (total number of unstained cells/total number of cells) × 100.

3.6 Determination of Cell Purity

Primary HSCs show some typical characteristics and express some typical markers that are not found in other hepatic cell types. The most typical feature of these cells is the occurrence of large cytoplasmic fat droplets that can be easily detected in microscopy by their high refraction under UV light exhibiting a striking rapidly fading blue–green autofluorescence when excited with 328 nm light. Moreover, these droplets are well represented in Nomarski differential interference-contrast microscopy. The high fat content in early cultures of HSCs can be identified in Oil Red O stain (for a detailed protocol see Ref. 20). In addition, the expression of glial acidic fibrillary protein (GFAP) and desmin is indicative of HSCs. Upon culturing, the expression of α-smooth muscle actin (α-SMA) is also a reliable marker to positively identify HSCs. Conversely, contaminating cells can be identified by staining for the surface markers F4/80, CD68, or CD11b that are present on resident macrophages (i.e., Kupffer cells) and RECA-1 (endothelial cell marker) or by determination of appropriate hepatocyte markers.

In our laboratory, we quantify the purity of cells post-sort using an aliquot (≥1000 events) and the same FACS conditions described above. For determination of purity in a culture, we stain the cells either with rhodamine phalloidin that specifically stains F-actin or with an antibody specific for desmin. For both procedures, the cells are grown on poly-L-lysine-pre-coated glass slides layered into 12-well plates with HSC culture medium. In the following, the two staining procedures for cultured HSC are briefly described.

3.6.1 Phalloidin Stain for Cultured HSCs

1. Remove the cell supernatant from the 12-well plates and wash the cells once with ice cold HBSS (without Ca^{2+}/Mg^{2+}).
2. Fix the cells in ice-cold 4% paraformaldehyde for 20 min on ice.
3. Remove the fixative and wash the cells with ice cold HBSS (without Ca^{2+}/Mg^{2+}).
4. Permeabilize the cells with ice cold PBS supplemented with 0.2% Triton X-100 for 4 min on ice.
5. Remove the solution and wash the cells with ice cold HBSS (without Ca^{2+}/Mg^{2+}).

6. Block the cells with PBS supplemented with 3% BSA for 5 min at room temperature.
7. Cover the cells with the rhodamine phalloidin conjugate (diluted 1:40 with PBS) and incubate at room temperature for 20 min.
8. Remove the staining solution and wash the cells three times with HBSS (without Ca^{2+}/Mg^{2+}).
9. For counterstaining of nuclei, incubate the cells with 0.1 µg/ml DAPI in HBSS (without Ca^{2+}/Mg^{2+}) for 5 min at room temperature.
10. Remove the staining solution and wash the cells three times with HBSS (without Ca^{2+}/Mg^{2+}).
11. Collect the glass slide using forceps, air-dry the cells, drop on an appropriate mounting medium onto the cell layer, place upside down on a microscope slide, and seal with nail polish. Keep the cells shielded from direct light to prevent photobleaching. At this stage, the slides can be stored at 4 °C for up to 6 months.
12. Documentation of successful staining is done under a fluorescent microscope using a red filter ("rhodamine filter") and appropriate objectives and oculars.

3.6.2 Desmin Stain for Cultured HSC

1. Wash, fix, permeabilize, and block the cells as described in **steps 1–6** of Subheading 3.6.1.
2. Cover the cells with a 1:100 dilution of the rabbit anti-desmin antibody prepared in PBS supplemented with 3% BSA. Incubate for 1.5 h at room temperature. As negative controls, you should use PBS with 3% BSA without the antibody and PBS with 3% BSA containing a rabbit isotype control immunoglobulin.
3. Discard the antibody solution and wash the cells with HBSS (without Ca^{2+}/Mg^{2+}).
4. Block the cells in PBS supplemented with 3% BSA for 5 min at room temperature.
5. Discard the blocking solution and add a 1:100 dilution of the Cy3-labeled donkey anti-rabbit antibody prepared in PBS supplemented with 3% BSA. Incubate for 30 min at 37 °C.
6. Remove the antibody solution and wash the cells three times with HBSS (without Ca^{2+}/Mg^{2+}).
7. For counterstaining of nuclei, incubate the cells with 0.1 µg/ml DAPI in HBSS (without Ca^{2+}/Mg^{2+}) for 5 min at room temperature.
8. Remove the DAPI solution and wash the cells three times with HBSS (without Ca^{2+}/Mg^{2+}).
9. Mount the cells and document the results as described in **steps 11** and **12**, Subheading 3.6.1 above.

3.7 Cell Culture

1. Dilute the purified cells (unsorted or sorted) in HSC culture medium and plate the cells at a density of 2×10^4 cells/cm^2 in tissue culture plates. These should be suitable for culturing of sensitive adherent primary cells.
2. Incubate the cells in a humidified incubator with 5% CO_2 at 37 °C.
3. Immediately after cell attachment (around 2 h or overnight), remove the plates to the incubator. As the quiescent HSCs are very fragile, carefully replace the medium with new prewarmed medium without damaging the cell monolayer.
4. The culture process on uncoated plastic will lead to "transdifferentiation," in which the HSCs lose their quiescence resulting in an activated phenotype, in which the cells slowly lose their vitamin droplets and acquire a typical star-shaped morphology. Cell activation is further accompanied by elevated expression of α-SMA and collagen type I.
5. After the cells reach confluence, they can be enzymatically detached from the plates by trypsin/EDTA or accutase and subcultured for four passages. The proteolytic detachment of the primary cells further promotes the activation process that finally results in a myofibroblast phenotype. Some representative images of isolated HSCs that were grown in culture for prolonged times on uncoated plastic are shown in Fig. 10a–c. The typical phenotypic alterations occurring during transdifferentiation are characteristic for primary HSCs and not observed in immortalized HSC cell lines (*see* **Note 6**). The results of a phalloidin stain (Fig. 10d) and a desmin immunocytochemistry (Fig. 10e) show the positivity of HSCs for filament-specific proteins (i.e., F-actin and desmin).
6. The cells that are prepared by this protocol are very homogenous in regard to their phenotypic appearance (*see* **Note 7**).

4 Notes

1. The activity of the necessary enzymes may significantly vary between different sources and preparations. If you attempt to perform HSC isolation on a regular basis, we strongly recommend that you reserve larger amounts of successfully tested enzymes from a specific batch (i.e., with fixed lot numbers). This will increase the reproducibility of this protocol.
2. There are other protocols available that use alternative reagents during density gradient centrifugation for isolation of HSCs. Most common are metrizamide, Stractan, OptiPrep, or Percoll. The structures and properties of these compounds are given in Fig. 11 and Table 1.

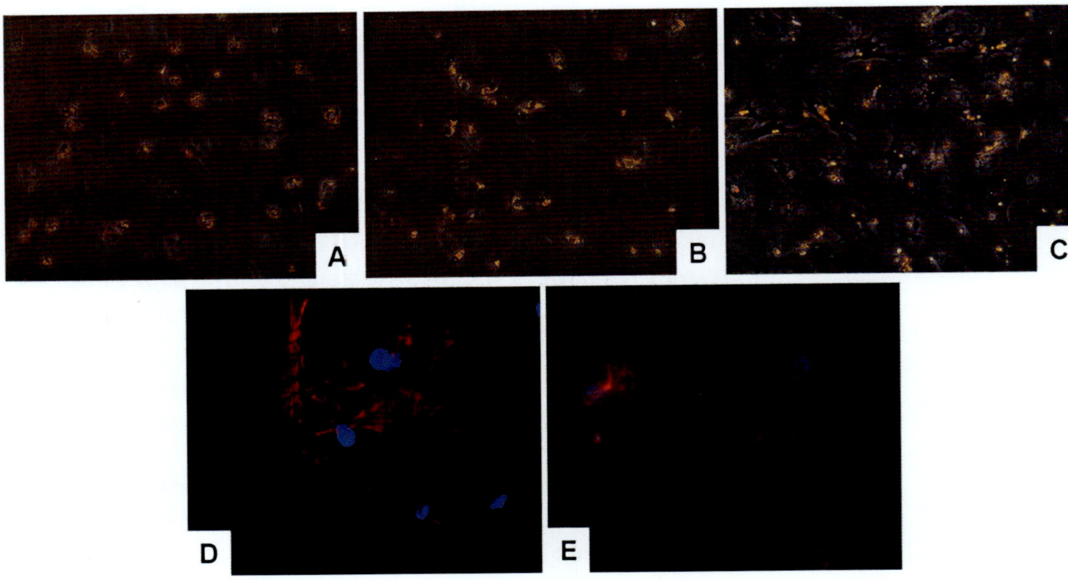

Fig. 10 Activation and transdifferentiation of primary HSCs in culture. Isolated HSCs were cultured on uncoated plastic for (**a**) 1 day, (**b**) 2 days, or (**c**) 5 days. Please note that during culturing, the content of vitamin A decreases and that the cells acquire a typical star-shaped phenotype. (**d**) HSCs were stained with a rhodamine phalloidin conjugate (*red*) and DAPI counterstaining (*blue*). (**e**) Desmin immunocytochemistry (*red*) of HSCs

3. There are increasing numbers of protocols available that report the simultaneous isolation of two or more different combinations of liver cells from rat, mouse, and men [21–23] during one batch.
4. We have established protocols for cryoconservation of rat HSCs [20]. Other laboratories have presented adequate protocols for cryopreservation of primary cultured human HSCs [24]. Although a precise protocol for freezing murine HSCs is not yet available, mouse HSCs are commercially available as cryopreserved stocks from many suppliers (e.g., from Innoprot, Cell Biologics, ScienCell Research Laboratories, iXCells Biotechnologies, and others). These are usually shipped in 0.5–1.0 × 10^6 cells per vial, and after thawing, there will be 30–50% dead cells.
5. Other cell counting chamber types are also acceptable but will require updating the cell calculation formulas given in this protocol.
6. There are several immortalized HSC lines from mice available that differ in morphology, growth characteristics, and chromosomal endowment. Although in these continuous and homogenous cell populations most phenotypic features remain constant for many passages, it is obvious that the results obtained in these cell lines may significantly differ from results obtained in experiments performed with primary results. In several aspects, they have limitations in mimicking the cellular dynamics of primary

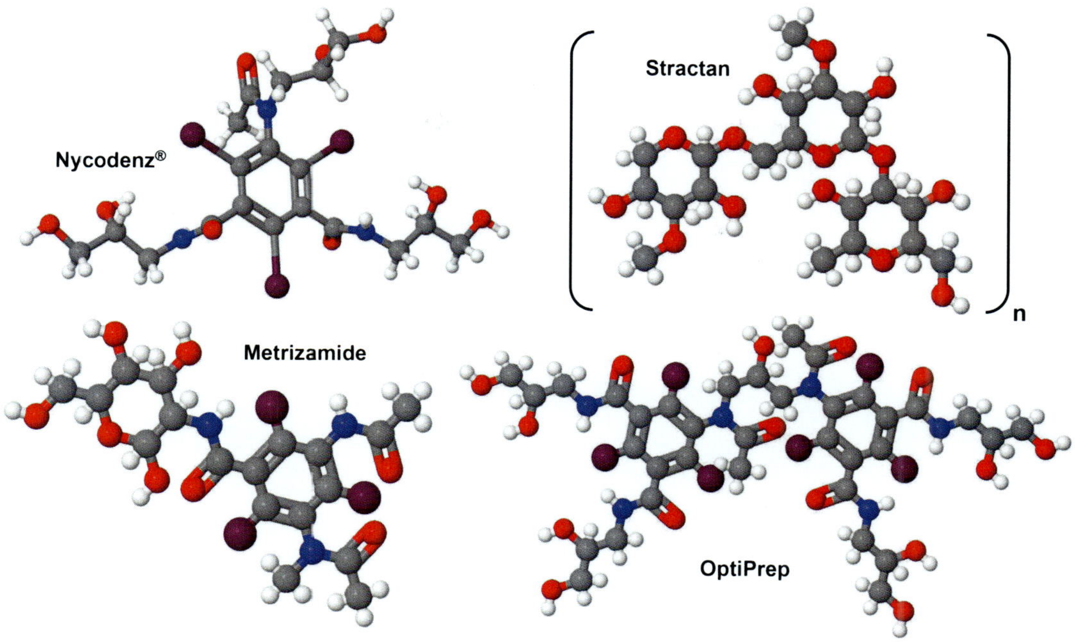

Fig. 11 Established density gradient compounds used for isolation of HSCs. The compound Nycodenz (CAS no., 66108-95-0), Stractan (arabinogalactan CAS no., 9036-66-2), metrizamide (CAS no., 31112-62-6), and OptiPrep (iodixanol, CAS no., 92339-11-2) are established density gradients in the purification of HSCs. In addition, Percoll (CAS no., 65455-52-9) consisting of 15–30 nm large silica particles that are coated with nondialyzable polyvinylpyrrolidone is a compound used for purification of HSCs. The depicted chemical structures were generated with the open-source software Jmol [26]. Please note that when using one of these substances, the optimal concentrations for gradient formation must be confirmed by appropriate experiments

HSCs that transdifferentiate upon culturing and are therefore not optimal to analyze fundamental biological processes such as apoptosis, necrosis, or pyroptosis. However, when trying to establish the purification of HSCs in your lab, these lines may serve as good positive controls when testing your primary cells for expression of typical HSC markers. Details about several murine HSC lines such as GRX, Sv68c-IS [25], A640-IS, M1-4HSC, and A7 that were established by different procedures are summarized in detail elsewhere [25].

7. Today it is well accepted that in healthy, uninjured livers, HSCs might be a heterogeneous cell population that differ in fat content and metabolism, activation status, marker gene expression, or many other biological features [12]. We admit that our protocol might preferentially purify a specific HSC fraction that is particularly rich in fat and vitamin A and has a similar activation status. However, continuous advancement in the field might allow adapting the current protocol, as the identification of new surface markers could be used to purify HSC subsets by FACS.

Table 1
Media used in gradient density centrifugation for enrichment of hepatic stellate cells

Medium	Other names	Composition	Molecular weight	Density	Remarks
Nycodenz	Iohexol, compound 545, Exypaque, Iohexol 350, Omnipaque, Histodenz (a copy product produced in China)	White, nonionic tri-iodinated derivative of benzoic acid with three aliphatic hydrophilic side chains that is used as contrast medium	821.14	10% (w/v): 1.052 20% (w/v): 1.105 80% (w/v): 1.426	Stock solution up to 80% (w/v) can be prepared that is stable for over 5 years when stored at room temperature and protected from light; stable to heat and autoclaving; very resistant to bacterial degradation; not metabolized by mammalian cells; concentration and density of solutions can be determined by measuring the refractive index [27]
Metrizamide	Amipaque, Amipak	Nonionic radiopaque, water-soluble contrast agent	789.10	10% (w/v): 1.051 40% (w/v): 1.216 80% (w/v): 1.436	Stock solutions up to 90% (w/v) can be prepared; stable in solution; can be used as a gradient medium over the pH range 2.5 to 12.5; susceptible to bacterial degradation; solutions should be sterilized by filtration and stored in the dark at −20 °C; not autoclavable; solution's density can be determined by its refractive index; large molar absorption in the ultraviolet region [28]

Stractan	(+)-Arabinogalactan, D-Galacto-L-arabinan, Larcoll, Galactoarabinan; Polyarabinogalactan	A nontoxic biopolymer consisting of arabinose and galactose monosaccharides; in microbial arabinogalactan, the galactan chain is linked with alternating 5-β-v- and 6-β-D-galactofuranosyl residues	500.49	28.5% (w/v): 1.12	When stored at room temperature, the powder is stable indefinitely; stock solutions are stable for at least 1 year at −20 °C; readily soluble in water, can be sterilized by filtration (0.45 μm) or autoclaving; not sensitive to changes in pH or dissolved salts; first introduced as a compound to separate erythrocytes by density gradient centrifugation [29]
OptiPrep	Iodixanol, Visipaque, Iodixanolum, Indixanol	A ready-made, sterile, nonionic, nontoxic, and endotoxin-tested 60% (w/v) solution of iodixanol in water; OptiPrep is approximately a dimer of Nycodenz	1550.18	60% (w/v): 1.32	Stable for 3 years when kept sterile and protected from light; should be stored between 4 and 24 °C; OptiPrep gradients have osmolalities approximately half that of Nycodenz solutions of the same density [30, 31]
Percoll		Nontoxic, low viscous compound consisting of colloidal silica particles of 15–30 nm diameter, coated with nondialyzable polyvinylpyrrolidone	NA	1.13 in a 23% (w/w) colloidal solution in water	Iso-osmotic throughout the gradient; will not penetrate biological membranes; pH of about 9.0 that is adjustable to pH 5.5–10-0; does not interfere with fluorescent activated cell sorting; solution can be stored at room temperature for at least 2 years; autoclavable at 120 °C for 30 min without any change in properties [32]

Acknowledgments

This work was supported by grants from the German Research Foundation (SFB/TRR 57 projects P09, P13, and Q3).

References

1. Tacke F, Weiskirchen R (2012) Update on hepatic stellate cells: pathogenic role in liver fibrosis and novel isolation techniques. Expert Rev Gastroenterol Hepatol 6(1):67–80. doi:10.1586/egh.11.92
2. Knook DL, Seffelaar AM, de Leeuw AM (1982) Fat-storing cells of the rat liver. Their isolation and purification. Exp Cell Res 139(2):468–471. doi:10.1016/0014-4827(82)90283-X
3. Friedman SL, Roll FJ (1987) Isolation and culture of hepatic lipocytes, Kupffer cells, and sinusoidal endothelial cells by density gradient centrifugation with Stractan. Anal Biochem 161(1):207–218. doi:10.1016/0003-2697(87)90673-7
4. Pinzani M, Gesualdo L, Sabbah GM et al (1989) Effects of platelet-derived growth factor and other polypeptide mitogens on DNA synthesis and growth of cultured rat liver fat-storing cells. J Clin Invest 84(6):1786–1793. doi:10.1172/JCI114363
5. de Leeuw AM, McCarthy SP, Geerts A et al (1984) Purified rat liver fat-storing cells in culture divide and contain collagen. Hepatology 4(3):392–403. doi:10.1002/hep.1840040307
6. Schafer S, Zerbe O, Gressner AM (1987) The synthesis of proteoglycans in fat-storing cells of rat liver. Hepatology 7(4):680–687. doi:10.1002/hep.1840070411
7. Weiskirchen R, Gressner AM (2005) Isolation and culture of hepatic stellate cells. Methods Mol Med 117:99–113. doi:10.1385/1-59259-940-0:099
8. Maschmeyer P, Flach M, Winau F (2011) Seven steps to stellate cells. J Vis Exp (51). doi:10.3791/2710
9. Elsharkawy AM, Wright MC, Hay RT et al (1999) Persistent activation of nuclear factor-kappaB in cultured rat hepatic stellate cells involves the induction of potentially novel Rel-like factors and prolonged changes in the expression of IkappaB family proteins. Hepatology 30(3):761–769. doi:10.1002/hep.510300327
10. Graham JM (2002) Fractionation of hepatic nonparenchymal cells. ScientificWorldJournal 2:1347–1350. doi:10.1100/tsw.2002.283
11. Blomhoff R, Berg T (1990) Isolation and cultivation of rat liver stellate cells. Methods Enzymol 190:58–71. doi:10.1016/0076-6879(90)90009-P
12. D'Ambrosio DN, Walewski JL, Clugston RD et al (2011) Distinct populations of hepatic stellate cells in the mouse liver have different capacities for retinoid and lipid storage. PLoS One 6(9):e24993. doi:10.1371/journal.pone.0024993
13. Geerts A, Niki T, Hellemans K et al (1998) Purification of rat hepatic stellate cells by side scatter-activated cell sorting. Hepatology 27(2):590–598. doi:10.1002/hep.510270238
14. Paik YH, Iwaisako K, Seki E et al (2011) The nicotinamide adenine dinucleotide phosphate oxidase (NOX) homologues NOX1 and NOX2/gp91(phox) mediate hepatic fibrosis in mice. Hepatology 53(5):1730–1741. doi:10.1002/hep.24281
15. Mederacke I, Dapito DH, Affo S et al (2015) High-yield and high-purity isolation of hepatic stellate cells from normal and fibrotic mouse livers. Nat Protoc 10(2):305–315. doi:10.1038/nprot.2015.017
16. Bartneck M, Warzecha KT, Tag CG et al (2015) Isolation and time lapse microscopy of highly pure hepatic stellate cells. Anal Cell Pathol (Amst) 2015:417023. doi:10.1155/2015/417023
17. Wang YQ, Ikeda K, Ikebe T et al (2000) Inhibition of hepatic stellate cell proliferation and activation by the semisynthetic analogue of fumagillin TNP-470 in rats. Hepatology 32(5):980–989. doi:10.1053/jhep.2000.18658
18. Davies D (2012) Cell separations by flow cytometry. Methods Mol Biol 878:185–199. doi:10.1007/978-1-61779-854-2_12
19. Donnenberg AD, Donnenberg VS (2007) Rare-event analysis in flow cytometry. Clin Lab Med 27(3):627–652, viii. doi:10.1016/j.cll.2007.05.013
20. Neyzen S, Van de Leur E, Borkham-Kamphorst E et al (2006) Cryopreservation of hepatic stellate cells. J Hepatol 44(5):910–917. doi:10.1016/j.jhep.2005.07.008
21. Riccalton-Banks L, Bhandari R, Fry J et al (2003) A simple method for the simultaneous

isolation of stellate cells and hepatocytes from rat liver tissue. Mol Cell Biochem 248(1-2):97–102. doi:10.1023/A:1024184826728

22. Werner M, Driftmann S, Kleinehr K et al (2015) All-in-one: advanced preparation of human parenchymal and non-parenchymal liver cells. PLoS One 10(9):e0138655. doi:10.1371/journal.pone.0138655
23. Mohar I, Brempelis KJ, Murray SA et al (2015) Isolation of non-parenchymal cells from the mouse liver. Methods Mol Biol 1325:3–17. doi:10.1007/978-1-4939-2815-6_1
24. Nakamura A, Ueno T, Yagi Y et al (2010) Human primary cultured hepatic stellate cells can be cryopreserved. Med Mol Morphol 43(2):107–115. doi:10.1007/s00795-009-0484-5
25. Herrmann J, Gressner AM, Weiskirchen R (2007) Immortal hepatic stellate cell lines: useful tools to study hepatic stellate cell biology and function? J Cell Mol Med 11(4):704–722. doi:10.1111/j.1582-4934.2007.00060.x
26. Jmol: an open-source Java viewer for chemical structures in 3D. http://jmol.sourceforge.net/. Accessed 26 Aug 2016
27. Lindgren E (1980) Iohexol, a non-ionic contrast medium: pharmacology and toxicology. Acta Radiol Suppl (Stockholm) 362:1–134
28. Rickwood D, Birnie GD (1975) Metrizamide, a new density-gradient medium. FEBS Lett 50(2):102–110. doi:10.1016/0014-5793(75)80467-4
29. Corash LM, Piomelli S, Chen HC et al (1974) Separation of erythrocytes according to age on a simplified density gradient. J Lab Clin Med 84(1):147-151. doi:0022-2143(74)90232-7 [pii]
30. Van Veldhoven PP, Baumgart E, Mannaerts GP (1996) Iodixanol (Optiprep), an improved density gradient medium for the iso-osmotic isolation of rat liver peroxisomes. Anal Biochem 237(1):17–23. doi:10.1006/abio.1996.0194
31. Graham JM (2002) OptiPrep density gradient solutions for mammalian organelles. ScientificWorldJournal 2:1440–1443. doi:10.1100/tsw.2002.840
32. Pertoft H, Laurent TC, Laas T et al (1978) Density gradients prepared from colloidal silica particles coated by polyvinylpyrrolidone (Percoll). Anal Biochem 88(1):271–282. doi:10.1016/0003-2697(78)90419-0

Chapter 12

Isolation and Culture of Adipose-Derived Stromal Cells from Subcutaneous Fat

Lawrence J. Liew, Huan Ting Ong, and Rodney J. Dilley

Abstract

Cells with mesenchymal stem cell characteristics can be isolated from human adipose tissue stroma. Relative ease of isolation in large numbers and their ability for expansion and differentiation means that they are becoming a preferred cell type for mesenchymal regenerative medicine applications. In addition to expansion and differentiation capacity, they also express valuable paracrine activities which promote tissue formation and wound healing, including pro- and anti-fibrotic mediators. Here we describe a method for routine isolation of adipose stromal cells, culture expansion, and characterization by differentiation and then production of conditioned media.

Key words Adipose, Mesenchymal stem cells, Cell culture, Characterization, Differentiation, Conditioned media

1 Introduction

Human adipose tissue contains mostly adipocytes by volume, but a range of other fibrous, vascular, and immune tissue cell types can be found in adipose stroma. Simple culture methods have allowed sorting based on adhesion and isolation of a homogeneous stromal cell population with multipotent mesenchymal stem cell (MSC) properties. The cells may be isolated from fat tissue obtained at surgery or from cell/tissue fragments in lipoaspirate after liposuction. These adipose-derived stem cells (ADSCs) may be particularly useful for regenerative cell therapies and tissue engineering due to the high yields from a minimally invasive procedure and a strong capacity for expansion ex vivo.

ADSC have been shown to differentiate to mesenchymal cell lineages [1], form colonies of fibroblast-like cells [2], and display MSC cell surface markers [3], similar to MSC grown from bone marrow [4]. The cells have been found to possess further beneficial properties for regeneration, expressing a range of growth factor and cytokine genes [5] and secreting a paracrine activity that

Laure Rittié (ed.), *Fibrosis: Methods and Protocols*, Methods in Molecular Biology, vol. 1627,
DOI 10.1007/978-1-4939-7113-8_12, © Springer Science+Business Media LLC 2017

supports angiogenesis [6, 7], promotes tissue formation [8] wound healing [9], and has a beneficial immunomodulation activity [10]. Hypoxic culture increases some of these paracrine activities [6].

Relevant to tissue fibrosis, the cells produce in culture many extracellular matrix (ECM) genes [5]; as cell therapy, they have an anti-fibrotic effect [11] and produce an ECM that regulates fibroblast behavior [12]. While the regulation of ECM has not been extensively examined, this capacity may prove beneficial for creating tissue engineering scaffolds [11] or to functionalize other scaffold materials. Furthermore the cells can have a modulating effect on cell biology of fibroblasts, including regulation of ECM production [13].

We describe here a method for isolation and characterization of MSCs from adipose tissue and the production of conditioned media in normoxic and hypoxic conditions.

2 Materials

2.1 Instruments and General Supplies

1. 4 in. dissecting forceps.
2. 4 in. iris scissors.
3. #21 blade steel scalpel.
4. 100 mm cell culture dish.
5. 50 ml conical tubes.
6. 100 μm nylon cell strainers.
7. 40 μm nylon cell strainers.
8. Tissue culture flask T75.
9. Benchtop centrifuge.
10. Reichert hemocytometer.
11. Flow cytometer (we use the FACSCanto from BD Biosciences).
12. Tissue culture plate, 12- and 24-well flat bottom.
13. Spectrophotometer for nucleic acid quantification (we use an Epoch™ microplate system from BioTek).
14. Real-time PCR detection system (we use a CFX Connect™ from Bio-Rad).
15. 0.3% (w/v) Trypan blue.
16. Cell culture setting, including cell culture incubator (37 °C with 95% air/5% CO_2, humid atmosphere), cell culture hood, sterile pipettes, and labware.
17. Atmospheric generator incubation system (we use the GENbox jar system including a jar, anaer indicator strips, and microanaer atmosphere generator sachet from BioMérieux).
18. Laboratory scale.
19. Water bath with shaker.

2.2 Tissue Digestion Reagents

1. 10X red blood cell lysis buffer: 1.5 M NH_4Cl, 0.1 M $KHCO_3$ (*see* **Note 1**), 1 mM EDTA. Dissolve in sterile distilled H_2O; store in 5 ml aliquots at 4 °C.
2. 10X collagenase II solution: dissolve 2.5% (w/v) collagenase II in sterile distilled H_2O; store in 1 ml aliquots at −20 °C.
3. 10X bovine serum albumin (BSA) solution: dissolve 5% (w/v) BSA in sterile distilled H_2O; store in 1 ml aliquots at −20 °C.
4. Dulbecco's modified Eagle's medium (DMEM)/Ham's F12 Nutrient Mixture (F12) (1:1).
5. Tissue digestion buffer: in a 10 ml tube, add 1 ml of 10X collagenase II solution and 1 ml of 10X BSA to 8 ml of serum-free DMEM/F12 medium.
6. Red cell lysis buffer: in a 50 ml tube, add 5 ml of 10X red blood cell lysis buffer to 45 ml of sterile distilled H_2O.

2.3 Cell Culture

1. Fetal bovine serum (FBS).
2. Complete DMEM/F12: mix DMEM/F12 and FBS at a 9:1 (v/v) ratio. Keep sterile.
3. Complete DMEM: mix DMEM and FBS at a 9:1 (v/v) ratio. Keep sterile.
4. Antibiotic-antimycotic.
5. Cell dissociation enzyme (we use TrypLE™ Express from Thermo Fisher Scientific).
6. Phosphate-buffered saline (PBS), pH 7.4.
7. Collagenase II (we use the one from Thermo Fisher Scientific).

2.4 Flow Cytometry

1. Phycoerythrin (PE)-conjugated mouse antihuman CD73.
2. PE-conjugated mouse antihuman CD34.
3. Fluorescein isothiocyanate (FITC)-conjugated mouse antihuman CD105.
4. FITC-conjugated mouse antihuman CD45.
5. Allophycocyanin (APC)-conjugated mouse antihuman CD90.
6. APC-conjugated mouse antihuman CD14.
7. Round bottom polystyrene flow tubes.
8. Flow buffer (PBS + 1% (w/v) BSA).

2.5 Trilineage Differentiation Reagents

1. 5 mg/ml insulin in PBS, store in 1 ml aliquots at 4 °C (*see* **Note 2**).
2. 0.5 M IBMX: dissolve IBMX in DMSO with gentle warming; store in 100 μl aliquots at −20 °C (*see* **Note 2**).
3. 50 mM indomethacin in absolute ethanol; store in 100 μl aliquots at −20 °C (*see* **Note 2**).

4. 20 mM β-glycerophosphate disodium salt hydrate in H_2O; store in 1 ml aliquots at −20 °C (*see* **Note 2**).
5. 0.5 mM dexamethasone in absolute ethanol; store in 100 μl aliquots at −20 °C (*see* **Note 2**).
6. 50 mM L-ascorbic acid in H_2O; store in 100 μl aliquots at −20 °C (*see* **Note 2**).
7. 0.1 mg/ml TGF-β1: dissolve TGF-β1 in 10 mM citric acid pH 3.0; store in 100 μl aliquots at −20 °C (*see* **Note 2**).
8. Adipogenic medium: DMEM/F12 with 10% FBS, 10 μg/ml insulin, 0.5 μM dexamethasone, 0.5 mM IBMX, and 50 μM indomethacin.
9. 10% (v/v) formalin.
10. Osteogenic medium: DMEM/F12 with 10% FBS, 0.01 μM dexamethasone, 2 mM β-glycerophosphate disodium salt hydrate, and 50 μM L-ascorbic acid.
11. Chondrogenic medium: complete DMEM/F12 containing 6.25 μg/ml insulin, 10 ng/ml TGF-β, and 50 nM L-ascorbic acid.

2.6 Preparation of Trilineage Histochemistry Staining Solution

1. 0.5% (w/v) Oil Red O stock solution in 100% isopropanol; syringe filter through 0.45um filter membrane, and store in 200 ml glass bottle at 4 °C. Prepare fresh working solution by diluting two parts of Oil Red O stock with three parts of PBS (*see* **Notes 3–5**).
2. 2.5% (w/v) silver nitrate working solution in sterile deionized H_2O. Store in 100 ml glass bottle at 4 °C, protected from light (*see* **Note 6**).
3. 1% (w/v) alcian blue working solution in 3% (v/v) acetic acid; adjust to pH 2.5, and store in a 100 ml glass bottle at room temperature.

2.7 Nucleic Acid Analysis

1. Total RNA extraction kit (we use FavorPrep Tissue Total RNA Mini Kit from Favorgen) (*see* **Note** 7).
2. Reverse transcription reagents (we use Omniscript® reverse transcription kit from Qiagen).
3. Reaction master mix for quantitative PCR (we use iQ™ SYBR Green Supermix from Bio-Rad).
4. PCR primers for the following genes (all human): peroxisome proliferator-activated receptor gamma (PPAR-γ), adiponectin (AdipoQ), collagen I (COL1A1), osteomodulin, collagen II (COL2A1), aggrecan, glyceraldehyde 3-phosphate dehydrogenase (GAPDH), beta-actin. Primers can be designed in-house or purchased in a ready-to-use format (we use QuantiTect primer assays from Qiagen).

3 Methods

3.1 Subcutaneous Fat Sample Isolation

1. Subcutaneous adipose tissue samples can be collected from theater or procedure rooms directly into sterile specimen jars (*see* **Notes 7** and **8**). Jars are transported to the cell culture facility where enzyme digestion and culture are performed under sterile conditions (Fig. 1).
2. Weigh subcutaneous adipose tissue before processing to determine total cell yield per gram (*see* **Note 9**).
3. Rinse tissue thoroughly with 5 ml of PBS containing 1% (v/v) antibiotic-antimycotic, and discard supernatant. Do not allow tissue to dry out.
4. Using sterile forceps, transfer tissue to a 100 mm cell culture dish.
5. Dissect off any skin and fibrous tissue and chop adipose tissue into fragments (1–2 mm) with scissors.
6. Transfer tissues to a 50 ml centrifuge tube containing 10 ml of tissue digestion buffer. Gently shake the tube to ensure all tissues are in the solution.
7. Incubate mixture in a 37 °C water bath with constant shaking for 2–3 h or until it reaches a homogeneous consistency.
8. Filter the mixture with a 100 μm cell strainer into a new 50 ml tube to remove debris and connective tissue remnants.

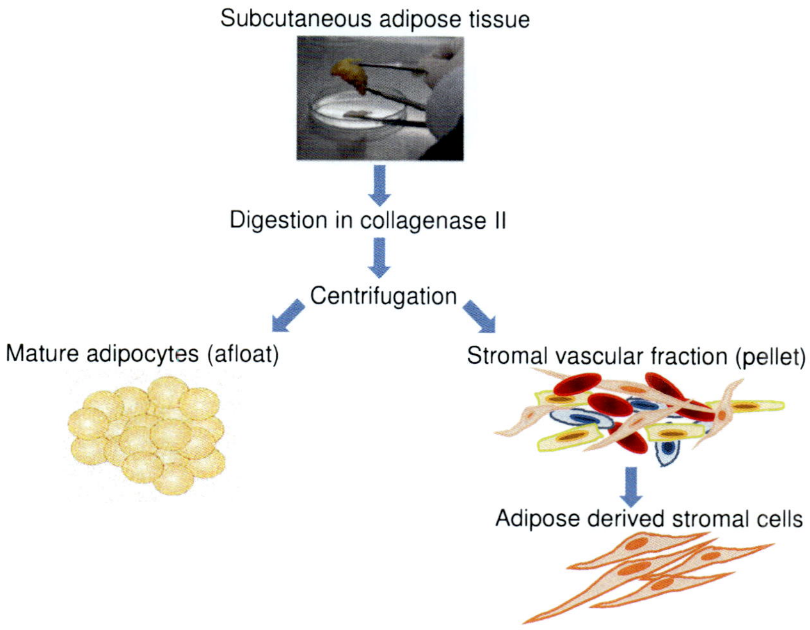

Fig. 1 Summary flow chart for isolating adipose-derived stem cells from subcutaneous adipose tissue samples

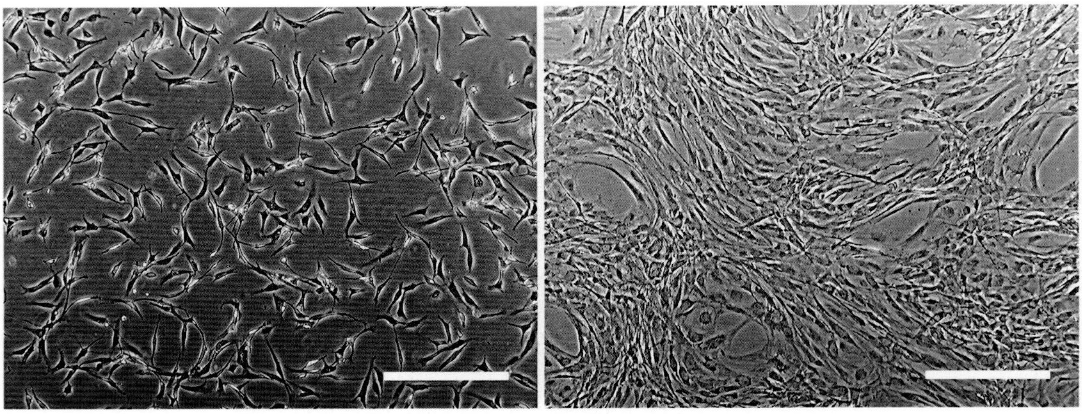

Fig. 2 Phase-contrast micrographs of adipose-derived stem cells soon after passaging (~40% confluence; *left panel*) and at 90% confluence for conditioned media production (*right*) (Scale bar = 500 μm)

9. Centrifuge at 300 *g* for 5 min to separate the mature adipocytes (floating upper layer) and stromal vascular fraction (cell pellet).
10. Remove mature adipocytes and supernatant via aspiration.
11. Add 5 ml of red blood cell lysis buffer to the cell pellet and incubate for 15 min at 37 °C.
12. Neutralize lysis buffer with 10 ml of PBS and centrifuge at 300 *g* for 5 min.
13. Discard supernatant and resuspend the cell pellet in 1 ml of complete DMEM/F12.
14. Perform a cell count (hemocytometer) to find total cell yield and seed cells in tissue culture flasks at a density of 2000 cells/cm^2 and complete DMEM/F12.
15. Incubate overnight to allow cells to adhere.
16. Aspirate spent medium to remove nonadherent cells. Add fresh complete DMEM/F12 to the adherent cell cultures and return to the incubator.
17. Feed cells with fresh complete DMEM/F12 twice weekly until ~80% confluent (Fig. 2).

3.2 Subculture of Adipose-Derived Stromal Cells

1. Subculture cells upon reaching 80% confluence.
2. Aspirate and discard medium, and rinse cell monolayer twice with PBS (5 ml for a T75 flask).
3. Incubate cells with 5 ml of pre-warmed dissociation enzyme solution at 37 °C for ~10 min and gently tap the bottom of flask to detach cells.
4. Add 10 ml of pre-warmed complete DMEM/F12 to neutralize the dissociation enzyme.
5. Centrifuge cells at 300 *g* for 5 min and decant supernatant.

6. Resuspend cells in 1 ml of complete DMEM/F12 and count cells with a hemocytometer.
7. Adjust volume with complete DMEM/F12 to reseed into fresh flasks at 2000 cells/cm^2.

3.3 Phenotyping of ADSCs by FACS Analysis

1. Harvest cells enzymatically at passage 2 using protocol described in Subheading 3.2.
2. Count cells with a hemocytometer and resuspend 2 × 10^5 cells in a flow tube with 200 μl of flow buffer.
3. Prepare an unstained ADSC control in a flow tube by resuspending 2 × 10^5 cells in 1 ml of flow buffer.
4. Prepare two cell suspensions for the identification of mesenchymal markers (CD73, CD90, and CD105) and the exclusion of hemopoietic markers (CD14, CD34, and CD45).
5. Add 1 μl (each) of CD73-PE, CD90-APC, and CD105-FITC to the first tube and CD14-APC, CD34-PE, and CD45-FITC to the second tube. Mix cell suspension by inverting tube and incubate at room temperature (in the dark) for 20 min.
6. Prepare separately single-stained cell suspensions for each fluorophore by staining 2 × 10^5 cells with 1 μl of positive antibody (i.e., CD73-PE, CD90-APC, CD105-FITC).
7. Add 800 μl of flow buffer to each tube and mix cell suspension by inverting tube.
8. Set flow cytometer by running an unstained control (ADSC) and adjust voltage to make sure cells are distributed in a forward scatter (FSC) vs. side scatter (SCC) plot. Set detectors to linear scale.
9. Run single-stained samples, and adjust the compensation between each channel to prevent overlap in fluorescent signals. Set all fluorescent channels to a logarithmic scale.
10. Define a gate on FSC and SCC plot (to exclude cell debris and doublets) and display the gated population on the following plots:
    (a) PE vs. FITC.
    (b) APC vs. FITC.
    (c) PE vs. APC.
11. Run analysis and collect a minimum of 10,000 events.
12. ADSCs are positive for CD73, CD90, and CD105 and negative for CD14, CD34, and CD45.

3.4 Trilineage Differentiation of ADSC

Cells are incubated in specific differentiation media and assessed by histochemistry or PCR to confirm their multipotency (Fig. 3). Control undifferentiated cell cultures are prepared in complete DMEM/F12 for comparison.

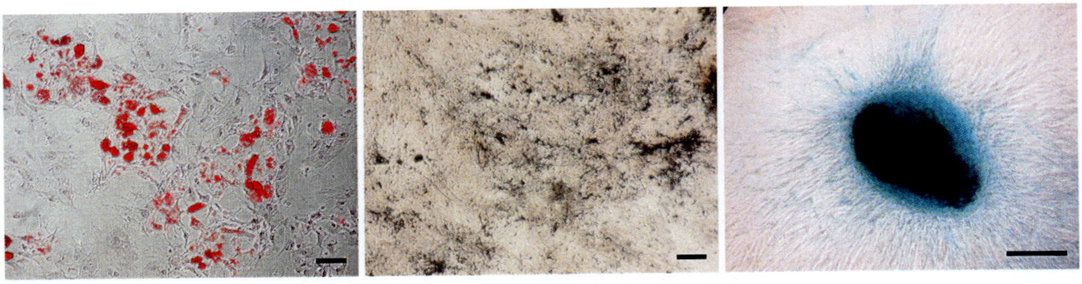

Fig. 3 Representative images of adipose-derived stem cells after trilineage differentiation protocols with histochemistry for adipogenesis (Oil Red O, *left panel*), osteogenesis (silver nitrate/von Kossa stain, *middle*), and chondrogenesis (alcian blue, *right panel*) (Scale bar = 100 μm)

3.4.1 Adipogenic Differentiation

1. Harvest sub-confluent cells at passage 2 as per protocol detailed in Subheading 3.2 and count cells using a hemocytometer.
2. Resuspend cells in complete DMEM/F12 and seed cells in a 12-well plate at 2 × 10^4 cells per cm^2. Allow cells to settle and adhere overnight in a cell culture incubator.
3. Aspirate medium and replace with adipogenic medium.
4. Replenish cells with fresh adipogenic medium (1.5 ml/well) twice weekly and check for the formation of cytoplasmic lipid droplets.
5. At day 14, aspirate medium and rinse well with 1 ml of PBS.
6. Fix cells in 10% formalin for 15 min and stain with freshly made Oil Red O working solution for 20 min.

3.4.2 Osteogenic Differentiation

1. Harvest sub-confluent cells at passage 2 as per protocol detailed in Subheading 3.2, and count cells using a hemocytometer.
2. Resuspend cells in complete DMEM/F12 and seed cells in a 12-well plate at 1 × 10^4 cells per cm^2 and leave cells to settle and adhere overnight in a cell culture incubator.
3. Aspirate medium and replace with osteogenic medium.
4. Replenish cells with fresh osteogenic medium (1.5 ml/well) twice weekly and check for the formation of calcium deposits.
5. At day 28, aspirate medium and rinse well with 1 ml of PBS.
6. Fix cells in 10% formalin for 15 min, rinse in deionized water, and stain with 2.5% silver nitrate solution for 30 min under UV light for color change.

3.4.3 Chondrogenic Differentiation

1. Harvest sub-confluent cells at passage 2 as per protocol detailed in Subheading 3.2 and count cells using a hemocytometer.
2. Resuspend 8 × 10^4 cells in 10 μl of complete DMEM/F12 and carefully pipet cell suspension onto the center of the well in a 12-well plate.

3. Allow cells to set for at least 3 h in a cell culture incubator.
4. Carefully pipet 1.5 ml of chondrogenic medium to each well, without disrupting the cell pellet.
5. Replenish cells with fresh chondrogenic medium (1.5 ml/well) twice weekly and check for the formation of spherical mass.
6. At day 14, aspirate medium and rinse well carefully with 1 ml of PBS.
7. Fix cells in 10% formalin for 15 min, rinse in PBS, and stain with 1% alcian blue solution for 30 min.

3.5 RNA Extraction and qRT-PCR

1. Extract total RNA using an RNA extraction kit according to manufacturer's instructions (*see* **Note 10**).
2. Determine RNA concentration using a spectrophotometer at 260 nm wavelength. 260:280 ratio for pure RNA should be 1.8–2.2 (*see* **Note 11**).
3. Synthesize cDNA using a reverse transcription kit according to manufacturer's instructions (*see* **Note 12**).
4. Mix a real-time PCR reaction consisting of reaction master mix, cDNA, primers, and RNase-free water.
5. Run real-time PCR according to corresponding primers used.
6. Quantification of gene expression for trilineage differentiation assays can be determined at the transcriptional level using the Ct values from the PCR results.

3.6 ADSC-Conditioned Medium Production

Cell density and serum depletion (starvation) are crucial in the preparation of ADSC-conditioned medium (*see* **Notes 13–15**).

1. Culture ADSCs in a T75 flask to near-confluent density using complete DMEM/F12.
2. Change medium to serum-free DMEM/F12 and incubate cells overnight at 37 °C.
3. Rinse cells with 10 ml of PBS and add an appropriate volume of serum-free DMEM/F12 (10 ml for a T75 flask or 25 ml for T175 flask).
4. Conditioned medium can be generated under different conditions, i.e., normoxic (20% air, 5% CO_2) and hypoxic (a three-gas incubator to produce 2% O_2, 5% CO_2, and balance with N_2) for 24, 48, or 72 h (*see* **Note 16**).
5. Collect conditioned medium and remove any cell debris using 0.2 μm filter membrane.
6. Use immediately for assays, or store conditioned medium at −80 °C until required.

4 Notes

1. Potassium bicarbonate may be replaced with 10 mM sodium bicarbonate ($NaHCO_3$).
2. Preparation of stock media additives for trilineage differentiation is aliquoted at 100 μl to make up 10 ml differentiation media. Make calculations for how much media is required corresponding to number of wells in use to determine beforehand the volume of stock to aliquot. This prevents repeated freeze-thaw cycles of media additives.
3. Oil Red O stock solution must be kept in a closed container since solvent evaporation will cause stain precipitation.
4. Oil Red O stock solution can be kept at room temperature, while working solution of Oil Red O should be made up fresh each time and be used immediately.
5. For quantification of lipid formation, Oil Red O stain can be eluted with 100% isopropanol and measured spectrophotometrically at 500 nm wavelength.
6. Silver nitrate solution should be kept at 4 °C and protected from light with a foil wrapping.
7. Patient tissues are collected with approval from local human research ethics committee and with informed consent from the patient.
8. Subcutaneous adipose tissue samples can be collected from various anatomical sites but abdominal and hip fat are commonly used.
9. For successful isolation and propagation of adipose-derived stromal cells, we use approximately 2–5 g of subcutaneous adipose tissue.
10. Recommended number of cells for RNA extraction using the FavorPrep Kit is approximately 1×10^6 cells per RNA extraction tube. Overloading tubes with cells may result in reduced RNA yield or poor RNA quality yield.
11. If RNA 260:280 ratio is below 1.8, it indicates a genomic DNA contamination. A column cleanup is recommended before proceeding to synthesizing cDNA.
12. The synthesis of cDNA from different samples should use the same amount of RNA so that Ct values are comparable and consistent.
13. For conditioned media production, the duration, cell density, and media volume of cultures can be titrated to optimize concentration of secreted products.
14. Serum depletion (starvation) is required in the preparation of ADSC-conditioned medium.

15. Cells should be used at lower passage number (2–8) to maintain the reproducibility of experiments as cellular aging may affect the secretory profiles of ADSCs.
16. There are many options for creating hypoxia, but a cost-effective and convenient system uses a GENbox jar (*see* Subheading 2) to produce anoxia (<0.1% O_2). The jar can be incubated simultaneously with a paired normoxic control culture.

References

1. Zuk PA, Zhu M, Mizuno H et al (2001) Multilineage cells from human adipose tissue: implications for cell-based therapies. Tissue Eng 7(2):211–228. doi:10.1089/107632701300062859
2. Zuk PA, Zhu M, Ashjian P et al (2002) Human adipose tissue is a source of multipotent stem cells. Mol Biol Cell 13(12):4279–4295. doi:10.1091/mbc.E02-02-0105
3. Dominici M, Le Blanc K, Mueller I et al (2006) Minimal criteria for defining multipotent mesenchymal stromal cells. The International Society for Cellular Therapy position statement. Cytotherapy 8(4):315–317. doi:10.1080/14653240600855905
4. Friedenstein AJ, Deriglasova UF, Kulagina NN et al (1974) Precursors for fibroblasts in different populations of hematopoietic cells as detected by the in vitro colony assay method. Exp Hematol 2(2):83–92
5. Katz AJ, Tholpady A, Tholpady SS et al (2005) Cell surface and transcriptional characterization of human adipose-derived adherent stromal (hADAS) cells. Stem Cells 23(3):412–423. doi:10.1634/stemcells.2004-0021
6. Moon MH, Kim SY, Kim YJ et al (2006) Human adipose tissue-derived mesenchymal stem cells improve postnatal neovascularization in a mouse model of hindlimb ischemia. Cell Physiol Biochem 17(5–6):279–290. doi:10.1159/000094140
7. Hsiao ST, Asgari A, Lokmic Z et al (2012) Comparative analysis of paracrine factor expression in human adult mesenchymal stem cells derived from bone marrow, adipose, and dermal tissue. Stem Cells Dev 21(12):2189–2203. doi:10.1089/scd.2011.0674
8. Matsuda K, Falkenberg KJ, Woods AA et al (2013) Adipose-derived stem cells promote angiogenesis and tissue formation for in vivo tissue engineering. Tissue Eng Part A 19(11–12):1327–1335. doi:10.1089/ten.TEA.2012.0391
9. Ebrahimian TG, Pouzoulet F, Squiban C et al (2009) Cell therapy based on adipose tissue-derived stromal cells promotes physiological and pathological wound healing. Arterioscler Thromb Vasc Biol 29(4):503–510. doi:10.1161/ATVBAHA.108.178962
10. Le Blanc K, Ringden O (2006) Mesenchymal stem cells: properties and role in clinical bone marrow transplantation. Curr Opin Immunol 18(5):586–591. doi:10.1016/j.coi.2006.07.004
11. Mazo M, Planat-Benard V, Abizanda G et al (2008) Transplantation of adipose derived stromal cells is associated with functional improvement in a rat model of chronic myocardial infarction. Eur J Heart Fail 10(5):454–462. doi:10.1016/j.ejheart.2008.03.017
12. Colazzo F, Sarathchandra P, Smolenski RT et al (2011) Extracellular matrix production by adipose-derived stem cells: implications for heart valve tissue engineering. Biomaterials 32(1):119–127. doi:10.1016/j.biomaterials.2010.09.003
13. Kim WS, Park BS, Sung JH et al (2007) Wound healing effect of adipose-derived stem cells: a critical role of secretory factors on human dermal fibroblasts. J Dermatol Sci 48(1):15–24. doi:10.1016/j.jdermsci.2007.05.018

Chapter 13

Isolation of Live Fibroblasts by Fluorescence-Activated Cell Sorting

Tripp Leavitt, Michael S. Hu, and Michael T. Longaker

Abstract

Flow cytometry is a powerful tool in cell biology in that it allows real-time characterization of cellular phenotypes. Additionally, through the process of fluorescence-activated cell sorting (FACS), living cells can be isolated for future in vitro experiments, including single cell analysis. Here we describe the isolation of live fibroblasts from the dermis of the skin in mice using FACS. This method circumvents the need for ex vivo expansion in cell culture, which can alter phenotypic and functional characteristics of cells.

Key words Fibroblasts, Skin, Flow cytometry, Fluorescence-activated cell sorting, Dermis, Dermal tissue harvest, Live cell isolation

1 Introduction

Flow cytometry and fluorescence-activated cell sorting (FACS) have helped to revolutionize the field of cell biology. They permit the characterization of cell populations harvested from living tissues or from cell culture. Simultaneous multiparametric analysis of thousands of particles per second is possible with current technologies. Additionally, data from this analysis can be utilized in "real time" through FACS, separating and isolating particular cells of interest. While virtually any mammalian tissue can be processed for flow cytometry, herein we focus on the characterization and isolation of fibroblast populations from the dermis of mouse skin.

Fibroblasts are fundamental components in the development and maturation of living organisms. While they are vital to our survival, they can also be the source of pathology, accumulating in fibrotic diseases. Therefore, these cells offer the potential for therapeutic targets in anti-fibrotic treatments. Development of such treatments necessitates the isolation and characterization of fibroblasts from living tissues. The vast majority of protocols for establishing primary fibroblast cultures involve directly plating tissues

Laure Rittié (ed.), *Fibrosis: Methods and Protocols*, Methods in Molecular Biology, vol. 1627,
DOI 10.1007/978-1-4939-7113-8_13,

following enzymatic digest. Cells are then given time to migrate out of the tissue and adhere to the cell culture dish. Such methods of harvest present several issues when extrapolating findings to in vivo processes. One potential issue with this methodology is that the cells that may exit the tissue are not necessarily all fibroblasts, which may thus affect downstream analyses. Additionally, fibroblasts demonstrate phenotypic changes when cultured in a dish as compared to in vivo [1]. In order to mitigate these issues, live fibroblasts can be isolated directly from dermal tissues through fluorescence-activated cell sorting [2]. The method presented here allows for the characterization of live fibroblasts based on cell-surface marker profile. The skin is mechanically and enzymatically digested to establish a cell suspension containing fibroblasts. This suspension is then incubated with fluorophore-conjugated antibodies that allow for non-fibroblast cells to be "gated out" during the FACS procedure. Subsequent analyses of sorted cells can provide insights into the physiological, transcriptional, and proteomic characteristics of these cells more closely aligned with fibroblasts in vivo [3].

2 Materials

1. Serially-diluted Betadine solutions in phosphate-buffered saline (1:5); equating to 20%, 4%, and 0.8% betadine in PBS (v/v).
2. Liberase DL (Dispase® Low) enzyme stock solution (5 mg/mL): per manufacturer instructions dissolve Liberase DL (Roche, 05466202001) in Dulbecco's Modified Eagle's Medium (DMEM) containing 25 mM HEPES, on ice for up to 30 min under gentle agitation. This can be aliquoted and stored at −20 °C for use in the enzyme dissociation buffer.
3. Enzyme dissociation buffer: 0.5 mg/mL Liberase DL in DMEM (25 mM HEPES). Dilute Liberase DL (Dispase® Low) enzyme stock solution in DMEM (1:10 dilution). Buffer should be made fresh with each harvest.
4. Wash medium: DMEM (25 mM HEPES), 10% fetal bovine serum (FBS), 1% penicillin–streptomycin (P/S). Store at 4 °C.
5. FACS buffer: phosphate-buffered saline (PBS), 1% FBS, 0.1% P/S, 1 mM ethylenediaminetetraacetic acid (EDTA, *see* **Note 1**), 25 mM HEPES. Filter at 0.22 μm and store at 4 °C.
6. Lineage antibodies (eBioscience San Diego, CA): *see* Table 1.
7. Streptavidin fluorochrome conjugates eFluor 450 (eBioscience 48-4317).
8. 3 μM DAPI solution for nuclear counter staining.

Table 1
Lineage antibodies used in isolation of live fibroblasts

Surface marker	Conjugate	Catalogue number	Amount (μg)
CD31	eFluor 450	48–0311-80	0.25
CD45	eFluor 450	48–0451-82	0.2
TIE-2 (CD202b)	Biotin	13–5987-81	0.5
TER-119	eFluor 450	48–5921-80	0.3
EpCAM CD326	eFluor 450	48–5791-80	0.4
CD324 (E-Cadherin)	Biotin	13–3249-80	0.25

This antibody cocktail is designed with a negative-gating strategy to select for fibroblasts based on the absence of these markers. The far right column indicates quantity of antibody to be added per 100 μl of cell suspension. All antibodies used in our protocol are purchased from eBioscience (San Diego, CA)

3 Methods

1. Sacrifice mice (*see* **Note 2**). Shave and depilate the dorsal and/or ventral dermis. Remove depilation cream with wet wipes. Spray with 70% ethanol and wipe clean.
2. Immediately harvest the dermis to preserve cell viability. Make full-thickness scalpel incisions around the region to be harvested. This region can then be lifted, starting at the cranial portion, with forceps and dissected bluntly along the fascial plane. Dissecting scissors can be used as needed. As the skin flap is lifted, a second set of forceps can also be used to remove subcutaneous fat which can interfere with the enzymatic digestion. The blunt side of a scalpel can also be used to scrape fat from the underside of the skin after it has been harvested.
3. Wash in three serial dilutions (1:5) of betadine starting with 20% betadine.
4. Wash in PBS.
5. Place the skin in DMEM in cell culture dish on ice until ready to begin mincing step (**step 6**).
6. Transfer the skin sample to tissue culture dish lid and finely mince with a scalpel (*see* **Note 3**).
7. Further break up samples using dissecting scissors. The tissue should achieve a uniform, paste-like consistency (Fig. 1).
8. Transfer samples to 50-ml conical tube containing 20 ml enzyme dissociation buffer. Shake tube to prevent clumping of tissue and increase surface area for enzymatic digest.

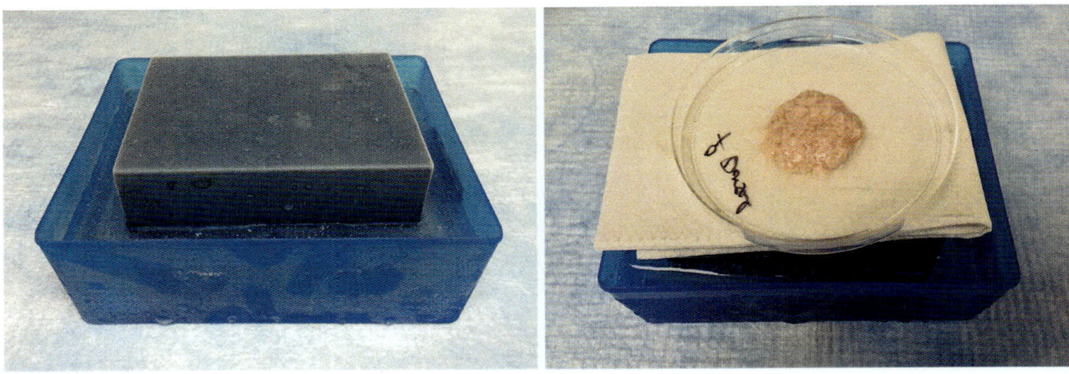

Fig. 1 Setup for mincing step and resulting tissue consistency. A heating block in a small container of water placed at −20 °C overnight (*left*) provides a solid, cold surface to perform mechanical digest while maintaining cell viability. Following mincing with both scalpel and scissors, tissue should achieve a uniform consistency as shown above (*right*)

9. Incubate at 37 °C in a water bath under vigorous agitation for 1.5 h.
10. Remove samples from the water bath shaker, and make up to 50 ml with wash medium to quench enzyme.
11. Centrifuge at 300 *g* for 5 min at 4 °C. If pellet appears small or loose, *see* **Note 4**.
12. Aspirate supernatant, leaving approximately 7.5 ml of medium. Take care to first remove the fat layer before remaining supernatant to reduce adipocyte contamination.
13. Resuspend the pellet with a 5-ml serological pipet. Triturate 5–10 times to achieve a homogeneous cell suspension that should not clog the pipette.
14. Filter cell suspension through a 100 μm cell strainer into a new 50-ml conical tube. Rinse original tube with 20–30 ml wash medium, and then filter as well.
15. Centrifuge filtered suspension at 300 *g* for 5 min at 4 °C.
16. Repeat **steps 12** and **13**, before passing cell suspension through a 40 μm cell strainer into a new 50-mL conical tube. Again, rinse tube with 20–30 ml of wash medium, filtering this as well.
17. Centrifuge filtered suspension at 300 *g* for 5 min at 4 °C.
18. Carefully aspirate entire supernatant.
19. Resuspend pellet in 500 μl FACS buffer and transfer to an Eppendorf tube (*see* **Note 5**). Rinse the conical tube with another 500 μl FACS buffer and add to cell suspension. Add

additional FACS buffer to fill the tube. If there are a large proportion of dead cells within the suspension, clumping can result. This can be circumvented by incubating with DNase for 15 min at room temperature (*see* **Note 6**).

20. Centrifuge cell suspension at 300 *g* for 5 min at 4 °C (*see* **Note 7**).
21. Carefully decant supernatant. Resuspend pellet in 500 μl FACS buffer.
22. Establish unstained control (*see* **Note 8**): transfer 20–50 μl (depending on expected yield) cell suspension to 200 μl FACS buffer in a separate tube, and place on ice under gentle agitation. Protect from light if cells express fluorescent reporter molecules.
23. Incubate remaining sample with fluorophore-conjugated lineage (Lin) antibodies: CD31, CD45, Tie2, Ter-119, EpCAM, and CD324 (E-cadherin) for 30 min under gentle agitation, protected from light (*see* **Note 9**). Relevant antibody concentrations are listed in Table 1.
24. If no secondary antibodies or streptavidin eFluor 450 are needed, skip to **step 28**. However, our protocol requires streptavidin eFluor 450 as TIE-2 and CD324 are currently only commercially available as biotin-conjugated, not eFluor 450-conjugated, antibodies.
25. Wash cell suspension by filling tube with FACS buffer and centrifuging cell suspension at 300 *g* for 5 min at 4 °C.
26. Carefully decant supernatant. Resuspend pellet in 500 μl FACS buffer.
27. Add 7.5 μl streptavidin eFluor 450 (eBioscience, 48-4317), and incubate on ice for 20 min under gentle agitation, protected from light.
28. Wash cell suspension with FACS buffer and centrifuge at 300 *g* for 5 min at 4 °C.
29. Decant supernatant and wash again.
30. Resuspend pellet in 500 μl FACS buffer. Transfer to round-bottom FACS tube through cell strainer cap as cell clumping may result in clogging of the flow cytometer. Rinse 2-ml tube with 500 μL FACS buffer and transfer as well.
31. Add viability dye of choice to sample such as DAPI (*see* **Note 10**).
32. FACS sort for Viability Dye$^-$/CD31$^-$/CD45$^-$/Tie2$^-$/Ter-119$^-$/EpCAM$^-$/CD324$^-$ cells. *See* Fig. 2 for representative sort layout when isolating fibroblasts.

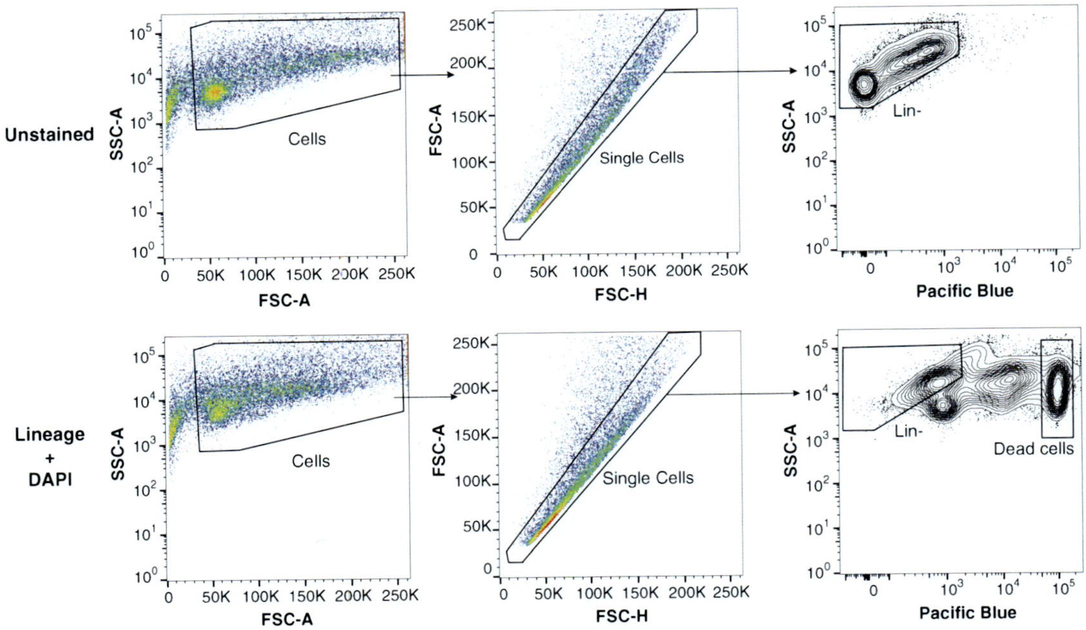

Fig. 2 Representative FACS plots for live fibroblast harvest. Generally, cellular debris is considered to be forward scatter (FSC) low, and thus the first gate is drawn around cells with higher FSC. Unstained controls are shown in the top row and are used to draw the lineage-negative gate. Fibroblasts can be isolated by sorting for Viability Stain⁻ (in this case DAPI) and lineage-negative (Lin⁻: CD31⁻/CD45⁻/Tie2⁻/Ter-119⁻/EpCAM⁻/CD324⁻) cells, after gating out doublets (*middle panels*). Our protocol relies on eFluor 450-conjugated antibodies, which, with DAPI, can collectively be analyzed in the Pacific Blue channel. In this example, ventral dermis was harvested from 4- to 6-week-old female C57/BL6 mice. While staining with Ter-119 excludes red blood cells (RBCs) from the Lin⁻ population, samples rich in RBCs, particularly fetal skin, may benefit from an ACK lysis buffer step (*see* **Note 5**). Shown here for reference, the RBC population is sometimes visible as a tight cluster of low foward- and side-scatter in the initial FACS plot (left panels). In samples stained with the Lin antibodies, this population can be seen just below the Lin⁻ gate, demonstrating a lower side-scatter compared to the cells of interest (bottom right)

4 Notes

1. EDTA is included to prevent cell clumping secondary to cell adhesion, which can be particularly important in generating a single cell suspension of fibroblasts. The EDTA concentration can vary between 1 and 5 mM in the FACS buffer. However, for mouse skin, 1 mM EDTA is suitable. Should this protocol be adapted for human skin, 5 mM EDTA may be appropriate.
2. Age of mice can vary, but mice aged 4 weeks demonstrate less subcutaneous fat which makes for a cleaner, easier harvest. Number of mice can vary, but in cases where only the dorsal skin is harvested, it is recommended that at least 3–5 mice be used to ensure suitable yield of fibroblasts. Insufficient yield

can result in smaller cell pellets, which become more difficult to work with at later steps. This issue also correlates with increased cell death.

3. During the mincing step, aim to keep the sample together to avoid it drying out. If needed, enzyme dissociation buffer can also be added to keep the tissue hydrated (e.g., an ~2-cm-diameter drop). Thoroughness of mincing correlates with yield, and therefore the sample should be broken up as finely as possible. The mincing step should also ideally be performed on ice or another cold surface to reduce cell death. An inverted heating block in a small container of water placed at −20 °C overnight is an excellent option (Fig. 1).

4. In some cases, during tissue processing, pellets following centrifugation may appear small or loose. This is likely due, at least in part, to adipose tissue contaminating the sample. In the isolation of live cells, centrifugation is recommended to not exceed 300 *g*. However, in our experience, centrifugation at 500 *g* allows for better pellet formation in such cases, without a noticeable increase in cell death.

5. If sample contamination with red blood cells (RBCs) is an issue (Fig. 2), ACK lysis buffer (Thermofisher, cat no. A1049201) can be used in transferring cells in step 19. Allow 3-5 min for RBC lysis prior to centrifugation. If the centrifuge to be used in later steps is equipped with swing-bucket rotor, 1.5-ml or 2-ml Eppendorf tubes can be used. Use of 2-ml Eppendorf tubes limits pellet loss when only a fixed-angle rotor is available. The size of the cell pellet should also be considered when selecting tube size.

6. If there is concern for cell clumping secondary to a large proportion of dead cells within the prep, the sample can be incubated for 15 min at room temperature with 100 μg/ml DNase (Sigma, St. Louis, MO; cat no. D-4513) in Hanks' balanced salt solution (HBSS, Sigma, cat no. H-6648) and 5 mM $MgCl_2$ [4]. If DNase is to be used, substitute the FACS buffer in **step 19** with HBSS (5 mM $MgCl_2$). Following the 15 min incubation, cells can then be washed in the FACS buffer, filling the tube and then continuing with the protocol at **step 20**. It is important to note that this protocol also incorporates EDTA into the FACS buffer to limit clumping of adherent fibroblasts, which will inhibit DNase activity by chelating divalent cations (Mg^{2+} and Ca^{2+}). Therefore, DNase is not incorporated into the FACS buffer.

7. Use of a swing-bucket rotor during centrifugation is recommended to limit loss of cells along the side wall of the tube.

8. Samples for compensation can also be established at this stage to control for fluorophore emission spectral overlap.

Compensation controls can be set up using either compensation beads or cells, which are stained with a single fluorophore-conjugated antibody. One compensation control sample is required for each fluorophore channel. This is unnecessary if only a single fluorophore is to be used.

9. Conjugated fluorophores should be selected based on channels available for flow cytometry analysis. In our studies we use eFluor 450 (formerly PacBlue). Also note that when using multiple fluorophores, fluorescence minus one (FMO) controls should be established.

10. Viability dye can be matched with the lineage antibody conjugates to preserve the range of available channels. In the case of eFluor 450, DAPI can be used to create a "dump channel" as the cells of interest will be Viability Dye$^-$/Lin$^-$.

References

1. Walmsley GG, Rinkevich Y, Hu MS et al (2015) Live fibroblast harvest reveals surface marker shift in vitro. Tissue Eng Part C Methods 21(3):314–321. doi:10.1089/ten.TEC.2014.0118
2. Walmsley GG, Maan ZN, Hu MS et al (2016) Murine dermal fibroblast isolation by FACS. J Vis Exp 107. doi:10.3791/53430
3. Rinkevich Y, Walmsley GG, Hu MS et al (2015) Skin fibrosis. Identification and isolation of a dermal lineage with intrinsic fibrogenic potential. Science 348(6232):aaa2151. doi:10.1126/science.aaa2151
4. Crissman HA, Mullaney PF, Steinkamp JA (1975) Methods and applications of flow systems for analysis and sorting of mammalian cells. Methods Cell Biol 9(0):179–246

Chapter 14

Detection of Infiltrating Mast Cells Using a Modified Toluidine Blue Staining

Nahum Puebla-Osorio, Seri N.E. Sarchio, Stephen E. Ullrich, and Scott N. Byrne

Abstract

Mast cells are part of the immune system and characteristically contain histamine- and heparin-rich basophilic granules. While these cells are usually associated with allergy and anaphylaxis, they also promote wound healing and angiogenesis and confer protection against pathogens. The presence of these cells is sometimes indicative of a poor prognosis, especially in skin cancer, pancreatic cancer, and lymphoma. Toluidine blue staining of acid-fast granules is an established method for the identification and quantification of mast cells. Generating detailed information on the location of mast cells within tissues is problematic using this technique and often requires serial sections from adjacent tissue to be separately stained with hematoxylin and eosin (H&E). Staining serial sections is not always possible, particularly if the sample is very small or rare. In such cases, a method of simultaneously identifying and localizing mast cells in a tissue would be advantageous. Toluidine blue and H&E are not commonly combined because H&E includes repetitive washes in water, which may affect the efficacy of the aqueous-soluble toluidine blue. We have developed and tested a novel staining technique that integrates toluidine blue between hematoxylin and eosin in one simple procedure. This protocol works on both frozen and formalin-fixed, paraffin-embedded tissue and readily allows for the identification of purple-stained mast cells against a clean H&E background. This facilitates a more accurate localization and proper counting of mast cells in normal and affected tissue.

Key words Toluidine blue, Hematoxylin and eosin, Mast cells, Skin, Inflamed intestine

1 Introduction

The identification of infiltrating mast cells is readily performed using antibody-based detection of endogenous proteins such as chymase and tryptase; however this is a time-consuming process and depends on high-quality detection antibodies. The histological staining with toluidine blue (TB) is a direct, rapid, highly effective, and efficient antibody-independent method to identify mast cells in tissue sections [1]. TB belongs to a set of dyes with metachromatic properties, conferred by its thiazine group, which stain tissues with differing degrees of intensity of the same color [1].

Laure Rittié (ed.), *Fibrosis: Methods and Protocols*, Methods in Molecular Biology, vol. 1627,
DOI 10.1007/978-1-4939-7113-8_14, © Springer Science+Business Media LLC 2017

Toluidine blue staining readily identifies mast cell metachromatic granules against a pale blue background.

However, while TB is a desirable stain for mast cells, it is often difficult to assess their precise location, as the surrounding tissue is barely distinguishable after the staining. This is particularly disadvantageous for the analysis of architecturally complex tissues like the intestine and skin. Mast cells play important roles in the cellular context, so it is often critical to localize them within a particular tissue compartment, as their location may correlate with disease outcomes.

Mast cells originate from a bone marrow progenitor and, under specific microenvironmental conditions, migrate to different tissues to complete their maturation [2]. They are rapidly recruited to sites of inflammation, damaged tissue, and tumors [3, 4] and respond in part by releasing the contents of their preformed granules (e.g., histamine and proteases) [5]. Mast cells can also produce a wide variety of other inflammatory mediators including prostaglandins, leukotrienes, cytokines, chemokines, growth factors (e.g., VEGF), reactive oxygen species, metalloproteinases, and neuropeptides [6, 7]. There is a strong prognostic association between changes in mast cell numbers and areas of tissue repair, chronic inflammation, and cancer. Aside from their role in type I (allergic) hypersensitivity responses [8], mast cells accumulate at sites of tumor growth in response to numerous chemoattractants [9]. Although their presence is considered beneficial under certain conditions [10], in certain cancers, mast cell infiltration is associated with a poor prognosis [11, 12]. Animal models of sunlight-induced skin [12, 13] and pancreatic [12] cancer show that pharmacologically targeting mast cells can be highly effective in both preventing and ameliorating already established cancer.

These factors have made identifying and quantitating mast cells in a particular tissue increasingly important for many disciplines. Current techniques rely on serial tissue sectioning in which one section is stained with TB for the detection of mast cells, while the contiguous section is stained with H&E to visualize the tissue architecture. This method depends on the ability to collect adjacent sections and the precision to which they can be paired to create "mirror" images for proper evaluation. However, this is a time-consuming process and could be problematic when dealing with scarce tissue samples such as tumor-bearing specimens. H&E staining requires repetitive washing through alcohols and water, which compromises acid-fast staining of mast cell granules because TB readily dissolves in water. Consequently TB integrated with H&E staining has not traditionally been performed on the same section, as incorporation of both stains has proved very challenging. Here we show that by combining TB and H&E in one single protocol, we are able to obtain high-quality images showing purple-stained mast cells against a clean H&E background.

To validate this protocol, we assessed the differences between tissue samples stained with TB only or with the combination of TB and H&E (TB-H&E). Briefly, we processed 5–7 μm formalin-fixed paraffin-embedded sections from $p53^{R1972P}Ku70^{-/-}$ inflamed intestine and skin and performed the respective staining procedures. Although TB makes it easy to recognize mast cells in the inflamed intestine, using TB alone not only prevents the visualization of the intestinal architecture (Fig. 1) but also impairs the identification of the tissue under study (Fig. 1). In contrast, using the combination TB-H&E staining allows for a clear definition of characteristic structures of the intestine including the mucosa, submucosa, and lamina propria (Figs. 2 and 3). This technique also facilitates the recognition of infiltrating immune cells other than mast cells within the inflamed tissue. In addition, this procedure facilitates the analysis of existing pathological changes observed in the affected tissue including edema, tissue degeneration, repair, and tumor formation, among others. TB-H&E also allowed us to recognize infiltrating mast cells within the dermis and epidermis (Fig. 4) and to detect mast cells in non-inflamed tissues including the adrenal gland, brain, kidney, and oviduct (Fig. 5). TB-H&E distinctively identifies mast cells in the tissue under study and allows the clear localization of these cells against the underlying structure. We have also used this technique to successfully identify and localize mast cells in frozen tissue from the brain, spinal cord, kidney, adrenal gland, and heart (data not shown) (*see* **Note 1**).

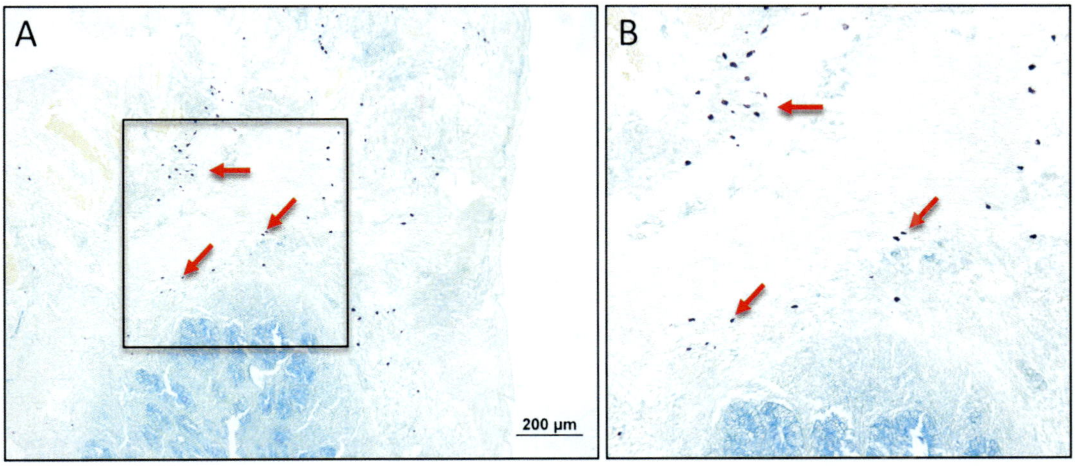

Fig. 1 Toluidine staining on inflamed colorectal tissue. (**a**) Toluidine blue (TB) makes readily evident infiltrating mast cells but provides little detail for the analysis of the affected tissue, and it is almost impossible to identify the type of tissue. (**b**) Enlarged frame from **a**. *Arrows* indicate representative TB-stained mast cells

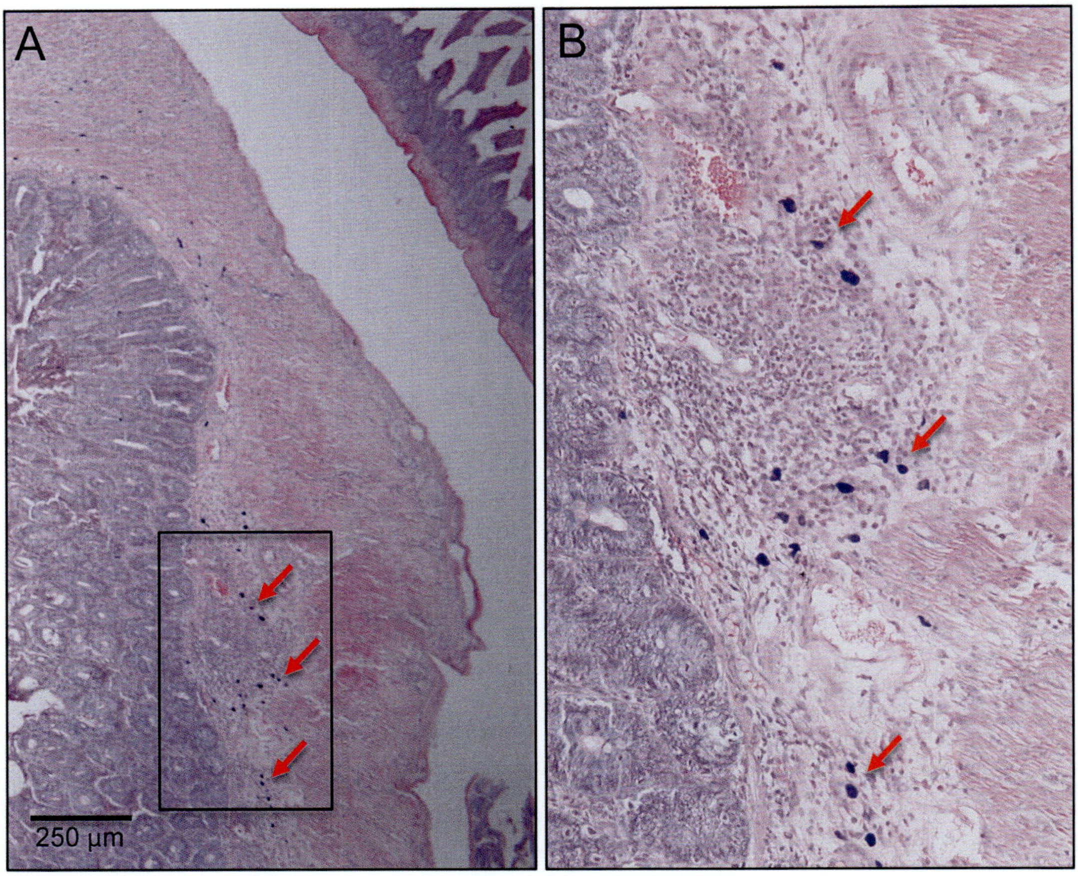

Fig. 2 Toluidine blue (TB) and hematoxylin and eosin (H&E) provide a clear picture of infiltrating mast cells and the tissue architecture. (**a**) The combination of both TB and H&E provides a clear location of mast cells and allows for a clean visualization of the intestinal tissue architecture; (**b**) detailed analysis of an enlarged segment showing a clear distinction between inflamed submucosa and infiltrating mast cells. *Arrows* indicate representative TB-stained mast cells

2 Materials

2.1 Reagents

1. 10% buffered formalin (w/v): mix 100 mL formaldehyde (36.5%, w/v), 4 g sodium phosphate monobasic (NaH_2PO_4), 6.5 g sodium phosphate dibasic (NaH_2PO_4), and distilled water to 1l.
2. M sodium acetate buffer pH 4: mix 13.6 g sodium acetate anhydrous and distilled water to 1 l. Stir until completely dissolved. Bring solution to pH 4 using glacial acetic acid. Store at RT or 4 °C for longer storage.
3. 0.4% toluidine blue solution (w/v): mix 0.4 g toluidine blue O with 100 ml 0.1 M sodium acetate buffer pH 4. Stir well. Adjust the pH to 2.0–2.5 by adding drops of 1 M hydrochloric

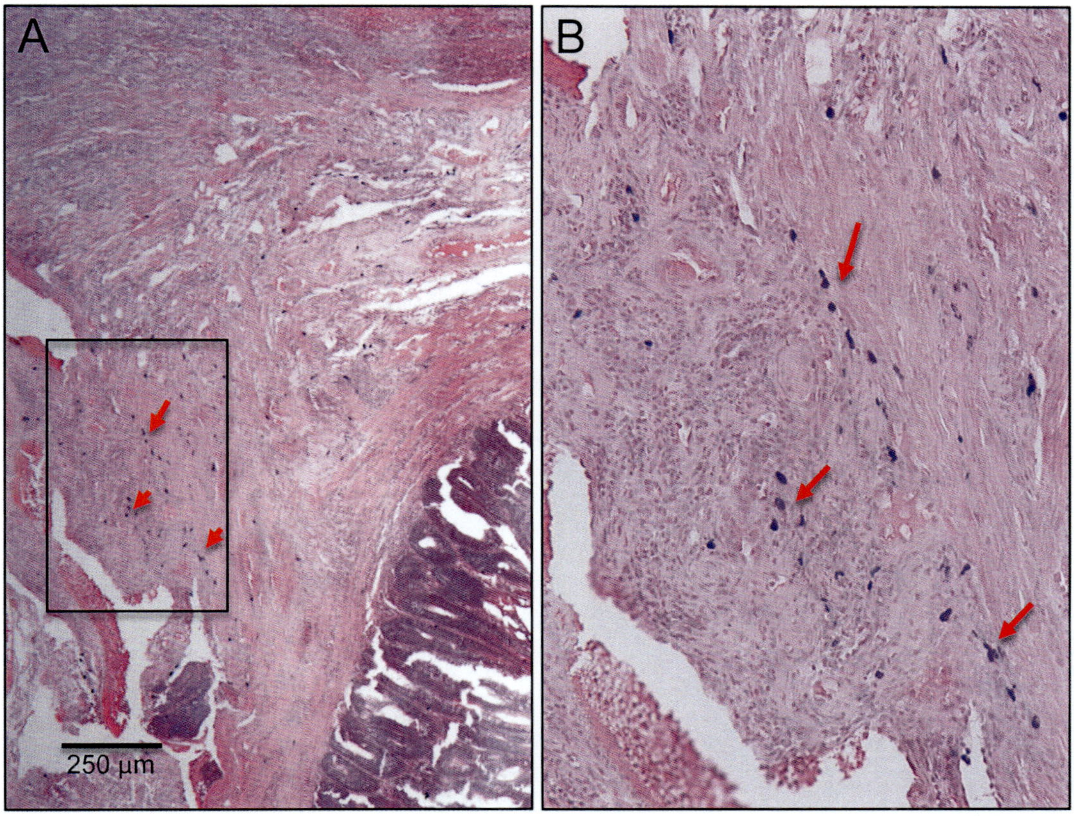

Fig. 3 The combination of toluidine blue (TB) and hematoxylin and eosin (H&E) allows for the analysis of severely affected colorectal tissue. (**a**) TB and H&E help to visualize the extent of damage of the affected intestine; (**b**) mast cells infiltrating severely damaged tissue that resulted from chronic inflammation. *Arrows* indicate representative TB-stained mast cells

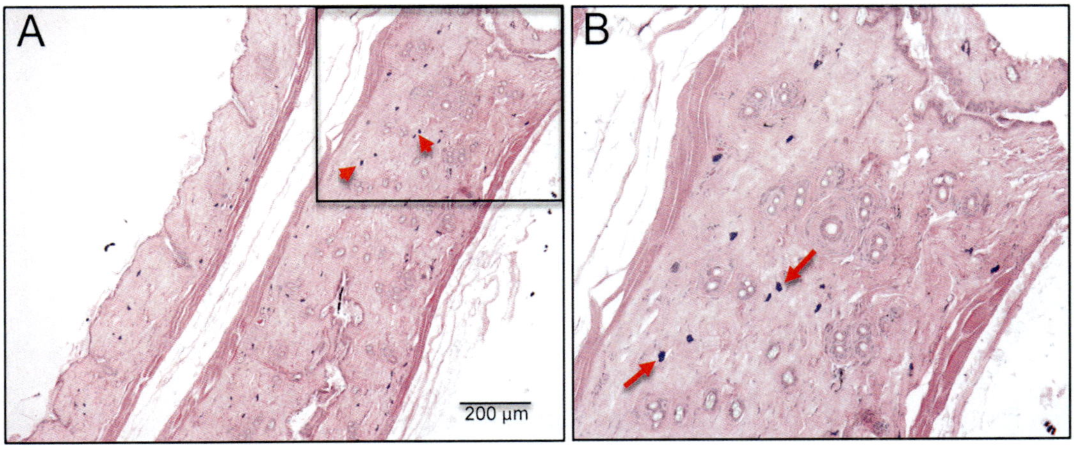

Fig. 4 The combination of toluidine blue (TB) and hematoxylin and eosin (H&E) can also be used for skin staining. (**a**) Detail of infiltrating mast cells in the dermis and epidermis and important structures of the skin; (**b**) enlarged picture from **a**. *Arrows* indicate representative TB-stained mast cells

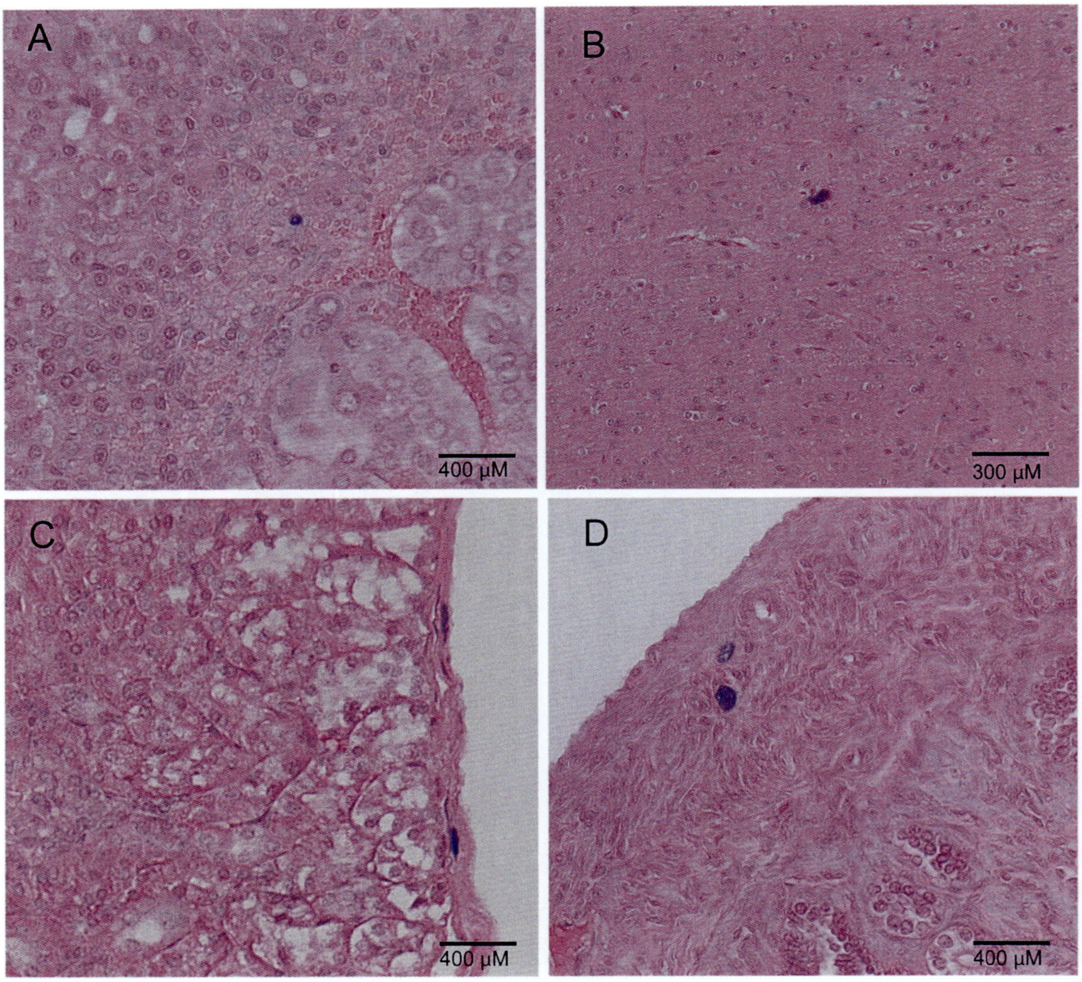

Fig. 5 The combination of toluidine blue (TB) and hematoxylin and eosin (H&E) can also distinguish mast cells in non-affected tissue. Mast cells were in low number in non-inflamed mouse tissues including the (**a**) adrenal gland, (**b**) brain, (**c**) kidney, and (**d**) oviduct

acid. Wrap bottle with aluminum foil and store at 4 °C. Equilibrate the solution to RT before use. Staining is performed at RT, protected from light.

4. TRIS base.
5. Organic mounting medium (e.g., Permount, Fisher Scientific, Hampton, NH).
6. Paraffin-embedding medium (e.g., Paraplast, McCormick, St. Louis, MO).
7. Histological clearing agent (e.g. Histo-Clear, National Diagnostics, Atlanta, GA).
8. Xylene.
9. Ethanol solutions: dilute ethyl alcohol 200 proof v/v with distilled water.

10. Harris' modified hematoxylin solution.
11. 5% eosin solution (w/v).
12. Scott's bluing solution.
13. Paper towels.
14. Tissue samples. We used murine tissue sections from the large intestine and skin obtained from $p53^{R1972P}$Ku70−/− mutant mice, which are prone to develop spontaneous colitis and colorectal cancer [14]. The University of Texas MD Anderson Cancer Center's Animal Care and Use Committee approved all experiments involving animals.
15. Coverslips thickness no. 1.5.

2.2 Equipment

1. Microscope and image collection devices (we used an Olympus DP70 digital color camera attached to an Olympus BX51 microscope (Olympus, Melville, NY)).
2. Tissue-processing carousel (e.g., Citadel 1000, Thermo Shandon, Waltham, MA).
3. Paraffin-embedding apparatus (e.g., Histocentre 2 model 6400012, Thermo Shandon).
4. Oven for slide drying (e.g., Isotemp Oven, Fisher Scientific).

3 Methods

3.1 Tissue Processing

1. Obtained tissue samples from desired organs.
2. Immersed tissue samples in 10% buffered formalin for 24 h.
3. Remove tissues from the fixative and place in 70% alcohol.
4. Embed in paraffin: sequentially incubate in 70, 85, 95, and 100% ethanol, xylene, and molten paraffin (30 min incubation each), and set tissues in paraffin blocks.
5. Cut paraffin-embedded tissue in 5–7 μm sections and place onto glass slides.
6. Bake the slides for a minimum of 1 h at 55 °C before use.

3.2 Tissue Staining

The following protocol works on both frozen and formalin-fixed paraffin-embedded tissue, facilitating the identification of mast cells according to their precise location without compromising the tissue architecture.

1. De-wax paraffin-embedded tissue sections by immersing slides 5 min in xylene (or Histo-Clear), and rehydrate tissue by sequential immersions (5 min each) in 100%, 95%, and 70% ethanol and a final 2 min immersion in distilled water.
2. Place the slides in Harris' hematoxylin solution for 70 s (*see* **Note 2**).

3. Briefly wash the excess of hematoxylin by immersing the slides two or three times in clean tap water. Briefly tap the slides on paper towels to remove excess water.
4. Immerse slides briefly three times in 70% alcohol, and wash again in clean tap water for 3 min. Remove excess water.
5. Place slides in Scott's bluing solution for up to a minute (*see* **Note 3**). This step gently transforms hematoxylin into an insoluble blue color within the nucleus.
6. Inspect the slides under the bright-light microscope to ensure the nuclei are properly stained (*see* **Note 4**).
7. Wash slides in clean tap water for 3 min, and remove excess water.
8. Immerse slides in clean 0.4% TB solution for 4 min (*see* **Note 5**).
9. Wash slides in clean tap water for 3 min (*see* **Note 6**) and remove excess water.
10. Quickly dip the slides three times in one batch of 70% ethanol and then dip them five times in 5% eosin solution.
11. Dehydrate the slides by successive immersion in 70% (2 min), 95% (twice, 2 min each), and 100% ethanol (twice, 2 min each); conclude this step by immersing the slides in xylene (or Histo-Clear) (twice, 3 min each) (*see* **Note 7**).
12. Permanently mount each slide with a clean coverslip using Permount or any other xylene-based mounting medium.
13. Let slides dry for a minimum of 60 min before analyzing them under the bright-light microscope.

4 Notes

1. Our results suggest that toluidine blue may still be the stain of choice if the aim is to simply quantitate absolute mast cell numbers. However, if detailed information regarding the location of mast cells in a particular tissue is required, or desired, then our new technique would be superior to toluidine blue alone.
2. The time may be changed between 30 and 70 s depending on the freshness of the hematoxylin. It is important to prevent hematoxylin over-staining as it could hinder the identification of mast cells. It will happen if the incubation is extended beyond the suggested time and if a new batch of hematoxylin is used.
3. The time could be shortened to 20–30 s depending on the intensity of blue nuclei.
4. If nuclei are not evenly stained, incubate slides in Scott's bluing solution for an additional time, but if the staining is too strong, immerse the slides briefly in 70% ethanol.

5. To prevent the deposit of insoluble debris on the slides, severely affecting the quality of the tissue section, make sure the TB solution is clean; a freshly made batch should be filtered using a 40 μm filter. The incubation time range may be 3.5–4.5 min.
6. Inspect one slide under the microscope to ensure mast cells are properly stained with the typical bright purple color.
7. To avoid xylenes contamination with water, often seen when cloudiness or multiple droplets appear while slides are permanently mounted, thoroughly dehydrate the slides by including an extra step in absolute alcohol.

Acknowledgments

This work was supported by the Cancer Institute NSW (Career Development and Support Fellowship to SNB; 07/CDF/01-07), the Multiple Sclerosis Research Australia (Project Grant: 12-007), the NSW Cancer Council (Project Grant: RG14-14), the National Health and Medical Research Council of Australia and the Sydney Medical School Foundation, and the Cancer Prevention and Research Institute of Texas (SEU; RP120777). Support was also provided by the histopathology facilities in the Discipline of Pathology, Sydney Medical School, University of Sydney, and Royal Prince Alfred Hospital. The animal and histology support facilities at the MD Anderson Cancer Center are funded in part by a core grant from the US National Cancer Institute (CA16672). We thank Bree Lege (RAII/MDACC) for insightful comments on the methodology.

References

1. Sridharan G, Shankar AA (2012) Toluidine blue: a review of its chemistry and clinical utility. J Oral Maxillofac Pathol 16(2):251–255. doi:10.4103/0973-029X.99081
2. Hanahan D, Coussens LM (2012) Accessories to the crime: functions of cells recruited to the tumor microenvironment. Cancer Cell 21(3):309–322. doi:10.1016/j.ccr.2012.02.022
3. Collington SJ, Williams TJ, Weller CL (2011) Mechanisms underlying the localisation of mast cells in tissues. Trends Immunol 32(10):478–485. doi:10.1016/j.it.2011.08.002
4. Ribatti D, Crivellato E (2012) Mast cells, angiogenesis, and tumour growth. Biochim Biophys Acta 1822(1):2–8. doi:10.1016/j.bbadis.2010.11.010
5. Galli SJ, Kalesnikoff J, Grimbaldeston MA et al (2005) Mast cells as "tunable" effector and immunoregulatory cells: recent advances. Annu Rev Immunol 23:749–786. doi:10.1146/annurev.immunol.21.120601.141025
6. Sarchio SN, Kok LF, O'Sullivan C et al (2012) Dermal mast cells affect the development of sunlight-induced skin tumours. Exp Dermatol 21(4):241–248.doi:10.1111/j.1600-0625.2012.01438.x
7. da Silva EZ, Jamur MC, Oliver C (2014) Mast cell function: a new vision of an old cell. J Histochem Cytochem 62(10):698–738. doi:10.1369/0022155414545334
8. Rodewald HR, Feyerabend TB (2012) Widespread immunological functions of mast cells: fact or fiction? Immunity 37(1):13–24. doi:10.1016/j.immuni.2012.07.007
9. Conti P, Pang X, Boucher W et al (1997) Impact of Rantes and MCP-1 chemokines on in vivo basophilic cell recruitment in rat skin

injection model and their role in modifying the protein and mRNA levels for histidine decarboxylase. Blood 89(11):4120–4127

10. Theoharides TC, Conti P (2004) Mast cells: the Jekyll and Hyde of tumor growth. Trends Immunol 25(5):235–241. doi:10.1016/j.it.2004.02.013
11. Molin D, Edstrom A, Glimelius I et al (2002) Mast cell infiltration correlates with poor prognosis in Hodgkin's lymphoma. Br J Haematol 119(1):122–124
12. Ma Y, Hwang RF, Logsdon CD et al (2013) Dynamic mast cell-stromal cell interactions promote growth of pancreatic cancer. Cancer Res 73(13):3927–3937. doi:10.1158/0008-5472.CAN-12-4479
13. Sarchio SN, Scolyer RA, Beaugie C et al (2014) Pharmacologically antagonizing the CXCR4-CXCL12 chemokine pathway with AMD3100 inhibits sunlight-induced skin cancer. J Invest Dermatol 134(4):1091–1100. doi:10.1038/jid.2013.424
14. Puebla-Osorio N, Kim J, Ojeda S et al (2014) A novel Ku70 function in colorectal homeostasis separate from nonhomologous end joining. Oncogene 33(21):2748–2757. doi:10.1038/onc.2013.234

Chapter 15

Cell-Populated Collagen Lattice Models

Beate Eckes, Fang Wang, Laure Rittié, Gabriele Scherr, and Paola Zigrino

Abstract

Investigation of cell function is often hampered by the complexity of the tissue context. This problem is circumvented by isolating cells from tissues and analyzing their behavior in culture. Most cell types are cultured as monolayers on planar, rigid Petri dishes, an environment that does not reflect the spatial, three-dimensional cellular environment in vivo. Culture in three-dimensional collagen lattices has been devised to optimize in vitro culture conditions and to provide a more physiologic "in vivo-like" environment. Collagen lattices can easily be manipulated to suit diverse cell types and to provide variable mechanical forces. Cells can be imaged in such surroundings, and gene expression as well as protein production and activity can be monitored.

Key words Fibroblast, Three-dimensional culture, Collagen-binding integrin, MMP, Morphology, Mechanical force

1 Introduction

Collagen lattices have been devised as early as 1979 to provide cells in culture with a three-dimensional environment and structural support made of extracellular matrix (ECM) that much better reflects their in vivo environment than planar, rigid tissue plastic [1]. In the latter, cells are traditionally induced to proliferate at maximal rate, often at the expense of their differentiated phenotype. Collagen lattice cultures consist of collagen type I that is one of the most abundant ECM proteins in vertebrate bodies, but they can be modified by addition of further ECM components such as other collagen types or proteoglycans in order to more closely reflect the composition of a given tissue. Three-dimensional collagen lattice cultures have been used to embed and analyze the behavior of connective tissue cells including fibroblasts, chondrocytes, and smooth muscle cells, as well as epithelial, immune, and tumor cells [2] and references therein [3, 4]. Fibroblasts are among the best characterized cell types in collagen lattice culture [5].

Laure Rittié (ed.), *Fibrosis: Methods and Protocols*, Methods in Molecular Biology, vol. 1627, DOI 10.1007/978-1-4939-7113-8_15, © Springer Science+Business Media LLC 2017

Collagen lattices are cast using a solution of collagen I monomers in dilute acid, which polymerize upon raising the pH to neutral values and increasing the temperature to 37 °C [1]. Cells are seeded either into the suspension of neutralized collagen or on top of the polymerized lattice. The original lattice type reported by E. Bell was a freely floating one, in which the embedded fibroblasts rearrange the collagen fibrils to a dense "tissue" in a process that depends on an intact cytoskeleton and either serum supplement or defined growth factors (e.g., TGFβ or PDGF) [1, 5, 6] (Fig. 1). This process is also termed contraction, retraction, or compaction of the lattice, depending on the author; contraction rate is directly proportional to cell density and inversely related to collagen concentration. Collagen lattice cultures were used as models reflecting tissue remodeling during wound contraction [7].

Besides the need for a more physiological environment, collagen lattices have been used as dermal transplants [1] and as the dermal compartment of complex coculture systems in which the lattices, populated by fibroblasts with or without endothelial cells, support the formation of a stratified epidermis built by keratinocytes; these cultures were used as full-thickness skin transplants [8].

Fibroblasts interact with the lattice environment through collagen-binding integrins [9], mainly $\alpha_2\beta_1$ [10, 11] and $\alpha_{11}\beta_1$ [12]. These transmembrane receptors bind to collagen by their extracellular domains while connecting to the actin/actomyosin cytoskeleton with their intracellular domains, thereby "integrating" the extracellular environment with the force-sensing cellular machinery and enabling bidirectional signal transduction. Among the most prominent signals induced by contracting collagen lattices is down-modulated ERK activity that results in a shutdown of fibroblast proliferation in comparison to monolayer culture [13].

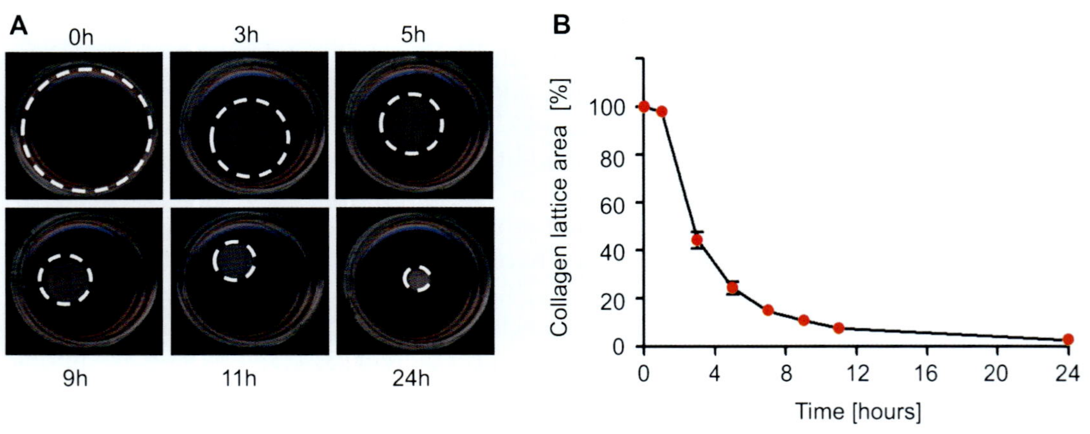

Fig. 1 Kinetics of contraction of floating collagen lattices by fibroblasts. Primary fibroblasts derived from mouse dermis were seeded into floating collagen lattices. Fibroblasts were seeded at 2×10^5 cells per ml into lattices with a final collagen concentration of 0.3 mg/ml. (**a**) Contraction was monitored over 24 h. *White circles* indicate the boundaries of the lattices. (**b**) Lattice area was plotted as a function of time

Fibroblast morphology also changes from spindle to stellate morphology, and their gene expression profile is altered: expression of collagens is strongly reduced [14], while that of matrix metalloproteinase (MMP) is highly elevated [15, 16].

In order to mimic the mechanical forces acting in a tissue, in which the collagen-rich connective tissue is not compacted but counteracts the contracting cellular force, a number of modifications of the original collagen lattice model have been introduced. Attached lattices are cast in tissue culture dishes in which the collagen lattice sticks to the bottom and wall of the dish [17]. Alternatively, the lattices are maintained in a non-contracted state by inserting posts [2, 18] or nylon threads [19] to which the lattices tether and remain extended (Fig. 2). In all these "stressed" conditions, fibroblasts are mechanically loaded, which is not the case in the floating lattices, introducing another level of gene regulation, namely, mechanoregulation. Tenascin-C and collagen XII have been reported early on as prime ECM components induced by mechanical forces [20], as well as α-smooth muscle actin (αSMA), the hallmark of myofibroblasts [21]. Using a comprehensive screen, comparing the gene expression profiles of fibroblasts grown in floating vs. stressed lattices later revealed two distinctly different fibroblast phenotypes

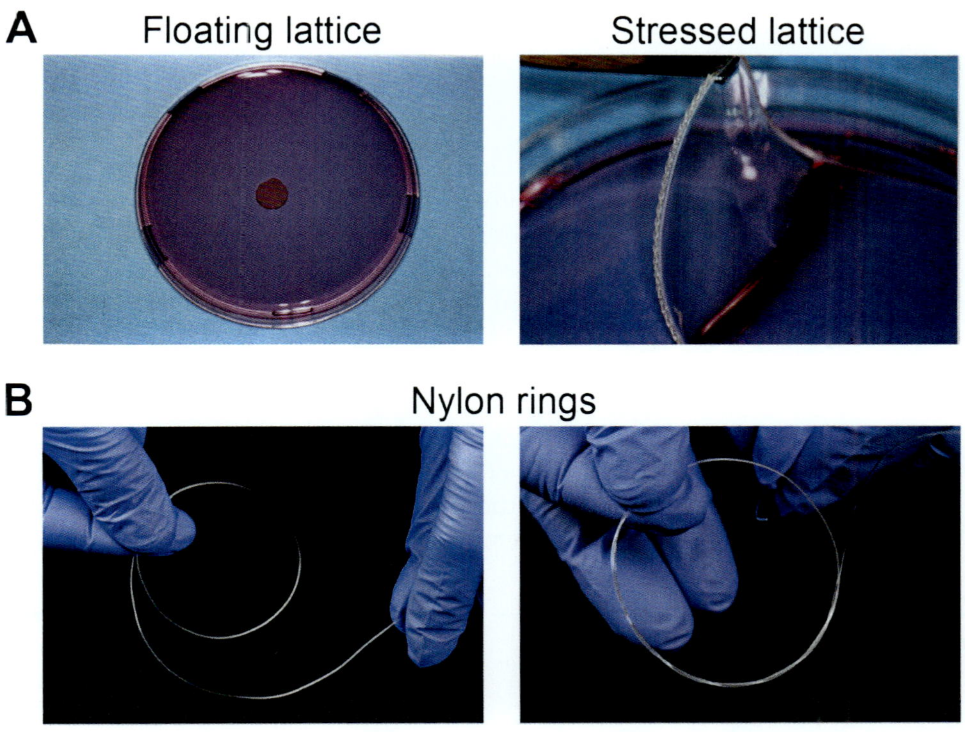

Fig. 2 Aspect of collagen lattices 24 h after seeding. (**a**) Primary human dermal fibroblasts were cultured as described in the text for 24 h in either floating or stressed conditions. The floating lattice is maximally contracted. The stressed lattice is attached to a braided nylon thread. (**b**) Images depict the procedure used to form the nylon thread holding the stressed lattice

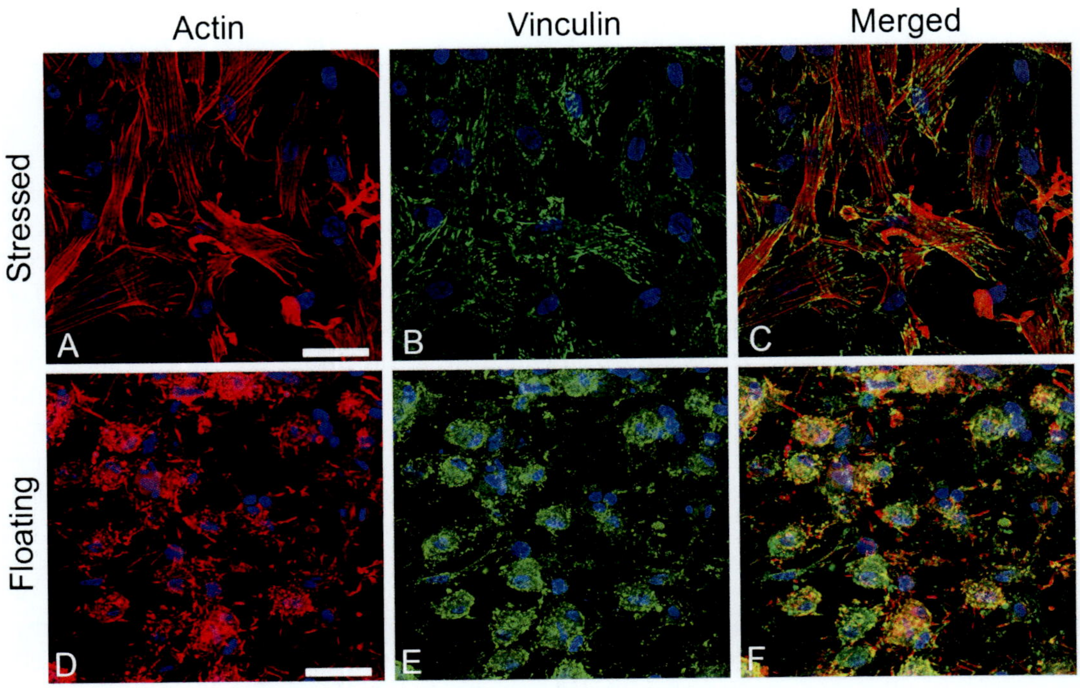

Fig. 3 Fibroblast morphology in collagen lattices. Primary human dermal fibroblasts were cultured for 20 h in stressed (**a**–**c**) or floating collagen lattices (**d**–**f**). Actin microfilaments and focal adhesion structures were visualized by phalloidin and vinculin staining, respectively. This research was originally published [19]. © The American Society for Biochemistry and Molecular Biology

[19]: Those in floating lattices do not proliferate and are quiescent in terms of ECM production but show high activity of MMP production and of various inflammatory mediators such as interleukin-6 and cyclooxygenase-2. In contrast, stressed fibroblasts proliferate and show abundant production of ECM components, protease inhibitors, and profibrotic mediators such as transforming growth factor-beta 1 (TGFβ-1) and monocyte chemoattractant protein-1 (MCP-1), while MMP production is low [16, 19]. The stressed environment induces the long spindle-shaped morphology also seen in monolayers (where the rigid substrate exerts even more force than the stressed lattice), and cells assemble well-defined focal adhesions which are not seen in floating lattices (Fig. 3).

2 Materials

2.1 Reagents

All culture reagents should be either purchased sterile or sterilized in the laboratory upon preparation by autoclaving or filtration (through 0.22 μm diameter pore filters). All sterile solutions should be kept sterile and manipulated in a biosafety cabinet (also known as "cell culture hood") only.

1. 3 mg/ml solution of collagen I (stock, sterile) in 0.1% (v/v) acetic acid (or 0.01 M HCl) (*see* **Notes 1** and **2**).
2. 0.1 M NaOH sterile solution.
3. 10X and 1X Dulbecco's modified Eagle's medium (DMEM) (*see* **Note 3**).
4. Phosphate-buffered saline (PBS).
5. Antibiotics stock (10,000 U/ml penicillin and 10,000 μg/ml streptomycin).
6. 200 mM L-glutamine stock.
7. (+)-Sodium L-ascorbate (*see* **Note 4**).
8. Fetal calf serum (FCS) or other type of serum adequate for chosen cells (e.g., fetal bovine serum).
9. Lattice supplements: mix 100 ml penicillin/streptomycin stock, 100 ml glutamine stock, 500 mg sodium L-ascorbate until homogeneous. Sterilize by filtration (0.22 μm), prepare 10 ml aliquots and store at −20 °C.
10. 1.76X lattice medium: dissolve 0.38 g $NaHCO_3$ in 10-ml H_2O, and add 17.6-ml 10X DMEM and 3.52 ml lattice supplements. Bring to 100 ml with H_2O. Sterilize by filtration (0.22 μm) and store at 4 °C for up to 4 weeks (*see* **Note 3**).
11. Complete DMEM: 1X DMEM containing 10% FCS, 100 U/ml penicillin, 100 μg/ml streptomycin, 2 mM glutamine, and 50 μg/ml sodium L-ascorbate (*see* **Note 4**).
12. Cultured fibroblasts (*see* **Note 5**).
13. Bacterial collagenase (for cell isolation after culture, if needed).

2.2 Equipment

1. 15-ml sterile plastic tubes.
2. Disposable 2-, 5-, and 10-ml pipettes.
3. 3-cm diameter bacteriological dishes (= not suited for tissue culture) for floating lattices.
4. 3-cm diameter tissue culture plastic for stressed lattices.
5. Nylon thread (approx. 0.45 mm in diameter).
6. Instant type glue.
7. Inverted phase contrast microscope with 10X or 20X objective.
8. Standard cell culture equipment (sterile hood, cell incubator, centrifuge, etc.).
9. Thin ruler or digital scanner and computer (for contraction measurements).

3 Methods

3.1 Casting Collagen Lattices

1. Trypsinize a fibroblast culture and prepare a 4.5–7.5 × 10^5 cell suspension (i.e., will contain 3–5 × 10^5 cells/0.67 ml) in complete DMEM (*see* **Note 5**).
2. Prepare lattice dishes (*see* **Note 6**):
   (a) For floating lattices, use sterile bacteriological-grade Petri dishes (to reduce cell adhesion to the dish) and proceed directly to **step 3** (*see***Note 7**).
   (b) For stressed lattices, use tissue culture plastic dishes, and insert nylon rings as follows: Bend one strand of nylon thread to form a ring, and adjust the circular size to the inner perimeter of the chosen lattice dish. Then wind the thread around itself as shown in Fig. 2b. Glue the ends with instant glue. Nylon rings cannot be autoclaved but need to be sterilized (immerse in 70% ethanol, incubate for ~5 min, discard ethanol, and let air dry under the hood).
3. Prepare lattice solution: the following protocol is suitable for making one 3-cm lattice (i.e., in a 3-cm dish), but triplicate lattices should always be used. Scale volumes up or down for differently sized dishes or for increasing the lattice number. Place a 15-ml sterile plastic tube on ice, and add chilled reagents by strictly adhering to the following order: 0.92 ml of 1.76X lattice medium, +0.2 ml collagen stock solution, +0.04 ml 0.1 M NaOH, +0.19 ml FCS, and + 0.67 ml cell suspension (from Subheading 3.1). Mix by pipetting up and down while avoiding forming bubbles, and quickly proceed to **step 4** (*see*-**Notes 8** and **9**).
4. Quickly dispense 2 ml of lattice solution in each 3-cm lattice dish.
5. Incubate at 37 °C (*see* **Notes 10** and **11**).
6. After 1–2 h when polymerization is well visible, floating gels that have not fully detached from the walls or bottom of the dish can be released by gentle tapping on the side of the dish.

3.2 Observing Cellular Changes

3.2.1 Observing Cell Morphology and Contraction

1. Changes in cell morphology can be documented by phase contrast microscopy using an inverted microscope (as for monolayer culture).
2. Lattice contraction can be documented either by measuring the lattice diameter with a thin ruler placed under the dish or by scanning dishes with a regular digital scanner (as for scanning documents). Translucent lattices are best visualized by placing them against a black background. Start with $t = 0$ (lag phase will last for 2–3 h), and then acquire images at 2 h intervals until $t = 7$ to 10 h. No change will be visible in stressed lattices, which only contract vertically. These lattices will remain clear (at the collagen concentrations used here).

3.2.2 Preparing Lattices for Immunofluorescence

Fibroblasts in floating as well as stressed collagen lattices can be visualized by immunofluorescence. Contracted lattices are more easily stained than stressed ones due to their compactness. Free-floating lattices can be cut into pieces like a pie and transferred to small tubes for fixation and subsequent staining according to standard techniques. Attached lattices should first be fixed with 2% paraformaldehyde or other fixative to prevent gel contraction upon ring removal (*see* **Note 12**). Lattices can then be removed from their dish or from the nylon ring for staining. We routinely employ these procedures to visualize the actin cytoskeleton and focal adhesion structures (Fig. 3) [19]. We recommend using a confocal microscope for imaging as lattices are typically thicker than monolayer cultures.

3.2.3 Preparing Lattices for Gene Expression Analysis

mRNA transcripts can be easily isolated by dissolving the complete lattice directly in RNAzol (available from Life Technologies, Sigma-Aldrich, or others) or RLT buffer (contained in Qiagen's RNA isolation kits). Homogenization can be assisted by mechanical disruption (e.g., using Mixer Mill (Retsch), ultraturrax, or polytron). RNA purification by column chromatography (Qiagen or other) is suggested to improve RNA quality. An example of such analysis is shown in Fig. 4a.

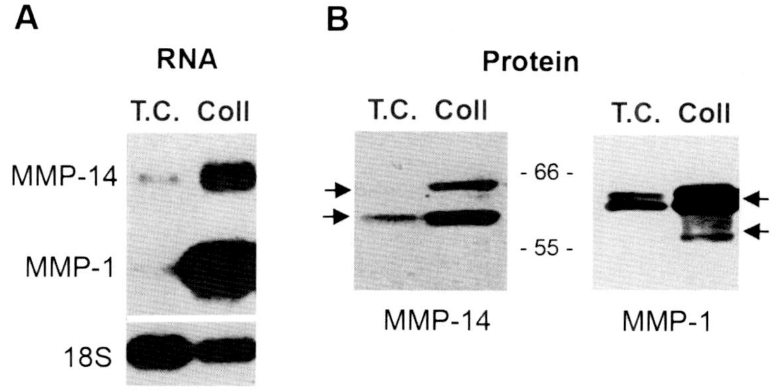

Fig. 4 MMP synthesis by fibroblasts in 2D and 3D cultures. Analysis of MMP mRNA and protein levels extracted from human skin fibroblasts grown as monolayers (T.C.) or in floating collagen lattices (Coll) for 48 h. (**a**). Northern blot analysis of RNA using ^{32}P–labeled cDNA probes for MMP-14 and MMP-1 detecting specific 4.5-kb and 2.2-kb mRNA species, respectively. 18S rRNA hybridization was used as loading control. (**b**) MMP-14 and MMP-1 proteins were analyzed in crude membrane preparations of fibroblasts extracted from collagen lattices (MMP-14) and in supernatants (MMP-1) of fibroblasts after 48 h of culture. SDS-PAGE-resolved proteins were transferred to nitrocellulose. Immunoblotting using a monoclonal antibody raised against human MMP-14 (clone 114-1F2, *Fuji* Chem., Toyama, Japan) and MMP-1 (kind gift of P. Angel, DKFZ, Heidelberg, Germany) identified bands corresponding to pro and active MMP enzyme forms (*arrows*). Molecular weight standards in kDa are shown on the *right*. Part of this figure is reprinted from [16] with permission from Elsevier

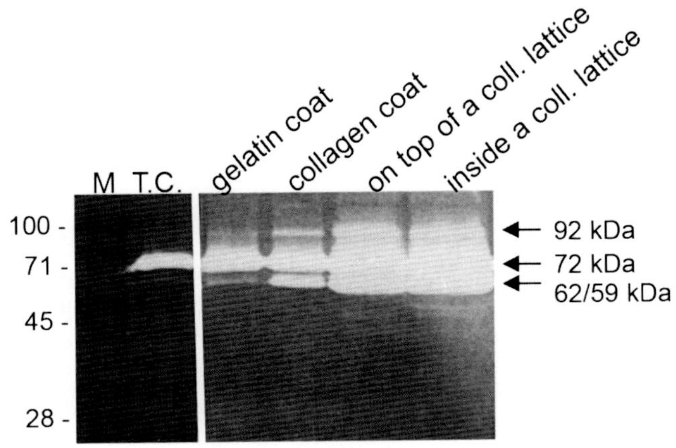

Fig. 5 MMP secretion and activity in fibroblast supernatants. Fibroblasts were grown on tissue culture plastic dishes (T.C.) and gelatin- and collagen-coated dishes, on top of or within a floating collagen lattice. To obtain fibroblast-conditioned media, after 24 h, cells and gels were washed with PBS and incubated for 24 h in serum-free media. Conditioned media, normalized to the cell number, were assayed by gelatin zymography to detect the expression and activation of the pro MMP-9 (92 kDa) and MMP–2 (72, 62/59 kDa forms). M, molecular weight standards

3.2.4 Preparing Lattices for Analysis of Protein Production

Analysis of secreted proteins is accomplished by collecting culture supernatants. In order to remove the proteins contained in serum, lattice cultures need to be washed gently (by swirling) three times with PBS and then placed in a serum-free medium for an additional 24 h (or required duration). We routinely employ this method to analyze secreted MMP-1 by Western blot (Fig. 4b) and MMP-2 and MMP-9 by zymography (Fig. 5) [3, 16].

Analysis of cell-associated proteins (intracellular and membrane bound) is hampered by the large amount of collagen I present in the lattices. To circumvent this problem, it is recommended first to liberate the cells from the lattice by digestion of collagen using bacterial collagenase as described in detail [16]. Cells can then be counted or processed using routine protocols. We used this procedure to analyze the abundance of the cell membrane-bound MMP-14 (pro and active forms) by Western blot (Fig. 4b).

4 Notes

1. Collagen is commercially available mostly as atelo-collagen, the form that lacks the telopeptides due to extraction by pepsin. As collagen fibril formation is enhanced by the presence of telopeptides, it is better to use an atelo-collagen, which is extracted from tissue using weak acid. It is, however, more difficult to find (Cell Systems is one company selling it).

2. Collagen solutions should be kept cold at all times as raising the temperature can initiate fibril formation. For long-term storage, keep collagen stock solution in a fridge; for use, transport collagen on ice and keep solution on ice at all times.
3. It is possible to also use different types of cell culture medium when using cells other than fibroblasts, e.g., 10X RPMI (Life Technologies) for melanoma cells [3].
4. Ascorbic acid addition is optional but required when analyzing collagen production. It is an essential cofactor of lysyl and prolyl hydroxylases but also impacts the transcription of collagen genes [22]. It is not stable in aqueous solutions and should be replenished daily when addressing collagen synthesis.
5. There are many sources of fibroblasts (primary or immortalized lines) available. The reader is referred to an earlier publication detailing the basics of fibroblast culture techniques [23].
6. Cell density and gel volumes can be adjusted to fit lattice cultures from 96-well format to any size Petri dish. We routinely use 3-cm dishes as they are well suited for monitoring contraction or 6-cm dishes if we extract RNA or proteins.
7. If bacteriological dishes are not available, tissue culture plasticware can be coated by poly-HEMA (poly(2-hydroxyethyl methacrylate)) to be repellant [24]. As the coating takes 24 h and may be variable, we prefer to use commercial bacteriological plastic.
8. Mixing of the collagen suspension on ice prevents rapid onset of polymerization.
9. When collagen stock is added to the 1.76X medium, the solution turns yellow (if DMEM contains the red pH indicator phenol red). When neutralizing with 0.1 M NaOH, the medium color will return to the usual red-pink color indicating neutral pH. If FCS is added to acidic collagen solution, it will precipitate. If cells are added before neutralization, they will not like it and show by a change in morphology.
10. As stressed lattices can detach from the ring, we recommend moving as little and as gently as possible.
11. Do not move plates in the initial 30 min while collagen polymerization proceeds. Polymerization is visible by a change from a clear to an opaque solution. A lag phase of about 2–3 h, in which no contraction is visible, is followed by an exponential decrease in lattice area (only floating lattices) until at about 10 h the minimal area is reached and does not change much more thereafter (Fig. 1). This is true for fibroblast-mediated lattice contraction, and kinetics may vary with different cell types.
12. Acetone fixatives should be avoided as they "melt" plasticware. It is good practice to test a fixative on an empty dish before using it on samples.

Acknowledgments

We thank all the members of the dermatology department in Cologne for their continued stimulating discussion; in particular we are grateful to Cornelia Mauch and Thomas Krieg for their constructive criticism and support. Work in the Eckes and Zigrino labs is supported by the German Research Foundation (Deutsche Forschungsgemeinschaft) through SFB 829.

References

1. Bell E, Ivarsson B, Merrill C (1979) Production of a tissue-like structure by contraction of collagen lattices by human fibroblasts of different proliferative potential in vitro. Proc Natl Acad Sci U S A 76(3):1274–1278. doi:10.1073/pnas.76.3.1274
2. Eckes B, Krieg T, Nusgens BV et al (1995) In vitro reconstituted skin as a tool for biology, pharmacology and therapy: a review. Wound Repair Regen 3(3):248–257. doi:10.1046/j.1524-475X.1995.30304.x
3. Kurschat P, Zigrino P, Nischt R et al (1999) Tissue inhibitor of matrix metalloproteinase-2 regulates matrix metalloproteinase-2 activation by modulation of membrane-type 1 matrix metalloproteinase activity in high and low invasive melanoma cell lines. J Biol Chem 274(30):21056–21062. doi:10.1074/jbc.274.30.21056
4. Zigrino P, Mauch C, Fox JW et al (2005) Adam-9 expression and regulation in human skin melanoma and melanoma cell lines. Int J Cancer 116(6):853–859. doi:10.1002/ijc.21087
5. Grinnell F, Petroll WM (2010) Cell motility and mechanics in three-dimensional collagen matrices. Annu Rev Cell Dev Biol 26:335–361. doi:10.1146/annurev.cellbio.042308.113318
6. Eckes B, Dogic D, Colucci-Guyon E et al (1998) Impaired mechanical stability, migration and contractile capacity in vimentin-deficient fibroblasts. J Cell Sci 111(Pt 13):1897–1907
7. Grinnell F (1994) Fibroblasts, myofibroblasts, and wound contraction. J Cell Biol 124(4):401–404. doi:10.1083/jcb.124.4.401
8. Smola H, Thiekotter G, Fusenig NE (1993) Mutual induction of growth factor gene expression by epidermal-dermal cell interaction. J Cell Biol 122(2):417–429. doi:10.1083/jcb.122.2.417
9. Barczyk M, Carracedo S, Gullberg D (2010) Integrins. Cell Tissue Res 339(1):269–280. doi:10.1007/s00441-009-0834-6
10. Zhang ZG, Bothe I, Hirche F et al (2006) Interactions of primary fibroblasts and keratinocytes with extracellular matrix proteins: contribution of alpha2beta1 integrin. J Cell Sci 119(Pt 9):1886–1895. doi:10.1242/jcs.02921
11. Zweers MC, Davidson JM, Pozzi A et al (2007) Integrin alpha2beta1 is required for regulation of murine wound angiogenesis but is dispensable for reepithelialization. J Invest Dermatol 127(2):467–478. doi:10.1038/sj.jid.5700546
12. Popova SN, Barczyk M, Tiger CF et al (2007) Alpha11 beta1 integrin-dependent regulation of periodontal ligament function in the erupting mouse incisor. Mol Cell Biol 27(12):4306–4316. doi:10.1128/MCB.00041-07
13. Rosenfeldt H, Grinnell F (2000) Fibroblast quiescence and the disruption of ERK signaling in mechanically unloaded collagen matrices. J Biol Chem 275(5):3088–3092. doi:10.1074/jbc.275.5.3088
14. Mauch C, Hatamochi A, Scharffetter K et al (1988) Regulation of collagen synthesis in fibroblasts within a three-dimensional collagen gel. Exp Cell Res 178(2):493–503. doi:10.1016/0014-4827(88)90417-X
15. Mauch C, Adelmann-Grill B, Hatamochi A et al (1989) Collagenase gene expression in fibroblasts is regulated by a three-dimensional contact with collagen. FEBS Lett 250(2):301–305. doi:10.1016/0014-5793(89)80743-4
16. Zigrino P, Drescher C, Mauch C (2001) Collagen-induced proMMP-2 activation by MT1-MMP in human dermal fibroblasts and the possible role of alpha2beta1 integrins. Eur J Cell Biol 80(1):68–77. doi:10.1078/0171-9335-00134
17. Grinnell F (2003) Fibroblast biology in three-dimensional collagen matrices. Trends Cell Biol 13(5):264–269. doi:10.1016/S0962-8924(03)00057-6
18. Chiquet M, Matthisson M, Koch M et al (1996) Regulation of extracellular matrix syn-

thesis by mechanical stress. Biochem Cell Biol 74(6):737–744. doi:10.1006/excr.1998.4363

19. Kessler D, Dethlefsen S, Haase I et al (2001) Fibroblasts in mechanically stressed collagen lattices assume a "synthetic" phenotype. J Biol Chem 276(39):36575–36585. doi:10.1074/jbc.M101602200

20. Trachslin J, Koch M, Chiquet M (1999) Rapid and reversible regulation of collagen XII expression by changes in tensile stress. Exp Cell Res 247(2):320–328. doi:10.1006/excr.1998.4363

21. Tomasek JJ, Gabbiani G, Hinz B et al (2002) Myofibroblasts and mechano-regulation of connective tissue remodelling. Nat Rev Mol Cell Biol 3(5):349–363. doi:10.1038/nrm809

22. Murad S, Grove D, Lindberg KA et al (1981) Regulation of collagen synthesis by ascorbic acid. Proc Natl Acad Sci U S A 78(5):2879–2882

23. Rittié L, Fisher GJ (2005) Isolation and culture of skin fibroblasts. Methods Mol Med 117:83–98. doi:10.1385/1-59259-940-0:083

24. Kuroda Y, Wakao S, Kitada M et al (2013) Isolation, culture and evaluation of multilineage-differentiating stress-enduring (muse) cells. Nat Protoc 8(7):1391–1415. doi:10.1038/nprot.2013.076

Chapter 16

Traction Force Measurement Using Deformable Microposts

Tianfa Xie, Jamar Hawkins, and Yubing Sun

Abstract

Recent findings suggest that mechanical forces strongly influence wound repair and fibrosis across multiple organ systems. Traction force is vital to the characterization of cellular responses to mechanical stimuli. Using hydrogel-based traction force microscopy, a FRET-based tension sensor, or microengineered cantilevers, the magnitude of traction forces can be measured. Here, we describe a traction force measurement methodology using a dense array of elastomeric microposts. This platform can be used to measure the traction force of a single cell or a colony of cells with or without geometric confinement.

Key words Traction force measurement, Micropost array, Mechanotransduction, Substrate rigidity, Extracellular matrix

1 Introduction

Recent findings suggest mechanical forces strongly influence wound repair and fibrosis across multiple organ systems [1, 2]. For example, mechanical stress has been demonstrated to promote tissue fibrosis and scarring by regulating inflammatory factors secretion and recruitment of inflammatory cells [3]. Traction forces exerted by cells, first measured in 1980, are important mechanisms that cells use to sense the surrounding extracellular matrix (ECM) environment [4, 5]. Therefore, there is a growing need for tools and in vitro systems to fully characterize cell traction forces in order to examine the functional involvement of mechanical cues in fibrosis.

The earliest and most prevailing traction force microscopy (TFM) uses elastic hydrogels embedded with fluorescent beads to measure forces exerted by adherent cells [6, 7]. Over the past few decades, tool sets for traction force measurement have been greatly expanded from low-resolution, two-dimensional, static traction force measurement to high-resolution, three-dimensional, dynamic measurement, as reviewed recently by Polacheck and Chen [8]. In this chapter, we will focus on a unique traction force measurement

Laure Rittié (ed.), *Fibrosis: Methods and Protocols*, Methods in Molecular Biology, vol. 1627,
DOI 10.1007/978-1-4939-7113-8_16,

methodology utilizing polydimethylsiloxane micropost array (PMA) system [9–11]. The PMA is a dense array of hexagonally spaced elastomeric microposts, which present identical surface geometry. Cells attached to the PMA pull the posts and result in a small, but measureable, deflection. When tip deflection is significantly smaller than the height of the posts, they can be modeled as linearly elastic beams subjected to pure bending. Thus, the force (F) applied at the tip and the resultant deflection (x) are described using *Euler–Bernoulli* beam theory as $F = 3EIx/L^3$, where E represents the elastic modulus of the polydimethylsiloxane (PDMS), I represents the area moment of inertia, and L represents the height of the posts. The discrete topography of the microposts prevents the force transmission through the substrate and thus is a preferred method to study the correlation between cytoskeleton tension and focal adhesions [12]. Moreover, because PMA is essentially a thin PDMS membrane, it can be easily integrated into most micromechanical or microfluidic devices for convenient quantification of the traction force of cells in complex microenvironment [13, 14].

The detailed protocol for generation PMA has been reported previously [15]. Here, we will focus on the traction force measurement by providing detailed protocols for post-surface functionalization, cell seeding, imaging, and data analysis.

2 Materials

2.1 Equipment

1. UV curing chamber (we use Electro-Cure 500, Electro-Lite Corporation, Bethel, CT).
2. Top-loading balance.
3. Two laboratory ovens.
4. Ultraviolet-ozone (UVO) cleaner (we use Jelight, model no. 342, Jelight, Irvine, CA).
5. Biosafety cabinet.
6. Chemical fume hood.
7. Tissue culture incubator.
8. Benchtop centrifuge.
9. Phase contrast, inverted microscope for tissue culture.
10. Inverted fluorescence microscope equipped with a 40X objective and a CCD camera.

2.2 Reagents and Supplies

1. Sylgard 184 polydimethylsiloxane (PDMS) silicone elastomer.
2. Ultrapure water.
3. Ethanol (200 proof).
4. 2% F127 Pluronic stock solution (w/v, in water).

5. Working solution of extracellular matrix (ECM) proteins to be coated on stamps (*see* **Note 1**). Prepare a 10X solution in PBS. Aliquot and store at −20 °C. Use fluorescently labeled extracellular protein if microposts are to be labeled this way in Subheading 3.2, **step 11**.
6. 500μg/ml DiI (1,1′dioleyl-3,3,3′,3′-tetramethylindocarbocyanine methane sulfonate) stock solution in ethanol (i.e., 10X solution).
7. Optical adhesive (we use Norland 61, cat. no. NOA 61, Norland Products, Cranbury, NJ).
8. Mammalian cells (e.g., HUVEC).
9. Cell culture medium (e.g., EGM2 BulletKit) (*see* **Note 2**).
10. Flat narrow tweezers and fine-tipped curved tweezers.
11. Compressed nitrogen gas.
12. Microscope glass slides (plain or charged).
13. Razor blades.
14. Borosilicate cover glass (no. 1 thickness).
15. 35 mm glass bottom Petri dishes with 20 mm holes (we use MatTek # P35-20-C-NON, Ashland, MA).
16. Tissue culture supplies: micropipette tips, serological pipettes, tissue culture flasks, conical tubes, and hemocytometer.
17. Petri dishes (100 or 150 mm diameter).
18. Vacuum desiccators.

3 Methods

3.1 Sample Preparation

1. Prepare polydimethylsiloxane micropost array (PMA) substrates on coverslips (25 mm, round) using the protocol described in reference [15] (*see* **Notes 3** and **4**).
2. To prepare flat PDMS stamps for microcontact printing:
   (a) Weigh 120 g of PDMS base prepolymer and 4 g of curing agent into a plastic cup, and mix them for 5 min (*see* **Note 5**).
   (b) Degas the mixed PDMS in a vacuum desiccator for 30 min until the mixture is both clear and free of air bubbles.
3. Transfer uncured PDMS mixture to a 150-mm Petri dish. Wait for 5–10 min to remove the bubbles introduced during pouring.
4. Carefully relocate the dish with PDMS to a leveled convection oven and cure the PDMS at 60 °C for 12 h.
5. Remove the dish containing PDMS from the oven, and let it cool to room temperature.

6. Use a razor blade to cut the slab of PDMS into stamps that fit the area of the PMA to be used. Store them in a Petri dish in room temperature, and clean them using a Scotch tape if needed.
7. Mount a flawless PMA substrate onto a glass bottom 35-mm Petri dish with a 20-mm hole for high-magnification imaging. Depending on the cell type and time available, either UV-curable adhesive (e.g., optical adhesive) or PDMS can be used for mounting (*see* **Note 6**).

3.2 Surface Functionalization of PMA

1. Sonicate stamps (from Subheading 3.1, **step 6**) in 100% ethanol in a Petri dish for 5 min to clean the surface of stamps.
2. Place the Petri dish containing PDMS stamps in a biosafety cabinet. Blow-dry the stamps with a stream of N_2 or compressed air, and transfer them to a new sterile Petri dish.
3. Prepare extracellular matrix (ECM) protein of choice to be coated on stamps (*see* **Note 1**). Typically, 100 μl of protein solution is sufficient to cover a 2 cm × 2 cm flat stamp.
4. Dispense droplets of the ECM protein solution on the top surface of each stamp (Fig. 1a). Pipet protein as a 5 × 5 array of droplets covering edge and corners (Fig. 1b), wait for 5 min to allow for initial wetting, and sweep over the droplets with a P200 micropipette tip to spread the solution to cover the whole surface (Fig. 1c).
5. Leave coated stamps at room temperature for 1 h to allow for protein absorption (*see* **Note 7**).
6. In biosafety cabinet, wash away excess ECM protein using deionized water, and dry the stamps with a stream of N_2.
7. Expose the PMA substrates to the ozone for 7 min in a UVO cleaner (*see* **Note 8**).

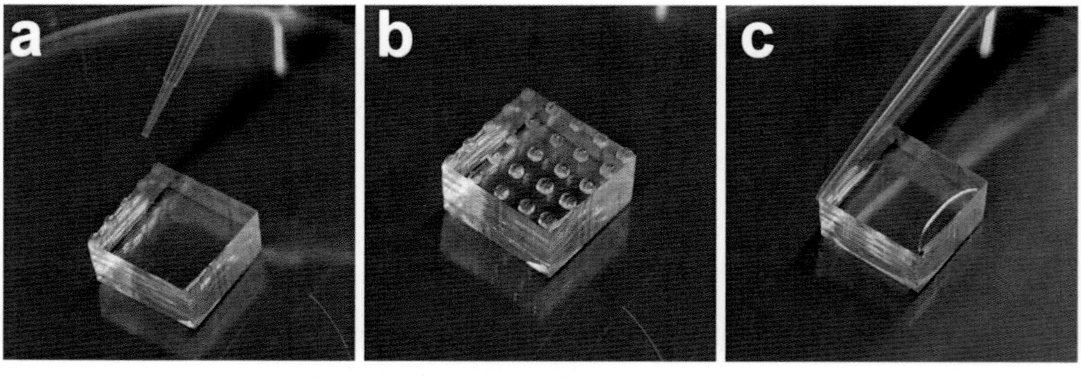

Fig. 1 Steps for coating a PDMS stamp with fibronectin. (**a**) The droplets of ECM protein solution were placed onto the top surface of each stamp. Start with the corners, then the edges, and lastly the interior regions. (**b**) A 5 × 5 array of protein droplets covering edges and corners. (**c**) A P200 micropipette tip was used to facilitate the solution to cover the whole surface

8. Within 30 min of ozone treatment, lay protein-coated stamps on top of the substrates, and apply gentle pressure to facilitate the protein transfer (*see* **Notes 9** and **10**).
9. Add 100% ethanol to the dish and gently peel away the stamps.
10. Gradually add deionized water to the dish to replace ethanol. Wash the dish with deionized water at least three times (*see* **Note 11**).
11. There are two ways to fluorescently label the microposts: (a) using DiI (or similarly, DiD if using far red channel) to stain the whole surface and (b) mixing fluorescently conjugated ECM protein (e.g., Alexa-Fluor 647 conjugated fibrinogen) with regular ECM protein in the microcontact printing steps (*see* **Note 12**).

    (a) DiI labeling:

    - Dilute DiI 10X stock solution to 1X working solution with deionized water.
    - Discard deionized water from the dish (Subheading 3.2, **step 10**), and add 2 ml DiI working solution.
    - Incubate for 1 h in the dark at room temperature.
    - Wash the substrates with deionized water five times. Store at 4 °C for no more than 1 week.

    (b) Fluorescently conjugated ECM labeling: in Subheading 3.2 **step 3**, prepare a mixture of fibronectin (50 μg/ml) and Alexa-Fluor 647-conjucated fibrinogen (25 μg/ml) instead of standard protein solution.

3.3 Cell Culture on PMAs

1. Warm cell culture medium and cell dissociation reagent (e.g., trypsin, collagenase, dispase, etc.) to 37 °C before cell seeding.
2. Discard deionized water from the dish (Subheading 3.2, **step 10** or Subheading 3.2, **step 11**a), and add a 2 ml fresh cell culture medium.
3. Detach cells from tissue culture plates or flasks using proper dissociation reagent, and count the resuspended cells using a hemocytometer.
4. Plate cells onto labeled PMA substrate (*see* **Note 13**).
5. Gently shake the dish to evenly disperse cells, and transfer the culture dish to an incubator to allow cells to attach.
6. Cells can be cultured on PMA substrates until ready to perform traction force measurement experiment.

3.4 Imaging and Data Analysis

1. Turn on the control modulus for environmental chamber of the microscope for at least 10 min before imaging to ensure the measurement can be done at 37 °C and 5% CO_2.

2. Use a low-magnification objective to locate the region of interest, and then switch to a 40X objective, and move the stage to locate the cell in the center of imaging area.
3. For each cell, both phase contrast images and fluorescent images of DiI should be taken to determine cell spreading area and post deflection.
4. A customized MATLAB program (available upon request to corresponding author) is used to analyze the position of deflected and freestanding microposts. Briefly, freestanding microposts are used as reference points to generate an ideal grid. The centroid of the post can be determined using two-dimensional (2D) Gaussian curve fitting. The deflection of the post is therefore determined by comparing the actual centroid and the centroid of the ideal grid. Traction force is then deduced by multiplying the spring constant with deflection. The traction force can be illustrated using either a heat or vector map (*see* **Note 14**).

3.5 Traction Force Measurement on Micropatterned Surface

Confining geometry of a single cell or a colony of cells using microcontact printing is widely used to confine cell migration in order to allow for more accurate and long-term monitoring of traction force dynamics, and decouple the effects of cell shape on traction forces [11]. Moreover, measuring the traction force of a monolayer of cell sheet is important for understanding collective mechanosensitive behaviors [16]. For measuring micropatterned single cell or a colony of cells using PMA, the protocol described above can be used, with the following three modifications:

1. Standard PDMS stamps used in Subheading 3.1 **step 2** should be replaced with micropatterned PDMS stamps made by replica molding (*see* **Note 15**).
2. From the two labeling methods described in Subheading 3.2 **step 11**, only the DiI post labeling method can be used because freestanding posts without cell attachment are needed as references (*see* **Note 16**).
3. In Subheading 3.3 **step 4**, the cell plating density should be carefully controlled because of the significantly reduced cell adhesion area. For single cell patterning, a lower seeding density is required in order to avoid having two cells occupying the same micropattern.

4 Notes

1. Frequently used ECM proteins include fibronectin (50 μg/ml), collagen I and IV (acid soluble, 50 μg/ml), vitronectin (20 μg/ml), and laminin (20 μg/ml). Complete transferring

proteins from stamps to PMAs is not always possible; therefore, it is recommended to use at least double the concentration used for tissue culture plates.

2. A cell culture medium without phenol red may help minimize the fluorescence background during imaging.
3. Because the rigidity of PMA substrate depends on post height, it is essential to select PMA substrate with proper geometry (Fig. 2). Typically, if the micropost diameter is 2 μm, a post height close to 9 μm is used for most cell types. For cell types that generate large traction forces such as cardiomyocytes, post height should be further reduced to 7–8 μm.
4. The rationale behind the choice of post height is threefold: first, an important assumption to use beam theory to deduce traction force is that the post deflection is small compared to the post height. Second, because both top surface and sidewall are labeled with fluorescent dye, image analysis of posts with large bending may involve extensive manual correction steps to avoid recognizing sidewall of posts as the tips of posts by the imaging analysis program. Last, the effective Young's modulus of PMA substrates with the post height of 9 μm is about 5 kPa, which is close to the in vivo modulus of the extracellular matrix for many tissues.

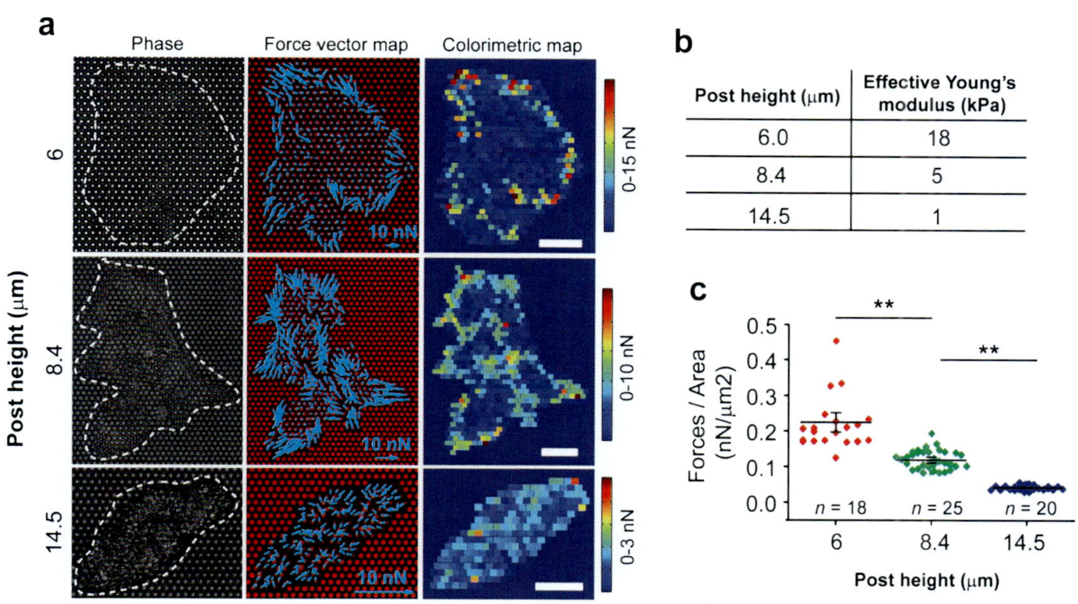

Fig. 2 Effects of micropost height on cell traction forces. (**a**) Phase images, fluorescence images, and vector and colorimetric maps showing the morphology and traction forces of clusters of human embryonic stem cells cultured on PMAs with different micropost heights. Scale bar = 25 μm. (**b**) Effective Young's moduli of PMA substrates with different post heights. (**c**) Average traction forces per unit area as a function of micropost height. Note that average forces per cell areas increase with rigidity. Data represents the means ± SEM. $^{**}P < 0.01$ (P-values calculated using unpaired t-test)

5. A 30:1 PDMS is recommended, because they are softer and can make firmer contact with PMA than a standard 10:1 PDMS.
6. UV-curable adhesive is convenient to use, and it only takes 1–2 min to complete the whole process. However, UV-curable adhesive is, to some degree, toxic to cells and should not be used for sensitive cell types such as human pluripotent stem cells. In contrast, PDMS is nontoxic if fully cured but requires a longer curing time (at least 4 h at 60 °C, curing overnight is recommended). In either approach, it is recommended to attach the coverslip from the outside of the Petri dish to allow for high-magnification imaging using objectives with short working distance.
7. For fibronectin and vitronectin, this process usually can lead to satisfactory results. However, for collagen, the solution normally will concentrate in the center of the stamp. Adding more collagen solution will help solve this issue.
8. Ozone temporarily and properly oxidizes the PDMS surface to allow ECM to bond covalently to PDMS. Oxygen plasma treatment is too strong and might change the surface topography and therefore is not recommended.
9. A successful contact will result in the complete absence of air bubbles trapped between the PMA and stamp.
10. If the microposts are pressed too hard, they can easily collapse. It is possible to rescue collapsed posts by submerging PMA substrates in 100% ethanol and sonicate for about 2 min. However, in this case, the side of microposts may also be coated with ECM proteins to allow cell attachment and therefore will result in underestimation of actual traction force.
11. If the microcontact printing in **step 8** is successful, PMA substrates now should be hydrophilic. However, the wash steps should be done as quickly as possible to avoid drying the substrates.
12. Each method has its own advantages and disadvantages. DiI staining is convenient and cost-effective and therefore is frequently used. The major pitfall of DiI staining is that some types of cells strongly absorb DiI and strong fluorescent signals in cell membrane may mask the microposts. Using a lower concentration and shorter incubation time (as short as 15 min) may help to solve this problem. Alternatively, fluorescently labeled ECM proteins, unlike DiI staining, only label the top surface of microposts and will not be absorbed by cells, resulting in a clean image of microposts, which also provides information pertained to quality of microcontact printing. However, this approach is expensive and cannot be used for a micropatterned surface (discussed in Subheading 3.5 below).

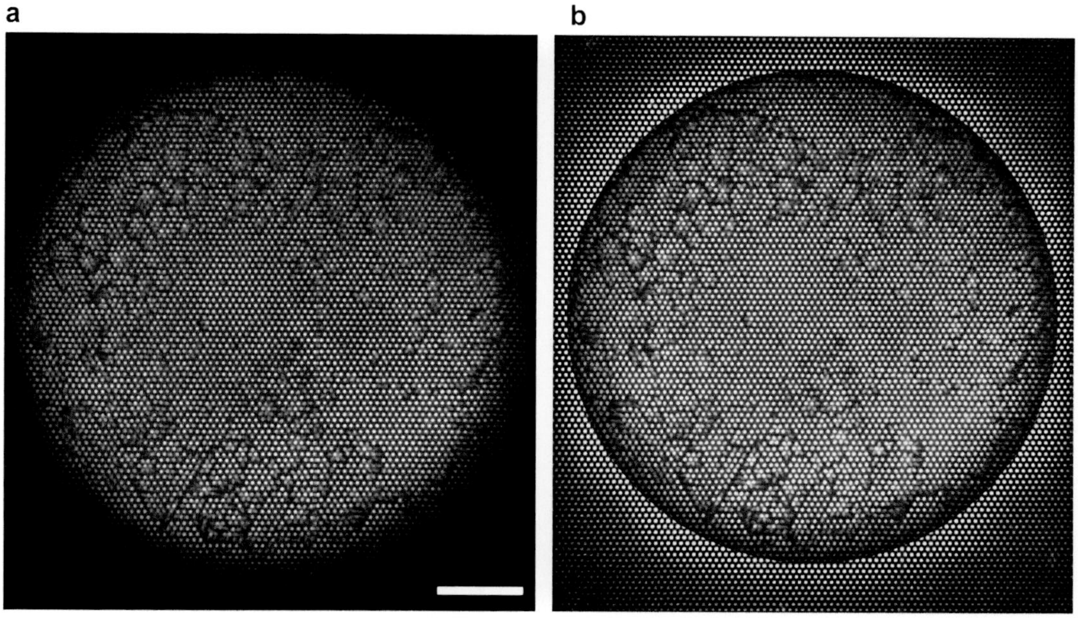

Fig. 3 Fluorescence images of micropatterned PMA substrates stained with DiI. (**a**) original and (**b**) contrast corrected. Scale bar = 50 μm

13. The plating density should be optimized based on the applications and cell type used. Typically, for single cell traction force measurement, 5,000 cells/cm^2 can be a good starting point.
14. The net traction force of a single cell should be close to zero because most of the time, the cell is stationary. This can be used to evaluate the accuracy of force measurement by adding together the net force in both x and y axes. A reliable traction force measurement should have an error less than 5%.
15. It is recommended to use a 10:1 ratio PDMS to prepare micropatterned stamps, especially for small features, to minimize the stamp deformation and collapse during microcontact printing.
16. DiI can form a stronger link to proteins than PDMS, so that the fluorescent intensity in the patterned/cell attached area is much stronger than unpatterned area (Fig. 3a). This may cause difficulty to select appropriate exposure time during imaging. This problem can be solved by taking images within 24 h after cell seeding; use a shorter DiI incubation time, or use imaging processing program (available upon request to corresponding author) to adjust contrast (Fig. 3b).

Acknowledgments

We acknowledge financial support from the Department of Mechanical and Industrial Engineering at the University of Massachusetts, Amherst.

References

1. Wong VW, Akaishi S, Longaker MT et al (2011) Pushing back: wound mechanotransduction in repair and regeneration. J Invest Dermatol 131(11):2186–2196. doi:10.1038/jid.2011.212
2. Duscher D, Maan ZN, Wong VW et al (2014) Mechanotransduction and fibrosis. J Biomech 47(9):1997–2005. doi:10.1016/j.jbiomech.2014.03.031
3. Aarabi S, Bhatt KA, Shi Y et al (2007) Mechanical load initiates hypertrophic scar formation through decreased cellular apoptosis. FASEB J 21(12):3250–3261. doi:10.1096/fj.07-8218com
4. Harris AK, Wild P, Stopak D (1980) Silicone rubber substrata: a new wrinkle in the study of cell locomotion. Science 208(4440):177–179
5. Sun Y, Chen CS, Fu J (2012) Forcing stem cells to behave: a biophysical perspective of the cellular microenvironment. Annu Rev Biophys 41:519–542. doi:10.1146/annurev-biophys-042910-155306
6. Dembo M, Oliver T, Ishihara A et al (1996) Imaging the traction stresses exerted by locomoting cells with the elastic substratum method. Biophys J 70(4):2008–2022. doi:10.1016/S0006-3495(96)79767-9
7. Dembo M, Wang Y-L (1999) Stresses at the cell-to-substrate interface during locomotion of fibroblasts. Biophys J 76(4):2307–2316. doi:10.1016/s0006-3495(99)77386-8
8. Polacheck WJ, Chen CS (2016) Measuring cell-generated forces: a guide to the available tools. Nat Methods 13(5):415–423. doi:10.1038/nmeth.3834
9. Tan JL, Tien J, Pirone DM et al (2003) Cells lying on a bed of microneedles: an approach to isolate mechanical force. Proc Natl Acad Sci U S A 100(4):1484–1489
10. du Roure O, Saez A, Buguin A et al (2005) Force mapping in epithelial cell migration. Proc Natl Acad Sci U S A 102(7):2390–2395. doi:10.1073/pnas.0408482102
11. Fu JP, Wang YK, Yang MT et al (2010) Mechanical regulation of cell function with geometrically modulated elastomeric substrates. Nat Methods 7(9):733–736. doi:10.1038/nmeth.1487
12. Weng S, Shao Y, Chen W et al (2016) Mechanosensitive subcellular rheostasis drives emergent single-cell mechanical homeostasis. Nat Mater. doi:10.1038/nmat4654
13. Lam RHW, Sun YB, Chen WQ et al (2012) Elastomeric microposts integrated into microfluidics for flow-mediated endothelial mechanotransduction analysis. Lab Chip 12(10):1865–1873. doi:10.1039/C2lc21146g
14. Mann JM, Lam RH, Weng S et al (2012) A silicone-based stretchable micropost array membrane for monitoring live-cell subcellular cytoskeletal response. Lab Chip 12(4):731–740. doi:10.1039/c2lc20896b
15. Yang MT, Fu J, Wang Y-K et al (2011) Assaying stem cell mechanobiology on microfabricated elastomeric substrates with geometrically modulated rigidity. Nat Protoc 6(2):187–213. doi:10.1038/nprot.2010.189
16. Brugues A, Anon E, Conte V et al (2014) Forces driving epithelial wound healing. Nat Phys 10(9):684–691. doi:10.1038/Nphys3040

Chapter 17

Mechanical Deformation of Cultured Cells with Hydrogels

Christal A. Worthen, Laure Rittié, and Gary J. Fisher

Abstract

Polyacrylamide hydrogels can be used to culture cells in a range of stiffness that can closer mimic physiological environments. Changes in environmental stiffness have been documented in conditions such as fibrosis, cancer, and aging. In this chapter, we describe a method in which we pour gels directly into multiwell plates using a plastic support that covalently binds to the polymerizing hydrogel. The hydrogel is then crosslinked to calfskin collagen using a crosslinker. The result is a thick hydrogel, scalable to any size plate, which covers the entire surface of the well with no edge effects. The gels can be routinely assembled and are easily reproducible. These scaffolds are used as in vitro models to study fibroblast reaction to variation in environmental stiffness.

Key words Hydrogels, Fibroblasts, Polyacrylamide, Stiffness, Multiwell, Cell culture

1 Introduction

Cells embedded in an extracellular matrix make connections with and exert force on their environment. The makeup and physical properties of the matrix in turn influence the cell shape and its ability to spread. Cells in a fragmented matrix attempt to make connections and exert force but collapse in the absence of the intact matrix [1–3]. These cells are rounded in shape and have a reduced capacity to spread or stretch, leading to functional differences in the cell signaling pathways and extracellular matrix production [4–8]. Cells grown on polyacrylamide hydrogels with varying degrees of crosslinking can mimic an environment in which cells are able to spread or stretch to varying degrees [9, 10]. "Stiffer" hydrogels, in which there is a higher ratio of bis-acrylamide to acrylamide, are resistant to deformation by cells and result in larger, spread out, or stretched cells. "Softer" hydrogels, in which there is a lower ratio of bis-acrylamide to acrylamide, deform easily and result in a collapsed cell phenotype in which cells are smaller, rounded, and unable to stretch or spread out. The hydrogels are easy to prepare and reproducible and have the ability to be tuned to a wide range of stiffness.

Laure Rittié (ed.), *Fibrosis: Methods and Protocols*, Methods in Molecular Biology, vol. 1627,
DOI 10.1007/978-1-4939-7113-8_17, © Springer Science+Business Media LLC 2017

We use an adaptation of a multiwell polyacrylamide hydrogel protocol [10] in which the gels are poured directly into the well, eliminating the need for dehydration and rehydration of the gels. The gels can easily be scaled up or down to fit the size of any plate or multiwell plate.

2 Materials

2.1 Plate Preparation

1. Cell culture plates. Plates of any well size can be used. We will describe this protocol with six well plates (just scale the given volumes up or down to account for volume changes if you need to use larger- or smaller-sized plates).
2. Polyacrylamide gel (PAG) film, i.e., sheets of transparent flexible polyester film designed to support polyacrylamide gels (we use 138 mm x 158 mm sheets of GelBond® PAG film for acrylamide gels from Lonza). This film covalently bonds with acrylamide monomers during the polymerization process resulting in a polyacrylamide gel that remains permanently adhered to the film. Protect from light.
3. Silicone elastomer kit (we use Sylgard® 184 from Dow Corning). Supplied as a two-part kit. When liquid components are thoroughly mixed, the mixture cures to a flexible silicone elastomer that cures at a constant rate regardless of sectional thickness and without exothermal heat production.
4. Paraffin film such as Parafilm®: Use quadruply-folded film to cut discs to the size of the well. These discs will be referred to as "paraffin coverslips" below.
5. Aluminum foil.

2.2 Polyacrylamide Hydrogels

1. 40% (w/v) acrylamide and 2% (w/v) bis-acrylamide solutions. Store at 4 °C.
2. 10% (w/v) ammonium persulfate solution is prepared fresh each time, using ultrapure water (*see* **Note 1**).
3. *N*,*N*,*N*,*N*-Tetramethylethylenediamine (TEMED) can be stored at room temperature (*see* **Note 2**).
4. Forceps.
5. Shaker plate.

2.3 Crosslinking and Coating

1. Long-arm crosslinker that contains an amine-reactive ester and a photoactivatable nitrophenyl azide (we use Sulfo-SANPAH (sulfosuccinimidyl 6-(4′-azido-2′-nitrophenylamino)-hexanoate) from ThermoFisher Scientific): Prepare a 50 mg/ml stock solution in DMSO. Snap freeze 40 μl aliquots in liquid nitrogen, and store at −80 °C until use. Just before use, dissolve 40 μl aliquots in 1.96 ml of ultrapure water (*see* **Note 3**).

2. Sterile phosphate-buffered saline (PBS), pH 7.4. The solution can be made, purchased, concentrated, or ready to use. PBS is used for solution preparation and washing of gels. The total amount needed will depend on the well size of the gels.
3. Type I collagen stock solution (we use calfskin collagen from Elastin Products Company). Prepare a 0.1 mg/ml working solution fresh each time in PBS.
4. 1% (w/v) bovine serum albumin (BSA) solution in PBS; sterilize via 0.22 μm filtration. Excess solution can be stored at 4 °C for subsequent use.

2.4 Additional Reagents and Equipment

1. Biosafety cabinet (tissue culture hood) with ultraviolet (UV) germicidal light.
2. UV lamp for the crosslinking of Sulfo-SANPAH (*see* **Note 4**).
3. Degassing chamber.
4. Fume hood.
5. Cell culture medium (we use Minimum Essential Media (MEM)-α containing 10% (v/v) fetal bovine serum (FBS) for primary fibroblasts) and standard cell culture reagents (such as sterile trypsin, PBS, etc.).
6. Standard cell culture utensils (sterile pipettes, tubes, etc.).

3 Methods

3.1 Plate Preparation

1. Cut some PAG film to the size of the wells you will be using (here 6-well plate = 34 mm diameter discs). It may be helpful to print and cut a paper template beforehand. Take care to expose to as little light as possible. Precut film can be stored away from light for future use (*see* **Note 5**).
2. Cut paraffin coverslips to the same size as the PAG films. Press the cut coverslips flat on the benchtop until use (*see* **Note 6**).
3. Prepare the silicone elastomer in the fume hood: Cut the tip off of a 1 ml pipet tip and pipette 1 ml of elastomer base and 100 μl of elastomer curing agent (10:1 ratio) in a disposable receptacle (we use the top of an old cap from a 50 ml conical tube). Mix the elastomer thoroughly with a pipette tip.
4. Add approximately 100 μl of elastomer mix to the bottom of each well. Using a droplet of water, determine which size of the precut PAG film is hydrophobic, and place the dry film hydrophobic side down into the well. Push the film down into the silicone elastomer until the elastomer is spread evenly under the entire surface of the film. Repeat for the remainder of the wells.
5. Wrap the plates in aluminum foil to protect the light-sensitive PAG film during curing of the elastomer. Place wrapped plates

Table 1
Reported Young's modulus and various ratios of bis-acrylamide to acrylamide for different stiffness gels [10]

Young's modulus (kPa)	% acrylamide	% bis-acrylamide	ml 40% acrylamide	ml 2% bis-acrylamide	ml H_2O	µl 10% APS
2.39[a]	5	0.03	1.25	0.15	8.60	50
10.64	5	0.1	1.25	0.50	8.25	50
29.14	8	0.1	2.00	0.50	7.50	50
66.01	8	0.25	2.00	1.25	6.75	50
112.25	12	0.25	3.00	1.25	5.75	50

[a]This modulus is extrapolated from reported data (*see* **Note 7**)

and leftover mixed elastomer in a dry 37 °C incubator to cure. Curing usually takes at least 4 h and can be prolonged overnight. Use the leftover mixed epoxy to validate curing time.

6. Glued plates can be used right away or stored at least a month at room temperature in the dark for later use.

3.2 Polyacrylamide Hydrogels

1. Prepare the acrylamide solutions corresponding to different stiffness by mixing 40% acrylamide, 2% bis-acrylamide, water, and 10% APS solution according to the stiffness of gel needed and using the volumes detailed in Table 1 (*see* **Note 7**).
2. Place the mixed solutions in a degassing chamber for at least 30 min.
3. Transfer the solutions to the fume hood and add 5 µl of TEMED for every 10 ml of polyacrylamide solution, one solution at a time.
4. Immediately transfer to wells, adding enough solution to cover the hydrophilic PAG film (previously glued and cured) at the bottom of the well. The thickness of the gel does not matter, as long as the entire well is covered (*see* **Note 8**). Keep leftover solution as a polymerization control.
5. Right after pouring, cover each hydrogel with a paraffin coverslip, taking care to avoid bubbles (*see* **Note 9**).
6. Allow the gels to polymerize at room temperature. Different percent gels will polymerize at different rates. Use any leftover solution to observe if gel is fully polymerized. Gels may be left overnight to polymerize and coated in the morning.

3.3 Crosslinking and Coating

1. Remove paraffin coverslips using forceps (*see* **Note 10**).
2. Quickly prepare working solution of crosslinker as described in Subheading 2.3 (*see* **Note 3**).
3. Cover hydrogels with crosslinker solution. Add enough solution to completely cover the gel (we use 1 ml per well of a 6-well plate).
4. Transfer plate to UV lamp for crosslinking and expose to appropriate dose of UV light (*see* **Note 4**).
5. Aspirate and discard crosslinking solution and wash three times (2 ml per well of a 6-well plate) for 20 min each with PBS under moderate shaking.
6. Discard the last rinsing solution, add 2 ml of fresh PBS to each well, and transfer to a tissue culture hood with germicidal light. Close the hood and turn on the light for 2 h to sterilize the plate.
7. Under sterile conditions, aspirate PBS, and add sterile collagen solution to each well (we use 1 ml per well of a 6-well plate). Ensure that the solution is evenly spread over the entire gel. Incubate for 2 h at room temperature.
8. Aspirate and discard the collagen solution and wash three times with sterile PBS.
9. Aspirate and discard PBS, and add sterile BSA solution. Incubate for 1 h at room temperature.
10. Aspirate and discard BSA solution and wash three times with sterile PBS. Hydrogels are now ready to be used. Alternatively, PBS can be added to each well and plates can be stored at 4 °C for 3 days.

3.4 Plating Cells

1. Trypsinize active primary fibroblast cultures and prepare a 100,000 cells/ml cell suspension using routine culture techniques [11] (*see* **Note 11**).
2. Plate cells in wells at no more than 70% confluency using medium that contains FBS using typical well volumes for the plate size used, i.e., 2 ml/well for a 6-well plate (*see* **Notes 12** and **13**). Cells plated on stiff gels will continue to divide and remain viable indefinitely. Collapsed cells grown on the softest gels (2.39 kPa) are good for 3 days, before they begin to lose viability. Morphological aspect of primary human fibroblasts grown on different stiffness polyacrylamide hydrogels is shown in Fig. 1.
3. Follow cells over time: Biochemical analysis can be performed after directly applying an RNA/DNA/protein extraction solution to the hydrogel, incubating, and harvesting. Histological analysis can be performed using routine staining techniques and an inverted microscope.

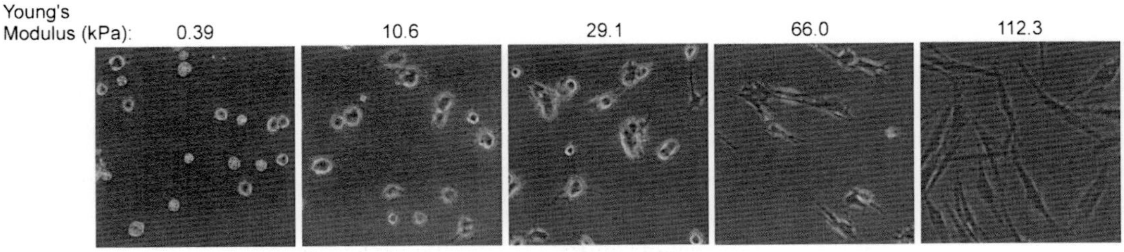

Fig. 1 Aspect of primary human fibroblasts grown on different stiffness polyacrylamide hydrogels for 24 h in MEM-α containing 10% FBS and observed with a phase-contrast microscope and 10X objective

4 Notes

1. Ammonium persulfate powder should be stored desiccated at room temperature and is good for 1 year.
2. TEMED is toxic and may cause respiratory irritation and should only be used under a fume hood.
3. Work quickly with Sulfo-SANPAH. Try to reconstitute, add to wells, and transfer to UV source within 10 min.
4. Sulfo-SANPAH can be crosslinked using a wide range of UV wavelengths and intensity [12]. Efficiency of crosslinking should be determined experimentally for each lamp. For our lab purposes, we use a UVB lamp (i.e., ~280–315 nm) with an output of 120 mJ/cm^2/min for 15 minutes.
5. For 96-well plates, a high-quality 1-hole punch can be used to cut the PAG film. We use the "crop-a-dile" hole punch (available at most craft stores) with 96-well plates that have a 0.34 cm growth area.
6. Ensure that there is no air caught between any of the parafilm layers, so that they remain flat.
7. Alternate ratios of bis-acrylamide to acrylamide can be used. However, surface creasing of the gel can occur when bis-acrylamide percentage is lower than 0.028% (w/v). A lower stiffness gel can still be achieved by lowering acrylamide percentage [13]. Surface creasing will negatively affect cell shape and attachment.
8. We use 2 ml acrylamide solution for one well of a 6-well plate.
9. If a bubble is formed, simply use thin forceps to lift one edge of the paraffin film and slowly re-lower the paraffin coverslip.
10. Paraffin coverslips may be reused if they are still in good condition.
11. This cell concentration is the one we use with primary fibroblasts. Cell concentration may need to be adjusted when working with other cell types.

12. If cells on soft gels are plated at a high confluency, they can form attachment to each other and stretch out instead of remaining collapsed. FBS-containing medium can be removed and replaced with serum-free medium once cells have attached.
13. Attachment to the hydrogels is not only a function of the stiffness of the hydrogel but also the concentration of crosslinker used to bind the collagen [14].

Acknowledgments

C.A.W. is supported by NIH award T32AR007197.

References

1. Varani J, Schuger L, Dame MK et al (2004) Reduced fibroblast interaction with intact collagen as a mechanism for depressed collagen synthesis in photodamaged skin. J Invest Dermatol 122(6):1471–1479. doi:10.1111/j.0022-202X.2004.22614.x
2. Fisher GJ, Varani J, Voorhees JJ (2008) Looking older: fibroblast collapse and therapeutic implications. Arch Dermatol 144(5):666–672. doi:10.1001/archderm.144.5.666
3. Quan T, Little E, Quan H et al (2013) Elevated matrix metalloproteinases and collagen fragmentation in photodamaged human skin: impact of altered extracellular matrix microenvironment on dermal fibroblast function. J Invest Dermatol 133(5):1362–1366. doi:10.1038/jid.2012.509
4. Smithmyer ME, Sawicki LA, Kloxin AM (2014) Hydrogel scaffolds as in vitro models to study fibroblast activation in wound healing and disease. Biomater Sci 2(5):634–650. doi:10.1039/C3BM60319A
5. Li Y, Lei D, Swindell WR et al (2015) Age-associated increase in skin fibroblast-derived prostaglandin E2 contributes to reduced collagen levels in elderly human skin. J Invest Dermatol 135(9):2181–2188. doi:10.1038/jid.2015.157
6. Xia W, Quan T, Hammerberg C et al (2015) A mouse model of skin aging: fragmentation of dermal collagen fibrils and reduced fibroblast spreading due to expression of human matrix metalloproteinase-1. J Dermatol Sci 78(1):79–82. doi:10.1016/j.jdermsci.2015.01.009
7. Fisher GJ, Shao Y, He T et al (2016) Reduction of fibroblast size/mechanical force down-regulates TGF-beta type II receptor: implications for human skin aging. Aging Cell 15(1):67–76. doi:10.1111/acel.12410
8. Purohit T, He T, Qin Z et al (2016) Smad3-dependent regulation of type I collagen in human dermal fibroblasts: impact on human skin connective tissue aging. J Dermatol Sci 83(1):80–83. doi:10.1016/j.jdermsci.2016.04.004
9. Sunyer R, Jin AJ, Nossal R et al (2012) Fabrication of hydrogels with steep stiffness gradients for studying cell mechanical response. PLoS One 7(10):e46107. doi:10.1371/journal.pone.0046107
10. Syed S, Karadaghy A, Zustiak S (2015) Simple polyacrylamide-based multiwell stiffness assay for the study of stiffness-dependent cell responses. J Vis Exp 97. doi:10.3791/52643
11. Rittié L, Fisher GJ (2005) Isolation and culture of skin fibroblasts. Methods Mol Med 117:83–98. doi:10.1385/1-59259-940-0:083
12. Thermo-Fisher TR001 Photoactivate-aryl-azides. https://tools.thermofisher.com/content/sfs/brochures/TR0011-Photoactivate-aryl-azides.pdf. Accessed 12 Dec 2016
13. Saha K, Kim J, Irwin E et al (2010) Surface creasing instability of soft polyacrylamide cell culture substrates. Biophys J 99(12):L94–L96. doi:10.1016/j.bpj.2010.09.045
14. Trappmann B, Gautrot JE, Connelly JT et al (2012) Extracellular-matrix tethering regulates stem-cell fate. Nat Mater 11(7):642–649. doi:10.1038/nmat3339

Chapter 18

Preparation of Decellularized Lung Matrices for Cell Culture and Protein Analysis

Franziska E. Uhl, Darcy E. Wagner, and Daniel J. Weiss

Abstract

The limited available treatment options for patients with chronic lung diseases, such as fibrosis, lead to poor prognosis after diagnosis and short survival rates. An exciting new bioengineering approach utilizes de- and recellularization of lung tissue to potentially overcome donor organ shortage and immune reactions toward the received transplant. The goal of decellularization is to create a scaffold which contains the necessary framework for stability and functionality for regenerating lung tissue while removing immunomodulatory factors by removal of cells. After decellularization, the scaffold could be re-functionalized by repopulation with the patient's own stem/progenitor cells to create a fully functional organ or can be used as ex vivo models of disease. In this chapter the decellularization of lung tissue from multiple species (i.e., rodents, pigs, and humans) as well as disease states such as fibrosis is described. We discuss and describe the various quality control measures which should be used to characterize decellularized scaffolds, methods for protein analysis of the remaining scaffold, and methods for recellularization of scaffolds.

Key words Biomaterial, Decellularization, Lung, Mass spectrometry, Proteomics, Scaffold, Tissue engineering

1 Introduction

Pulmonary fibrosis is a devastating disease characterized by a marked increase in lung stiffness, mainly due to excessive deposition of collagen and loss of alveolar surface area, and thereby leads to declining lung function. While two pharmaceutical treatments have recently become available for the treatment of pulmonary fibrosis, they only serve to halt disease progression and cannot reverse disease pathogenesis. Thus, at end-stage disease, the only option is lung transplantation.

While mouse models can be used to study certain aspects of fibrosis, they incompletely recapitulate the heterogeneity seen in human disease. The most common mouse model is the intratracheal instillation of bleomycin which leads to fibrosis development after a short period of time (about 14 days) but resolves after

Laure Rittié (ed.), *Fibrosis: Methods and Protocols*, Methods in Molecular Biology, vol. 1627,
DOI 10.1007/978-1-4939-7113-8_18, © Springer Science+Business Media LLC 2017

longer periods (about 28–56 days) [1–5]. Other models include irradiation, intratracheal administration of fluorescein isothiocyanate (FITC), instillation of mineral fibers like silica, as well as diverse transgenic and viral induced fibrosis but all of them are only capable of recapitulating some of the features of the human disease [1]. New models are thus needed to help close the gap between promising in vitro and in vivo studies and the clinic. An exciting new bioengineering approach utilizes de- and recellularization of lung tissue to generate three-dimensional scaffolds.

The initial goal of decellularization technologies was to use these scaffolds to overcome donor organ shortage and provide a scaffold purported to be devoid of immune reactions in the transplant recipient. After initial proof-of-concept studies in rodents [6, 7], several groups scaled these processes up to more clinically relevant lung tissue from pigs, nonhuman primates, and human [8–14]. Although clinical application of recellularized lungs is still many years away, the use of decellularized preclinical and patient tissue has provided a powerful tool for expanding our knowledge of human disease onset and pathogenesis. Lungs from both normal and diseased murine and human lungs have been successfully decellularized. Emphysematous lungs from murine and human chronic obstructive pulmonary disease (COPD) patients can be decellularized and retain pathologic appearances such as distal airspace enlargement. Strikingly, immortalized murine epithelial cells recellularized onto these scaffolds did not survive as long as those recellularized on normal lung scaffolds [3]. In an emphysematous model with aging superimposed, cell survival was further reduced. In a follow-up study, it was found that epithelial cells seeded onto scaffolds derived from aged mice have decreased laminin expression, and thus this might be one reason for changes in epithelial cell survival and proliferation [15]. Interestingly, we observed comparable trends of decreased cell survival on human scaffolds derived from patients with emphysema and COPD as compared to healthy patients, indicating that there may be something fundamentally deranged with emphysematous scaffolds [10].

Murine lungs derived from bleomycin-treated animals were found to retain their characteristic fibrotic appearance by histological assessment as well as have an increase in a range of extracellular matrix (ECM) components as compared to murine lungs decellularized from healthy mice [3]. While their ECM composition seemed to differ, there were no detectable differences in cell survival or proliferation by any of the endpoints utilized for two different cell types (immortalized distal epithelial cells and murine bone marrow-derived mesenchymal stem cells).

With regard to human studies related to fibrosis, recellularization of decellularized fibrotic human lung tissue with healthy human fibroblasts led to activation to myofibroblasts with increased smooth muscle actin expression, a feature typically seen in fibrotic tissue [8]. This indicates that the composition of the ECM and environment is a critical factor and might be critically involved in disease progression. In an additional study, cultivation of primary lung fibroblasts from healthy and idiopathic pulmonary fibrosis (IPF) patients on decellularized lungs from healthy and IPF patients resulted in significant differential expression of pro-fibrotic genes. Notably, the origin of the scaffold had a greater effect on gene expression than did origin of the cells [16]. Another study identified chitinase 3-like 1 (CHI3L1), a prototypic chitinase-like protein that is elevated in IPF patients, to be sufficient to induce myofibroblast transformation in human fibroblasts when cultured on decellularized normal lung tissue [17]. De- and recellularization approaches have also been used to study the effect of the ECM of scleroderma patients on the differentiation capacity of peripheral blood mononuclear cells into fibrocytes [5]. A netrin-1-dependent pathway was identified which is involved in bleomycin-induced fibrosis in mice and may therefore be a possible treatment target [5]. These examples all demonstrate good correlation with hallmarks of the human disease and point out the important knowledge that can be gained by studying the ECM composition of and cell behavior on diseased decellularized lungs. Further analyses of the protein composition of normal vs. diseased decellularized lungs with advanced proteomic methods such as mass spectrometry will provide valuable additional insight into specific pathogenic changes in the ECM and help with the identification of novel treatment candidates. In summary, decellularized scaffolds have been invaluable tools for furthering our understanding of lung biology and disease.

In this chapter the induction of fibrosis in a rodent model and a protocol for decellularization of lung tissue from multiple species like rodents, pigs, and humans is described. Further, quality controls and methods for protein analysis of the remaining scaffold are discussed, including mass spectrometry. In addition, recellularization techniques for high-throughput studies from single murine lungs or single human patients are discussed. These tools can be used as new technologies for researchers to deepen understanding of human fibrosis pathology.

2 Materials

2.1 Induction of Fibrosis in Mice via Bleomycin

1. Adult mice (usually 8 weeks of age).
2. Anesthesia: a mixture of medetomidine (0.5 mg/kg mouse), midazolam (5.0 mg/kg mouse), and fentanyl (0.05 mg/kg mouse) (MMF).
3. Anesthesia antagonist: a mixture of atipamezole (2.5 mg/kg mouse), flumazenil (0.5 mg/kg mouse), and naloxone (1.2 mg/kg mouse).

4. Bleomycin (3.6 U/kg mouse), prepared in 75 μl of sterile 1X PBS.
5. Scale capable of weighing in a range of 10–100 g.
6. Respiratory assessment system to evaluate lung function and determine fibrosis severity (we use FlexiVent from SCIREQ).

2.2 Solutions and Materials for Decellularization

Prepare solutions sterile or sterile filter (0.22 μm) before usage. All solutions should be prepared with deionized (di) or ultrapure water. An overview of the amount of the solutions needed for different species on each day and steps of the decellularization protocol is shown in Table 1. The following solutions and materials are used in the decellularization process:

1. Sterile environment (cell culture hood) and dissection utensils (sterilized, i.e., autoclaved or rinsed with 70% ethanol—forceps, scissors, petri dishes, beakers, plastic bins, syringes, and cannulas).
2. Wash solution: 5X penicillin/streptomycin (PS), i.e., 500 U/ml penicillin, 500 μg/ml streptomycin in diH_2O.
3. Triton solution: 0.1% (w/v) Triton X-100, 5X PS.
4. Sodium deoxycholate (SDC): 2% SDC (w/v) (*see* **Note 1**).
5. NaCl solution: 1 M NaCl, 5X PS.
6. DNAse solution: 30 μg/ml porcine pancreatic DNAse, 1.3 mM $MgSO_4$, 2 mM $CaCl_2$, 5X PS (*see* **Note 2**).
7. Peracetic acid (PAA) solution: 0.1% peracetic acid, 4% ethanol.
8. Storage solution: 5X PS, 2.5 μg/ml amphotericin-B, 50 μg/ml gentamicin, in PBS.
9. Roller pump (i.e., Stockert Shigley) capable of a flow rate of 2 l/min.

2.3 Solutions and Materials for Mass Spectrometry

1. 4X lysis buffer: 250 mM Tris, pH 6.8, 8% (w/v) sodium dodecyl sulfate (SDS), 400 mM dithiothreitol (DTT).
2. Running buffer for SDS-PAGE: 50 mM Tris base, pH 8.3, 380 mM glycine, 0.22% (w/v) SDS.
3. 100 mM NH_4HCO_3.
4. 50 mM NH_4HCO_3 in 50% (v/v) acetonitrile (ACN).
5. 100% (v/v) ACN.
6. 10 mM DTT in 100 mM NH_4HCO_3.
7. 55 mM (10 mg/ml) iodoacetamide (IAA) in 100 mM NH_4HCO_3.
8. Trypsin solution: 6–12 ng/μl trypsin, 5% (v/v) ACN in 40 mM NH_4HCO_3.

Table 1
Details of the decellularization protocol for different species

			Mouse	Rat	Pig	Human
			Each via trachea and right ventricle	Each via trachea and right ventricle	Each via trachea/main bronchus and pulmonary artery/main vessel	Each via trachea/main bronchus and pulmonary artery/main vessel
Day 1			Manually	Manually	Perfusion pump 2 l/min	Perfusion pump 2 l/min
Solution		Incubation time	Amount (ml) × times	Amount (ml) × times	Amount (l) × times	Amount (l) × times
diH_2O 5X PS	Washing	–	3, 5X	20–30, 5X	2–3, 3X	2–3, 3X
0.1% Triton	Washing	–	–	–	2–3	2–3
0.1% Triton	Filling	24 h, 4 °C, shaking	3	20–30	2–3	2–3
Day 2						
diH_2O 5X PS	Washing	–	3, 5X	20–30, 5X	2–3, 3X	2–3, 3X
2% SDC	Washing	–	–	–	2–3	2–3
2% SDC	Filling	24 h, 4 °C, shaking	3	20–30	2–3	2–3
Day 3						
diH_2O 1X PS	Washing	–	3, 5X	20–30, 5X	2–3, 3X	2–3, 3X
1 M NaCl	Washing	–	–	–	2–3	2–3
1 M NaCl	Filling	1 h, RT, shaking	5	20–30	2–3	2–3
diH_2O 1X PS	Washing	–	3, 5X	20–30, 5X	2–3, 3X	2–3, 3X

(continued)

Table 1
(continued)

			Mouse	Rat	Pig	Human
DNAse	Washing	–	–	–	2–3	2–3
DNAse	Filling	1 h, RT, shaking	3	20–30	2–3	2–3
diH_2O 1X PS	Washing	–	–	–	2–3, 3X	2–3, 3X
Peracetic acid	Washing	–	–	–	2–3	2–3
Peracetic acid	Filling	1 h, RT, shaking	–	–	2–3	2–3
diH_2O 1X PS	Washing	–	3, 5X	20–30, 5X	2–3, 3X	2–3, 3X
Storage solution	Washing	–	–	–	2–3, 2X	2–3, 2X
Storage solution	Filling	Storage, 4 °C	3	20–30	2–3	2–3

9. 4 mM NH_4HCO_3.
10. 5% (v/v) formic acid (FA) in 50% (v/v) ACN.
11. Loading solution: 2.5% (v/v) ACN in 2.5% (v/v) FA.
12. SDS-polyacrylamide gel electrophoresis (SDS-PAGE): To clean the protein lysate from salts and detergents of the lysis buffer, it should be run on a denaturing gel (*see* **Note 3**) permitting the sample to run until it is located in the separation gel. The bands should not separate in order to minimize the amount of gel to be excised for trypsin digestion. In our setup, we have found that running at 80 V for around 10–15 min is sufficient with the use of 20–50 mg per lane.
13. Sample homogenizer (e.g., Polytron PT2100 from Kinematica; Ball mill such as Mikro-Dismembrator S from Sartorius).
14. Centrifuge.
15. Protein assay reagents such as BCA, Bradford, etc. (we use the DC detergent compatible protein detection Kit from Bio-Rad).
16. 70% (v/v) ethanol.
17. Razorblades to excise protein bands.
18. Microcentrifuge tubes.
19. Vortex.
20. Speed vac.
21. Heat block for incubations at 56 °C.
22. Conventional ultrahigh-pressure liquid chromatography (UHPLC) or high-pressure liquid chromatography (HPLC) equipment.
23. Capillary fused silica column (12 cm × 100 μm inner diameter) packed with HALO C18 2.7 μm particle size, 90 A (from Michrom Bioresources).
24. Gradient of 0–35% ACN/0.1%FA (Fisher Chemical, Optima, LC/MS grade), 35–100% ACN/0.1% FA, 100% ACN, and 0.1% FA in H_2O.
25. Mass spectrometer (we use a Q-Exactive mass spectrometer from Thermo Fisher Scientific).
26. Proteome Discoverer 1.4 software (Thermo Fisher Scientific).

2.4 Lung Histology

1. 4% paraformaldehyde (20 cm H_2O pressure).
2. Xylene.
3. Graded ethanol series.
4. Paraffin.
5. Glass slides.
6. Cover slips.

7. Microtome.
8. Deparaffinization station.
9. Histological stain as needed (e.g., hematoxylin and eosin, DAPI, Verhoeff's Van Gieson, Masson's Trichrome, Alcian Blue).
10. Normal light or fluorescence microscope.

2.5 Electron Microscopy

1. 0.1 M cacodylate buffer, pH 7.2.
2. Karnovsky's fixative: 2.5% (w/v) glutaraldehyde, 1.0% (w/v) paraformaldehyde in 0.1 M cacodylate buffer, pH 7.2.
3. 1% (w/v) osmium tetroxide.
4. Graded ethanol series.
5. Propylene oxide.
6. Spurr's epoxy resin.
7. Glass knife or diamond knife on an ultracut microtome.
8. Methylene blue-azure II.
9. 200 mesh thin bar nickel grids.
10. Uranyl acetate: 2% (w/v) uranyl acetate in 50% ethanol.
11. Lead citrate.
12. Transmission electron microscope (TEM, we use a JEOL 1400 from JEOL USA Inc.).

2.6 Immunohistochemistry (IHC)

1. Standard deparaffinization station.
2. Sodium citrate buffer: 10 mM citrate buffer pH 6 (we use the one from Dako).
3. 0.1% (w/v) Triton X-100.
4. Wash solution: 1% (w/v) BSA in PBS.
5. Blocking solution: 10% goat serum.
6. Primary antibody. Antibodies routinely used in our lab include anti-fibronectin (#610077 from BD Transduction Laboratories, used at 1:100), anti-laminin (#ab11575 from Abcam, used at 1:100), anti-alpha elastin (#ab21607 from Abcam, used at 1:100), anti-smooth muscle myosin heavy chain 2 (#ab53219 from Abcam, used at 1:100), anti-collagen I (#ab292 from Abcam, used at 1:100), anti-proliferation marker Ki67 (#ab16667 from Abcam, used at 1:50), anti-cleaved caspase-3 (#Asp175 from Cell Signaling Technology, used at 1:100), antihuman actin (#1A4 from Dako, used at 1:10,000).
7. Secondary antibody. Secondary antibodies routinely used in our lab include Alexa Fluor 568 goat anti-rabbit IgG (H + L) (1:500, Invitrogen), Alexa Fluor 568 F(ab')2 fragment of goat anti-mouse IgG (H + L) (1:500, Invitrogen) [10, 12, 18–20].

8. 4′,6-diamidino-2-phenylindole (DAPI) nuclear stain.
9. Mounting medium (we use Aqua-Poly/Mount from Polysciences Inc.)

2.7 Assessment of Residual DNA

1. Tissue paper (e.g., Kimwipe®).
2. DNA extracting kit (we use the DNeasy Blood & Tissue Kit from Qiagen).
3. 0.8% (w/v) agarose gel and agarose gel running apparatus.
4. SYBR Safe DNA Gel Stain.
5. UV light or molecular imager (we use a Versa Doc from Bio-Rad).
6. 100 bp ladder and salmon sperm DNA.
7. dsDNA quantitation assay (we use the Quant-iT™ PicoGreen® dsDNA Assay kit from Thermo Fisher Scientific)

2.8 Gelatinase Assay

1. Gelatinase activity measuring kit (we use the EnzChek Gelatinase Assay from Molecular Probes) as previously described [21].
2. Tris-buffered saline (TBS): 50 mM Tris–HCl, pH 7.4, 150 mM NaCl.
3. Gelatin standard (we use DQ™ gelatin from Life Technologies).

2.9 Assessment of Residual Detergent

1. 0.0125% (w/v) methylene blue (MB) in diH_2O.
2. Chloroform.
3. Vortex.
4. Spectrophotometer to read absorbance at 630 nm (plate reader is recommended).
5. Polypropylene 96-well plates.
6. Pure diH_2O or PBS for blanks.
7. Triton, SDC, NaCl, or DNAse for standard curve preparation [22].

2.10 Cell Survival

1. Cell counting chamber or viability assays like WST/MTT or LDH release.

2.11 Cells and Cultivation Media for Recellularization

A variety of different cell types can be used for recellularization studies, depending on the experimental questions. We have also found that different cell types have different thresholds for detergent-induced cytotoxicity, and therefore testing of different cell types is advantageous in assessing cytocompatibility of acellular scaffolds [22]. Although in disease models or diseased human tissue, assessment of cytotoxicity may be complicated to interpret due to potential differences in residual proteins or toxic components.

1. For recellularization of rodent, nonhuman primate, pig, and human scaffolds, we have generally utilized four different cell lines (*see* **Note 4**):
   (a) Human mesenchymal stem cells (i.e., hMSC, University of Minnesota, NHLBI Production Assistance for Cell Therapy program [23]).
   (b) Human lung fibroblasts (HLF) (ATCC, CCL 171).
   (c) Human bronchial epithelial cells (HBE, courtesy of Albert van der Vliet, University of Vermont, originally from Dr. J. Yankaskas [24]).
   (d) Pulmonary endothelial colony-forming cells (CBF, courtesy of Mervin Yoder, Indiana University—Purdue University Indianapolis) [3, 10, 12, 14, 19, 20, 25].
2. Cell culture-treated plastic (i.e., petri dishes, T-flasks, multiwall plates).
3. Incubator capable of 37 °C and 5% CO_2.
4. hMSC medium: Modification of Eagle's Medium-Earle's Balanced Salt Solution (MEM-EBSS), 20% fetal bovine serum, 100 IU/ml penicillin/100 μg/ml streptomycin, 2 mM L-glutamine (*see* **Note 5**).
5. HLF medium: DMEM/F-12 (1:1, v/v) with 10% (v/v) fetal bovine serum, 100 IU/ml penicillin/100 μg/ml streptomycin, 2 mM L-glutamine.
6. HBE medium: DMEM/F-12 (1:1, v/v) with 10 ng/ml cholera toxin, 10 ng/ml epidermal growth factor, 5 μg/ml insulin, 5 μg/ml transferrin, 0.1 μM dexamethasone, 15 μg/ml bovine pituitary extract, 0.5 mg/ml bovine serum albumin, and 100 IU/ml penicillin/100 μg/ml streptomycin.
7. CBF medium: EGM-2 (Lonza), 5% fetal bovine serum, 0.04% hydrocortisone, 0.4% hFGF-B, 0.1% VEGF, 0.1% R3-IGF-1, 0.1% ascorbic acid, 0.1% hEGF, 0.1% gentamicin sulfate amphotericin-B, 100 IU/ml penicillin/100 μg/ml streptomycin. These cells are grown and expanded on collagen type I-coated tissue culture surfaces.

3 Methods

3.1 Induction of Fibrosis in Mice via Bleomycin

There are several different models for the induction of fibrosis in mice. One common method is intratracheal administration of bleomycin (*see* Chap. 2 for detailed protocols and tips). Other mouse models of fibrosis such as radiation, silicosis, or adeno-TGFβ could also be used.

1. Anesthetize mice (usually 8 weeks of age) according to local IACUC protocols.

2. Instill 3.6 U/kg of bleomycin by oropharyngeal or intratracheal administration (*see* **Note 6**).
3. Allow mice to recover from anesthesia or antagonize the narcosis.
4. Monitor mouse weight and health during the next 14 days. Anticipated weight loss is approximately 5–10%. If the mice lose too much weight or exhibit other symptoms of distress, follow your local protocols for euthanasia.
5. Harvest heart-lung blocs 14 days post-bleomycin instillation and subsequently decellularize as described below [1, 3, 5, 26].

3.2 Decellularization of Rodent Lungs

1. Perform all works in a sterile environment (cell cultivation hood) using sterilized utensils. A typical hood setup is shown in Fig. 1.
2. Euthanize the rodents according to your local animal regulations.
3. Extract the heart and lung en bloc.
4. Cannulate the trachea with a blunted 18 gauge cannula with (for rats) or without silicone tubing (for mice) to account for trachea size (Fig. 1d), and immediately clear the lung vasculature of blood by injecting 10 ml wash solution into the right ventricle.

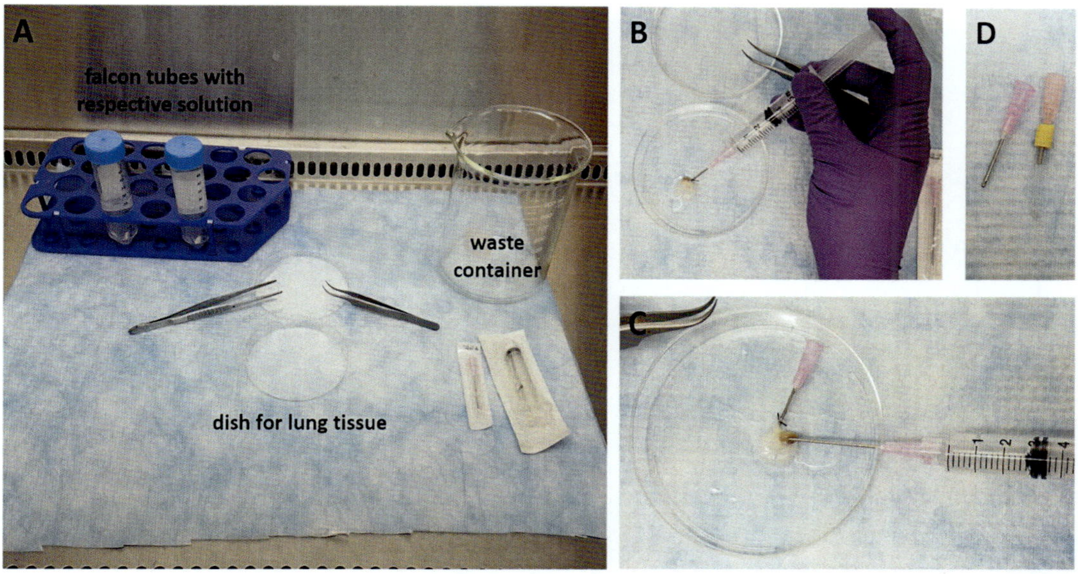

Fig. 1 Rodent lung decellularization. (**a**) Hood setup with indication of the dish for the rodent lung tissue, waste container, and conical polypropylene tubes with solutions used during the decellularization; (**b**) flushing of a mouse lung via the tracheal cannula; (**c**) flushing of a mouse lung vasculature via the right ventricle; (**d**) cannulas used for rodent lung decellularization; *left*, cannula for mouse lungs, 18 gauge cannula with blunted edge and groove for attachment of the surgical thread; *right*, cannula for rat lungs, a silicone tube is used over a blunted 18 gauge cannula to increase diameter of the cannula and fit rat trachea size

5. Flush the lungs slowly and carefully using a syringe; flush five times, each alternating via the trachea and right ventricle with the amounts indicated in Table 1 [3, 18, 19, 25]. Between each filling the lung should be cleared of the respective solution as much as possible by passive drainage due to elastic recoil of the lung (*see* **Note 7**). At the conclusion of each filling and draining cycle (immediately before the next filling), take a sample to evaluate effluent contents, such as detergent or proteins. We have found that proper removal of detergents, in particular anionic detergents, is critical for producing cytocompatible acellular scaffolds [22].
6. At the conclusion of the decellularization protocol, take samples/biopsies as desired (*see* **Note 8**). Store the decellularized lung tissue in a sterile container filled with storage solution, covered and placed at 4 °C until further processing or usage for reseeding (*see* **Note 9**).

3.3 Decellularization of Pig and Human Lungs

1. Perform all works in a sterile environment (cell cultivation hood) using sterilized (autoclaved or rinsed with 70% ethanol) plastic basins/4 l-pyrex beakers, tubings, forceps, and scissors. A typical hood setup is shown in Fig. 2.
2. Take photographs of the lungs after each decellularization step to document loss of coloration and gross morphology. During decellularization the lungs should lose red coloration and should result in a glossy, white looking tissue (Fig. 3). Thermography, a method that is used to study heat distribution in structures or regions with the help of an infrared camera, can also be used to assess the distribution of perfused fluids

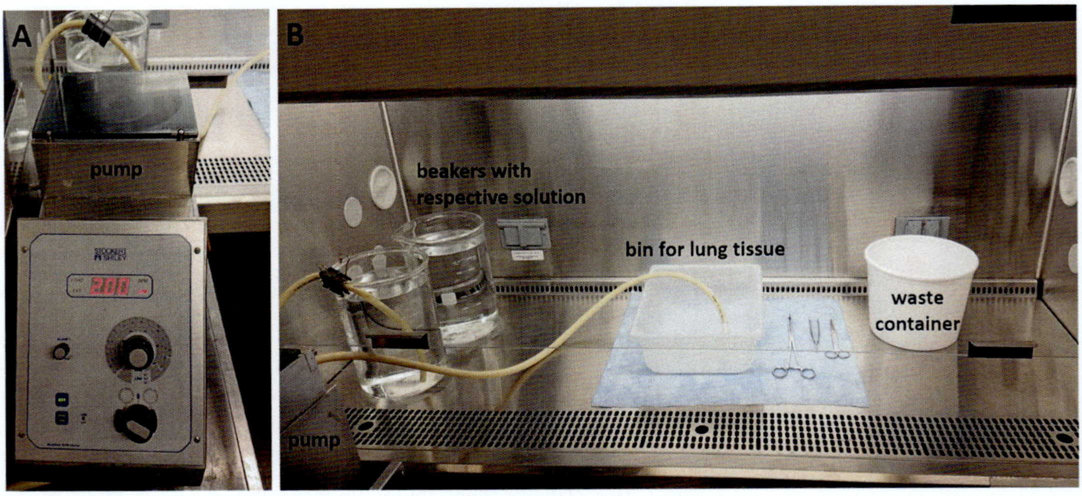

Fig. 2 Human and porcine lung decellularization. (**a**) Pump used for volume-controlled decellularization; (**b**) hood setup with indication of the pump, bin for the lung tissue, waste container, and beakers with solutions used during the decellularization

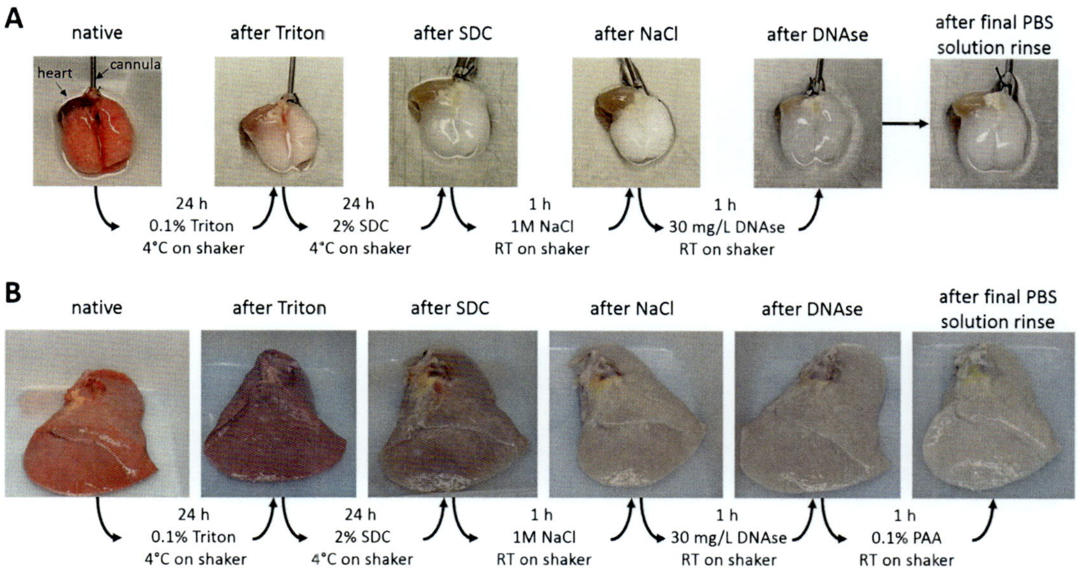

Fig. 3 Overview of loss of tissue coloration during decellularization. (**a**) Murine lungs at the different steps of the protocol; (**b**) human lung lobe at the different steps of the protocol

during the decellularization protocol. We have found by the use of thermography that decellularization solutions are not evenly distributed in IPF lungs [10] (Fig. 4). This is most likely due to the heterogeneity in the lungs in fibrotic versus normal areas and the derangement of the normal perfusion pathways.

3. On day 1, dissect a single lobe by retaining as much of the main bronchi and vasculature as possible.
4. Flush the lungs by using a roller pump at a flow rate of 2 l/min with wash solution alternating via trachea/main bronchi and pulmonary artery/main vessel (*see* **Note 10**) [3, 12, 14, 18, 19, 25]. During the vascular flushing, clamp the trachea/main bronchus to allow for tissue inflation. Fluids will flow out of both the pulmonary artery and veins by passive drainage. At the conclusion of each filling and draining cycle (immediately before the next filling), take a sample of the effluent to evaluate effluent contents, such as detergent or protein content [22].
5. After the tracheal flushing is completed and the liquid is drained from the tissue (*see* below), connect the pump and tubing to the vasculature.
6. Typical volumes and the order of the solutions used for decellularization can be found in Table 1. Inflate lungs carefully (*see* **Note 11**). The inflation volume required for full inflation depends on the size of the lung/lobe and underlying disease. Between each filling, clear the lung from the respective solution as much as possible by a combination of elastic recoil and

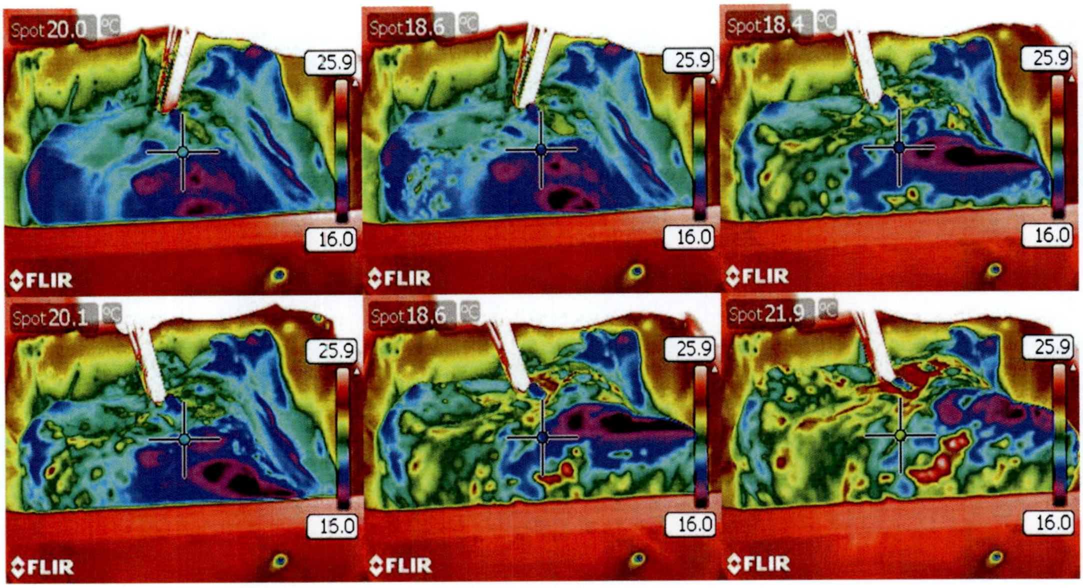

Fig. 4 Thermographic imaging of the liquid distribution during decellularization of a human idiopathic pulmonary fibrosis (IPF) lung lobe. Representative still images from thermographic analysis demonstrate nonhomogenous liquid distribution during decellularization of a human IPF lung lobe indicated by color changes. Regions that were limited or not accessible remained *blue*/*violet*. The human lobe was chilled at 4 °C in PBS after completion of the decellularization protocol. diH_2O was warmed to 37 °C to create a thermal gradient (temperature scale bar shown) for detection by the FLIR camera

light manual manipulation, (i.e., gently kneading) to help drain the liquid (*see* **Note 7**).

7. Since fibrotic tissue is denser and not as accessible for decellularization reagents as healthy tissue due to obliterated vasculature and airways, a second cycle or decellularization via immersion of excised smaller segments may be necessary [12]. For this, repeat all the steps described above. Immerse tissue in the respective decellularization agent (detergent, NaCl, DNAse, PAA) for the time periods indicated in Table 1 with 3 diH_2O wash steps of 10 min each (instead of the diH_2O flushes) under agitation to facilitate mixing and distribution of the solutions.
8. At the conclusion of the decellularization, take samples/biopsies (*see* **Note 8**). Store the decellularized lung tissue covered with storage solution in a sterile container and at 4 °C until further processing or usage for reseeding. Change the storage solution every 3 weeks to minimize the risk of contamination (*see* **Note 9**).

3.4 Scaffold Evaluation

3.4.1 Evaluation of Fibrosis Severity

It is known that the bleomycin model for fibrosis in rodents resolves over time and that fibrotic change peaks are established by day 14 after intratracheal bleomycin instillation with a peak around days 21–28 [27]. Lung function generally declines during fibrosis development, and a reduction in lung compliance and increase in lung elastance are seen and can be assessed using a device like the flexiVent [4]. Lung fibrosis is further characterized by excessive deposition of ECM proteins (like collagen, fibronectin, alpha smooth muscle actin, elastin, and tenascin C) [1, 28]. These changes can be evaluated in native tissue either by qPCR; quantitative protein assays such as Sircol™ (*see* Chap. 22 for detailed protocol and tips), Fastin™ Elastin, BioColor, etc.; Western blotting; histology (e.g., Masson Trichrome staining); or immunohistochemistry. After establishing and evaluating the preferred model of fibrosis in your laboratory, these lungs can then be decellularized and evaluated for fibrotic markers using the quantitative protein assays above and histological, immunofluorescence, or mass spectrometric proteomics assessment to evaluate changes as compared to healthy decellularized lungs. As the cells have been removed, normalization for quantitative Western blotting with cell-associated loading controls cannot be performed. Alternatively, prior to beginning decellularization, the right lungs can be removed after ligating the right bronchus. The right lung lobes can be used for traditional quantitative readouts as to the extent of fibrosis, and the left lobe could be used for decellularization. However, volumes would need to be adjusted as just the left lobe would be filled.

3.4.2 Tissue Morphology and Integrity

Lung Histology

1. Fix native or decellularized rodent lungs by gravity in 4% paraformaldehyde (20 cm H_2O pressure) for at least 3 h at room temperature. Fix tissue samples of native and decellularized pig and human lungs (about 1 cm^3) by immersion in 4% paraformaldehyde for at least 3 h at room temperature.
2. Embed samples in paraffin, and cut 5 μm sections on glass slides.
3. Deparaffinize and stain sections with any standard histological stain.
4. Assess sections using normal light or fluorescence microscopy (Fig. 5). Use H&E staining to determine overall tissue integrity.
5. Assess proper decellularization by the absence of nuclear material in the H&E and loss of DAPI staining [29]. The presence of visible red cellular material or "ghost cells" in H&E or in Masson's Trichrome staining indicates incomplete cell removal.
6. Assess the retention/loss of elastin and proteoglycans by Verhoeff's Van Gieson and Alcian Blue staining.

Electron Microscopy

For electron microscopic analyses, small segments (about 10 mm^3) of native or decellularized lung tissue can be processed as follows:

1. Fix tissue overnight at 4 °C in Karnovsky's fixative.
2. Rinse in cacodylate buffer.
3. Mince the tissue into approximately 1 mm^3 pieces.

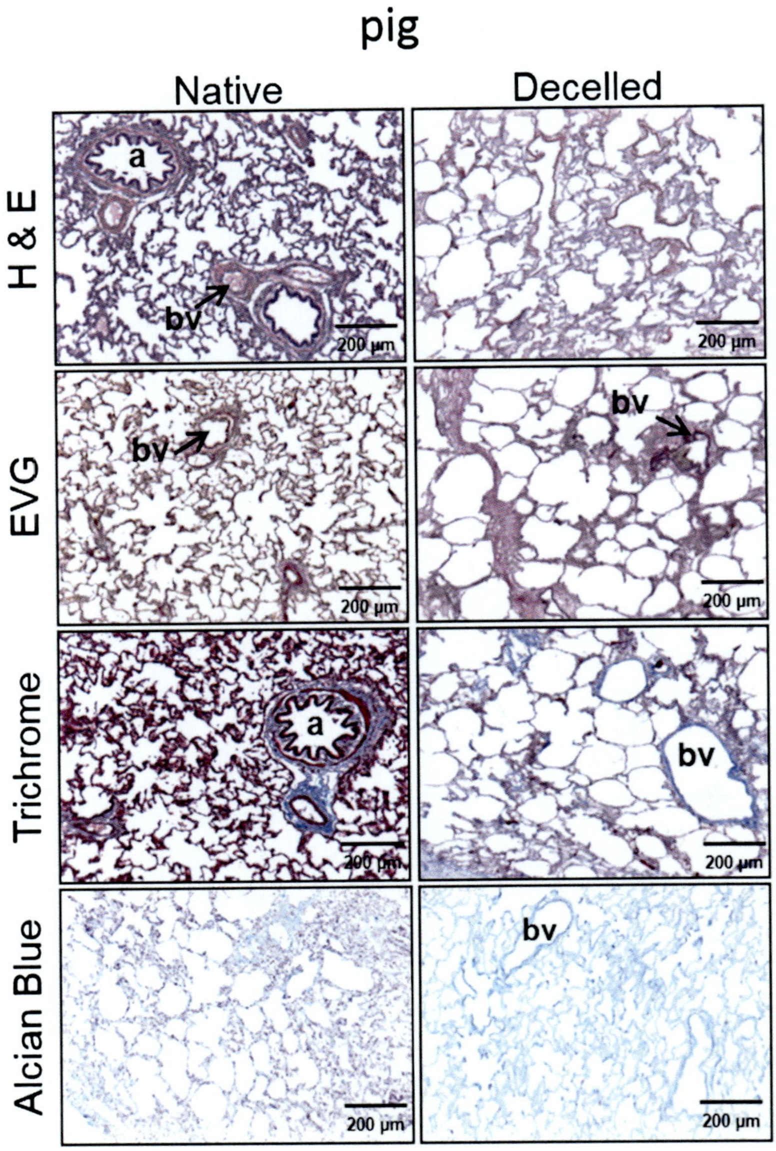

Fig. 5 Evaluation of lung morphology using histology. Hematoxylin and eosin (H&E), Masson Trichrome, Verhoeff's Van Gieson (EVG), and Alcian Blue staining of a native and decellularized pig lung lobe (Reprinted with permission from Ref. 14)

4. Fix in osmium tetroxide for 2 h at 4 °C.
5. Rinse the pieces again in cacodylate buffer.
6. Dehydrate through a graded ethanol series.
7. Clear in propylene oxide.
8. Embed in Spurr's epoxy resin.
9. Cut semi-thin sections (1 μm) using glass knives on a Reichert ultracut microtome.

10. Stain with methylene blue-azure II and then evaluate for areas of interest (proximal and distal alveolar septa, large/small airways, blood vessels).
11. Cut ultrathin sections (60–80 nm) with a diamond knife.
12. Retrieve on 200 mesh thin bar nickel grids.
13. Contrast with uranyl acetate and lead citrate.
14. Examine with a TEM operating at 60 kV [12].
15. Use electron microscopy images to compare the native and decellularized tissue morphologies, assess the integrity of the alveolar-capillary barrier, and determine whether the ultrastructure of fibers like collagen and elastin is retained (Fig. 6).

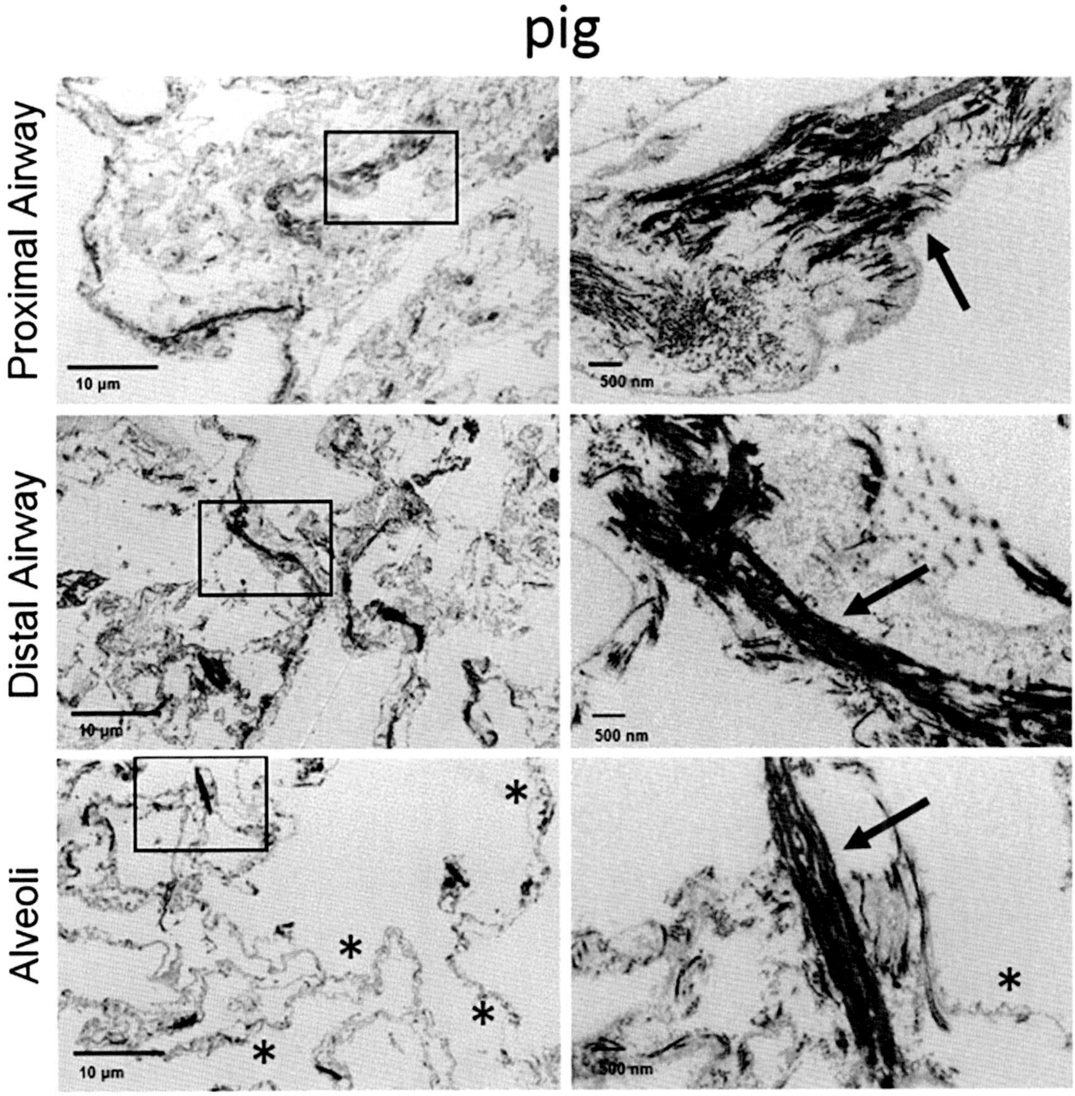

Fig. 6 Scanning electron microscopy images from a decellularized pig lung lobe. Collagen fibrils are pointed out by *arrows* and intact alveolar barrier can be observed next to the *stars* (Modified with permission from Ref. 14)

Immunohistochemistry (IHC)

1. Perform standard deparaffinization with three separate 10 min incubations in xylene.
2. Rehydrate in a descending series of ethanol and finally in water.
3. Perform antigen retrieval by heating tissue in 1X sodium citrate buffer at 98 °C for 20 min followed by a brief 20 min cool at room temperature.
4. Permeabilize tissue sections in Triton X-100 solution for 15 min.
5. Remove Triton X-100 with two 10 min washes in wash solution.
6. Block with blocking solution for 60 min.
7. After blocking, add primary antibody and incubate tissue sections overnight at 4 °C in a humidified chamber.
8. Wash tissues three times with wash solution for 5 min each.
9. Add secondary antibody and incubate for 60 min at room temperature in a dark humidified chamber.
10. Wash tissues again three times in wash solution for 5 min each in the dark.
11. Add DAPI nuclear stain for 5 min at room temperature in the dark followed by two washes in wash solution for 5 min each.
12. Mount the sections in Aqua-Poly/Mount and image with a fluorescence microscope. Typical staining is shown in Fig. 7.

3.4.3 Assessment of Residual DNA

1. Dry native and decellularized lung tissue on a tissue paper until no more liquid is visibly released and weigh the tissue.
2. Extract DNA by using a DNA extraction kit following the instructions provided by the manufacturer.
3. Run the isolated DNA on a 0.8% agarose gel and visualized under UV light or molecular imager with SYBR Safe DNA Gel stain dsDNA quantitation assay.
4. Use a 100 bp ladder and salmon sperm DNA as DNA size marker and positive control (Fig. 8). Ideally no DNA fragments will be visible on the gel.
5. Quantify the amount of double stranded (ds) DNA using a dsDNA quantitation assay following the instructions of the manufacturer. The threshold for adequate decellularization is less than 50 ng/mg dry tissue weight [29] (*see* **Note 12**).

3.4.4 Gelatinase Assay

1. Determine net gelatinolytic activity using a gelatinase activity measuring kit as previously described [21].
2. Homogenize the decellularized lung tissue in TBS and report gelatinolytic activity (in 80 mg protein) as the rate of fluores-

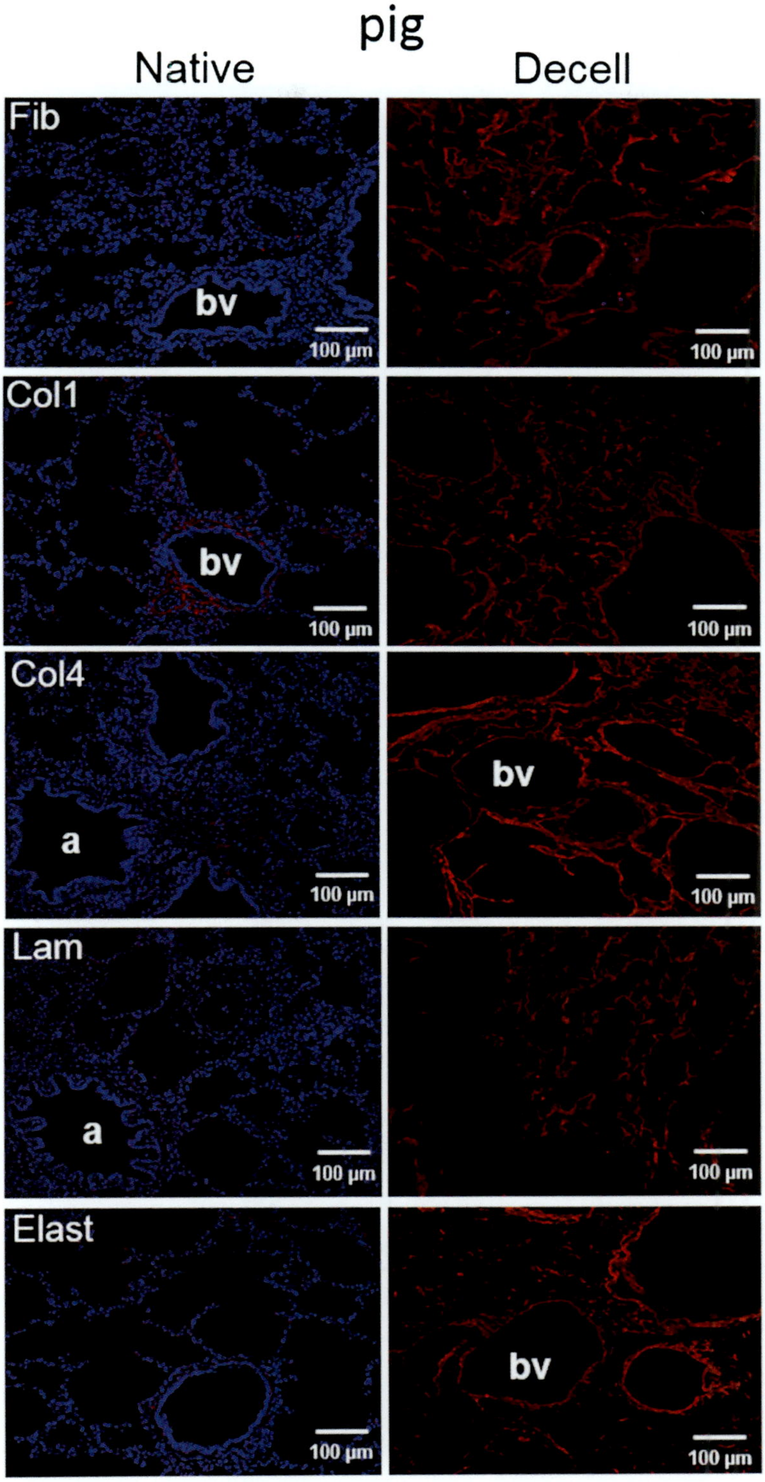

Fig. 7 Decellularization preserves major extracellular matrix (ECM) proteins in wild-type pig lungs. Representative photomicrographs are depicted and demonstrate qualitative retention of ECM proteins. Nuclear DAPI staining is depicted in *blue* and the stains of interest are depicted in *red*. Original magnifications: 100X. Col1, type I collagen; Col4, type 4 collagen; Elast, elastin; Fib, fibronectin; Lam, laminin (Reprinted with permission from Ref. 14)

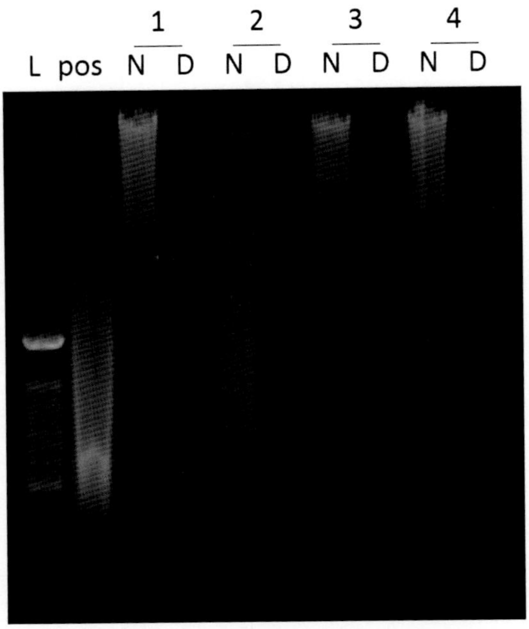

Fig. 8 Agarose gel for visualization of residual DNA in the decellularized lung tissue. Bands from *left* to *right*: L, 100 bp ladder; pos, salmon sperm DNA used as positive control; N, DNA from native human tissue; D, DNA from decellularized human tissue; 1–4, sample number

cence increase over 4 h normalized to assay reagent containing DQTM gelatin alone [18].

3. Use native lung tissue as a control.

3.5 Scaffold Cytotoxicity

3.5.1 Assessment of Residual Detergent

Concentrations of SDC in wash effluents can be determined using a modified MB assay we recently developed [22]:

1. Mix effluent samples with MB at a ratio of 1:10 (w/v) and vortex.
2. Add chloroform at a ratio of 1:2 (sample: chloroform, v/v) and vortex for 1 min.
3. Incubate 30 min at room temperature.
4. Extract 150 μl from the bottom chloroform layer and collect in a polypropylene 96-well plate (*see* **Note 13**).
5. Add wells with diH_2O or PBS containing no detergent for blanks.
6. Add SDC standards (concentration range—0–5 mg/ml, i.e., 0–0.5% (w/v)) prepared in either diH_2O (for Triton, SDC, NaCl, and DNAse effluents) or storage solution (for PBS effluents).
7. Read the absorbance at 630 nm with a plate reader.

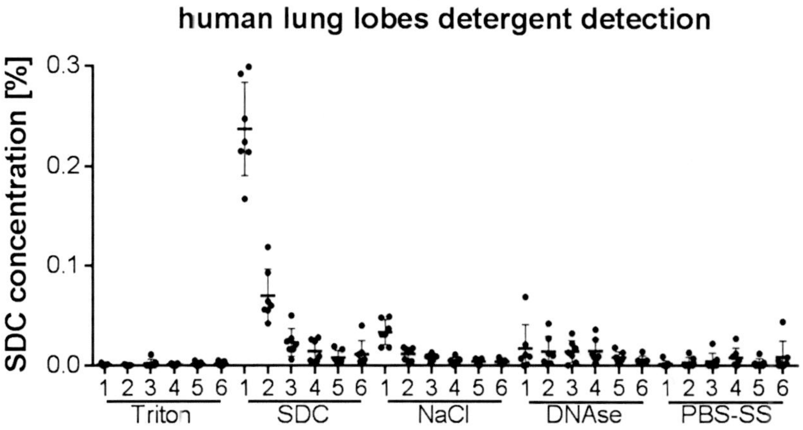

Fig. 9 Detergent detection in human lung lobes shows removal of detergent with consecutive diH_2O washes. Calculated sodium deoxycholate (SDC) concentration is displayed from seven human lung lobe decellularizations after detergent quantification in the respective effluents. Data are displayed as mean ± standard deviation

8. Calculate SDC concentration based on SDC standard curve. An example graph from several human lung lobe decellularizations is shown in Fig. 9.

3.5.2 Cell Survival

1. Determine the survival of cells on acellular lung scaffolds via indirect or direct contact with the scaffold by simple cell counting or viability assays like WST/MTT or LDH release in accordance to the ISO 10993-5:2009(E) standard.
2. For indirect determination incubate small pieces of the tissue in PBS for a fixed period of time (e.g., 24 h) to generate effluents and treat different cell lines with it for 24 h before evaluating cell survival. For direct contact seed the cells into/onto tissue pieces/slices (*see* **Note 14**) and evaluate cell survival 24 h later. Both methods were used in a recently published study from our group, and details about the assays can be found there [22]. In general we suggest the use of multiple different cell types rather than just one as each cell type may have different thresholds for detergent-induced cytotoxicity (*see* Subheading 2.4). An example of the seeding of cells into the different compartments (airway and vasculature) can be seen in Fig. 10.

3.6 Protein Analysis

3.6.1 General Considerations

Residual proteins in the decellularized tissue can be analyzed in multiple ways. An easy qualitative method is immunohistochemical stainings for specific proteins. Standard Western blotting [18, 19] can also be used to quantitate differences; however normalization in decellularized scaffolds can be difficult since there is loss of cellular proteins normally used for quantification and normalization. Both methods are limited to the availability and expense of antibodies and can only detect a small number of proteins at once. Proteins of

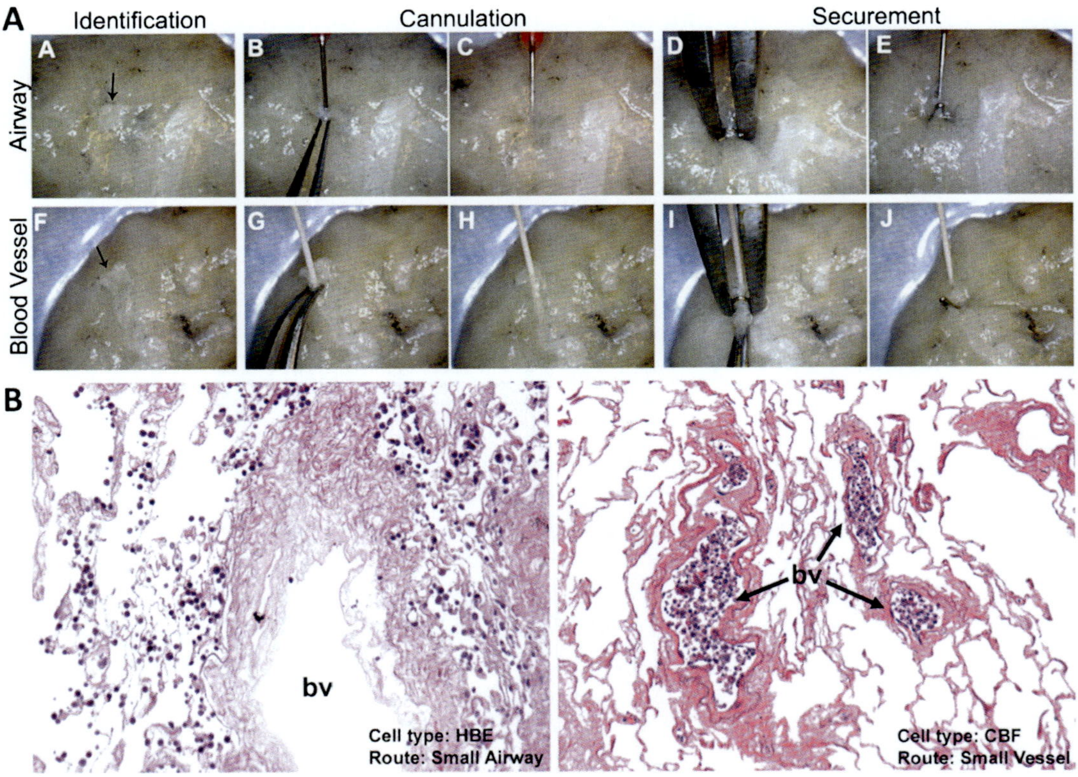

Fig. 10 Recellularization of different compartments of decellularized human lung lobes. Excised segments of acellular human lung were selectively seeded through airways or vasculature with the use of a calcium alginate coating. (**a**) Identification of small airways and vessels, cannulation and securement with surgical clips for controlled cellular inoculation. (**b**) Human bronchial epithelial (HBE) and pulmonary endothelial colony-forming (CBF) cells were retained in their respective compartment after 24 h of culture (Reprinted with permission from Ref. 12)

interest need to be identified beforehand for these techniques, and thus techniques such as mass spectrometry proteomics offer a more unbiased and general approach to determine the protein composition of the decellularized scaffold. There are both targeted and nontargeted approaches as well as quantitative and semiquantitative approaches. Targeted approaches offer the benefit of being able to quantitate differences between native and decellularized lungs or between disease states, but standards must be generated beforehand. Thus these methods, while powerful, can be costly and are limited to known proteins of interest. In nontargeted, semiquantitative approaches, the composition of the scaffolds, including previously unknown proteins, has the potential to be detected. Thus, there are pros and cons for each approach depending on the experimental questions. Here, we present our approach for nontargeted, semiquantitative mass spectrometry proteomics.

3.6.2 Semiquantitative Mass Spectrometry Proteomics

Sample Preparation

1. Obtain three samples of about 125 mg wet weight from different locations of the decellularized lung tissue. In the case of murine lungs, we typically take one single lobe from each animal following decellularization.
2. Homogenize each sample for 30 s using a sample homogenizer at maximal speed in 800 μl of 1X lysis buffer.
3. Centrifuge for 5 min at 15,000 *g* at 4 °C.
4. Separate supernatant and pellet.
5. Determine the protein content of the supernatant with a protein assay kit.
6. Run the protein lysate (20–50 mg per lane) on an SDS-PAGE gel to clean it from salts and detergents (*see* **Note 3**) letting the sample run until it is located in the separation gel. The bands should not separate in order to keep the amount of gel for the trypsin in-gel digestion small. At 80 V this will take about 10–15 min.
7. Submit the whole band of each sample to trypsin in-gel digestion.

Trypsin In-Gel Digestion

1. Clean all surfaces and tools with 70% ethanol to avoid sample contaminations.
2. Excise protein spot/band and cut into small cubes (~1 mm^3) with razorblades. Transfer to a clean microcentrifuge tube and incubate with 200 μl water for at least 15 min (*see* **Note 15**).
3. Remove water and destain three times by adding 50 mM NH_4HCO_3 in 50% ACN, incubate for 15–30 min with occasional vortexing, and discard the liquid with each wash (*see* **Note 16**).
4. Remove destaining solution and add enough 100% ACN to fully cover gel piece, incubate for 5 min, and discard ACN (*see* **Note 17**).
5. Dry gel pieces for 5 min using a SpeedVac (*see* **Note 18**).
6. Add 10 mM DTT in 100 mM NH_4HCO_3 to the dried gel piece and incubate for 1 h at 56 °C (*see* **Note 19**).
7. Let the gel pieces cool to room temperature and discard DTT solution. Add 55 mM IAA in 100 mM NH_4HCO_3 until gel pieces are covered. Incubate gel pieces in the dark for 45 min at room temperature (*see* **Note 20**).
8. Remove IAA/NH_4HCO_3 solution and discard to waste.
9. Add 100 mM NH_4HCO_3 and incubate for 5 min at room temperature.
10. Remove and discard solution.
11. Dehydrate with 100% ACN. Remove and discard solution when gel pieces are white/opaque. Repeat this step to ensure gel pieces are fully dehydrated.

12. Re-swell in 100 mM NH_4HCO_3 for 5 min. Remove and discard solution.
13. Dehydrate with 100% ACN. Remove and discard solution when gel pieces are white/opaque. Repeat this step to ensure gel pieces fully dehydrated.
14. Evaporate remaining solvents in a SpeedVac for 5 min.
15. Add 30 µl of trypsin solution to re-swell gel pieces completely at 4 °C for 30 min. If after 30 min, gel pieces are uncovered, add more NH_4HCO_3 buffer to cover gel pieces (*see* **Note 21**).
16. Digest 16–18 h at 37 °C in trypsin solution (*see* **Note 22**).
17. Transfer the solution to a new vial and add 5% FA in 50% ACN to the gel pieces; incubate for 1 h at room temperature (*see* **Note 23**).
18. Transfer the solution to the same vial as in **step 17**.
19. Add ACN and dehydrate. Transfer the solution to the same vial as **step 17** (*see* **Note 24**).
20. Dry the solution using a SpeedVac. and store at −80 °C until used for mass spectrometry.

Mass Spectrometry

1. Add 50 µl loading solution and load 5 µl of sample onto a capillary fused silica column packed with HALO C18 at a flow rate of 300 nl/min.
2. Separate peptides by a gradient of 0–35% ACN/0.1% FA over 120 min, 35–100% ACN/0.1% FA for 1 min, and a hold of 100% ACN for 8 min, followed by an equilibration 0.1% FA in H_2O for 21 min.
3. Introduce the peptides to the mass spectrometer via a nanospray ionization source and a laser pulsed ~3 µm orifice with a spray voltage of 2.2 kV.
4. Acquire mass spectrometry data in a data-dependent "Top 10" acquisition mode, in which a survey scan from m/z 360–1600 is followed by ten higher-energy collisional dissociation tandem mass spectrometry (MS/MS) scans of the most abundant ions. Acquire MS/MS scans with the following parameters: isolation width = 1.6 m/z and normalized collision energy = 26.
5. Search product ion spectra using the SEQUEST HT engine implemented on the Proteome Discoverer 1.4 software against the respective species-specific UniProt/NCBI protein database. Search parameters are as follows: (1) full trypsin enzymatic activity, (2) two missed cleavages, (3) peptides between the MW of 350–5000, (4) mass tolerance at 20 ppm for precursor ions and 0.02 Da for fragment ions, (5) dynamic modifications on methionine (+15.9949 Da: oxidation), (6) three

maximum dynamic modifications allowed per peptide, and (7) static modification on cysteine (+57.0215 Da: carbamidomethylation). Filter the combined data set to contain less than 1% false positive (with the Target Decoy PSM Validator node).

6. Assign proteins positively identified with two or more distinct peptide hits manually to one of six groups: ECM, cytoplasm, cytoskeletal, nuclear, membrane-associated, secreted, and uncharacterized in case no subcellular location is specified.
7. Generate heatmaps with the log2 transformation of peptide hits from each positively identified protein [3, 10, 12]. We have found that the log2 transformation is beneficial due to the non-normality of the data. If any of the proteins is matched to more than one category, choose its predominant subcellular location for functional grouping.

4 Notes

1. SDC solution should not be stored long term at 4 °C since this may cause precipitation or gelation, resulting in a weakening of the SDC solution. We have also found that the SDC must be at neutral or basic conditions as acidic conditions lead to the formation of precipitates. Other groups have reported the usage of the ionic detergents SDS or CHAPS as decellularization agents [11, 13]. The hydrophile-lipophile balance (HLB) is a value used to determine the hydrophilic character of a detergent. While a detergent with a low value is regarded as a water in oil emulsifier, detergents with higher values (>16) are regarded as solubilizer [30]. SDC (ionic detergent) and Triton X-100 (nonionic detergent) both have an HLB in the non-denaturing range, while SDS is a harsher solubilizer. CHAPS is a zwitterionic, non-denaturing detergent [31] (Table 2). Different decellularization protocols and detergents have been previously compared by different groups in different species (mouse and rat) analyzing differences in ECM composition, residual enzyme activity (e.g., matrix metalloproteinases), and initial viability of cells seeded onto the scaffolds. While matrix composition, total peptide amounts detected via mass spectrometry, and residual enzyme activity varied, no obvious differences were observed in initial recellularization studies [11, 18]. To date, there has been no comparison of the method of decellularization in fibrotic tissue. Due to the differences in cross-linking and composition of fibrotic tissue, usage of different decellularization techniques may also preferentially alter the remaining scaffold:

Table 2
Properties of different detergents commonly used in whole-organ decellularization

Agent	CMC (mM)	HLB	Properties
Triton X-100	0.2–0.9	13.5	Nonionic detergent used to solubilize proteins; mild non-denaturing detergent
Sodium deoxycholate (SDC)	4–8	16	Water-soluble anionic detergent used for disrupting and dissociated protein interaction
Sodium dodecyl sulfate (SDS)	7–10	40	Anionic surfactant used for lysing cells and unraveling proteins
3-[(3-cholamidopropyl) dimethylammonio]-1-propanesulfonate (CHAPS)	6–10	–	Non-denaturing zwitterionic detergent used to solubilize proteins

CMC critical micelle concentration, *HLB* hydrophile-lipophile balance

2. DNAse solution should always be either prepared fresh or stored in aliquots at −20 °C. The magnesium and calcium in the solution are necessary for the activity of the enzyme.
3. Gels for SDS-PAGE should be in the range of 10–15% polyacrylamide.
4. Other investigators have used a range of other cells and cell types including human umbilical vein endothelial cells [11, 32], small airway epithelial cells [11], pulmonary alveolar epithelial cells [11], rat distal lung epithelial cells [33], induced pluripotent stem cells [32, 34, 35], mouse A9 fibroblast cells [36], human lung fibroblasts [8], human peripheral blood mononuclear cells (PBMC) [5], and bone marrow-derived mesenchymal stem cells [37].
5. hMSCs have previously been extensively characterized for cell surface marker expression and differentiation capacity [23] and should not be used past passage 7.
6. Amounts of bleomycin administration vary between laboratories. Usually a single dose of 1.25–4 U/kg is administered [1, 3–5, 17]. It should be noted that different mouse strains have different susceptibilities to bleomycin [1]. Chapter 2 of this volume provides ample details for this method.
7. The lung volume should decrease significantly before the next filling. For mouse and rat lungs, this takes up to 1 min. Pig and human lungs need manual handling which means gently kneading the lung tissue in order to drain the liquid. Having the trachea/main bronchi at the lowest point of the tissue increases draining efficiency. Especially when the lung is filled, handling of the tissue should be done carefully. Kneading needs to be done more carefully with the pig lungs due to the lack of alveolar interconnectivity (lack of pores of Kohn).

Therefore pig lungs are more likely to form pleural blebs which will significantly reduce decellularization efficiency and should be avoided.

8. Samples for quality control from pig and human lungs should be taken from at least three different locations of the tissue to account for local variations. Quality control samples include but are not limited to pieces for histology/IHC and DNA determination.

9. Based on our experience, acellular lungs should not be stored longer than 3 months due to degradation and loss of biological activity [25].

10. Pump-aided inflation (pig and human lungs) should start with a low flow rate slowly increasing to 2 l/min. A lower flow rate was shown to not properly clear the lungs from debris, while a higher flow rate negatively impacted tissue integrity [12]. Other groups reported different flow rates and the usage of pressure-controlled decellularization protocols [7, 11, 38–40]. An overview of different protocols used for decellularization is given in [41]. We believe that the decellularization is not only based on the membrane-disrupting action of the detergents to lyse the cells but also on the shear stresses imposed by flushing the tissue. For this reason a pressure-controlled decellularization protocol may need higher volumes to achieve a similar clearance of cellular debris.

11. Do not under- or overinflate the lungs. Underinflation will lead to improper decellularization and can be noticed by visual and manual examination. If the tissue feels soft at the edges or is still expanding while filling it is not filled completely. Proper filling volume should be recorded with the initial wash solution washes and be used as a guide for later fillings. During the decellularization process, the lungs will become leaky due to the loss of cells, and inflation volumes may need to be increased at later stages to achieve full tissue inflation and distribution of solutions to the alveoli and capillaries. Great care should be taken to not overinflate since this will result in damage and may lead to pleural blebbing (dislocation of the pleura from the lung tissue with fluid entrapment and bubble formation) especially in pig lungs. As soon as all parts of the lung are filled, you can proceed with draining/manual manipulation of the lung to empty the tissue from the fluid.

12. Absorbance measurements (e.g., using a Nanodrop) can be used to evaluate DNA content, but it is not as accurate as methods like the Quant-iT™ PicoGreen® dsDNA assay since it will additionally detect single-stranded DNA as well as RNA. It was found that this overestimates the amount of dsDNA in the sample since the amount of dsDNA detected by PicoGreen was found to be in the range of 25–40% of the amount determined via Nanodrop [42].

13. Transfer only eight samples at once and measure the absorbance in order to prevent inaccuracy due to chloroform evaporation.
14. To seed the cells into/onto the tissue, slices of about 1 mm thickness can be cut with sterile razorblades and trimmed to a diameter of 6 mm with a standard biopsy punch to fit the tissue into a 96-well plate. Cells can then directly be seeded onto the tissue for incubation and viability evaluation.
15. Ensure that gel pieces are completely covered with each reagent.
16. Destain until gel pieces are clear (~30 min or overnight if the dye has not diffused out).
17. ACN shrinks the gel pieces and dehydrates them by extracting H_2O. Gel pieces should be white/opaque and shrunken after incubation with acetonitrile. Repeat ACN step if gel pieces are not completely white.
18. When using the SpeedVac, it is important to first turn on the centrifuge before turning on the vacuum in order to not lose the sample. After drying, first turn off the vacuum and then the centrifuge.
19. DTT reduces the disulfide bonds and makes the protein linear. Make sure all the gel pieces are covered.
20. IAA leads to alkylation by binding covalently with the thiol group of cysteine so the protein cannot form disulfide bonds.
21. Trypsin should be 6 ng/μl for silver stain and 12 ng/μl for Coomassie blue stained gels. The trypsin to protein ratio should be 1:20–1:100 (w/w).
22. Do not digest longer than 18 h. Trypsin cuts at lysine (Lys) and arginine (Arg) locations. It is important to have predictable peptide fragments for proper identification in mass spectrometry proteomic databases. Proteins are trapped in the gel, but when you introduce the enzyme, they are cleaved into peptides and diffuse out of the gel as peptides ending in Lys or Arg.
23. This step will extract the peptides from the gel pieces.
24. This step may have to be done twice to fully dehydrate the gel pieces.

Acknowledgments

The authors are grateful to Douglas Taatjes Ph.D. and Nicole Bishop of the UVM Microscopy and Imaging Center for assistance with IHC staining, transmission electron microscopy imaging, and image interpretations. We would like to thank Caroline Andrews, Nicholas Bonenfant, Zachary Borg, Amy Coffey, Amanda Daly, Jacob Dearborn, Nathan Gasek, Ethan Griswold, Zachary Phillips, Joseph Platz, Alexander Riveron, Dino Sokocevic, John Wallis,

Sean Wrenn, and Basa Zvorova for the assistance with lung decellularizations, microscopy, and analysis of the detergent effluents. Studies were supported by the NIH RO1 HL127144-01 (DJW), Vermont Lung Center CoBRE grant (P20RR15557), NIH PACT program (contract HHSN268201000008C), NHBLI Lung Biology Training grant T32 HL076122, NIH Institutional Development Award (IDeA) NIGMS grant P20GM103449, and NCRR grant P40RR017447.

References

1. Moore BB, Hogaboam CM (2008) Murine models of pulmonary fibrosis. Am J Physiol Lung Cell Mol Physiol 294(2):L152–L160. doi:10.1152/ajplung.00313.2007
2. Mouratis MA, Aidinis V (2011) Modeling pulmonary fibrosis with bleomycin. Curr Opin Pulm Med 17(5):355–361. doi:10.1097/MCP.0b013e328349ac2b
3. Sokocevic D, Bonenfant NR, Wagner DE et al (2013) The effect of age and emphysematous and fibrotic injury on the re-cellularization of de-cellularized lungs. Biomaterials 34(13):3256–3269. doi:10.1016/j.biomaterials.2013.01.028
4. Schiller HB, Fernandez IE, Burgstaller G et al (2015) Time- and compartment-resolved proteome profiling of the extracellular niche in lung injury and repair. Mol Syst Biol 11(7):819. doi:10.15252/msb.20156123
5. Sun H, Zhu Y, Pan H et al (2016) Netrin-1 regulates fibrocyte accumulation in the decellularized fibrotic sclerodermatous lung microenvironment and in bleomycin-induced pulmonary fibrosis. Arthritis Rheumatol 68(5):1251–1261. doi:10.1002/art.39575
6. Price AP, England KA, Matson AM et al (2010) Development of a decellularized lung bioreactor system for bioengineering the lung: the matrix reloaded. Tissue Eng Part A 16(8):2581–2591. doi:10.1089/ten.TEA.2009.0659
7. Petersen TH, Calle EA, Zhao L et al (2010) Tissue-engineered lungs for in vivo implantation. Science 329(5991):538–541. doi:10.1126/science.1189345
8. Booth AJ, Hadley R, Cornett AM et al (2012) Acellular normal and fibrotic human lung matrices as a culture system for in vitro investigation. Am J Respir Crit Care Med 186(9):866–876. doi:10.1164/rccm.201204-0754OC
9. Gilpin SE, Guyette JP, Ren X et al (2013) Up-scaling decellularization and whole organ culture for human lung regeneration. J Heart Lung Transpl 32(4):S69–S70. doi:10.1016/j.healun.2013.01.172
10. Wagner DE, Bonenfant NR, Parsons CS et al (2014) Comparative decellularization and recellularization of normal versus emphysematous human lungs. Biomaterials 35(10):3281–3297. doi:10.1016/j.biomaterials.2013.12.103
11. Gilpin SE, Guyette JP, Gonzalez G et al (2014) Perfusion decellularization of human and porcine lungs: bringing the matrix to clinical scale. J Heart Lung Transplant 33(3):298–308. doi:10.1016/j.healun.2013.10.030
12. Wagner DE, Bonenfant NR, Sokocevic D et al (2014) Three-dimensional scaffolds of acellular human and porcine lungs for high throughput studies of lung disease and regeneration. Biomaterials 35(9):2664–2679. doi:10.1016/j.biomaterials.2013.11.078
13. Balestrini JL, Gard AL, Liu A et al (2015) Production of decellularized porcine lung scaffolds for use in tissue engineering. Integr Biol (Camb) 7(12):1598–1610. doi:10.1039/c5ib00063g
14. Platz J, Bonenfant NR, Uhl FE et al (2016) Comparative study to the use of decellularized alpha-Gal KO pig lungs for xenogeneic lung transplantation. Tissue Eng Part C Methods. doi:10.1089/ten.TEC.2016.0109
15. Godin LM, Sandri BJ, Wagner DE et al (2016) Decreased laminin expression by human lung epithelial cells and fibroblasts cultured in acellular lung scaffolds from aged mice. PLoS One 11(3):e0150966. doi:10.1371/journal.pone.0150966
16. Parker MW, Rossi D, Peterson M et al (2014) Fibrotic extracellular matrix activates a profibrotic positive feedback loop. J Clin Invest 124(4):1622–1635. doi:10.1172/jci71386
17. Zhou Y, Peng H, Sun H et al (2014) Chitinase 3-like 1 suppresses injury and promotes fibroproliferative responses in mammalian lung fibrosis. Sci Transl Med 6(240):240ra276. doi:10.1126/scitranslmed.3007096
18. Wallis JM, Borg ZD, Daly AB et al (2012) Comparative assessment of detergent-based protocols for mouse lung de-cellularization and re-cellularization. Tissue Eng Part C

Methods 18(6):420–432. doi:10.1089/ten.TEC.2011.0567

19. Daly AB, Wallis JM, Borg ZD et al (2012) Initial binding and recellularization of decellularized mouse lung scaffolds with bone marrow-derived mesenchymal stromal cells. Tissue Eng Part A 18(1–2):1–16. doi:10.1089/ten.TEA.2011.0301
20. Bonvillain RW, Danchuk S, Sullivan DE et al (2012) A nonhuman primate model of lung regeneration: detergent-mediated decellularization and initial in vitro recellularization with mesenchymal stem cells. Tissue Eng Part A 18(23–24):2437–2452. doi:10.1089/ten.TEA.2011.0594
21. Lluri G, Langlois GD, McClellan B et al (2006) Tissue inhibitor of metalloproteinase-2 (TIMP-2) regulates neuromuscular junction development via a beta1 integrin-mediated mechanism. J Neurobiol 66(12):1365–1377. doi:10.1002/neu.20315
22. Zvarova B, Uhl FE, Uriarte JJ et al (2016) Residual detergent detection method for nondestructive cytocompatibility evaluation of decellularized whole lung scaffolds. Tissue Eng Part C Methods 22(5):418–428. doi:10.1089/ten.TEC.2015.0439
23. Reed W, Noga SJ, Gee AP et al (2009) Production Assistance for Cellular Therapies (PACT): four-year experience from the United States National Heart, Lung, and Blood Institute (NHLBI) contract research program in cell and tissue therapies. Transfusion 49(4):786–796. doi:10.1111/j.1537-2995.2008.02027.x
24. Yankaskas JR, Haizlip JE, Conrad M et al (1993) Papilloma virus immortalized tracheal epithelial cells retain a well-differentiated phenotype. Am J Phys 264(5 Pt 1):C1219–C1230
25. Bonenfant NR, Sokocevic D, Wagner DE et al (2013) The effects of storage and sterilization on de-cellularized and re-cellularized whole lung. Biomaterials 34(13):3231–3245. doi:10.1016/j.biomaterials.2013.01.031
26. Melo E, Cardenes N, Garreta E et al (2014) Inhomogeneity of local stiffness in the extracellular matrix scaffold of fibrotic mouse lungs. J Mech Behav Biomed Mater 37:186–195. doi:10.1016/j.jmbbm.2014.05.019
27. Moeller A, Ask K, Warburton D et al (2008) The bleomycin animal model: a useful tool to investigate treatment options for idiopathic pulmonary fibrosis? Int J Biochem Cell Biol 40(3):362–382. doi:10.1016/j.biocel.2007.08.011
28. Fernandez IE, Amarie OV, Mutze K et al (2016) Systematic phenotyping and correlation of biomarkers with lung function and histology in lung fibrosis. Am J Physiol Lung Cell Mol Physiol 310(10):L919–L927. doi:10.1152/ajplung.00183.2015
29. Crapo PM, Gilbert TW, Badylak SF (2011) An overview of tissue and whole organ decellularization processes. Biomaterials 32(12):3233–3243. doi:10.1016/j.biomaterials.2011.01.057
30. Griffin WC (1954) Calculation of HLB values of non-ionic surfactants. J Soc Cosmet Chem 5:249–256
31. Hjelmeland LM (1980) A nondenaturing zwitterionic detergent for membrane biochemistry: design and synthesis. Proc Natl Acad Sci U S A 77(11):6368–6370. doi:10.1073/pnas.77.11.6368
32. Ren X, Moser PT, Gilpin SE et al (2015) Engineering pulmonary vasculature in decellularized rat and human lungs. Nat Biotechnol 33(10):1097–1102. doi:10.1038/nbt.3354
33. Calle EA, Mendez JJ, Ghaedi M et al (2015) Fate of distal lung epithelium cultured in a decellularized lung extracellular matrix. Tissue Eng Part A 21(11–12):1916–1928. doi:10.1089/ten.TEA.2014.0511
34. Ghaedi M, Calle EA, Mendez JJ et al (2013) Human iPS cell-derived alveolar epithelium repopulates lung extracellular matrix. J Clin Invest 123(11):4950–4962. doi:10.1172/JCI68793
35. Gilpin SE, Ren X, Okamoto T et al (2014) Enhanced lung epithelial specification of human induced pluripotent stem cells on decellularized lung matrix. Ann Thorac Surg 98(5):1721–1729. doi:10.1016/j.athoracsur.2014.05.080
36. Sun H, Calle E, Chen X et al (2014) Fibroblast engraftment in the decellularized mouse lung occurs via a beta1-integrin-dependent, FAK-dependent pathway that is mediated by ERK and opposed by AKT. Am J Physiol Lung Cell Mol Physiol 306(6):L463–L475. doi:10.1152/ajplung.00100.2013
37. Sun Z, Gong X, Zhu H et al (2014) Inhibition of Wnt/beta-catenin signaling promotes engraftment of mesenchymal stem cells to repair lung injury. J Cell Physiol 229(2):213–224. doi:10.1002/jcp.24436
38. Ott HC, Clippinger B, Conrad C et al (2010) Regeneration and orthotopic transplantation of a bioartificial lung. Nat Med 16(8):927–933. doi:10.1038/nm.2193
39. Nichols JE, Niles J, Riddle M et al (2013) Production and assessment of decellularized pig and human lung scaffolds. Tissue Eng Part A 19(17–18):2045–2062. doi:10.1089/ten.TEA.2012.0250

40. Price AP, Godin LM, Domek A et al (2015) Automated decellularization of intact, human-sized lungs for tissue engineering. Tissue Eng Part C Methods 21(1):94–103. doi:10.1089/ten.TEC.2013.0756

41. Wagner DE, Uhl FE, Weiss DJ (2015) Acellular lung scaffolds in lung bioengineering. In: Bertoncello I (ed) Stem cells in the lung: development. Repair and Regeneration. Springer International Publishing, Cham, pp 309–347. doi:10.1007/978-3-319-21082-7_18

42. Huleihel L, Hussey GS, Naranjo JD et al (2016) Matrix-bound nanovesicles within ECM bioscaffolds. Sci Adv 2(6):e1600502. doi:10.1126/sciadv.1600502

Part III

ECM Proteins: Purification, Quantification, and Analysis

Chapter 19

Type I Collagen Purification from Rat Tail Tendons

Laure Rittié

Abstract

Type I collagen, or collagen I, is the most abundant protein in the human body and provides strength and resiliency to tissues such as bone, tendons, ligaments, and skin. Collagen I forms macromolecular networks in which resident mesenchymal cells are embedded. Cell-extracellular matrix interactions are critical not only for maintenance of tissue properties but also for guiding and orienting the phenotype of resident cells. Cues from the extracellular matrix have been shown to be critical in pathophysiologies such as fibrosis, aging, and cancer. Hence, the details of these interactions are being scrutinized to better understand the mechanisms of such diseases and conditions. Many in vitro assays, such as cell-embedded collagen lattices, preparation of hydrogels, adhesion assays, etc., have been developed to study various aspects of cell-extracellular matrix interactions. All these in vitro models rely on utilizing high-quality purified collagen I. Here, we provide state-of-the-art collagen I extraction protocol and useful tips to produce high-quality purified collagen I solutions. We also provide a detailed protocol for pepsin digestion of collagen I, for a highly reliable collagen concentration assay, and guidelines for conducting quality controls to validate purified collagen solutions. Collagen I prepared with these procedures is highly suitable for many in vitro applications.

Key words Collagen, Purification, Precipitation, Lyophilization, SDS-PAGE, Concentration assay

1 Introduction

Collagens are a family of proteins that comprise the bulk of the network of macromolecules that form extracellular matrices (ECMs) throughout the body. There are currently 28 known collagen proteins (or "types"). Collagen types are designated by roman numerals from I to XXVIII in order of discovery and encoded by distinct genes. Type I collagen, or collagen I, is the most abundant protein in the human body and accounts for 30% of total proteins [1]. Collagen I is made within cells by the assembly of three chains (two α1 chains and one α2 chain) into "procollagen," a triple helix that ends in short non-helical telopeptides followed by globular propeptides at both the N- and C-termini. Once secreted, the N- and C-terminal globular propeptides are rapidly and enzymatically cleaved, and the resulting "tropocollagen"

Laure Rittié (ed.), *Fibrosis: Methods and Protocols*, Methods in Molecular Biology, vol. 1627,
DOI 10.1007/978-1-4939-7113-8_19,

helices assemble into fibrils. Collagen I fibrils further assemble with other macromolecules (e.g., other collagens such as collagens III, V, XII, XIV, proteoglycans) to form collagen fibers. Hence, although collagen fibers are often called "type I collagen fibers," they are actually made of more proteins than just collagen I. Collagen fibers are stabilized by intra- and interchain enzymatic cross-links catalyzed by extracellular enzymes [2]. Many cross-link sites reside in the telopeptides. Collagen fibers are responsible for the functional integrity of tissues such as bone, teeth, tendons, ligaments, and skin. The concentration of collagen I fibrils within a connective tissue varies depending on the tissue and its intended physical properties. For example, addition of mineral to the bone ECM during bone mineralization is responsible for the tissue typical hardness. Tendons and ligaments are relatively rich in collagen I, skin contains relatively more non-collagenous proteins such as elastin and lipids than tendons, and human lungs contain almost as much elastin as collagen [3]. Relative collagen concentration is not only important for the biomechanical properties of a tissue but also key when considering extracting collagen I from tissue samples.

Tendons are a tissue of choice for collagen extraction because of their relatively high collagen I concentration compared to other tissues. In addition, tendons are easy to isolate, which makes the starting material fairly uncontaminated. Lastly, tendon-rich anatomical structures are readily available as surgical remnants of animal experimentation (e.g., mouse or rat tails) or from slaughterhouses (e.g., cow or pig feet). Skin can also be used, though it contains much more non-collagenous proteins (e.g., blood- and appendage-derived proteins) and lipids than tendons. These two contaminants thus need to be removed during the collagen purification protocol (the former by solubilization and the latter by adipose tissue dissection or chemical delipidation or both). Interestingly, small variations of protein sequence have been noted, not only between species but also between tissues of the same species. For example, collagen I molecules extracted from rat tendon and rat skin were shown to differ in the amount of 3-Hyp residues they contain (3–4 per chain vs. 0–1, respectively) [4]. This difference was thought to guide a tighter packing of collagen I in tendons vs. skin [5]. Although the species of origin for collagen extraction is often overlooked—collagen I is exceptionally conserved—small variations do exist and may influence the extracted molecule's properties. Thus, I strongly recommend being consistent in your choice of collagen source, avoiding changing species or tissue of origin during the course of a project. In this chapter, we will focus on the most common source of type I collagen for laboratory use: rat tail tendons.

The aim of this chapter is to provide the state-of-the-art collagen I extraction protocol together with useful tips that I learned hands-on during my training in Biochemistry [6–8] (protocol itself derived from pioneer methods [9, 10]). In essence, the process involves (a) manual dissection of the rat tail tendons, (b) elimination of the soluble non-collagenous proteins, (c) solubilization of acid-soluble collagens in weak acid solutions, (d) purification of type I collagen from other collagen types by salt precipitation, (e) elimination of salt by dialysis against water, and (f) elimination of water (dehydration) by lyophilization, which also allows concentration, preservation, and further sterilization for cell culture applications (*see* **Note 1**). The resulting purified collagen I will be suitable for many applications such as producing cell-embedded collagen lattices (see [11] and Chapter 15), preparation of hydrogels (Chapter 17), adhesion assays [7, 8], in vitro fibrillation experiments (Chapter 24), etc.

We also detail a method to prepare pepsin-digested collagen I. Pepsin is used on collagen I to remove the non-triple helical telopeptides at both ends of the triple helix [12]. Telopeptide release may be sought for cross-link removal [13] or for differentiating specific telopeptide-dependent interactions such as in adhesion studies and thereby enhance collagen solubilization [7]. Pepsin treatment of collagen will also alter the molecule's antigenicity and aggregation properties [12]. We have noticed that at equal collagen concentration, pepsin-digested collagen lattices were softer than those made of nondigested collagen (unpublished observations).

Many different collagen extraction protocols have been used and published and sometimes differ from the above by lacking one or more steps. We will detail the importance and role of each step below, but, in all cases, biochemical analysis of the end product (i.e., purified collagen I) should be documented to validate any extraction method. The best analysis to be performed is denaturing polyacrylamide gel electrophoresis (SDS-PAGE) in reducing condition, as collagen I has a very unique pattern of migration (Fig. 1). Collagen I run on a SDS-PAGE in reducing conditions should produce two monomeric α-chains (α1 and α2), three dimeric β-chains (β11, β12, and variant β11), and one trimeric γ-chain (the term "β-chain" is used to describe a collagen dimer and "γ-chain" a trimer). It is also common to see an additional band stuck at the stacking gel and consisting of more complex cross-linked aggregates that are unable to enter the concentrating gel. Beta-11 chains are homodimers of α1 chains, and β12 chains are heterodimers of α1 and α2 chains. β11 and β12 dimers are both cross-linked at the N-terminal telopeptide. Variant β11 chains are homodimers of α1 chains cross-linked both at the N- and C-terminal telopeptides. As seen on Fig. 1, presence of cross-links readily alters the apparent molecular weight (MW) of β-chains (e.g., compare migrations of β11 and variant β11). Posttranslational modifications of α-chains also cause differences between calculated and apparent MWs. As shown on Fig. 1, the α1 and α2 chain monomers migrate with apparent MW of >116 kDa and <116

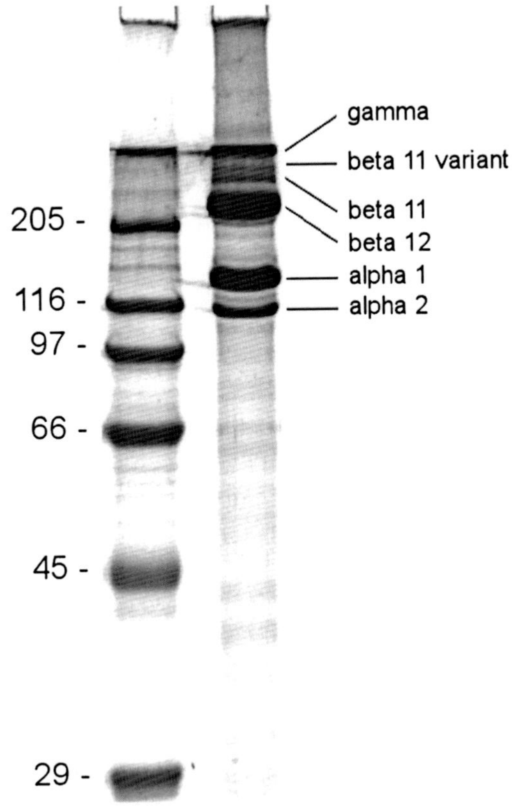

Fig. 1 SDS-PAGE migration pattern of type I collagen. Coomassie brilliant blue-stained 8% SDS-polyacrylamide gels run under reducing conditions reveals the typical migration pattern of collagen I. *Left lane* is molecular weight markers (with corresponding MW on the *left*). *Right lane* is collagen I and its typical six migration bands (from *bottom* to *top*): two monomeric α-chains (α1 and α2), three dimeric β-chains (β11, β12, and variant β11), and one trimeric γ-chain (see text for details)

kDa, respectively (much different from their calculated MWs of 91.7 and 94.9 kDa, respectively [14, 15]). Practically, the α2 chain is lighter not only in apparent MW but also in intensity (because a collagen I triple helix is made of two α1 chains and one α2 chain). In all, a good-quality purified collagen solution should produce six bands when run on a SDS-PAGE under reducing conditions. These bands can be resolved on an 8% acrylamide separation gel (Fig. 1), but are separated even better on a 5% gel (e.g., [16]). Presence of major bands migrating faster than the α2 chain is indicative of suboptimal preparation (either due to contaminant proteins or degraded collagen chains). I recommend that such quality control be regularly performed to validate the nature of a purified collagen I preparation, whether it is extracted by the methods detailed herein or from commercial source (*see* **Notes 2** and **3**).

2 Materials

2.1 Extraction of Acid-Soluble Collagen I

1. Rat tails from adult animals (typically from a sacrificed experimental cohort) (*see* **Notes 4** and **5**).
2. 70% (v/v) ethanol in diH_2O.
3. A 7 or 10 in. pliers wrench.
4. Gloves and personal protection equipment according to local regulations (wear gloves at all times).
5. Scalpel or sharp razor blade.
6. Scissors and tweezers.
7. 100 mm-diameter glass Petri dish.
8. Autoclaved flasks: at least one 2 l Erlenmeyer flask, one 2 l beaker, and two 1 l beakers.
9. Two autoclaved 60 × 10 mm (i.e., 6 cm-long) magnetic stirrers and stirring plate. You can get by with two stirrers if you can wash and autoclave one stirrer every day. You will also need another stirrer, a magnet, or a magnetic wand to remove stirrer from large vessels without touching solutions.
10. Working station: wrap a flat piece of Styrofoam in heavy-duty aluminum foil. This makes a compliant working surface that can be easily disposed of when experiment is complete (just remove and discard the foil with biohazard waste).
11. Buffer A: mix ~900 ml diH_2O and 1.21 g of Tris base (10 mM final), 8.77 g of NaCl (0.15 mM), 1.9 g EDTA·4H_2O (5 mM), 0.626 g *N*-ethylmaleimide (5 mM), 0.174 g phenylmethanesulfonyl fluoride (PMSF, 1 mM), and 0.783 g benzamidine (5 mM) in a 2 l beaker. Stir with a magnetic stirrer. Once solubilized, adjust the pH to 7.5 using 1 M HCl. Transfer solution to a 1 l volumetric flask and adjust volume to 1 l with diH_2O. Transfer to a storage bottle and store at 4 °C for up to 3 months.
12. NaCl salt.
13. Glacial acetic acid (i.e., 17.4 M; handle under a fume hood) for the following solutions:
    (a) 0.5 M acetic acid: prepare 500 ml of solution by adding ~450 ml diH_2O and 14.4 ml glacial acetic acid to a beaker. Mix, adjust volume to 500 ml, and store at 4 °C.
    (b) 18 mM acetic acid: prepare 500 ml of solution by adding 0.5 ml of glacial acetic acid to 500 ml of diH_2O. "18 mM" concentration is traditionally used because it is easy to prepare (i.e., ~1‰ ("one per mille") dilution).
14. Freezers (−80 and −20 °C). A shell freezer to prepare samples for lyophilization is also highly recommended.

15. Cold room (or at the very least, refrigerated cabinet).
16. Laboratory scale.
17. Centrifuge compatible with 10,000 *g* centrifugation of large vessel (we use a Sorvall™ centrifuge with an SS-34 fixed-angle centrifuge head).
18. Four to six autoclaved 250 ml capped bottles that allow ≥10,000 *g* centrifugal force (we use Nalgene™ polypropylene copolymer centrifuge bottles with polypropylene screw closures #3120-0250).
19. Seamless cellulose dialysis tubing: we use a roll that we cut to length. Membranes have 4.8 nm-diameter pores that retain materials with 12,000 and higher molecular weight. Store at room temperature in a dry location.
20. Small plastic funnel.
21. Airtight, moisture-resistant polypropylene vials.
22. Two 16 l buckets filled with diH_2O for dialysis. Each bucket needs to be filled and refrigerated at least 24 h prior to use.
23. Lyophilizer (we use an old Labconco FreeZone Freeze Dry System with a 12-port drying chamber attached to a general vacuum pump and a vacuum gage).
24. Freeze-dry flasks (our lyophilizer system requires 3/4″ flask adapters) and rubber lids.

2.2 Miscellaneous

1. Pepsin powder (generally prepared from the gastric mucosa of pigs, cattle, or sheep). Use lyophilized powder of at least 2500 units/mg of protein (1 unit defined as producing a change in A_{280} of 0.001 per min at pH 2.0 at 37 °C, measured as trichloroacetic acid-soluble products using hemoglobin as substrate, a final volume of 16 ml, and a 1 cm-long absorption path).
2. SDS-PAGE apparatus (mini-gels or large gels), with 5–10% acrylamide separation gel, migration box, power supply, Coomassie blue G-250 for staining, and 10% acetic acid for destaining.

2.3 Sterilization for Cell Culture Applications

1. Sterile 50 ml conical centrifuge tubes.
2. 70% (v/v) ethanol in diH_2O.
3. Sterile 10 ml Luer lock syringes.
4. Sterile long needles such as a lumbar puncture needle (the purpose here is to reach the bottom of a 15 ml tube without entering the syringe in the tube).
5. Sterile and chilled 18 mM acetic acid (*see* **item 13b** in Subheading 2.1).
6. Rotating wheel.

2.4 Collagen Concentration Assay

1. Heat block pre-heated to 50 °C.
2. Laboratory scale.
3. Vortex.
4. Spectrophotometer to read absorbance at 650 nm.
5. Spreadsheet program (LibreOffice Calc or similar) for preparation of standard curve and assessment of test samples.
6. 1.5 ml polypropylene microtubes.
7. 50 and 15 ml conical tubes.
8. 18 mM acetic acid (*see* **item 13b** in Subheading 2.1).
9. Collagen preparation of known concentration, commercial or not (<1 ml needed, concentration ≥1.2 mg/ml).
10. Solution A: in a 50 ml conical tube, add ~30 ml of diH_2O, 0.16 g of potassium sodium tartrate tetrahydrate, and 4 g of Na_2CO_3. Add 2 ml of 10 M NaOH and vortex until solubilization is complete. Adjust volume to 40 ml with diH_2O. Store at room temperature for up to 6 months.
11. Solution B: in a 50 ml conical tube, add ~30 ml of diH_2O, 0.8 g of potassium sodium tartrate tetrahydrate, and 1.2 g of $CuSO_4{\cdot}5H_2O$. Add 0.4 ml of 10 M NaOH and mix until solubilization is complete. Adjust volume to 40 ml with diH_2O. Store at room temperature for up to 6 months.
12. Folin-Ciocalteu reagent (used as Folin solution, i.e., 1:15 (v/v) dilution in water, just before use).

3 Methods

3.1 Important Considerations

1. Always wear protective gloves.
2. Always work with clean vessels: although most of the extraction will be done in non-sterile conditions, I recommend thoroughly cleaning all supplies (vessels, magnetic stirrers, etc.) and autoclaving them when possible.
3. Always work on ice or at 4 °C: because collagen will start the fibrillogenesis process leading to formation of insoluble polymers even in the presence of salts [17], it is important to keep all solutions cold at all times. All buffers need to be prechilled before use, and all the incubations are done at 4 °C. The use of a cold room will greatly facilitate your task as some of the vessels used are quite bulky. In the absence of cold room, a refrigerated cabinet may be used (it needs to be large enough to store two 16 l buckets).
4. Beware of harsh agitation: agitation is a common cause of protein degradation, and all agitation systems cause some degree of denaturation [18]. Keep in mind that the stir bar system we

elected to use here produces intense shear near the stir bar surface. Agitation should be as gently as possible (i.e., selecting the lowest speed that creates slight liquid movement on the periphery of the vessel). Vortexing should be avoided unless stipulated.

3.2 Extraction of Acid-Soluble Collagen I

1. Harvest rat tails from adult animals (typically from a sacrificed experimental cohort) and store the tails in a plastic bag at −20 °C until extraction day (*see* **Notes 4** and **5**).
2. On extraction day, prepare a 2 l Erlenmeyer flask containing 1 l of chilled buffer A, and thaw rat tails at room temperature for 5–10 min (*see* **Note 6**).
3. Transfer tails into a 100 mm-diameter glass Petri dish containing 70% ethanol until completely thawed (~10 min). Meanwhile, prepare a working surface as described in Subheading 2.1.
4. Transfer a thawed tail onto the working surface.
5. Use a 7–10 in. pliers wrench to grab the most caudal vertebrae of the tail, and break the intravertebral joint by holding the tail firmly in one hand and making a couple of back and forth motions with the wrench with the other hand (you want to fold/unfold the vertebrae over until it breaks).
6. While maintaining your grab with the wrench, hold firmly the tail down against the working surface and pull the vertebrae with the wrench: the tail tendons, which are attached to the vertebrae, will detach from their sheath and come out. Pull until the tendons are totally extracted from the rest of the tail (*see* **Note 7**).
7. Cut the tendon flush at the vertebrae using a scalpel or a sharp razor blade, discard the skin-covered vertebrae, and use tweezers to transfer the tendons into a 2 l Erlenmeyer flask containing 1 l of chilled buffer A (*see* **Note 8**).
8. Repeat **steps 5–7** with the next vertebrae on the same tail, and continue until most of the vertebrae are used (*see* **Notes 9–11**).
9. Process the other tails similarly; mix all tendons together in the same Erlenmeyer flask (*see* **Notes 12** and **13**).
10. Add a large magnetic stirrer to the Erlenmeyer flask and incubate overnight at 4 °C under moderate agitation (*see* **Notes 14–16**).
11. On day 2, remove magnetic stirrer using another stirrer, a magnet, or a magnetic wand (*see* **Note 17**).
12. Discard buffer A by decantation (*see* **Notes 18** and **19**).
13. Add 200 ml of 0.5 M acetic acid to the flask and a clean magnetic stirrer to the Erlenmeyer flask and incubate 24 h at 4 °C under moderate agitation (*see* **Notes 15** and **20**).

14. On day 3, collect the supernatant by transferring it to an even number of sterile 250 ml centrifuge bottles by decantation (*see* **Note 21**).
15. Balance the centrifugation tubes (*see* **Note 22**) and centrifuge at 10,000 *g* for 30 min at 4 °C (*see* **Note 23**).
16. Collect the supernatant in a 1 l beaker by decantation. Estimate the total volume of supernatant using the beaker graduations in ml (= *V*) (*see* **Note 24**).
17. Calculate the amount of NaCl needed to bring the final NaCl concentration to 0.7 M: the molecular weight of NaCl is 58.443, which means that a 1 M solution contains 58.443 g/l NaCl. Thus, the mass of NaCl ("M" in g) necessary to make a 0.7 M solution based on the volume measured in **step 16** ("V" in ml) is:

$$M = \frac{58.443 \times 0.7 \times V}{1000}$$

18. Weight "M" grams of NaCl in a weighing dish.
19. In the cold room, add a clean magnetic stirrer to the beaker from **step 16** and agitate the supernatant. While maintaining a moderate-to-vigorous agitation, slowly add the salt to the supernatant (*see* **Note 25**).
20. Slow down the agitation to low speed, and agitate 24 h at 4 °C (*see* **Note 26**).
21. Transfer the supernatant to an even number of large centrifuge tubes and centrifuge at 10,000 *g* for 30 min at 4 °C (*see* **Notes 22** and **27**).
22. Solubilize the pellets in chilled 18 mM acetic acid: add 10–15 ml acetic acid to one pellet, agitate by hand to detach the pellet, and transfer to a 1 l beaker. Repeat with all the tubes, and rinse each tube with a small amount of acetic acid and top beaker with acetic acid to the desired final volume. Experience will help estimate the volume needed, which is typically based on the viscosity of the solution collected in **step 14**. If the solution was noticeably viscous, use 150–200 ml of acetic acid total. If the solution was only somewhat viscous, use 80–150 ml of acetic acid (*see* **Note 28**). In all cases, solubilization will take several hours to overnight.
23. Add a clean magnetic stirrer to the collagen solution and incubate under moderate agitation at 4 °C for several hours to overnight (*see* **Note 29**).
24. Once the collagen pellets are totally dissolved: if pepsin digestion is desired, follow the steps described in Subheading 3.3 before proceeding to **step 25**. If pepsin digestion is not needed, proceed directly to **step 25**.

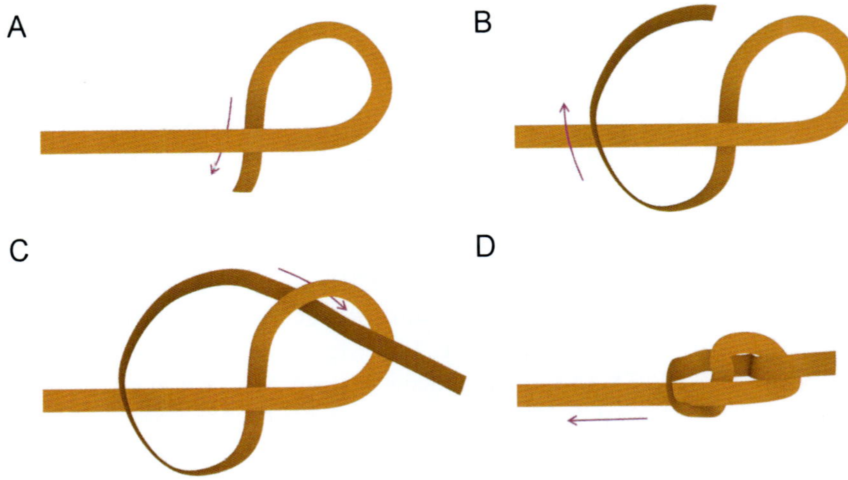

Fig. 2 The stopper knot used for securing dialysis tubing. Tie a knot by looping under (**a**) then over (**b**) the standing part of the tubing, forming an "eight"-shaped loop at one extremity. Pass the end of the tubing under the start of the loop and through the loop (**c**), and pull the standing part of the tubing to tightly secure the knot (**d**). Place the knot approximately 2 cm (3/4 in.) from the end of the dialysis tube

25. Dialyze the collagen solution against cold diH_2O according to the following steps:
    (a) Cut dialysis tubing into several ~40 cm (~16 in.) sections and soak the pieces in a clean container filled with diH_2O for at least 5 min (*see* **Note 30**).
    (b) Take a piece of dialysis tubing, squeeze it between index and middle fingers to remove excess water, and tie a stopper knot at one end (Fig. 2) (*see* **Note 31**).
    (c) Open the other end of the tubing by rolling it between your thumb and finger (*see* **Note 32**).
    (d) Fill the dialysis tubing with collagen solution using a small funnel until at least ~10 cm (4 in.) below the top of the tube (*see* **Note 33**).
    (e) Close the tube by squeezing out as much air as possible, and tie a stopper knot at the end of the piece of tubing (*see* **Note 34**). Check for leaks, retie a knot, or change the piece of tubing if needed.
    (f) Attach a piece of string with a simple knot noosed below the stopper knot (long enough to be able to fold over the side of the bucket), and place the tubing in the bucket full of diH_2O (prechilled in **step 23**).
    (g) Prepare as many dialysis tubing as needed to hold the entire volume of the collagen solution.
26. Return the bucket to 4 °C for 24 h, and prechill another bucket filled with diH_2O for the following day.

27. Transfer the dialysis tubes to a fresh bucket of cold water every day, until dialysis is complete (*see* **Notes 35** and **36**).
28. Collect the dialysate in a clean 1 l beaker: hold the dialysis tube in the beaker and use scissors to cut a very small slit just above the bottom knot (be prepared for the dialysate to spill right out). Squeeze the tube to collect the entire dialysate into the beaker. Discard the used dialysis tube and repeat with all remaining tubes.
29. Lyophilize the collagen (*see* **Note 37**):
    (a) Transfer the aqueous collagen solution in freeze-dry flasks (*see* **Notes 38** and **39**).
    (b) Cover the flasks with their rubber lids and freeze the collagen solution at −80 °C in a slanted way using a shell freezer (*see* **Notes 40–42**). Once sample are completely frozen, they can be kept at in a −80 °C freezer for several days until next step.
    (c) Proceed to lyophilization. As a general rule of thumb, use a primary drying temperature set at −5 °C (the collagen solution is an aqueous sample, and the shelf temperature is set to just below the sample's eutectic temperature of 0 °C) and a standard −50 °C collector (*see* **Note 43**).
30. When the lyophilization is complete, the collagen looks and feels like dense cotton fibers. Weigh collagen samples from each flask and transfer them in airtight containers (samples may be combined; *see* **Note 44**). Ensure the container is as airtight as possible, write the weight and date on it, and store at −80 °C until use (*see* **Note 45**).
31. Subheading 3.4 will detail important tips to prepare a collagen solution, whether you need it sterilized or not. Also, Subheading 3.5 will detail a useful method to perform collagen assays for quantification of purified type I collagen solutions.

3.3 Pepsin Digestion

1. The pepsin will be added to the acid solution of collagen with a target concentration of 1% (i.e., 1 g pepsin for 100 g collagen) (*see* **Note 46**). As the collagen concentration is unknown at this point, it is recommended to take an aliquot of the solution and test the collagen concentration:
    (a) Pipette a known volume of acid solution of collagen with a positive displacement pipette (*see* **Note 47**).
    (b) Perform nine 1:2 serial dilutions of the acid solution of collagen in 0.5 M acetic acid.
    (c) Assess collagen concentration in the ten samples (*see* method in Subheading 3.4) (*see* **Note 48**). Draw a standard curve based on standard results and plot the ten samples on the curve. Only the results in the linear range of the assay should

be considered (i.e., a 1:2 dilution should result in half the concentration) and other sample points eliminated.

(d) The collagen concentration of the initial acid solution of collagen can be estimated as the average of the concentrations obtained from the samples deemed technically valid (*see* **Note 49**).

2. Calculate the mass (=M, in mg) of pepsin needed based on the estimated collagen concentration determined in **step 1d** (=C, in mg/ml), the volume of acetic acid used in **step 22** (=V, in ml), and the following formula:

$$M = \frac{C \times V}{100}.$$

3. Weight "M" mg of pepsin in a weighing dish.
4. In the cold room, start agitating the collagen solution from **step 24**, Subheading 3.2. While maintaining a moderate agitation, slowly add the pepsin to the solution (*see* **Note 25**).
5. Agitate on low speed 24 h at 4 °C.
6. Upon pepsin digestion, the α1 chain will release the two N- and C-telopeptides made of 15 and 25 amino acid, respectively [14]. The telopeptides for the α2 chain are slightly shorter than those of α1 (e.g., 9 and 15 amino acids for the α2 N- and C-telopeptides of bovine collagen I [16]; rat not ascertained [15]). These peptides will be eliminated by dialysis, by resuming the collagen purification method at **step 25** of Subheading 3.2.

3.4 Sterilization for Cell Culture Applications

1. Transfer up to 250 mg of dried collagen in an empty 50 ml conical centrifuge tube (*see* **Note 50**). Record the exact weight of collagen used (= W, in g).
2. Fill the tube with 70% ethanol and incubate on ice or at 4 °C for 20 min.
3. In a sterile hood, aspirate the ethanol using a 10 ml syringe and a long needle (*see* **Note 51**) and discard it. The collagen has now a spongy appearance.
4. Use your long needle to press the collagen against the wall of the tube to squeeze out any remaining ethanol, and discard the ethanol.
5. When virtually all the ethanol is removed, repeat **steps 2–4** twice for a total of three washes, with the third wash lasting overnight instead of 20 min.
6. When virtually all the ethanol is removed after the third wash, leave the tube open in the sterile cabinet for ~30 min to allow evaporation of the ethanol remnants.

7. Add X ml of 18 mM of cold sterile acetic acid, with $X = W/5$ (for a targeted 5 mg/ml collagen solution) (*see* **Note 52**).
8. Close the tube very tightly and place on a slow-rotating wheel at 4 °C for solubilization (*see* **Note 53**). Solubilization may take anywhere from overnight to 3 days, depending on the quality of the purified protein and the accuracy of the weighing process.
9. Determine the exact concentration of the collagen solution by Hyp measurement (high-performance liquid chromatography or colorimetric assay) or by using the collagen concentration assay detailed in Subheading 3.5.

3.5 Collagen Concentration Assay

We have extensively and successfully used the method first reported by Komsa-Penkova et al. [19] for determining the collagen concentration of our purified solutions:

1. Turn on a heat block to 50 °C.
2. Prepare the first standard in a microtube by diluting a commercial collagen solution or previous collagen preparation of known concentration in 18 mM acetic acid to obtain 500 μl of solution at 1.2 mg/ml collagen I.
3. Make five 250 μl, 1:2 serial dilutions of the first standard to obtain the following five standards (0.6, 0.3, 0.15, 0.075, and 0.0375 mg/ml).
4. Add 200 μl of each standard (**steps 2** and **4**) to six fresh microtubes.
5. Add 200 μl of 18 mM acetic acid to a seventh microtube for the "zero."
6. Prepare the first test sample (i.e., 1:5) by diluting 100 μl of the collagen I solution with 400 μl 18 mM acetic acid (*see* **Note 54**).
7. Make three 250 μl, 1:2 serial dilutions of the first sample to obtain the following test samples: 1:10, 1:20, and 1:40 (*see* **Note 55**).
8. Add 200 μl of each sample (**steps 6** and **7**) to four fresh microtubes. You should now have 11 test tubes: seven standards (including the "zero") and four test samples. Discard all the tubes that were used to make dilutions.
9. Add 180 μl of solution A to all tubes.
10. Add 20 μl of solution B to all tubes.
11. Close all the tubes, vortex, and place tubes on a heat block at 50 °C for 20 min.
12. Transfer all microtubes to a rack and allow slow cooling to room temperature (~10 min). Meanwhile, prepare the Folin solution: in a 15 ml conical tube, mix 6.53 ml of diH_2O and

467 μl of Folin-Ciocalteu reagent (*see* **Note 56**). Mix by vortexing.

13. When all microtubes are cooled down to room temperature, centrifuge briefly to collect the moisture from caps, open the lids, and add 600 μl of Folin solution to each tube.
14. Close all microtubes, vortex, and place tubes on a heat block at 50 °C for 10 min.
15. Transfer all test tubes to a rack and allow slow cooling to room temperature (~10 min).
16. Centrifuge briefly to collect the moisture from caps before opening the lids, and read absorbance at 650 nm. Use standards to generate a standard curve and to calculate the collagen concentration of each test samples. Figure 3 and accompanying legend provide an example of how to perform these calculations.
17. You may want to adjust the concentration of your collagen solution. For example, we like to further dilute our sterile solution to 4 mg/ml final to simplify volume calculations down the road. To do so, add the desired volume of sterile 18 mM acetic acid to your solution, and place under low agitation as described in **step 8** of Subheading 3.4 at least overnight at 4 °C.
18. Before utilizing your collagen solution, run a 5 or 8% SDS-PAGE in denaturing conditions (i.e., in the presence of denaturing agent such as β-mercaptoethanol or dithiothreitol) for quality control, loading 2 μg collagen I on a mini-gel or 10 μg on a large gel. *See* Subheading 1 for details on interpretation.

4 Notes

1. "Lyophilization" and "freeze-drying" are interchangeable terms.
2. Commercial solutions are often sterilized by ultrafiltration, and, depending on the quality and maintenance of the equipment, this treatment may damage the integrity of the collagen protein (which is a long fibrillar protein and therefore very susceptible to damage when forced though small filtration pores). If you notice that a collagen solution (commercial or not) does not form expected gel-like structures in your experiments, run a quality control as described in Subheading 1: damaged collagen will produce more than six bands, the bulk of additional bands migrating faster (i.e. lower) than the α2 chain.
3. Performing a quality control to each batch of collagen preparation can save you a lot of time by revealing potential molecular damage or contamination that may alter your experimental results.

A

Abs (650 nm)	Coll I (mg/ml)
0.0002	0
0.0722	0.0375
0.1036	0.075
0.1892	0.15
0.3376	0.3
0.6020	0.6
1.0874	1.2

B

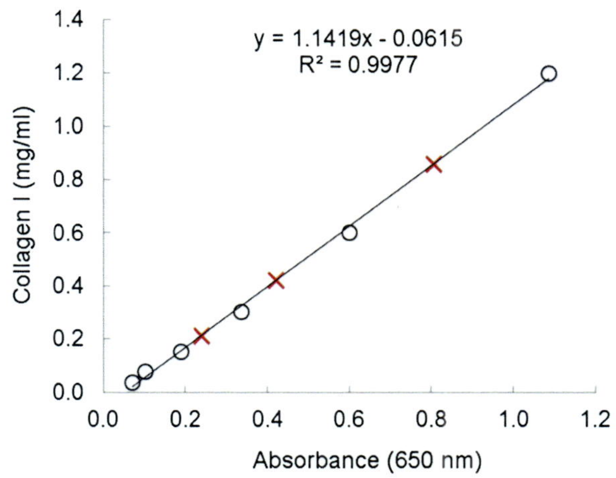

C

tested sample ID	Abs (650 nm)	calculcated concentration	dilution factor	Coll I (mg/ml)
1:2	0.8075	0.861	2	1.721
1:4	0.4265	0.426	4	1.702
1:8	0.2411	0.214	8	1.710

Fig. 3 Calculations for the collagen concentration assay. (**a**) Collagen I concentration of each Standard (*right column*) and corresponding Absorbance readings (*left column*) were entered in a spreadsheet program and used to draw a scatter plot (**b**, *black circles*). The "zero" values (from the blank) were not included in the scattered plot because we intended to discard any data point that would have a smaller value than the lowest standard (i.e., less than 0.07 absorbance value). A linear trend line was added over the scatter points, selecting the options to display the "R-squared value" (i.e., the assay quality control) and the "trend line equation" on the chart. The closest to 1 the R-squared value is, the more accurate the assay is. If R-squared value is <0.9, I recommend to rerun the entire assay paying particular attention to pipetting accuracy and repeatability. The trend line equation will allow calculating the collagen concentrations (y) from the absorbance values (x) of the tested samples. (**c**) Four dilutions (undiluted, 1:2, 1:4, and 1:8) of a collagen solution were run in parallel with the standards. We discarded the results from the undiluted solution because it had a greater absorbance value than the highest standard (i.e., >1 absorbance value). The remaining three tested samples were plotted with *red crosses* on chart in **b** for reference. (**c**) Absorbance readings of the three tested samples were entered in the second column and used to calculate respective collagen concentrations (third column) using the standards' trend line equation. In the last column, the final concentrations of collagen I were calculated taking into consideration the initial dilutions of the three tested samples. In all, we obtained three measurements that were very close (as it should be if the assay is run with good laboratory practices). The collagen I concentration of the original solution will be identified as the average of the three measurements (i.e., 1.71 mg/ml)

4. Acquisition of animal remnants must comply with local regulations.
5. When obtaining rat tails from a sacrificed experimental cohort, ensure you only select the tails of the animals from the control group.
6. We typically process 3–4 adult rat tails at a time.
7. Tendons look like whitish glossy strings, as shown in Fig. 1 of reference [20].

8. Make sure you place tendons in the buffer, not on the side of the flask where they will strongly stick and dry out.
9. The first few vertebrae, which are relatively small, are relatively easy to pull. As you go along, it will become harder and harder to (1) break the vertebrae and (2) pull out the tendons (mostly because the remainder of the tail gets shorter). Try to collect as many tendons as possible, but keep the task reasonably doable (we usually process ~2/3 of each tail).
10. It could be tempting to attempt to slit the skin along the tail and somehow dissect the tendons out. I recommend against it as the extraction by pulling will ensure good separation of the tendons from their protective sheaths and from other structures such as blood vessels. This will certainly increase the quality of the overall purification.
11. It could also be tempting to select more tails and dissect only the first few vertebrae on each tail. I recommend collecting as many "thicker" tendons as possible to increase the overall yield.
12. Take your time. The entire procedure, with 3–4 tails, typically takes 30–60 min.
13. If you decide against processing all the tails, do not refreeze the unused tails, but discard them as freezing and thawing cycles are known to alter ECM protein integrity (and you want the best possible starting material).
14. This step will solubilize all the soluble proteins (i.e., blood-derived material, most proteoglycans, immature collagen, etc.)
15. Agitation is meant to maintain movement in the flask to allow buffer access to all areas. I recommend against a too harsh agitation that might break the tendons or generate heat.
16. It is common that the tendons end up curled around the magnetic stirrer, which is fine. Reducing agitation speed may help mitigate the problem.
17. If tangled in the middle of tendons, gently isolate the stirrer with gloved hands, and make sure to return the tendons to the buffer, not to the side of the flask where they will strongly stick and dry out. Change your gloves before proceeding to next step.
18. Always proceed with extreme caution when decanting: you want to slowly pour out the supernatant and get a feel of how likely your desired material will stay in the vial. In this case, you want to remove as much buffer as possible without losing the tendons.
19. At this stage, the tendons appear much whiter in color than on day 1. If old buffer A appears very cloudy and tendons do not look totally white, it might be necessary to repeat the overnight incubation with 1 l of chilled fresh buffer A.

20. This step will solubilize mostly collagens I and III. Insoluble material and highly cross-linked collagens will not be solubilized and remain insoluble.
21. If the supernatant appears extremely viscous, it might be useful to repeat the acetic acid extraction step: harvest and store the supernatant in a tight container at 4 °C, add 100 ml of 0.5 M acetic acid to the tendon-containing flask, and incubate 24 h at 4 °C under moderate agitation. The following day, mix the new supernatant with the old one, and proceed to centrifugation. In all cases, discard what is left of the tendons as biohazard material.
22. Safe centrifugation requires balanced loading of the centrifuge rotor to avoid equipment damage. Use an even number of tubes and weight-balance your tubes in pairs: use a scale and a transfer pipette to homogenize the weight between the tubes of a given pair, and load paired tubes in the centrifuge across from each other. I do not recommend using an odd number of tubes with a water-filled balance tube because balancing should be done between liquid of similar density (balancing by mass alone is not correct). In this case, the collagen solution is very dense, and I find it easier to use an even number of tubes rather than to find a density match for balancing.
23. This step will "clear" the supernatant from insoluble material.
24. I recommend against trying being perfect when estimating this volume (e.g., using a graduated cylinder) as the supernatant is quite viscous. Changing vials twice would result in a non-negligible loss of material.
25. Aim at the side of the swirling liquid rather than the center of the vortex to ensure proper mixing. Also, add the salt little by little, ensuring each bit is dissolved before adding more salt.
26. This step will precipitate collagen I (not collagen III).
27. This step is to separate the collagen I-containing pellet from other proteins in the supernatant.
28. The goal here is to use enough acetic acid to solubilize the pellet but not too much to keep the concentration relatively high (and volume relatively low). When unsure, the experimenter should start with a low volume (75–100 ml) and estimate the state of solubilization after several hours of incubation (i.e., whether the pellet disappears overtime and how viscous the solution is). Remember: you can always add more acetic acid, but you cannot remove it if you added too much.
29. Ensure the pellet is completely dissolved and the solution homogenized (not globs) before proceeding to next step. If globs are present after overnight incubation, add a little more chilled 18 mM acetic acid and incubate the collagen solution under low agitation at 4 °C for another several hours to overnight.

30. The dialysis tubing is ready when flexible but can stay in diH_2O for prolonged periods of time.
31. I find the stopper knot ideal for this application and fairly easy to perform with a little practice. In addition, this knot is a "crossed" knot and thus cannot be unfolded if the tube is swirled in one direction. If you choose to use simple knots (i.e., the first components of a shoelacing knot), I recommend you perform two knots, one dexter and one sinister (or vice versa).
32. You may blow in the opening to open the tube but avoid direct contact with the mouth.
33. We typically use a small funnel to pour the solution into the tube, squeezing the tube and funnel together with one hand and pouring the solution with the other hand. Alternatively, one can use a 10 or 25 ml sterile plastic pipette (be careful not to puncture the dialysis tube with the pipette tip) although you may lose some material this way. In all cases, ensure you hold the tube tight because it will become heavier as it gets filled with solution.
34. The rate of dialysis is directly proportional to the surface area of the membrane. The "flatter" a sample can be (i.e., the less volume per length of tube), the faster its dialysis will be (mostly because all molecules in the sample will be closer to the membrane and more available for exchange). Although it may seem more work to fill the dialysis tubes only halfway, it may increase the quality of the purification process or decrease the dialysis time.
35. For static dialysis (i.e., without agitation or flow), we typically estimate that the buffer/water volume needs to be 200 times the volume of the dialysate. For instance, for 200 ml of collagen solution, you will need a minimum of 40 l of water (2.5 × 16 l), i.e., three changes of 16 l bucket, 24 h each, to complete the dialysis. The amount of collagen solution per tube, as discussed in **Note 34**, will greatly influence this estimation.
36. While standard static dialysis is good enough in the laboratory, other techniques such as dynamic or flow dialysis are also acceptable. Ensure the solution is kept between 0 and 4 °C the entire time.
37. Lyophilization is a common freeze-drying process that allows long-term protein preservation without deterioration. Lyophilization may be considered costly because it involves investing in relatively expensive equipment but is important for more than preservation. Without the step of dialysis, your collagen solution will contain high concentration of salt (from NaCl precipitation). With dialysis but without lyophilization, the extracted collagen will be in suspension in water and thus very likely to fibrillate, of unknown (and most often than not

too low) concentration, and will not be sterile (sterilization method for cell culture application below). Lyophilization will allow preparing high-quality, repeatable, and stable collagen solutions.

38. Freeze-dry flasks are designed to handle the temperature change during freezing and the deep vacuum pressures required for lyophilization. They should be purchased with the lyophilization system.

39. To avoid freeze-dry flask breakage, flasks should not be filled more than one third of their capacity.

40. Shell freezers are designed to rotate the flask during freezing. Thus, the collagen solution freezes a thin coating of sample at a time, homogeneously covering the inside walls of flask. This freezing method greatly enhances the overall quality of the lyophilization. Using a shell freezer is highly recommended here.

41. If you don't have access to a shell freezer, you may freeze your sample in a −80 °C freezer (this technique is suboptimal). In this case, do not cover the flasks with their rubber lids and use aluminum foil instead as the rubber can get damaged during freezing. Also, avoid placing your flasks in an upright position as the increase of volume that accompanies the freezing process may break the flask. Favor a 30–45° slanted position in the −80 °C freezer, preferably rotating the flask one fourth turn every 10 min during freezing. Alternatively, use dry ice or liquid nitrogen to freeze the solution while regularly rotating the flasks (wear suitable protection and prechill the flasks before placing them in very cold temperatures).

42. The freezing step of the lyophilization process is very important for quality and stability. The reader is encouraged to learn more about this step [20].

43. The rate (and thus total time) of lyophilization depends on the quality of the equipment and the freezing method used. In most cases, our collagen samples were lyophilized in approximately 48 h. You will know that all of the water is extracted from the sample when the sample volume no longer visually decreases overtime (you may also break the vacuum, weigh a sample-containing flask, restart the lyophilization process, and control the weight a few hours later).

44. Although samples may be combined to save space, we found that storing dried collagen in small aliquot is helpful because it allows us to use the "true" dry weight noted on the container as opposed to have to reweigh the dry collagen on the day of use. Collagen always undergoes some level of rehydration during storage. Using the lyophilization day weight minimizes errors due to potentially weighing added water. We tend to use 250 mg at a time (*see* **step 1** in Subheading 3.4 and **Note 50**).

45. Ensure you promptly weigh and store the dried collagen protein and minimize the protein air exposure time. Also ensure the container used for −80 °C storage is airtight as collagen will capture the moisture in the air/freezer and increase its water content over time.
46. Pepsin is most active under acidic conditions and inactive at pH >6.5; it will thus be active in the 0.5 M acetic acid solution obtained from **step 23** of Subheading 3.2.
47. Using a positive displacement pipette (such as Microman® from Gilson) will ensure accuracy and precision when pipetting a viscous liquid such as this collagen solution. The overall collagen concentration will be calculated based on this sample amount, so precision at this stage is paramount. Glass microsyringe pipettes (from Hamilton Company or similar) are also acceptable. Alternatively, use an air-displacement pipette (Pipetman® from Gilson or similar) with a wide orifice pipette tip and a very slow pipetting motion. This latter option is not as good as the other two options as it reduces pipetting accuracy and repeatability.
48. The ten samples have a dilution factor of 1 (pure, not diluted), 2 (i.e., one half the initial concentration), 4, 8, etc. until 512. Therefore, concentration result of the corresponding sample will have to be multiplied by 1, 2, 4, 8, etc. until 512 to reflect the concentration of the initial solution.
49. The samples deemed technically valid should yield pretty similar concentration results. If they differ between them by more than 10%, this may indicate technical error, the most common of which being pipetting (either pipetting technique or accuracy of the pipette itself).
50. If using the original weigh as recommended in **Note 44**, no correction is needed. If you opted for freezing larger quantities at a time, it may be useful to reweigh the total dry collagen sample for which you have a lyophilization day weight and calculate a weigh correction factor to correct for added moisture. For example, if lyophilization day weight was 1 g and today's weigh is 1.2 g, then weigh 20% more than what you need (i.e., 250 × 1.2 = 300 g). The so-called exact weight of collagen remains 250 g.
51. Depending on the needle used, a portion of the syringe may enter the tube when you try to reach the very bottom. Avoid touching the lower part of the syringe with your hands.
52. Although some commercial collagen solutions are sold at concentrations as high as 10 mg/ml, we find that good-quality collagen is hard to solubilize at concentrations higher than 5 mg/ml. We typically use 4 mg/ml stock solutions.

53. Avoid forming bubbles at all costs as they will be hard to remove. Bubbles form when agitation is too strong or cap is not airtight. If the speed of your rotating wheel is not adjustable, you may use an oscillation shaker. If you find your collagen solubilized but full of bubbles, do not try to shake the tube. Instead, leave your tube vertical and at 4 °C for a week or 2 (or longer), and bubbles will slowly but surely migrate toward the surface.
54. This dilution was done to obtain and estimate collagen I concentration of 1 mg/ml based on what was done in **step 7** of Subheading 3.4. Change these volumes if you added a different amount of acetic acid than what was suggested for **step 7**.
55. This approach will allow to: (1) ascertain samples are within the linear range of the assay and (2) average results to even out any potential pipetting inaccuracies.
56. Folin-Ciocalteu reagent is corrosive and can cause damage to the skin and the eyes. Please wear protective gloves, protective clothing, eye and/or face protection.

Acknowledgments

I thank Drs. Roselyne Garnotel, Jean-Claude Monboisse, and George Bellon for teaching me the ropes of collagen biochemistry.

References

1. Nimni ME (1983) Collagen: structure, function, and metabolism in normal and fibrotic tissues. Semin Arthritis Rheum 13(1):1–86. doi:10.1016/0049-0172(83)90024-0
2. Yamauchi M, Sricholpech M (2012) Lysine post-translational modifications of collagen. Essays Biochem 52:113–133. doi:10.1042/bse0520113
3. Balestrini JL, Gard AL, Gerhold KA et al (2016) Comparative biology of decellularized lung matrix: implications of species mismatch in regenerative medicine. Biomaterials 102:220–230. doi:10.1016/j.biomaterials.2016.06.025
4. Piez KA, Eigner EA, Lewis MS (1963) The chromatographic separation and amino acid composition of the subunits of several collagens. Biochemistry 2(1):58–66. doi:10.1021/bi00901a012
5. Eyre DR, Weis M, Hudson DM et al (2011) A novel 3-hydroxyproline (3Hyp)-rich motif marks the triple-helical C terminus of tendon type I collagen. J Biol Chem 286(10):7732–7736. doi:10.1074/jbc.C110.195768
6. Rittié L, Berton A, Monboisse JC et al (1999) Decreased contraction of glycated collagen lattices coincides with impaired matrix metalloproteinase production. Biochem Biophys Res Commun 264(2):488–492. doi:10.1006/bbrc.1999.1519
7. Garnotel R, Rittié L, Poitevin S et al (2000) Human blood monocytes interact with type I collagen through alpha x beta 2 integrin (CD11c-CD18, gp150-95). J Immunol 164(11):5928–5934. doi:10.4049/jimmunol.164.11.5928
8. Monboisse JC, Rittié L, Lamfarraj H et al (2000) In vitro glycoxidation alters the interactions between collagens and human polymorphonuclear leucocytes. Biochem J 350(Pt 3):777–783. doi:10.1042/0264-6021:3500777
9. Chandrakasan G, Torchia DA, Piez KA (1976) Preparation of intact monomeric collagen from rat tail tendon and skin and the structure of the nonhelical ends in solution. J Biol Chem 251(19):6062–6067
10. Vogel KG, Paulsson M, Heinegard D (1984) Specific inhibition of type I and type II colla-

gen fibrillogenesis by the small proteoglycan of tendon. Biochem J 223(3):587–597. doi:10.1042/bj2230587

11. Bell E, Ivarsson B, Merrill C (1979) Production of a tissue-like structure by contraction of collagen lattices by human fibroblasts of different proliferative potential in vitro. Proc Natl Acad Sci U S A 76(3):1274–1278. doi:10.1073/pnas.76.3.1274
12. Rubin AL, Drake MP, Davison PF et al (1965) Effects of pepsin treatment on the interaction properties of tropocollagen macromolecules. Biochemistry 4(2):181–190. doi:10.1021/bi00878a001
13. Woodley DT, Yamauchi M, Wynn KC et al (1991) Collagen telopeptides (cross-linking sites) play a role in collagen gel lattice contraction. J Invest Dermatol 97(3):580–585. doi:10.1111/1523-1747.ep12481920
14. NCBI Collagen alpha-1(I) chain precursor [Rattus norvegicus] – Protein – NCBI. https://www.ncbi.nlm.nih.gov/protein/NP_445756.1. Accessed 7 Dec 2016
15. NCBI Collagen alpha-2(I) chain precursor [Rattus norvegicus] – Protein – NCBI. https://www.ncbi.nlm.nih.gov/protein/NP_445808.1. Accessed 7 Dec 2016
16. Qian J, Okada Y, Ogura T et al (2016) Kinetic analysis of the digestion of bovine type I collagen telopeptides with porcine pepsin. J Food Sci 81(1):C27–C34. doi:10.1111/1750-3841.13179
17. Gross J, Kirk D (1958) The heat precipitation of collagen from neutral salt solutions: some rate-regulating factors. J Biol Chem 233(2):355–360
18. Bai G, Bee JS, Biddlecombe JG et al (2012) Computational fluid dynamics (CFD) insights into agitation stress methods in biopharmaceutical development. Int J Pharm 423(2):264–280. doi:10.1016/j.ijpharm.2011.11.044
19. Komsa-Penkova R, Spirova R, Bechev B (1996) Modification of Lowry's method for collagen concentration measurement. J Biochem Biophys Methods 32(1):33–43. doi:10.1016/0165-022X(95)00046-T
20. Rajan N, Habermehl J, Cote MF et al (2006) Preparation of ready-to-use, storable and reconstituted type I collagen from rat tail tendon for tissue engineering applications. Nat Protoc 1(6):2753–2758. doi:10.1038/nprot.2006.430

Chapter 20

Purification of Human Plasma/Cellular Fibronectin and Fibronectin Fragments

Giampiero Pietrocola, Simonetta Rindi, Giulia Nobile, and Pietro Speziale

Abstract

A method is described for the purification of plasma fibronectins based on a combination of gelatin- and arginine-Sepharose chromatography steps. Cellular fibronectin can be purified from an osteosarcoma fibroblast cell line by affinity chromatography using a monoclonal antibody anti-fibronectin as ligand. Furthermore, we also provide a protocol for the purification of fibronectin domains obtained by fractionation of thermolysin-digested plasma fibronectin on ion-exchange/gel filtration chromatography columns. Assessment of the fibronectin purity is performed by SDS-PAGE, while the ligand binding activities of specific fibronectin domains are determined by ELISA.

Key words Fibronectin, Fibronectin purification, Affinity chromatography, Fibronectin domain, Ion-exchange chromatography, Gel filtration chromatography, SDS-PAGE, ELISA

1 Introduction

Fibronectin (Fn) is a multifunctional glycoprotein found in the extracellular matrix (ECM) and body fluids of higher organisms [1]. In the ECM, Fn plays a critical role in numerous processes such as cell adhesion, cell spreading, migration, growth, and differentiation. Other important functions attributed to Fn include a role in physiological processes such as embryogenesis, wound healing, hemostasis, and thrombosis [2]. Fn exists in two main forms: cellular Fn, which is localized and assembled in a fibrillar matrix in tissues, and soluble Fn synthesized and secreted by hepatocytes and found at 300 μg/ml in human plasma [3].

Human Fn is composed of two polypeptides (α and β chains) with a molecular weight of 220–250 kDa each and joined by two disulfide bonds near the carboxyl termini to form a dimer. The chains are primarily made up of three different repeating modules of <100 amino acids, termed type I, II, and III repeats. In addition, sets of adjacent modules concur to the formation of a variety of discrete globular domains connected by flexible segments (Fig. 1).

Laure Rittié (ed.), *Fibrosis: Methods and Protocols*, Methods in Molecular Biology, vol. 1627, DOI 10.1007/978-1-4939-7113-8_20, © Springer Science+Business Media LLC 2017

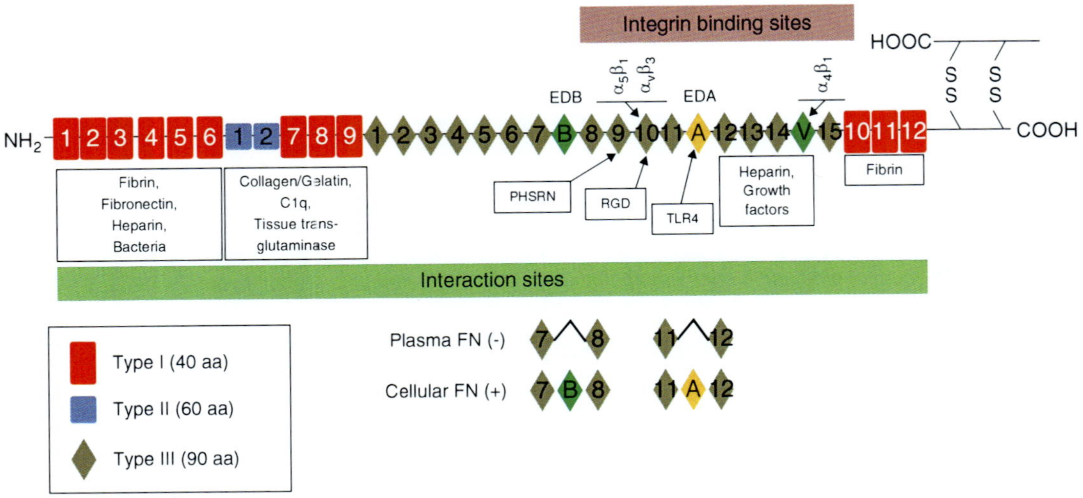

Fig. 1 Schematic representation of fibronectin. The scheme shows a representation of a Fn dimer and its interaction with specific ligands. The different types of homologies (12 type I, two type II, and 15 type III) are also reported. Numbering of type III homologies does not include EDA and EDB subdomains. Type I, II, and III domains are constituted of 40, 60, and 90 amino acids, respectively. Constitutive (RGD) and synergy (PHSRN) sites are indicated, together with their integrin receptors

Partial protease digestion of Fn was used to isolate these globular domains that retain their function and shown to be useful to map the location of major structural features of the protein. The different domains specifically interact with various biological molecules including heparin, fibrin, collagens/gelatin, and glycosaminoglycans of the ECM and integrins on the surface of the cells. Fn also binds to a wide variety of microorganisms, most particularly bacteria. The N-terminal domain (modules I_{1-5}) can be released and isolated as an early fragment of 25–30 kDa by a variety of proteases. It binds among others to heparin, fibrin, and Gram-positive bacteria (*S. aureus* and streptococci) and participates in folding of Fn in matrix assembly and can be cross-linked via factor XIII to collagen and bacteria [2]. Adjacent to the N-terminal domain is the 40–45 kDa glycosylated, intrachain disulfide bond-rich gelatin-binding domain [4]. This domain also binds the collagen-like domain of the complement factor C1q [5]. The region following the gelatin-binding site is made up of 15 constitutive type III repeating units and serves as a natural ligand for several integrins [6].

Alternative spliced type III repeats extra domains A (FnIII EDA) and B (FnIII EDB) are expressed during embryogenesis [7], wound healing [8], and tumor progression [9] and at sites of chronic inflammation such as psoriatic lesions [10]. One of the most interesting functions attributed to FnIII EDA is its ability to act as ligand for the pattern recognition toll-like receptor (TLR) 4 [11] that leads to the activation of NF-kB. Through TLR4 signaling FnIII EDA promotes chronic cutaneous fibrosis in conditions such as scleroderma [12]. A segment connecting two other type

III repeats, called type III connecting segment (IIICS) or variable V region, also exists between the 14th and 15th type III module that contains the binding site for α4β1 integrin [13]. It is present in most cellular fibronectin, but only one of the two subunits in a plasma fibronectin dimer contains a V-region sequence. Modules III_{9-10} correspond to the "cell-binding domain" of Fn. The RGD sequence (Arg-Gly-Asp) located in III_{10} is the site of cell attachment via α5β1 and αVβ3 integrins on the cell surface [6]. Some integrins require a "synergy sequence" (PHSRN, Pro-His-Ser-Asn) in repeat III_9 for maximal interaction of integrins with Fn [14]. This central domain contains also sites for fibrin (III_{10-12}), heparin, and syndecan binding (III_{12-14}). Small fragments (21–37 kDa) comprising three repeats of type I disulfide-bonded loop structure are released from plasma Fn by thermolysin or plasmin and show a fibrin-binding activity [1].

Plasma Fn has been purified through standard methods of protein chemistry including precipitation steps, gel filtration chromatography, and ion-exchange chromatography. These procedures produce reasonably pure Fn, although the yields are relatively low and Fn purified in this way usually contains contaminants. Presently, the most used procedure is based on the gelatin-Sepharose affinity chromatography method developed by Engvall and Ruoslahti [15, 16]. This procedure allows isolation of large quantities of Fn, although several contaminants such as fibrinogen and plasminogen co-elute with the protein. A development of the above strategy includes a combination of gelatin-affinity column with heparin affinity chromatography. With this procedure, Fn is initially purified on gelatin-Sepharose column and then adsorbed on heparin-Sepharose column pre-equilibrated with 4 M urea. The Fn is then eluted from the column by 0.5 M NaCl [17]. In this work, we propose plasma Fn purification protocol based on gelatin-affinity chromatography combined with arginine-affinity chromatography, as previously reported by Vuento and Vaheri [18]. The yield of purified Fn obtained by this method is about 60%. We also report on a rapid analytical method to isolate cellular Fn by immunoaffinity chromatography. Furthermore, we describe a protocol for the purification of Fn domains following digestion of the protein with thermolysin and fractionation on a hydroxyapatite column as described by Zardi et al. [19]. Assays to test the functionality of the purified fragments, based on their ability to recognize appropriate ligands, are also described.

2 Materials

All buffers should be prepared using double distilled and sterile filtered (0.2 μm) water and analytical grade reagents. Prepare and store all concentrated reagents at 4 °C for 2–3 weeks and dilute to 1X before use.

2.1 Preparation of Human Plasma

1. 0.2 M PMSF (phenyl-methyl-sulfonyl fluoride) in 95% (v/v) ethanol. PMSF will be used at a final concentration of 1 mM (1:200 dilution).
2. Citrate phosphate dextrose (CPD) solution (we use the one from Sigma).
3. Human citrated plasma (*see* **Notes 1** and **2**).

2.2 Chromatography Analyses

Different types of chromatography equipment can be used, from automated systems to simpler alternatives such as peristaltic pump connected to an absorbance measuring unit that can follow protein elution and a fraction collector.

2.3 Affinity Columns

1. Glass columns: size: 3 × 7.5 cm; volume:~ 50 ml.
2. Vacuum pump.
3. Sintered glass filter.
4. End-over-end mixer.
5. Ice-cold 1 mM HCl.
6. Ultrafiltration apparatus.
7. Washing solution for gelatin treatment: 3 M NaCl, 10 mM EDTA.
8. Porcine skin gelatin (*see* **Note 3**).
9. 200 mM EDTA stock solution (*see* **Note 4**).
10. L-Arginine.
11. CNBr-activated Sepharose 4B Fast Flow.
12. Coupling buffer: 0.1 M $NaHCO_3$, 0.5 M NaCl, pH to 8.3 with 1 M HCl.
13. 0.2 M glycine solution, pH 8.0.
14. 0.1 M sodium acetate, 0.5 M NaCl, pH 4.
15. Tris buffer saline (TBS): 50 mM Tris/HCl, 0.15 M NaCl, pH 7.4.
16. 95% (v/v) ethanol in ultrapure water (*see* **Note 5**).
17. 0.2% (w/v) sodium azide stock solution in ultrapure water (*see* **Note 6**).
18. Bradford protein assay reagents (we use the BCA kit from Bio-Rad).
19. Anti-plasma Fn mouse monoclonal antibody (we use clone IST-9 from Abcam) (*see* **Note 7**).
20. Cellular Fn eluting buffer: 20 mM CAPS (*N*-cyclohexyl-3-aminopropanesulfonic acid), 0.15 M NaCl, 10 mM EDTA, pH 11.
21. Dialysis tubes, buckets, and beakers.

2.4 Fibroblast Culture

1. Osteosarcoma fibroblasts MG-63 cell line (*see* **Note 8**).
2. Eagle minimum essential medium.
3. Fetal bovine serum.
4. Nonessential L-amino acids.
5. Penicillin.
6. Streptomycin.

2.5 ELISA

1. EIA/RIA microtiter plates.
2. Bovine serum albumin (BSA).
3. Heparin.
4. Porcine gelatin (*see* **Note 3**).
5. Recombinant human $\alpha 5\beta 1$ integrin (we use the one from R&D Systems).
6. Human fibrinogen.
7. Thrombin (purified from human plasma).
8. Immobilization buffer: 50 mM Na_2CO_3, pH 9.5.
9. Phosphate buffer saline (PBS).
10. Washing solution (PBST): PBS containing 0.5% (v/v) Tween 20.
11. Blocking solution: 2% (v/v) bovine serum albumin (BSA) in PBS.
12. *o*-Phenylenediamine dihydrochloride (OPD) solution: mix four tablets with 12 ml of distilled water and 5 μl of 30% hydrogen peroxide (*see* **Note 9**).
13. Anti-human fibrinogen antibody.
14. Anti-human plasminogen antibody.
15. Anti-human Fn antibody.
16. Horseradish peroxidase (HRP)-conjugated secondary antibody (*see* **Note 10**).
17. Stop solution: 0.5 M H_2SO_4.

2.6 Purification of Fn Fragments

1. Thermolysin (protease type X) (we use the one from Sigma).
2. Thermolysin digestion buffer: 25 mM Tris buffer containing 0.5 mM EDTA, 50 mM NaCl, and 2.5 mM $CaCl_2$, pH 7.6.
3. Hydroxyapatite DNA grade Bio-Gel.
4. Gel equilibrating buffer: 0.5 mM sodium phosphate buffer pH 6.8, with 0.1% (w/v) sodium azide.
5. Bio-Gel P-30 (fractionation range: 2,500–40,000 Da).
6. Superdex 75 (fractionation range: 3,000–75,000 Da).
7. Sephadex G-150 Superfine (fractionation range: 4,000–150,000 Da).

2.7 Sodium Dodecyl Sulfate Polyacrylamide Gel Electrophoresis (SDS-PAGE)

1. Electrophoresis unit.
2. Gel casting system.
3. Water bath.
4. Benchtop centrifuge.
5. Reducing loading buffer: 50 mM Tris/HCl, pH 6.8, 20% (v/v) glycerol, 0.1% bromophenol blue, 2% (w/v) sodium dodecyl sulfate (SDS), and 20 mM dithiothreitol (DTT).
6. Running buffer: dissolve 3 g Tris base, 14.04 g glycine, and 1 g SDS in 1 l of distilled water.
7. Coomassie blue staining solution: dissolve 0.4 g Coomassie brilliant blue R250 in 60 ml 2-propanol, 40 ml of glacial acetic acid, and 100 ml distilled water.
8. Protein molecular weight standard (full range, MW 10–250 kDa).
9. Destaining solution: methanol/water/glacial acetic acid (45:45:10, v/v/v) (*see* **Notes 5** and **11**).

3 Methods

3.1 Coupling of Gelatin and Arginine to Sepharose 4B Fast Flow and Preparation and Packing of Affinity Columns

1. Suspend 15 g of freeze-dried powder of CNBr-activated Sepharose 4B Fast Flow in 3 l of 1 mM ice-cold HCl.
2. Wash the slurry on a sintered glass filter with 1 mM HCl for 20 min.
3. Transfer slurry to a beaker and equilibrate with 80–100 ml of coupling buffer.
4. Add 100 ml of gelatin or arginine dissolved in coupling buffer (2–3 mg/ml).
5. Incubate the gel suspension at room temperature in an end-over-end mixer for 2 h.
6. To block remaining reactive groups, centrifuge the mixture at 1,000 *g* for 5 min; resuspend the slurry with a 0.2 M glycine solution, pH 8.0; and incubate for 2 h.
7. Wash the gel with 250 ml coupling buffer followed by 250 ml of 0.1 M sodium acetate buffer, pH 4, containing 0.5 M NaCl (*see* **Note 12**). Repeat this two-step wash for a total of three times to wash away excess of uncoupled ligand in the slurry.
8. Resuspend and equilibrate the slurry in TBS and store at 4 °C until use.
9. To prepare and pack the affinity columns (gelatin- or arginine-Sepharose 4B Fast Flow), allow the slurries in TBS to equilibrate at room temperature for at least 2 h.
10. Degas the suspension under vacuum.

11. Slowly pour the slurry into a column and permit settling of the matrix bed under gravity.
12. Pack the column by running TBS at a flow rate of 2–3 ml/min for at least 60 min.

3.2 Purification of Plasma Fibronectin on Affinity Columns

3.2.1 Gelatin-Sepharose Chromatography

1. Pour 100 ml of cleared plasma through a 50 ml column of gelatin-Sepharose Fast Flow, previously equilibrated with TBS containing 1 mM PMSF and 0.02% (w/v) sodium azide (*see* **Note 13**).
2. *Important*: For each step below, set aside 50–100 μl of sample from each flow through obtained from column washes and elutions for later SDS-PAGE and other analyses.
3. Wash the column with TBS until no material appears in the eluent, as monitored by absorption at 280 nm (*see* **Note 12**) (Fig. 2a).
4. Wash sequentially the slurry with 100 ml of 1 M NaCl and 100 ml of 0.2 M arginine.
5. Elute bound Fn from the column with 1 M arginine.
6. Dialyze pooled fractions against ~5 l of TBS for 48 h at 4 °C.
7. Clarify the above dialyzed solution by centrifugation at 10,000 *g* for 10 min.
8. Collect supernatant and concentrate by ultrafiltration.

3.2.2 Arginine-Sepharose Fast Flow Chromatography

1. Apply the concentrated, clarified material to a column containing 50 ml arginine-Sepharose Fast Flow equilibrated with TBS.
2. Wash the column with 150 ml of TBS.
3. Elute bound Fn with TBS containing 0.3 M NaCl (Fig. 2b).
4. Dialyze Fn at 4 °C against 5 l of TBS.
5. Determine the concentration of purified protein by UV measurement at 280 nm, based on a value of 12.8 for the absorbance of a 1% Fn solution. Alternatively, protein concentration can be determined by BCA protein assay kit, using bovine serum albumin as reference protein.
6. Purified Fn can be aliquoted and stored in polyethylene tubes at 4 °C for several weeks without apparent degradation. For long-term storage, freeze aliquots in containers at −20 °C or colder. To thaw Fn samples, place the containers at room temperature with occasional agitation. Where formation of cryoprecipitates is observed in the Fn solution, it is advisable to subject the Fn solution to centrifugation (10,000 *g* for 10 min).

3.3 Culturing of Human Osteosarcoma Fibroblasts MG-63 Cell Line

Grow MG-63 fibroblast cell line in Eagle minimum essential medium supplemented with 10% heated (56 °C, 30 min) fetal bovine serum, nonessential amino acids, penicillin (200 U/ml), and streptomycin (100 μg/ml) using standard cell culture methods.

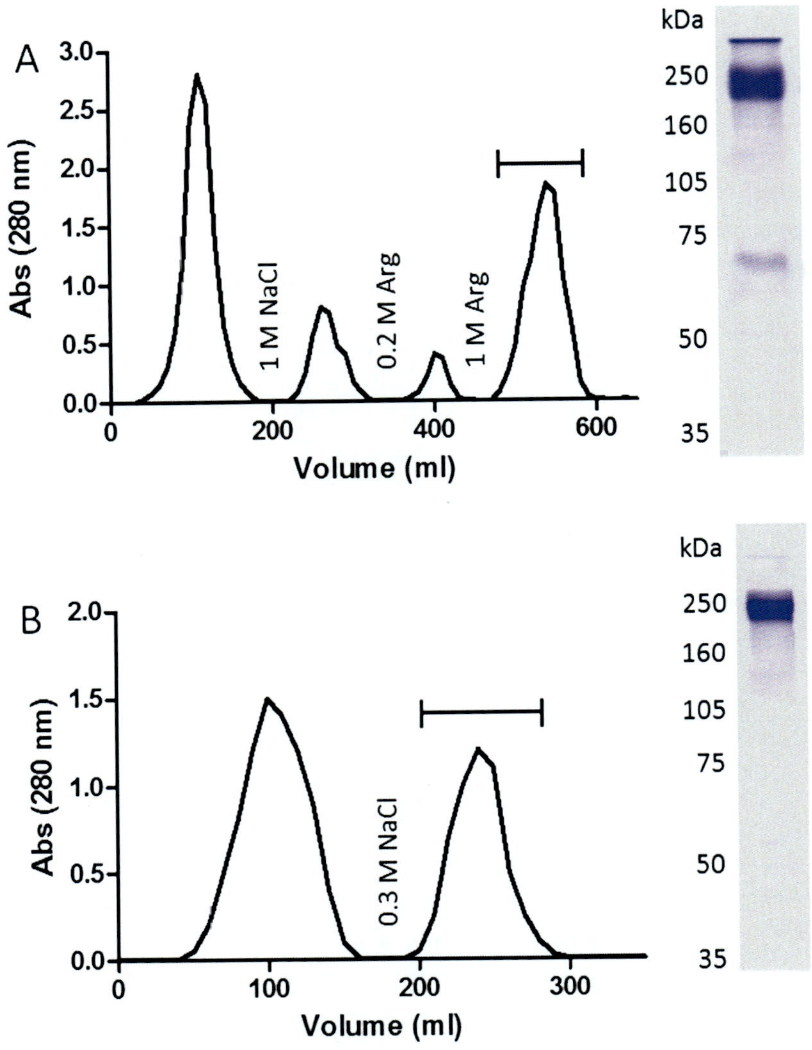

Fig. 2 Purification steps of fibronectin from human plasma. (**a**) Chromatography on gelatin-Sepharose column. Human plasma is loaded on gelatin-Sepharose column. After removing nonspecifically adsorbed proteins to the slurry by washing with equilibrating buffer, the column is sequentially washed with 1 M NaCl and 0.2 M arginine. Fn is eluted from the column with 1 M arginine. (**b**) Affinity chromatography on arginine-Sepharose column. The material obtained from gelatin-Sepharose column is dialyzed and after concentration by ultrafiltration applied to a column of arginine-Sepharose. The column is washed with equilibrating buffer and fibronectin eluted from the gel with 0.3 M NaCl. The pooled fraction are dialyzed and quantitated for protein content. In the *insets*, the 7.5% SDS-PAGE analysis under reducing conditions of Fn eluted with 1 M arginine from gelatin-Sepharose column (**a**) and with 0.3 M NaCl from arginine-Sepharose (**b**) column is reported. On the *left* of each gel, molecular masses (in kDa) of standard proteins are indicated

3.4 Purification of EDA (+) Fn

EDA(+) Fn can be purified on IST-9 mouse monoclonal antibody conjugated to Sepharose 4B Fast Flow from the culture medium of human osteosarcoma fibroblasts MG-63 cell line.

1. Prepare a 1–2 ml column of anti-Fn monoclonal antibody IST-9 coupled to Sepharose 4B.

2. Equilibrate the column with 10 ml TBS containing 1 mM PMSF and 0.02% (w/v) sodium azide.
3. Clear 100 ml of conditioned cultured medium by centrifugation at 5,000 *g* for 5 min.
4. Collect supernatant and pour it onto the equilibrated column.
5. Wash the column with TBS until no material appears in the eluent, as monitored by absorption at 280 nm (*see* **Note 12**).
6. Elute EDA(+) Fn from the affinity column with 10 ml elution buffer.
7. Dialyze against 2 l TBS containing 0.5 mM PMSF at 4 °C for 24 h.
8. Store the dialysate at −20 °C.

3.5 Isolation of Plasma Fn Fragments by Ion-Exchange Chromatography Column

Plasma Fn can be cleaved into five domains [20], and we refer to these discrete domains as N-terminal heparin/fibrin-binding domain-1 (HBD-1/FBD-1), gelatin-binding domain (GBD), cell-binding domain (CBD), heparin-binding domain-2 (HBD-2), and C-terminal fibrin-binding domain-2 (FBD-2).

3.5.1 Digestion of Fibronectin

1. Digest approximately 40 mg of intact fibronectin at 1 mg/ml with 2.5 μg/ml thermolysin at room temperature for 4 h in thermolysin digestion buffer.
2. Add 200 mM EDTA stock solution (to 5 mM final concentration) to terminate the digestion. This treatment inactivates thermolysin [20].

3.5.2 Fractionation of Fibronectin Proteolytic Fragments on Hydroxyapatite Chromatography Column

Fractionation of Fn fragments is performed as previously reported by Zardi et al. [19].

1. Hydrate 20 g of dry powder of Bio-Gel hydroxyapatite with 120 ml of 0.5 mM sodium phosphate buffer, pH 6.8, containing 0.1% (w/v) sodium azide with gentle swirling. Avoid the use of magnetic stir bars or stirring rods, as these will damage the powder.
2. Allow the slurry to settle for 30 min at room temperature.
3. Decant the fine particles present at the top of the settled bed.
4. Degas the suspension under vacuum and pack the gel in a 20 × 1.6 cm glass column.
5. Equilibrate the column with gel equilibrating buffer.
6. Dialyze the total thermolysin Fn digest (~ 40 mg in 40 ml thermolysin digestion buffer) against 4 l of gel equilibrating buffer at 4 °C for 48 h.
7. Load the whole fibronectin thermolysin onto the hydroxyapatite column.

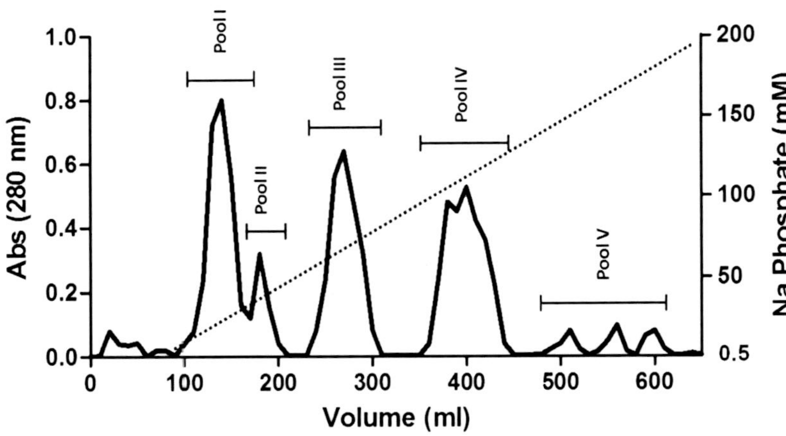

Fig. 3 Elution profile of thermolysin digest of Fn from hydroxyapatite chromatography column. Forty milligrams of Fn subjected to thermolysin digestion and equilibrated with 0.5 mM Na phosphate buffer, pH 6.8, are loaded onto a chromatography column of hydroxyapatite. Fragments of Fn were sequentially eluted with a linear Na phosphate (0.5–200 mM) gradient. Five main peaks are observed in the eluate of hydroxyapatite column, and the pooled fractions were analyzed for molecular weight on a 4–20% SDS-PAGE gradient. The main pooled factions are pool I, 40 kDa; pool II, 20 kDa; pool III, 110 kDa; pool IV, a mixture of 150 + 28 kDa polypeptides; and pool V, 38/30 kDa

8. Wash the column with 60 ml of the above buffer.
9. Elute bound fragments with 600 ml of a linear gradient of 0.5–200 mM sodium phosphate buffer, pH 6.8, at room temperature with a flow rate of 16 ml/h.
10. Check the concentration of the fragments in the eluent buffer by absorbance at 280 nm measurements (Fig. 3).

3.5.3 Purification of Fibronectin Binding Domains by Gel Filtration Chromatography

Each pool obtained from the ion-exchange chromatography of hydroxyapatite can be further fractionated by gel filtration chromatography as follows:

1. Suspend Bio-Gel P-30, Superdex 75, and Sephadex G-150 Superfine slurries in gel equilibration buffer. Fine particles can be removed by decantation.
2. Degas the suspensions under vacuum.
3. Mount 90 × 2 cm columns on a laboratory stand, and pour the well-mixed gel suspension into the vertical mounted column using a glass road. All the gel required should be poured in a single step.
4. Load the individual pools on the appropriate column and elute with the gel equilibration buffer.
5. Pool I (40 kDa, gelatin-binding domain) is purified on Superdex 75 (Fig. 4a).
6. Pool II (20 kDa, fibrin-binding domain) is fractionated on Bio-Gel P30 chromatography column (Fig. 4b).

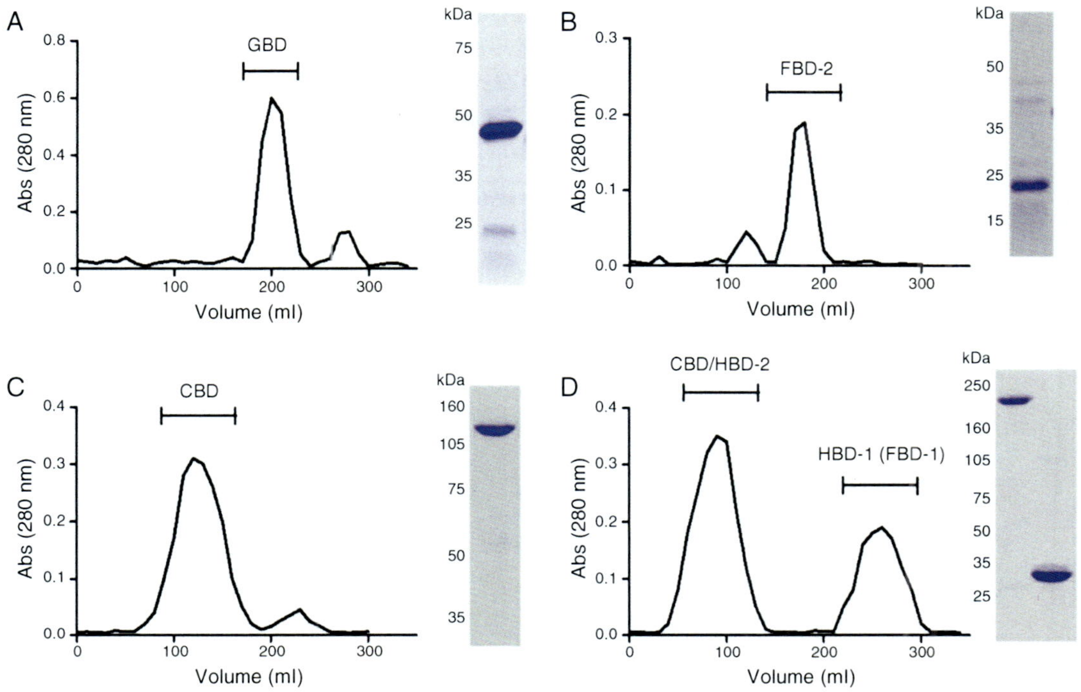

Fig. 4 Purification of fibronectin fragments by gel filtration chromatography. (**a**) Elution profile of hydroxyapatite pool I from a Superdex 75 chromatography column (100 × 2.5 cm). (**b**) Elution profile of hydroxyapatite pool II obtained from a Bio-Gel P30 chromatography column. (**c**) Elution profile of hydroxyapatite pool III resulting from a Sephadex G-150 Superfine chromatography column. (**d**) Elution profile of hydroxyapatite pool IV from a Superdex 75 chromatography column. Pooled fractions obtained by gel filtration chromatography columns were concentrated, analyzed for protein content, and subjected to 10% SDS-PAGE under unreduced conditions (*insets*). Each fragment is also identified by ELISA on the basis of the binding properties for specific ligands (*see* Table 1)

7. Pool III (110 kDa, cell-binding domain) is purified on Sephadex G-150 Superfine chromatography column (Fig. 4c).
8. Pool IV loaded on a Superdex 75 chromatography column separate 150 kDa Cell/hep-2 region from a 29 kDa fragment (Fig. 4d).
9. The heparin-binding domain-2 (HBD-2) (pool V) elutes as a pure polypeptide directly from the hydroxyapatite column and does not need to be further fractionated by gel filtration chromatography.

3.6 Analysis of Fn and Fn Fragments by SDS-PAGE

The purity of all preparations (full-length Fn and Fn fragments) is checked by electrophoresis analysis, using SDS-PAGE.

1. Pour a gel-casting system with a 7.5% (for full length Fn) or 12% (for Fn fragments) acrylamide separating gel and a 4–5% acrylamide stacking gel.

2. Remove the well-forming comb and fill the sample wells with running buffer. Place the gel into the electrophoresis unit and fill the unit with 900 ml of running buffer.
3. Mix 10 μg (at 1 μg/μl) of the appropriate fraction obtained from purification steps with 10 μl reducing loading buffer, and incubate at 99 °C for 3 min in a water bath, and centrifuge for 20 s at 10,000 *g* on a benchtop centrifuge.
4. Load the samples into the wells of the stacking gel within the running buffer.
5. Load 5 μl of molecular weight standard into one lane.
6. Close the tank with its lid, and carry out the electrophoresis at a constant voltage of 100 V for 10 min to allow uniform penetration of the samples in the separating gel.
7. Increase the voltage to 125 V until the dye front reaches the bottom of the gel.
8. Turn off the power; disconnect the cassette from the electrodes.
9. Gently remove the gel from the glass plates and transfer into Coomassie blue stain to visualize protein bands. Stain under gentle agitation for 30 min.
10. Discard the stain and wash 3–4 times with tap water for 10 min each.
11. Destain by immersing gel in 20 ml destaining solution. Maintain gentle agitation until the background staining is reduced and the protein bands appear clear.
12. Transfer gel into tap water for storage.

3.7 ELISA of Purified Fibronectin and Fragments

To validate the absence of trace amounts of fibrinogen and/or plasminogen in the final purified Fn preparation, the arginine-Sepharose purified Fn samples are subjected to ELISA-type assay.

3.7.1 Assessment of Fn Purity

1. Coat microtiter wells with 1 μg/well of isolated Fn in immobilization buffer.
2. Prepare standards in parallel: one "zero" well with immobilization buffer alone and five additional wells with pure Fn (range between 50 and 1,000 ng/well).
3. Incubate the plate overnight at 4 °C.
4. Discard the coating solution by reverting the plate, and wash the plates with 200 μl/well of PBST. Discard the washing solution. Repeat wash for a total of three washes.
5. Block additional protein-binding sites in the wells by treatment of the plates with 200 μl/well of blocking solution for 1 h at room temperature.
6. Discard blocking solution.

7. Incubate the plates for 1 h with 100–200 μl of 5 μg/ml primary anti-Fn, anti-fibrinogen, or anti-plasminogen antibody.
8. Discard antibody and wash the plates three times with PBST.
9. Incubate the plates for 1 h with 100 μl of 1:1000 dilution HRP-conjugated secondary antibody.
10. Discard antibody and wash the plates three times with PBST.
11. Add 100 μl of OPD solution to each well and follow development of yellow color.
12. When a suitable color has developed (~1–5 min), stop the enzymatic reaction by adding 100 μl of stop solution.
13. Quantify the binding of the secondary antibody measuring the absorbance at 490 nm in an ELISA plate reader.
14. Use the standard curve to translate OD value to Fn concentration.

3.7.2 Identification of the Isolated Fn Fragments by Assessment of the Binding Properties

Single isolated pools obtained by the combination of hydroxyapatite chromatography and gel filtration chromatography columns are analyzed for the binding to surface-coated ligands heparin, gelatin, fibrin (*see* **Note 14**), and $\alpha_5\beta_1$ integrin as it follows:

1. Coat microtiter wells with 1 μg/well of the appropriate Fn ligand diluted at 10 μg/ml in immobilization buffer at 4 °C overnight.
2. Wash the plates with 200 μl/well of PBST.
3. Block additional protein-binding sites in the wells by treatment of the plates for 1 h at room temperature with blocking solution.
4. Discard blocking solution.
5. Incubate the plates for 1 h with 1 μg of each isolated Fn fragment (typically in 100 μl).
6. Discard the samples and wash the plates with 200 μl PBST per well.
7. Add 100–200 μl of 5 μg/ml anti-Fn primary antibody in 1% (w/v) BSA to the wells, and incubate for 90 min at room temperature.
8. Wash the plates with PBST.
9. Add 100 μl of 1:1,000 dilution HRP-conjugated secondary antibody, and incubate for 1 h at room temperature.
10. The quantification of the secondary antibody binding to the wells can be determined as reported in **step 13** of Subheading 3.7.1.
11. On the basis of molecular weight determined by SDS-PAGE and the binding properties determined by ELISA (Table 1), a correlation between the isolated pools and the identity of each purified fragment can be established (*see* **Note 15**).

Table 1
Analysis of binding properties of Fn fragments

	Ligand			
Fn fragment	**Heparin**	**Gelatin**	**$\alpha5\beta1$**	**Fibrin**
GBD		+		
CBD			+	
CBD/HBD-2	+		+	
HBD-1 (FBD-1)	+			
FBD-2				+
HBD-2	+			

Microtiter wells are coated overnight at 4 °C for 1 μg of the heparin, gelatin, $\alpha5\beta1$ integrin in 0.1 M sodium carbonate, and pH 9.5. For binding analysis of Fn fragments to fibrin, fibrinogen was immobilized and cleaved with thrombin as reported in **Note 14**. After washing with 0.5% Tween 20 in PBS (PBST), the wells are treated for 1 h at 22 °C with 2% BSA dissolved in PBS. The wells are then incubated with the 1 μg of the appropriate Fn fragment. After several washings with PBST, 1 μg of anti-Fn rabbit IgG in BSA is added to the wells and the mixture incubated for 90 min. After washing, the plates are incubated for 1 h with goat HRP-conjugated anti-rabbit IgG. After washing, o-phenylenediamine dihydrochloride is added to the wells and the absorbance at 490 nm determined using an ELISA plate reader

4 Notes

1. Human blood is potentially hazardous, so treat any sample according to health and safety standards.
2. Human plasma can be obtained by centrifugation of whole blood. The usual starting material for Fn purification is outdated human plasma, although the fresh citrated plasma is better in order to avoid some degree of proteolysis. To prevent Fn degradation, plasma should be stored at −20 °C, and all purification steps have to be carried out at 4 °C. Protease inhibitors such PMSF should be also included during the process of purification, particularly in the early steps of purification when proteases are still present in the crude preparations. It is recommended to use as starting material citrated plasma (15 ml CPD for 100 ml of blood) which has been supplemented with PMSF (add 1/200 of blood volume of 0.2 M stock solution to the plasma with stirring to reach a final PMSF concentration of 1 mM).
3. To prepare and solubilize porcine skin gelatin, wash 100 mg of dry gelatin with several changes of distilled water at 4 °C over a period of 24 h, with occasional shaking and a final centrifugation at 1,000 *g* for 10 min. Then, wash the gelatin for 1 h

with 3 M NaCl solution containing 10 mM EDTA, followed by three washes with distilled water. The protein is finally solubilized in gelatin-dissolving solution and by heating at 65 °C under continuous and vigorous stirring for 1 h. The concentration of the proteins is estimated using a value for absorbance at 235 nm of $E_{1mg/ml} = 0.8$.

4. EDTA is difficult to dissolve when the pH is below 7.0. To ensure an easy dissolution, mix 29.22 g of EDTA and 12.5 g of NaOH pellets in 500 ml of deionized water, which yield a 200 mM solution, pH 7.8.
5. Ethanol, methanol, and propanol are highly flammable. Store and handle according to appropriate health and safety requirements
6. Sodium azide (NaN_3) is very toxic. If contact with skin occurs, wash immediately with tap water. The stock solution (0.2%, w/v) should be prepared under ventilated hood.
7. Anti-Fn antibody IST-9 is a monoclonal antibody raised against a region in the EDA domain of human cellular fibronectin.
8. It is important to ascertain the origin and health of the cell line. Purchasing a new vial at a cell culture depository (such as the American Tissue Culture Collection (ATCC)) and keeping track of passages will ensure good cell culture practices.
9. OPD tablets are light sensitive. Store the vial containing the tablets at 4 °C protected from light with the lid tightly closed.
10. Repeated freezing and thawing of antibody solutions reduces the activity of the proteins. Thawed solutions that are not completely used can be kept at 4 °C for several weeks.
11. Glacial acetic acid is strongly corrosive and may cause severe burns. Ensure safety glass or face mask and nitrile gloves are worn.
12. To wash the gel, resuspend in appropriate buffer, homogenize, and centrifuge at 1,000 *g* for 5 min.
13. Due to the tendency of gelatin-Sepharose column to gel in the cold, it is advisable that this step is performed at room temperature.
14. To analyze the binding of purified fragments to immobilized fibrin, microtiter 96-well plates are coated with 100 μl of 0.34 g/l fibrinogen for 1 h at room temperature. Fibrin clot in the wells is generated by adding 0.05 U/ml thrombin in 20 mM Tris–HCl, pH 7.4, 150 mM NaCl, and 5 mM $CaCl_2$ overnight at room temperature.
15. The identification of the isolated domains can be also achieved assessing the immunological reactivity of each fragment for specific monoclonal or polyclonal antibodies, where available, by ELISA-type assay.

Acknowledgments

This work was supported in part by Fondazione CARIPLO Grant Vaccines 2009-3546 to P.S.

References

1. Hynes RO (1990) Structure of Fibronectins. In: Fibronectins. Springer, New York, NY, pp 113–175. doi:10.1007/978-1-4612-3264-3_6
2. Henderson B, Nair S, Pallas J et al (2011) Fibronectin: a multidomain host adhesin targeted by bacterial fibronectin-binding proteins. FEMS Microbiol Rev 35(1):147–200. doi:10.1111/j.1574-6976.2010.00243.x
3. Tamkun JW, Hynes RO (1983) Plasma fibronectin is synthesized and secreted by hepatocytes. J Biol Chem 258(7):4641–4647
4. Katagiri Y, Brew SA, Ingham KC (2003) All six modules of the gelatin-binding domain of fibronectin are required for full affinity. J Biol Chem 278(14):11897–11902. doi:10.1074/jbc.M212512200
5. Carsons SE, Schwartzman S, Diamond HS et al (1988) Interaction between fibronectin and C1q in rheumatoid synovial fluid and normal plasma. Clin Exp Immunol 72(1):37–42
6. Leiss M, Beckmann K, Giros A et al (2008) The role of integrin binding sites in fibronectin matrix assembly in vivo. Curr Opin Cell Biol 20(5):502–507. doi:10.1016/j.ceb.2008.06.001
7. Ffrench-Constant C, Hynes RO (1989) Alternative splicing of fibronectin is temporally and spatially regulated in the chicken embryo. Development 106(2):375–388
8. Jarnagin WR, Rockey DC, Koteliansky VE et al (1994) Expression of variant fibronectins in wound healing: cellular source and biological activity of the EIIIA segment in rat hepatic fibrogenesis. J Cell Biol 127(6 Pt 2):2037–2048. doi:10.1083/jcb.127.6.2037
9. Rybak JN, Roesli C, Kaspar M et al (2007) The extra-domain A of fibronectin is a vascular marker of solid tumors and metastases. Cancer Res67(22):10948–10957.doi:10.1158/0008-5472.CAN-07-1436
10. McFadden JP, Baker BS, Powles AV et al (2010) Psoriasis and extra domain A fibronectin loops. Br J Dermatol 163(1):5–11. doi:10.1111/j.1365-2133.2010.09737.x
11. Okamura Y, Watari M, Jerud ES et al (2001) The extra domain A of fibronectin activates Toll-like receptor 4. J Biol Chem 276(13):10229–10233. doi:10.1074/jbc.M100099200
12. Bhattacharyya S, Tamaki Z, Wang W et al (2014) Fibronectin EDA promotes chronic cutaneous fibrosis through Toll-like receptor signaling. Sci Transl Med 6(232):232ra250. doi:10.1126/scitranslmed.3008264
13. Mostafavi-Pour Z, Askari JA, Whittard JD et al (2001) Identification of a novel heparin-binding site in the alternatively spliced IIICS region of fibronectin: roles of integrins and proteoglycans in cell adhesion to fibronectin splice variants. Matrix Biol 20(1):63–73. doi:10.1016/S0945-053X(00)00131-1
14. Redick SD, Settles DL, Briscoe G et al (2000) Defining fibronectin's cell adhesion synergy site by site-directed mutagenesis. J Cell Biol 149(2):521–527. doi:10.1083/jcb.149.2.521
15. Engvall E, Ruoslahti E (1977) Binding of soluble form of fibroblast surface protein, fibronectin, to collagen. Int J Cancer 20(1):1–5. doi:10.1002/ijc.2910200102
16. Ruoslahti E, Hayman EG, Pierschbacher M et al (1982) Fibronectin: purification, immunochemical properties, and biological activities. Methods Enzymol 82(Pt A):803–831. doi:10.1016/0076-6879(82)82103-4
17. Hynes RO (1990) Methods for identification of fibronectins. In: Fibronectins. Springer, New York, NY, pp 7–23. doi:10.1007/978-1-4612-3264-3_2
18. Vuento M, Vaheri A (1979) Purification of fibronectin from human plasma by affinity chromatography under non-denaturing conditions. Biochem J 183(2):331–337. doi:10.1042/bj1830331
19. Zardi L, Carnemolla B, Balza E et al (1985) Elution of fibronectin proteolytic fragments from a hydroxyapatite chromatography column. A simple procedure for the purification of fibronectin domains. Eur J Biochem 146(3):571–579. doi:10.1111/j.1432-1033.1985.tb08690.x
20. Sekiguchi K, Fukuda M, Hakomori S (1981) Domain structure of hamster plasma fibronectin. Isolation and characterization of four functionally distinct domains and their unequal distribution between two subunit polypeptides. J Biol Chem 256(12):6452–6462

Chapter 21

Laser Capture Microdissection of Tissue Sections for High-Throughput RNA Analysis

Julia Hoffmann, Jochen Wilhelm, and Grazyna Kwapiszewska

Abstract

The heterogeneous nature of most human organs and tissues represents a common challenge when analyzing specific structures or cells. Laser capture microdissection (LCM) enables isolation of pure cells from a mixed population of cells or tissue samples via usage of laser energy. Combined with high-throughput gene or protein techniques, compartment specific analysis elucidating the role of specialized cell types in physiological or pathophysiological activity can be performed. This chapter describes the crucial steps that have to be taken into consideration when designing and conducting a LCM project. Detailed protocols describing the workflow from project planning to high-throughput analysis of LCM material used in our laboratory are provided. Routinely occurring challenges and appropriate solutions, e.g., when working with fibrotic tissue are described.

Key words Laser capture microdissection, RNA extraction, Preamplification, Microarray analyses

1 Introduction

In response to pathological stimuli, altered properties of each cell type in any given tissue may be unique and relevant to disease progression. The heterogeneous nature of most tissue samples containing a multitude of diverse cell populations results in imprecise findings when analyzing homogenates. A clean molecular signature of a disease-related specific cell type can be masked or even be lost. Increased specificity and sensitivity of cell-specific molecular profiling from tissue sections can be achieved by applying laser capture microdissection (LCM). It presents a simple, fast, flexible, and reliable method to investigate specific cell populations or regions within tissue samples. Via laser energy, the region of interest can be excised [1]. LCM material can then be subjected to various analyses such as real-time PCR [2, 3], microarrays [4, 5], or protein analysis [6–8] (Fig. 1).

The LCM procedure itself and analysis of microdissected material can be challenging. The amounts of isolated nucleic acids and

Laure Rittié (ed.), *Fibrosis: Methods and Protocols*, Methods in Molecular Biology, vol. 1627,
DOI 10.1007/978-1-4939-7113-8_21, © Springer Science+Business Media LLC 2017

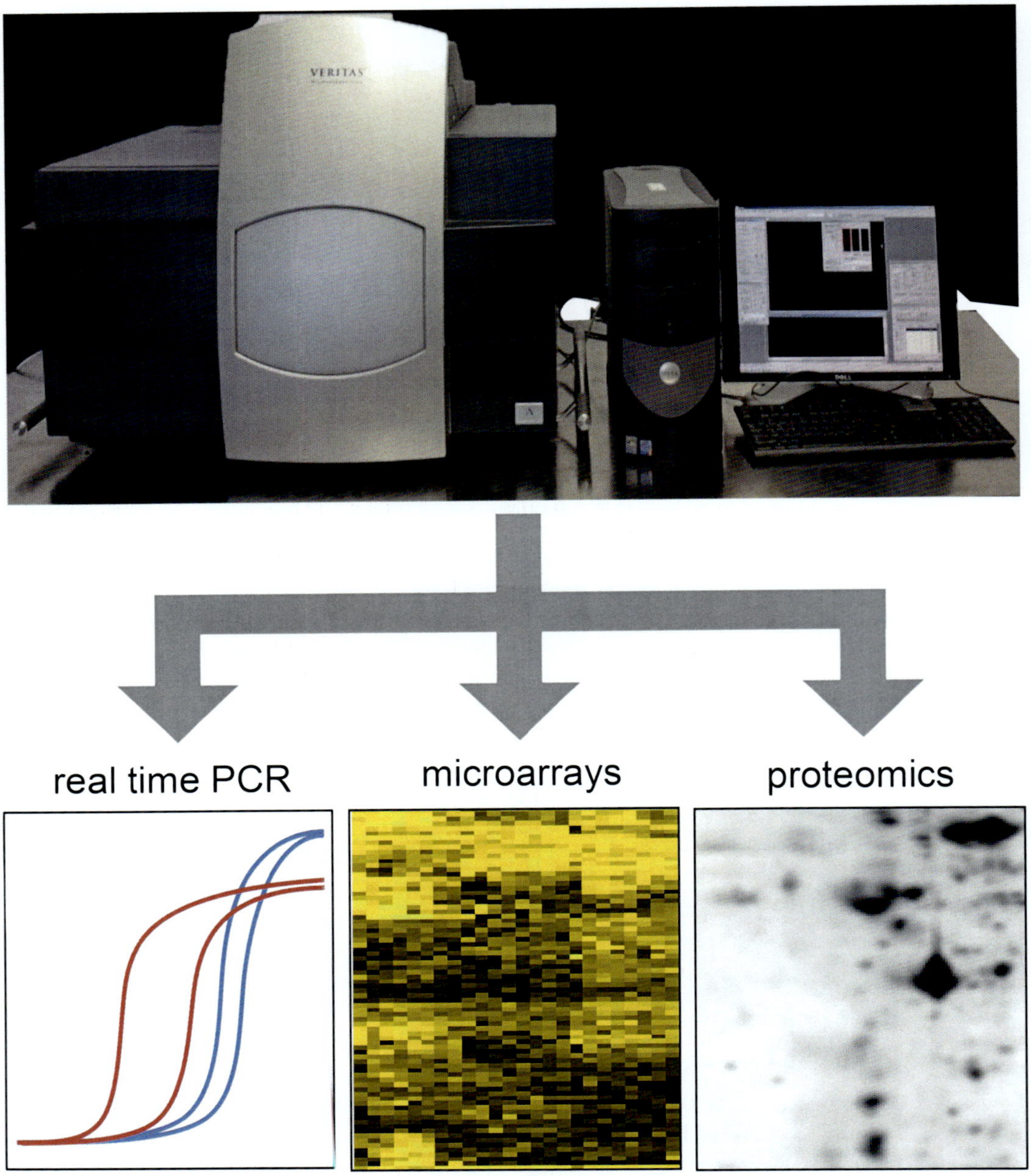

Fig. 1 Setup of the Arcturus Veritas™ combined IR/UV LCM system. LCM material can be subjected to several subsequent analyses such as real-time PCR, microarrays, or proteomics

proteins are very small, and the quality is far from optimal. Both problems limit the sensitivity and the precision of quantitative analyses. For instance, the RNA degradation has a pronounced impact on quantitative analyses [9–11]. This led to the suggestion that only high-quality RNA should be used, especially for microarray studies, to get meaningful and reliable results. However, it is usually impossible to acquire high-quality RNA from LCM samples, and the only chance to get some insights is to analyze such samples despite their limited quality. However, the problem is not as severe as often promoted. When comparisons are made only between samples of similar (suboptimal) quality, it can be shown that the analysis of low-quality RNA in microarray studies can reveal biologically relevant information [12].

The application of formalin-fixed, paraffin-embedded (FFPE) material can be particularly challenging. The fixation process causes cross-linkage between nucleic acids and proteins and covalently modifies RNA by the addition of monomethyl groups to the bases. As a result, the molecules are rigid and susceptible to mechanical shearing, and the cross-links may compromise the use of RNA as a substrate for reverse transcription. Formalin residuals inhibit enzyme activity during extraction, enzymatic amplification, and labeling reactions. Degradation and fragmentation of RNA molecules may further impede getting sufficient amounts of quantifiable molecules. Preparation of the samples requires additional de-paraffinization and de-fixation steps and thus takes a longer time and is more laborious as compared to the preparation of cryo-material.

The present chapter describes key practical aspects of tissue handling and sample preparation for LCM and subsequent applications utilizing the LCM material. A focus is placed on the workflow executed in our laboratory. Figure 2 depicts the crucial steps as well as common pitfalls of this workflow.

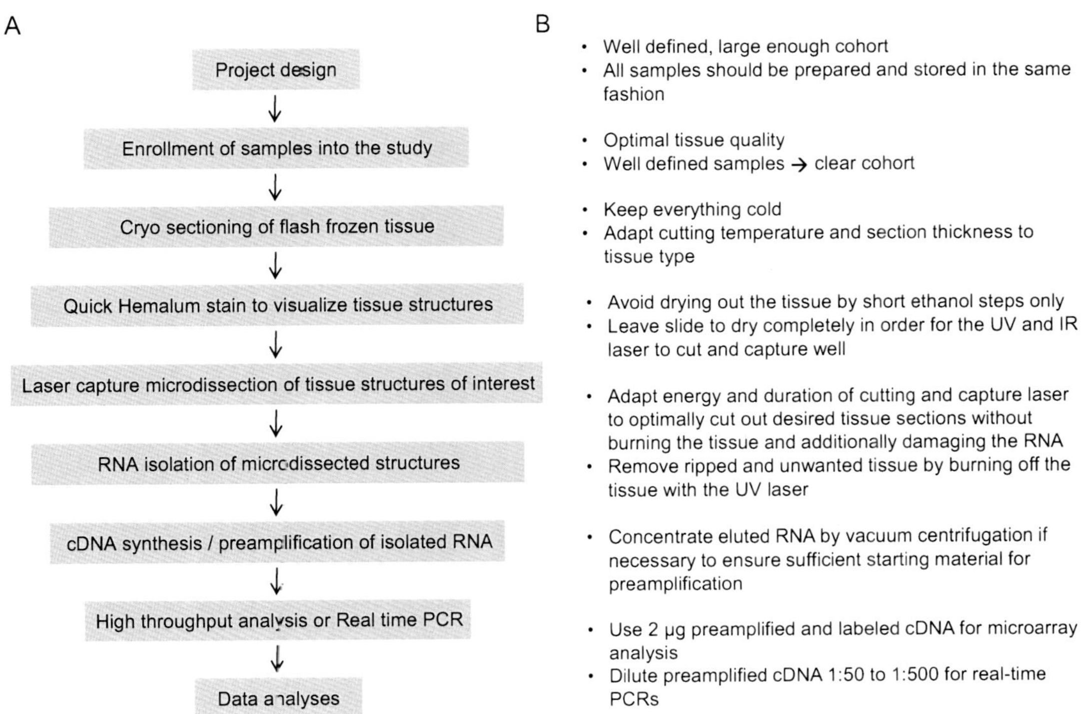

Fig. 2 (**a**) Workflow of laser capture microdissection (LCM) from tissue sections; (**b**) CAVE for single steps in workflow

2 Materials

2.1 Instruments

1. Pipettes.
2. Centrifuges.
3. Vortexers.
4. LCM system (we use Arcturus Veritas™ combined IR/UV, Thermo Fisher Scientific) (*see* **Note 1**).
5. Real-time PCR system.
6. Three Dri-block heaters (e.g., PN 022031, Kisker Biotech).
7. PCR instrument (LifeTouch, Biozym Scientific).
8. UV/VIS nano-spectrophotometer (such as NanoDrop®).
9. Agilent hybridization chambers.
10. Microscopic slide staining dishes.
11. Two hybridization ovens (one with rotisserie).
12. Magnetic stirrer.
13. Microarray scanner (such as InnoScan is900, Innopsys).

2.2 Tissue Sectioning, Staining, and LCM

1. Cryo-microtome and disposable microtome blades.
2. PEN membrane-based laser microdissection slides (Leica Microsystems Cat# 11505158).
3. Optimal cutting temperature (OCT) compound, clear (such as Tissue-Plus®, Cryomatrix).
4. Small paint brush.
5. Glass cuvettes or any other system for staining.
6. Mayer hemalum.
7. Absolute ethanol (≥99.8% p.a).
8. Ethanol 70% and ethanol 50% (dilute absolute ethanol with RNase-free water in suitable RNase-free glass staining dishes under the hood).
9. Arcturus CapSure Macro LCM Caps (Cat# LCM0211, Thermo Fisher Scientific).
10. Liquid nitrogen and −80 °C storage.

2.3 RNA Isolation, RT-PCR, and Real-Time PCR

1. RNeasy Micro Kit (Qiagen) for frozen tissues or RNeasy FFPE Kit (Qiagen) for FFPE tissues.
2. RNase decontamination solution (e.g., RNaseZap® Wipes and Spray, Ambion).
3. Nuclease-free water.

4. Reverse transcriptase cDNA synthesis kit [e.g., iScript (Bio-Rad Laboratories) or Ovation PicoSL WTA System V2 (NuGEN Technologies)].
5. Real-time SYBR Green PCR Kit [e.g., QuantiFast SYBR PCR Kit (Qiagen) or SYBR® Green PCR Master Mix (ABI)].

2.4 Microarray

1. PCR purification kit (e.g., QIAquick, Qiagen).
2. DNA labeling kit (e.g., SureTag, Agilent Technologies).
3. SurePrint G3 8 × 60K Microarrays (Agilent Technologies).
4. Hybridization backings for eight microarrays per slide (PN G2534, Agilent Technologies).
5. One-Color RNA Spike-in Kit (Agilent Technologies).
6. Hi-RPM Gene Expression Hybridization Kit (Agilent Technologies).
7. Gene Expression Wash Buffer Kit (Agilent Technologies).
8. Stabilization and Drying Solutions (Agilent Technologies).

3 Methods

The following steps describe how crucial processes are performed in our laboratory. Alternatives to our procedures are possible, partly provided (mostly as notes) and briefly discussed.

3.1 Project Design

Irrespective of the subsequent analysis that will be applied to the LCM samples, care has to be taken that samples in the comparison groups (e.g., fibrotic samples to non-fibrotic samples) are not systematically different in any way except in the experimental factor (e.g., the presence of fibrotic structures). This includes preparation, processing, and measurement of the samples. Importantly, if the samples are prepared or processed in batches, the batches should always contain samples from all groups. Otherwise, differences that will be identified between groups cannot be unambiguously attributed to a group-specific difference.

When using commercially available microarrays, it is better to use as many biological replicates as possible and not technical replicates. In other words, there is usually no need for mere technical replications when using commercially available microarrays, as the correlation of technical replicates is much higher than the correlation between different biological samples. Hence, the available resources on microarray hybridizations should be used with as many biological replicates as possible.

Human microdissected material is very heterogeneous and one of the most difficult materials to generate reliable conclusions from screening experiments. The required sample size depends on the variability of the samples as well as on the expected sizes of the effects that should be investigated. As a rule of thumb, in an optimal case, a sample size of at least $n = 16$ per group should usually be sufficient. It will likely produce confidence intervals of the log fold changes with a width smaller than 3 (±1.5). On the scale of the fold changes, these intervals range from 35 to 280% of the mean estimate. If interactions should be analyzed, a minimum of $n = 32$ samples per group should be considered to get a similar precision for the interaction estimates. However, in most cases, much lower numbers of samples are assigned to sample groups due to difficult access to samples, large costs, and time-consuming technology of LCM. To our experience, if the samples are well characterized and of good quality, $n = 8$ per group might be sufficient for subsequent analyses [5]. However, it should be considered to estimate the sample variability in preliminary experiments and use this information for a more rigorous sample size calculation.

3.2 Tissue Preparation

3.2.1 Collection and Storage

1. Prepare and snap freeze tissue samples in liquid nitrogen directly upon receiving tissue biopsies or transplant tissue (*see* **Note 2**).
2. Transfer tissue into a cryo-vial. The size of the tissue for LCM procedure should not be larger than the cryo-vial (the sample should not be squeezed into cryo-vial).
3. Store samples at −80 °C until use (*see* **Note 3**).

3.2.2 Sectioning

1. Thoroughly clean the working space with RNase inhibitors. All tools should be clean, and gloves should be worn all the time as skin is a potent source of RNases. Additionally, care should be taken not to subject the cryo-frozen sample to room temperature longer than necessary in order to preserve RNA quality.
2. Set temperature of the microtome-cryostat, knife holder, and specimen to −20 °C (*see* **Note 4**).
3. Clean the knife holder with absolute ethanol.
4. Deposit samples and brushes in the microtome-cryostat.
5. Wait at least 5 min for the sample to equilibrate with the temperature of the cryostat.
6. Mount the samples to the metal specimen holder with Tissue-Plus® compound, orientate, and fixate them according to region of interest (*see* **Note 5**).
7. Trim Tissue-Plus® from the block until tissue becomes visible using a clean blade. For cuts that will be utilized for LCM, set cutting thickness to 10 μm (*see* **Note 6**).
8. To prevent tissue folding or curling, use a small clean brush to straighten out the sections.

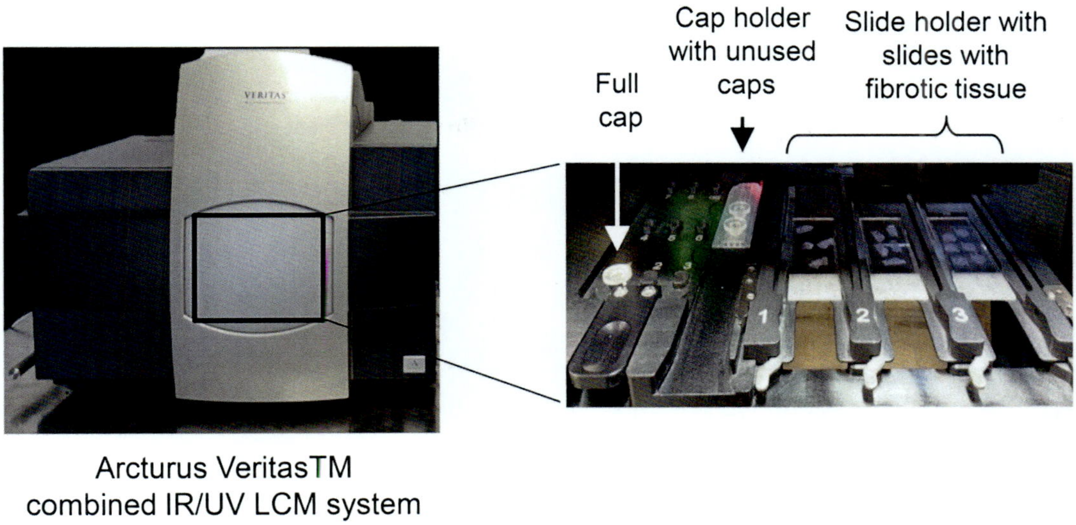

Fig. 3 Image of the Arcturus Veritas™ combined IR/UV LCM system with zoomed interior. Cap and slide holders are presented

9. Place cut sections on room temperature PEN membrane-based laser microdissection slides, making sure that Tissue-Plus® and adjacent tissue do not overlap.

3.3 Staining

1. Stain slide with hemalum stain for 30 s (*see* **Note 7**).
2. Wash slide with nuclease-free water.
3. Wash slide with 50% ethanol for 5 s.
4. Wash slide with 70% ethanol for 5 s.
5. Wash slide with absolute ethanol for 5 s.
6. Allow slide to air dry (approx. 5 min).
7. Continue directly with LCM.

3.4 LCM

1. Place slides in designated slide holders in the Arcturus Veritas™ instrument (Fig. 3).
2. Place Arcturus CapSure® Macro LCM Caps in the appropriate cap holders.
3. Locate the area of interest.
4. Cut the area of interest with UV laser.
5. Place a CapSure® LCM Cap over the target area. Pulsing the laser through the cap causes the thermoplastic film to form a thin protrusion that bridges the gap between the cap and tissue and adheres to the target cell. Lifting of the cap removes the target cell(s) now attached to the cap. The isolated cells are now available for extraction of biomolecules (*see* **Note 8**).

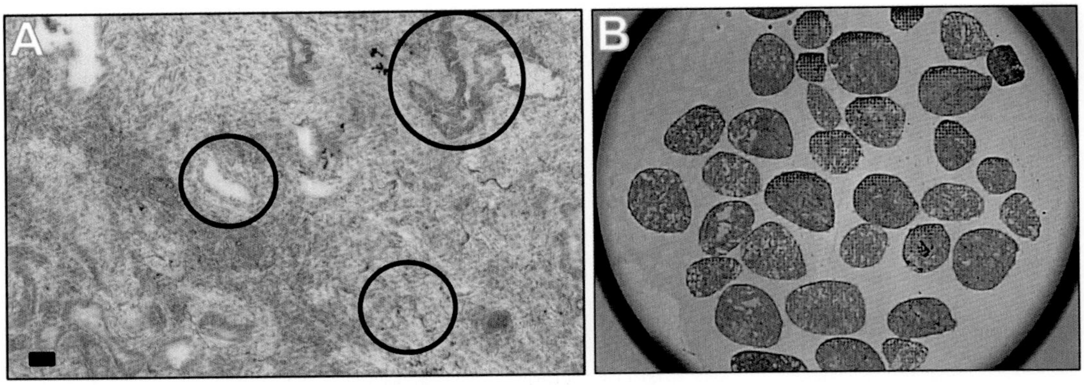

Fig. 4 General example of LCM. (**a**) Fibrotic flash-frozen, cryo-cut, and hemalum-stained lung tissue, selected structures for LCM, scale bar: 50 μm; (**b**) dissected structures on the cap

6. The IR laser activates the transfer film on a cap placed on the tissue sample, adhering the film to the underlying cells of choice. The cells of interest are then lifted away from the tissue section, leaving all unwanted cells behind and providing a pure population for cell-specific molecular analysis (*see* **Note 9**).
7. In order to retrieve sufficient amounts of RNA, the cap should be at least 50–80% covered with compartment/cells of choice. Exemplary images are provided in Figs. 4 and 6.
8. After finishing microdissection, dissolve the dissected areas on the membrane cap into lysis buffer provided by the RNeasy Micro Kit by capping and inverting the tube. The amount of lysis buffer is dependent on collection vessel used for microdissection and the amount of expected RNA (*see* **Note 10**).
9. Flash freeze the RNA immediately in liquid nitrogen and store at −80 °C.

3.5 RNA Isolation

As RNA is highly susceptible to degradation by RNases in the environment, several precautions should be taken. All equipment, laboratory benches, pipette tips, tubes, reagents, and other consumables must be RNase-free. Gloves should be worn at all times and changed frequently. Material should be processed quickly, and care should be taken to avoid contamination during tissue collection, processing, RNA isolation, and following applications. Well-purified RNA is relatively stable and can be stored for months at −80 °C or in liquid nitrogen without a relevant loss of quality.

3.5.1 RNA Isolation from LCM Frozen Tissue

1. Use the RNeasy Micro Kit and follow the manufacturer's instructions.
2. Elute RNA in minimum amount of buffer (*see* **Note 11**).
3. RNA quantity (small number of cells) and quality (degradation) from LCM samples are difficult to be measured as com-

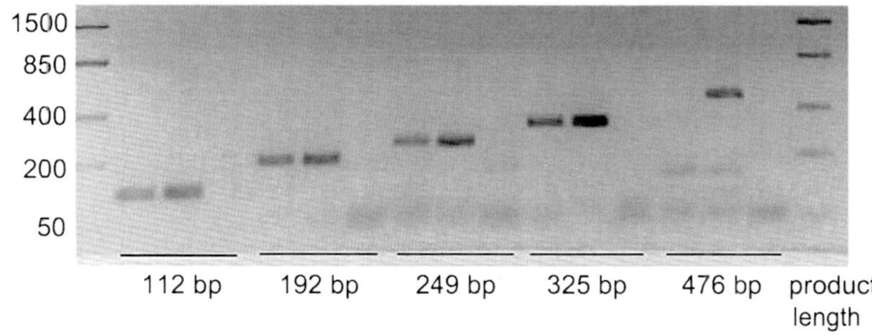

Fig. 5 RNA integrity test; LCM samples are checked for quality and quantity via real-time PCR and subsequent gel analysis; primer pairs resulting in different product lengths are designed and applied; *bp* base pairs; for every product length, two samples and one non-template (NT) control are displayed

monly used RNA quantification techniques might be too insensitive and unreliable. Recently, new methods have been developed to determine concentrations from small amount of the material such as Qubit® 3.0 Fluorometer (Thermo Fisher) or Agilent RNA 6000 Pico Kit (Agilent). However, also without special equipment, the RNA quantity and integrity can be estimated by running a real-time PCR with PCR primers producing products of different lengths. The amplification of long products indicates intact RNA and therefore indirectly reflects RNA quantity (Fig. 5).

3.5.2 RNA Isolation from LCM FFPE Tissue

Use the RNeasy FFPE Kit and follow the kit instructions. Afterward, the steps for frozen and FPPE material are the same.

3.6 Real-Time PCR

We generally use SYBR Green I for the signal generation during real-time PCR and perform relative quantifications using the expression of "reference genes" as internal calibrator (loading control). Any available real-time PCR system can be used, and the described protocol should work with all instruments.

3.6.1 cDNA Synthesis for Real-Time PCR

For real-time PCR analysis, several commercially available kits can be used. The kit we use (iScript) generates sufficient amounts of cDNA from LCM material to perform several real-time PCRs. Although preamplification of cDNA is not obligatory for real-time PCR, preamplified material can be used as well. The RNA can be preamplified with the SPIA protocol described for the microarrays (*see* Subheading 3.7.1). For use in real-time PCR, the amplified dscDNA should be diluted (depending concentration from 1:50 to 1:500). Application of preamplified material allows investigating more genes of interest (GOI) than classical cDNA synthesis protocol.

3.6.2 Real-Time PCR Primer Validation

Valid real-time PCR results will be obtained only when the primer systems are well optimized. It should be confirmed in assay validation experiments that the amplification efficiency of all primers is close to 100% and that no unspecific products are amplified. The reference genes should be selected as genes that are expressed in the selected tissue or cell types and supposedly not differentially expressed between the conditions that shall be compared (*see* **Note 12**). As RNA quality and quantity are low in LCM samples, primers generating a small PCR product, e.g., lower 100 bp, should be applied. Also, highly expressed genes are more suitable. In our workflow, beta-2 microglobulin is a reliable reference gene (*see* **Note 12**). Remember to use respective negative controls such as no reverse transcription control and no cDNA control.

3.6.3 Cycling Conditions for Real-Time PCR

1. Set up PCR reactions using QuantiFast SYBR PCR Kit and follow the kit instructions (handbook for QuantiFast SYBR Green PCR, Qiagen). We recommend performing duplicate reactions per sample.
2. Try to place all PCRs from diverse samples on the same plate when you want to compare the difference between the groups. If possible, try not to measure some genes of a sample on one plate and other genes on another plate.
3. Cycling conditions used are as follows: 5 min 95 °C [5 s 95 °C, 5 s 60 °C, 10 s 72 °C] × 45. A final melting curve analysis can be made to check for contaminations and specific amplification.

3.6.4 Analysis of Real-Time PCR Data

1. Check the amplification curves. Do not consider Ct values for quantification from curves that show an uncommon pattern or that have a different slope in the log linear phase. You can set the threshold specific for each gene. Do not use Ct values from samples with differences from replicate PCRs greater than 0.5 cycles.
2. Average the Ct values of the replicate PCRs, and average the Ct values of all reference genes (ref) for each sample. The resulting averaged Ct values will be denoted as $Ct_{(ref)}$.
3. Calculate the normalized ΔCt value as normalized measure for the expression of the gene of interest as $\Delta Ct = Ct_{(ref)} - Ct_{(GOI)}$ (*see* **Note 13**). Calculated this way, higher ΔCt values indicate a higher (normalized) expression of the gene of interest.

3.7 Microarrays

Several microarray platforms from different companies are available on the market (Affymetrix, Exiqon, Agilent, etc.). The following protocol will describe the workflow we used for Agilent platform together with the InnoScan 900 scanner. Our protocol is optimized for relatively low amounts of samples/hybridizations and allows the processing of up to 32 samples in parallel. If more samples need to be processed on a regular basis, we recommend using a pipetting robot system and the Agilent scanner system.

Some microarray slides, e.g., from Agilent, contain several arrays spotted on one slide. These arrays are processed in parallel. In this case, a single slide should be seen as a "batch of hybridizations," and one should make sure to distribute samples from all groups on all slides to avoid systematic batch effects between experimental groups. It is therefore advisable to first collect all samples and start any further processing when all samples are available.

3.7.1 Generation and Amplification of dscDNA for Microarray

RNA preamplification is required prior to microarray analysis. Depending on the starting amount of RNA, several methods and kits can be used. Arcturus RiboAmp for in vitro transcription (IVT) and Ovation Kits from NuGEN are the most commonly used. The NuGEN kit Ovation PicoSL WTA System V2 is used in our workflow [13]. The kit includes reagents for cDNA synthesis, second-strand synthesis, and amplification of dscDNA based on the Ribo-SPIA technology (single-primer isothermal amplification using RNA/DNA hybrid primers and pol-II DNA polymerase). This kit allows the reliable amplification of 0.5–50 ng total RNA yielding sufficient amounts of dscDNA for microarray hybridizations.

1. Utilize the Ovation PicoSL WTA System V2 and follow the kit instructions (user guide PN 3312).
2. Add a no template (NT, no RNA) control.
3. Perform purification of SPIA dscDNA using the QIAquick PCR Purification Kit according to the kit instructions (step H).
4. Measure product yield (OD_{260}) and purity (OD_{260}/OD_{280}) using 1 μl cDNA (*see* **Note 14**).

3.7.2 Fluorescence Labeling

The dscDNA obtained in the previous section will next be fluorescently labeled using the SureTag DNA labeling kit. You can use either Cy3 or Cy5 as fluorescent dye (*see* **Note 15**).

The Agilent labeling and hybridization protocols include the use of spike-in controls. These controls may be useful as positive controls and to calibrate signal intensities between slides and experiments, but they are not essential. Valid relative quantifications are possible without spike-in controls, so you can consider omitting preparation and use of these controls (then just add water instead of the prepared spike-in RNAs, or use the additional volume to add a higher volume of sample).

1. Use 2 μg of the purified dscDNA as sample and follow the kit instructions.
2. Determine the quantity of the labeled material and the dye incorporation according to the kit instructions. Expected yields and incorporation rates are provided in the manual.

3.7.3 Hybridization, Washing, Scanning, and Gridding

Hybridization to Agilent whole genome microarrays is carried out as described in the Agilent hybridization protocol, with slight modifications. Although dual-color hybridizations are possible, we recommend single-color hybridizations on high-density arrays (e.g., 8 × 60K).

1. Use 2 μg of the labeled dscDNA for hybridization.
2. Mix the hybridization solution according to the Agilent user manual for dual- or single-color hybridizations (e.g., PN G4140-90040 [14], following Chapter 2 [Procedures]: Hybridization) without fragmentation step; add water instead of fragmentation buffer.
3. Omit the 30 min incubation at 60 °C and pipet the "fragmentation mix" directly into the hybridization buffer.
4. Hybridize and wash the slides according to the Agilent user manual. Be aware that the dyes are degraded by ozone (*see* **Note 16**).
5. Scan the slides. The Agilent user manual describes the procedure for the Agilent scanner and its extraction software. Follow the manual of your scanner. High-density slides need to be scanned with a resolution of at least 3 μm/pixel. If possible, adjust the sensitivity of the scanner to get intensities of at least 214 for bright corner features. The intensities of the dark corner features should be lower than 25.
6. Grid the arrays. Gridding finds the spots, evaluates the spot properties (intensity, homogeneity, etc.), and creates delimited text files with this information. The scanners usually have specialized software for scanning and gridding/image analysis (e.g., GeneSpring for Agilent scanners, GenePix for Axon scanners, Mapix for Innopsys scanners, etc.). Agilent provides gene annotation lists (GAL files) that stipulate annotation information for their arrays that can be used by most software. Agilent arrays come in different "designs" (spot layouts), as specified by the design ID (e.g., 072363 for a human v3 whole genome gene expression array). Make sure to use the appropriate GAL file for the design of the arrays you are using.

3.7.4 Analysis of Microarray Data

There are plenty of options and software available to analyze microarray data, and many procedures are still being further developed or optimized. It is therefore impossible to provide a detailed procedure to analyze microarrays. We recommend involving a bioinformatician or biostatistician with experience in the analysis of "omics data" in the project.

A rich source of up-to-date analysis tools is available through the Bioconductor project (www.bioconductor.org). The tools are based on the free statistical software and environment R (www.r-project.org). We use the limma package [15] from Bioconductor [16] for most of the analysis, according in principle to the following analysis pipeline (for more details and options, see the limma user guide).

The basic steps of the analysis comprise quality checks (visualization of the distributions of spot intensities and histograms or box plots and as spatial maps, analysis of the correlation of the intensity distributions), background correction, normalization, calculation and visualization of the interesting comparisons, and the ranking or selection of genes. All statistical analyses such as averaging and comparisons between groups are done based on the (background-corrected and normalized) log2 signal intensities. Further analyses may include, among many other methods, clustering of expression profiles across genes and/or across samples, principle component analyses, overrepresentation analyses of selected genes, and gene set enrichment analyses.

4 Notes

1. Different classes of LCM systems that use infrared (IR) and/or ultraviolet (UV) lasers are available [17]. They differ mainly by way of sample collection. An example of a combined IR/UV system is the Arcturus Veritas™ instrument which will be explained in this chapter. The Arcturus system consists of an inverted microscope, a solid-state near-infrared laser diode, a laser control unit, a software controlled microscope stage, a camera, and a monitor (Fig. 3). The powerful UV laser is used for dissecting the structure/cells of interest from the rest of the tissue, while the gentle IR laser helps to capture the cells of interest onto a special thermoplastic film placed on a plastic cap (Figs. 4 and 6). Alternative LCM systems are available from Zeiss (PALM MicroBeam, Carl Zeiss, MicroImaging GmbH, Bernried, Germany) and Leica (LMD7000, Leica Microsystems Inc., Bannockburn, USA). Both systems apply laser power to cut around the sample. The difference is that the Zeiss instrument catapults the region of interest into a vial, while in the Leica system, the sample falls into a vial.

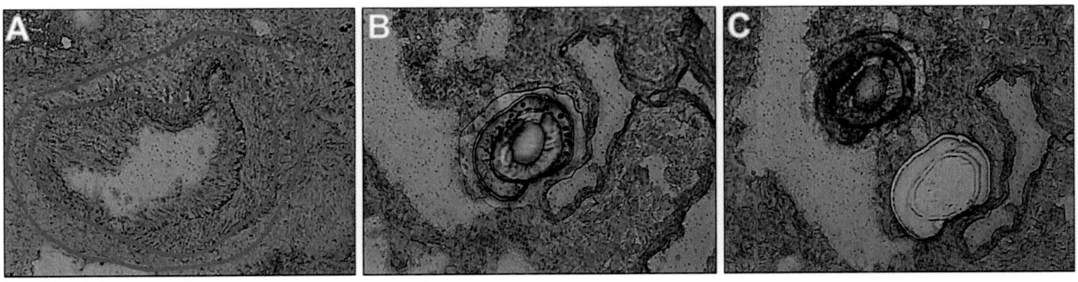

Fig. 6 Specific example of LCM. (**a**) Fibrotic flash-frozen, cryo-cut, and hemalum-stained lung tissue, selected structures for LCM; *blue rings* mark laser cutting lines; (**b**) dissected tissue; (**c**) dissected tissue on the cap, cap above tissue slide with cutout structure

2. The LCM technique may be applied to (a) histological specimens, (b) living cells, and (c) cell cultures. The histological specimen can be either formalin-fixed paraffin-embedded (FFPE) or snap-frozen tissue. In general, it is possible to use stained or unstained tissues. Here, we explain how to work with fresh-frozen samples.
3. After several months of tissue storage, RNA quality decreases drastically; however, it is still satisfactory for further analysis. All samples should be processed the same way to avoid intra-preparation variations.
4. The temperature of the blade, knife holder, and specimen stage should be adapted depending on the tissue composition and desired cutting properties. If the tissue breaks while cutting (e.g., when cutting fibrotic tissue), the temperature might have to be elevated by a few degree Celsius.
5. Flash-frozen tissue has to be embedded in Tissue-Plus® in order for it to be cut. The samples have to be fully covered by Tissue-Plus® and are ready for cutting when the compound is solidified and the Tissue-Plus® has turned white in color.
6. Cutting thickness depends on the laser system used for LCM. For the Arcturus system, a maximal sample thickness of 12 μm is recommended. If the tissue is thicker, precise cutting properties might be lost, and tissue might be ripped. When cutting fibrotic tissue, lower sample thickness is recommended as tissue is typically dense and difficult to cut and specific structures might be found in a thin but dense cell layer only.
7. Visualization of cells and structures within the tissue sections is an important step as it helps distinguishing diverse tissue compartments and cell types. However, the staining procedure should be as fast as possible as it is performed at room temperature, and longer procedure will lead to worse RNA quality. If possible, all solutions should be prepared fresh every day.
8. IR and UV laser energy can be adapted to specific needs. Laser power should be strong enough to reliably and specifically cut and capture region of interest without burning the sample completely. When cutting fibrotic tissue or FFPE tissue, higher laser power might be required in order to precisely dissect the area of interest without tearing any unwanted tissue. Additionally, capture spot size and quantity should be optimized depending on individual needs.
9. In case of tissue rupture, unwanted material on cap can be eliminated by burning it off with the UV laser.
10. A sufficient volume of lysis buffer should be used in order to fully dissolve the collected tissue off the caps. However, it should not exceed 65 μl (Leica instruments) or 300 μl (other instruments).

11. In order to maximize RNA concentration, RNA should be eluted in 12 μl (as described as minimal amount by manufacturer) or concentrated by vacuum centrifugation to 5 μl.
12. Not every housekeeping gene is a permissive reference gene, and not every useful reference gene needs to be a housekeeping gene. It is generally advisable to use a set of reference genes to get an improved average estimate for the loading control value that is less likely different between the compared conditions. In our experience with our tissue (human lungs), we find the human beta-2 microglobulin is a reliable housekeeping gene (b2m; forward primer: TGGAGGCTATCCAGCGTACT, reverse primer: TGTCGGATGGATGAAACCCA; product size: 111 base pairs).
13. Livak and Schmittgen [18] proposed $\Delta Ct = Ct_{(GOI)} - Ct_{(ref)}$, which is the expression of the reference gene normalized to the expression of the gene of interest (because the Ct value is proportional to − log(conc); mind the minus sign!). This is counterintuitive, and we therefore do not recommend this.
14. The expected product yield will be in the ng range. The ratio OD_{260}/OD_{280} represents sample purity. A ratio of ~1.8 is generally accepted as "pure" for DNA; a ratio of ~2.0 is generally accepted as "pure" for RNA. If the ratio is appreciably lower in either case, it may indicate the presence of protein, phenol, or other contaminants that absorb strongly at or near 280 nm. Such samples should be discarded.
15. Cy3 typically gives brighter signal but also higher noise. From our experience, the signal-to-noise ratio on Agilent arrays is similar for both dyes. However, skin oils, fluff, and dust particles that may accidentally contaminate the microarray will fluoresce at wavelengths similar to those of Cy3.
16. The ozone concentration in the lab should be low. Avoid running laser printers or copiers in the lab. We recommend following the supplemental procedures "Preventing Ozone-Related Problems" in the user manual, even if ozone is not a problem. This procedure includes additional immersion steps after the washing of the slides in acetonitrile and drying and stabilization solution. When only few slides are processed, we use Falcon tubes instead of staining dishes for this purpose.

References

1. Datta S, Malhotra L, Dickerson R et al (2015) Laser capture microdissection: big data from small samples. Histol Histopathol 30(11):1255–1269. doi:10.14670/HH-11-622
2. Fink L, Seeger W, Ermert L et al (1998) Real-time quantitative RT-PCR after laser-assisted cell picking. Nat Med 4(11):1329–1333. doi:10.1038/3327
3. Bidarimath M, Edwards AK, Tayade C (2015) Laser capture microdissection for gene expression analysis. Methods Mol Biol 1219:115–137. doi:10.1007/978-1-4939-1661-0_10

4. Kwapiszewska G, Wilhelm J, Wolff S et al (2005) Expression profiling of laser-microdissected intrapulmonary arteries in hypoxia-induced pulmonary hypertension. Respir Res 6:109. doi:10.1186/1465-9921-6-109
5. Hoffmann J, Wilhelm J, Marsh LM et al (2014) Distinct differences in gene expression patterns in pulmonary arteries of patients with chronic obstructive pulmonary disease and idiopathic pulmonary fibrosis with pulmonary hypertension. Am J Respir Crit Care Med 190(1):98–111. doi:10.1164/rccm.201401-0037OC
6. Kwapiszewska G, Meyer M, Bogumil R et al (2004) Identification of proteins in laser-microdissected small cell numbers by SELDI-TOF and Tandem MS. BMC Biotechnol 4:30. doi:10.1186/1472-6750-4-30
7. Fink L, Kwapiszewska G, Wilhelm J et al (2006) Laser-microdissection for cell type- and compartment-specific analyses on genomic and proteomic level. Exp Toxicol Pathol 57(Suppl 2):25–29. doi:10.1016/j.etp.2006.02.010
8. Liu NQ, Braakman RB, Stingl C et al (2012) Proteomics pipeline for biomarker discovery of laser capture microdissected breast cancer tissue. J Mammary Gland Biol Neoplasia 17(2):155–164. doi:10.1007/s10911-012-9252-6
9. Fink L, Bohle RM (2005) Laser microdissection and RNA analysis. Methods Mol Biol 293:167–185. doi:10.1385/1-59259-853-6:167
10. Barcala M, Fenoll C, Escobar C (2012) Laser microdissection of cells and isolation of high-quality RNA after cryosectioning. Methods Mol Biol 883:87–95. doi:10.1007/978-1-61779-839-9_6
11. Kolijn K, van Leenders GJ (2016) Comparison of RNA extraction kits and histological stains for laser capture microdissected prostate tissue. BMC Res Notes 9(1):17. doi:10.1186/s13104-015-1813-5
12. Fink L, Kohlhoff S, Stein MM et al (2002) cDNA array hybridization after laser-assisted microdissection from nonneoplastic tissue. Am J Pathol 160(1):81–90. doi:10.1016/S0002-9440(10)64352-0
13. NuGEN Ovation® PicoSL WTA System V2. http://www.nugen.com/sites/default/files/M01226_v4%20-%20User%20Guide,%20Ovation%20PicoSL%20WTA%20System%20v2.pdf. Accessed 6 Apr 2016
14. Technologies a one-color microarray-based gene expression analysis. http://www.agilent.com/cs/library/usermanuals/Public/G4140-90040_GeneExpression_OneColor_6.9.pdf. Accessed 6 Apr 2016
15. Ritchie ME, Phipson B, Wu D et al (2015) limma powers differential expression analyses for RNA-sequencing and microarray studies. Nucleic Acids Res 43(7):e47. doi:10.1093/nar/gkv007
16. Huber W, Carey VJ, Gentleman R et al (2015) Orchestrating high-throughput genomic analysis with Bioconductor. Nat Methods 12(2):115–121. doi:10.1038/nmeth.3252
17. Vandewoestyne M, Goossens K, Burvenich C et al (2013) Laser capture microdissection: should an ultraviolet or infrared laser be used? Anal Biochem 439(2):88–98. doi:10.1016/j.ab.2013.04.023
18. Schmittgen TD, Livak KJ (2008) Analyzing real-time PCR data by the comparative C(T) method. Nat Protoc 3(6):1101–1108. doi:10.1038/nprot.2008.73

Chapter 22

Collagen Quantification in Tissue Specimens

João Quintas Coentro, Héctor Capella-Monsonís, Valeria Graceffa, Zhuning Wu, Anne Maria Mullen, Michael Raghunath, and Dimitrios I. Zeugolis

Abstract

Collagen is the major extracellular protein in mammals. Accurate quantification of collagen is essential in the biomaterials (e.g., reproducible collagen scaffold fabrication), drug discovery (e.g., assessment of collagen in pathophysiologies, such as fibrosis), and tissue engineering (e.g., quantification of cell-synthesized collagen) fields. Although measuring hydroxyproline content is the most widely used method to quantify collagen in biological specimens, the process is very laborious. To this end, the Sircol™ Collagen Assay is widely used due to its inherent simplicity and convenience. However, this method leads to overestimation of collagen content due to the interaction of Sirius red with basic amino acids of non-collagenous proteins. Herein, we describe the addition of an ultrafiltration purification step in the process to accurately determine collagen content in tissues.

Key words Collagen quantification, Colorimetric assay, Biological specimens, Ultrafiltration purification, Sirius red

1 Introduction

The accurate determination of collagen content is essential in tissue engineering and regenerative medicine for the fabrication of reproducible scaffolds [1, 2], the characterization of cellular activity in cell and tissue culture [3, 4], and the study of pathophysiologies [5, 6], such as fibrosis [7, 8]. Although quantitative (e.g., hydroxyproline assay [9–11]) and semiquantitative (e.g., sodium dodecyl sulfate-polyacrylamide gel electrophoresis followed by densitometric analysis [12–14]) methods are widely used, the required time of the former and the qualitative nature of the latter have triggered investigations into more convenient methods.

Authors João Quintas Coentro and Héctor Capella-Monsonís contributed equally to this work.

Laure Rittié (ed.), *Fibrosis: Methods and Protocols*, Methods in Molecular Biology, vol. 1627,
DOI 10.1007/978-1-4939-7113-8_22, © Springer Science+Business Media LLC 2017

Sircol™ Collagen Concentration Assay (SCA) has been introduced as a convenient methodology for the quantification of collagen in cell and tissue culture [15, 16]. SCA is based in the binding of Sirius red F3B dye (SR) with the basic amino acids of collagen [17, 18]. Unfortunately, SR binds to both collagenous and non-collagenous basic amino acids present in serum, resulting in erroneously overestimated collagen quantification, imposing the need for the introduction of an ultrafiltration purification step [19]. Herein, we present a detailed methodology to accurately quantify collagen content in tissue specimens using a modified SCA protocol with the introduction of an ultrafiltration purification step prior to quantification.

2 Materials

Prepare all solutions using ultrapure water (or in case this is not available, deionized water) and analytical grade reagents. Prepare and store all reagents at room temperature, unless stated otherwise. Diligently follow all waste disposal regulations, when disposing waste materials.

2.1 Sircol™ Collagen Concentration Assay

1. Sircol™ Collagen Concentration Assay kit (we use the one from Biocolor Ltd., UK) can be stored at room temperature for up to 1 year, with exception of the collagen standard solution and the acid-salt wash reagent, which should be kept at 4 °C or in ice once opened.
2. Acid-salt wash reagent: dilute the concentrated acid-salt wash reagent in the Sircol™ kit in distilled water in a ratio of 1:4 (v/v).
3. Collagen solution: if testing commercially available collagen preparations, it is essential that they are acid soluble (or acid-pepsin soluble); otherwise precipitates will occur, which can influence the obtained results. Purified collagen preparations are recommended, as they are almost entirely acid soluble, resulting in clear solutions. Always keep the collagen samples at 4 °C or in ice to prevent denaturation.
4. 0.5 M acetic acid: dilute 28.57 ml of glacial acetic acid 99 % with distilled water and adjust the volume to 1 l. The solution can be stored at room temperature for 1 year.
5. 3,500–4,200 U/mg pepsin from porcine gastric mucosa: prepare 0.1 mg/ml pepsin solution in 0.5 M acetic acid (i.e., 350–420 U/ml final). Always prepare this solution fresh as pepsin can have autolytic activity, effectively neutralizing its activity after a few hours in solution. Store the lyophilized pepsin at −20 or −80 °C to prevent self-digestion.
6. pH meter.

7. Laboratory scale.
8. 50 ml tubes.
9. 15 ml tubes.
10. 1.5 ml micro-tubes: it is recommended to use low protein binding micro-centrifuge tubes to prevent the formation of albumin films on the surface of the tubes, to which the Sircol™ dye can attach, thus influencing the absorbance results.
11. 6 mm biopsy punches.
12. Cotton wool buds.
13. Benchtop vortex mixer.
14. 96-well tissue culture plate.
15. Spectrophotometer plate reader.

2.2 Modified Sircol™ Collagen Concentration Assay for Tissue Samples

1. Same reagents used for the normal SCA.
2. Ultrafiltration centrifugal filters (we use Amicon® Ultra—0.5 ml 100 kDa from Merck Millipore).

3 Methods

Carry out all procedures at room temperature unless otherwise specified.

3.1 Sircol™ Collagen Concentration Assay

1. Prepare reagent blanks using 100 μl of deionized water, 0.5 M acetic acid, and extraction buffer, using the same solution as the testing samples.
2. Prepare collagen standards using 0–50 μg of the collagen reference standard, and complete the volume of solution up to 100 μl using the same solvent as the reagent blanks according to Table 1 (*see* **Note 1**).

Table 1
Sircol™ standard curve preparation

Collagen concentration (μg/100 μl)	50	30	20	15	10	5	1	0
Volume (μl) of 0.5 mg/ml collagen standard stock to prepare 100 μl of standard	100	60	40	30	20	10	2	0

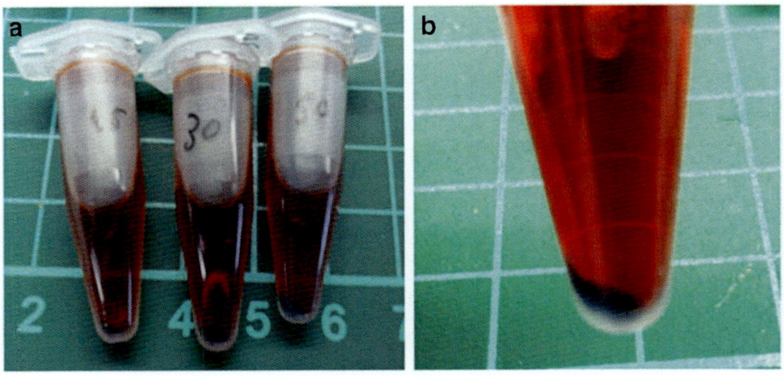

Fig. 1 Pellet formation after first centrifugation step. (**a**) Pellet formation at different values of collagen (μg). (**b**) Formed pellet in detail

3. Prepare test samples using volumes between 10 and 100 μl, and make up to 100 μl using the same solvent as the reagent blanks (*see* **Notes 2–4**).
4. To each tube, add 1 ml of Sircol™ dye reagent. This is the required volume to fully saturate the collagen molecules in 100 μl of solution (*see* **Notes 5** and **6**).
5. Cap the tubes and mix the contents by inverting the tubes and placing them in a gentle mechanical shaker for 30 min (*see* **Note 7**).
6. Centrifuge the samples at 13,600 *g* for 10 min.
7. Carefully discard the supernatants by draining the tubes (Fig. 1 and *see* **Note 8**).
8. Gently add 750 μl of acid–salt wash reagent (ice cold) on the collagen pellet to remove unbound dye (*see* **Note 9**).
9. Centrifuge at 13,600 *g* for 10 min.
10. Discard the wash by draining it into a waste container, and remove any excess fluid from the lips of the tubes using cotton wool buds (*see* **Note 10**).
11. Add 250 μl of alkali reagent to blanks, standards, and test samples (*see* **Note 11**).
12. Recap the tubes and release the collagen into solution using a vortex mixer (*see* **Notes 12** and **13**).
13. Transfer 200 μl of each sample to individual wells in a 96-well plate, and measure the absorbance at 555 nm or the closest matching blue–green filter. Measurements should be conducted against water (*see* **Notes 14** and **15**).

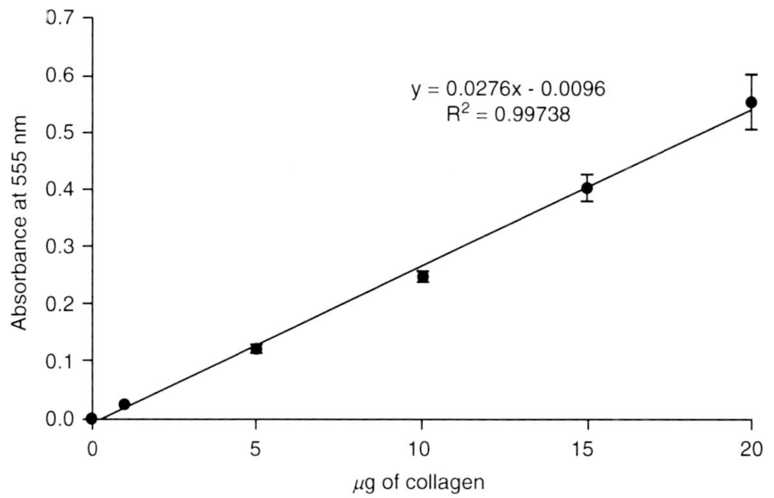

Fig. 2 Standard curve for the quantification of collagen samples obtained by plotting the absorbance at 555 nm against different collagen contents

14. Calculate the collagen concentrations in the tested samples from the standard concentration curve (Fig. 2 and *see* **Note 16**).

3.2 Modified Sircol™ Collagen Concentration Assay for Tissue Samples

For assaying tissue samples, an acid-pepsin extraction and an ultrafiltration purification step are required to remove proteins that might interfere with the collagen quantification results.

3.2.1 Acid-Pepsin Collagen Extraction

1. Use 6 mm biopsy punches to cut approximately 70 mg of sample tissue (e.g., tendon, skin).
2. Weigh the samples in order to normalize results accordingly to sample weight.
3. Suspend the tissue pieces in 2 ml of 0.1 mg/ml pepsin in 0.5 M acetic acid solution, and incubate overnight at 4 °C using gentle mechanical agitation (*see* **Note 17**).
4. Store the supernatant resultant from the acid-pepsin at −20 °C for future use.

3.2.2 Ultrafiltration Purification

1. As the ultrafiltration centrifugal filter contains trace amounts of glycerine, a rinsing step with buffer or ultrapurified water should be conducted (*see* **Note 18**).
2. Insert the ultrafiltration filter into one of the provided microcentrifuge tubes.
3. Add up to 500 μl of sample to the ultrafiltration filter and cap the tube.

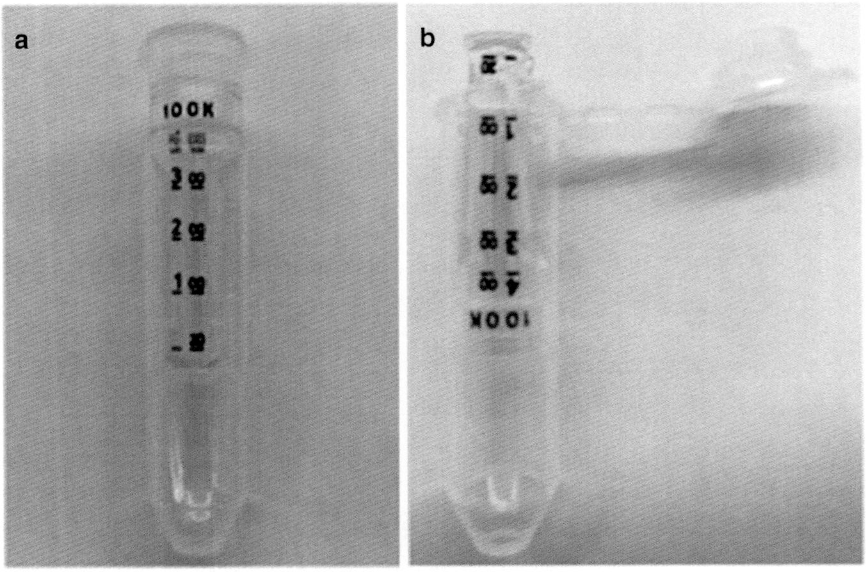

Fig. 3 Ultrafiltration 100 kDa 0.5 ml centrifugal filter. (**a**) Ultrafiltration device in position for purification step. (**b**) Ultrafiltration device in position for recovery of purified sample

4. Place the capped filter device into the centrifuge rotor, aligning the cap toward the center of the rotor, and counterbalance it with a similarly loaded device.
5. Centrifuge the device at 13,000 *g* for 10 min.
6. Discard the flow through, and wash the retentate adding 500 μl of 50 mM acetic acid to the ultrafiltration filter.
7. Cap the tube and centrifuge again at 13,000 *g* for 10 min.
8. Repeat **steps 6** and 7 three times (*see* **Note 19**).
9. Remove the assembled device from the centrifuge and separate the ultrafiltration filter from the micro-centrifuge tube.
10. To recover the concentrated solute (collagen), place the ultrafiltration filter upside down in a clean micro-centrifuge tube (Fig. 3). Place in centrifuge, aligning the cap toward the center of the rotor, and counterbalance it with a similarly loaded device.
11. Immediately spin the samples for 2 min at 1,000 *g* to transfer the concentrated sample from the device to the tube.
12. The ultrafiltrate can be stored in the centrifuge tube (*see* **Note 20**).

3.2.3 Sircol™ Collagen Concentration Assay on Tissue Samples

After the steps described in Subheadings 3.2.1 and 3.2.2, it is possible to follow the normal protocol for the SCA (Fig. 4 and [19]).

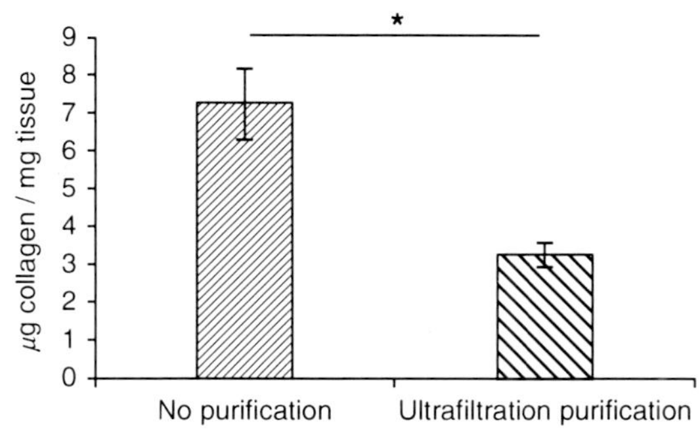

Fig. 4 Collagen quantification of rabbit skin tissue using conventional Sircol Collagen Concentration Assay (no purification) and modified Sircol Collagen Concentration Assay (ultrafiltration purification). In the conventional protocol, a significant overestimation of twofold can be observed ($*p < 0.05$). This overestimation is solved with the addition of a purification step using a 100 kDa ultrafiltration membrane, which discards proteins that react with the Sirius red dye, resulting in a purified collagen solution that leads to accurate collagen quantification

4 Notes

1. The collagen standard solution should not be used if it is cloudy or has impurities/insoluble collagen, as the collagen concentration of the sample would be off.
2. When transferring the sample solution into the micro-centrifuge tube, make sure that the solution is homogenized (vortex mixing followed up by pipette mixing are recommended) as this might compromise the reproducibility of the results.
3. If there is no way to estimate the concentration range of collagen present in the test sample, 50 or 100 μl of test material should be used for a trial run. This trial run should also be used to determine if the collagen standards are appropriate for the intended concentration or if higher concentrations should be used to make the collagen concentration reference curve.
4. Samples can be kept frozen at −20 °C for up to 1 week.
5. When using a large number of samples, the use of a repetitive pipette is recommended for time efficiency.
6. Sirius red dye easily stains clothing and biological tissues; wear protective clothing and gloves at all times.
7. Instead of using a mechanical shaker, you can manually mix the solutions every 5 min.
8. When discarding the excess dye, compaction of the formed pellet on the bottom of the tube is essential to prevent loss of collagen, as this might lead to the absence of collagen pellet or very low quantities of pellet. It is recommended to partially

block the tube opening with a low porosity filter or sieve or even a spatula to prevent the escape of the centrifuged pellet.

9. To prevent pellet detachment, making the next draining step easier, it is recommended to very gently add the acid-salt wash reagent (ice cold) on top of the formed collagen-dye pellet.
10. When discarding the excess dye, take extra care to prevent pellet loss. If the pellet is well deposited on the bottom of the tube, carefully discard excess dye in one movement. For smaller concentrations of collagen, the pellet might not be deposited. In this case the same precautions of the previous draining step apply. Remove any excess fluid from the inside and lips of the tubes using cotton wool buds in order to minimize the influence of unbound Sircol™ dye on the final absorbance readings.
11. If the values of measured absorbance are too high for the obtained calibration curve, the assay should be repeated with higher standard concentrations (15, 30, and 50 μg) and using 1,000 μl of alkali reagent.
12. All of the bound dye should be dissolved before measuring the absorbance; otherwise, the measured results will be altered.
13. In case the collagen pellet does not dissolve completely after thorough vortex mixing, possibly due to excessive quantity of collagen-dye complex exceeding the solubility in the provided volume, it is recommended to increase the volume of alkali reagent to a maximum of 1,000 μl or decrease the initial volume of sample tested. If the problem persists, a dilution of the original sample is recommended.
14. When transferring the sample solution into the well plate, make sure that the solution is homogenized (vortex mixing followed by pipette mixing are recommended), as this might compromise the reproducibility of the results, originating observable color differences between replicates. Also try to avoid the formation of bubbles by pipetting the solution slowly into the well plate, as air bubbles might interfere with light diffraction.
15. Measurement of the absorbance should be conducted within 2–3 h of adding the alkali reagent for optimal results, as the intensity will slightly fade as a function of time. The tubes should also be kept capped until ready to be measured.
16. Duplicates should be within 5 % of their mean value. If values greatly differ from each other, the assay should be repeated. Also, absorbance values should read between 0.1 and 0.8, as values outside this range are not reliable. For values higher than 0.8, the assay should be repeated with lower volumes of sample or with sample dilutions, if this problem persists (Fig. 5). If the collagen concentration is too low to be accurately measured (absorbance values close to the blank or outside the calibration curve), a collagen isolation and

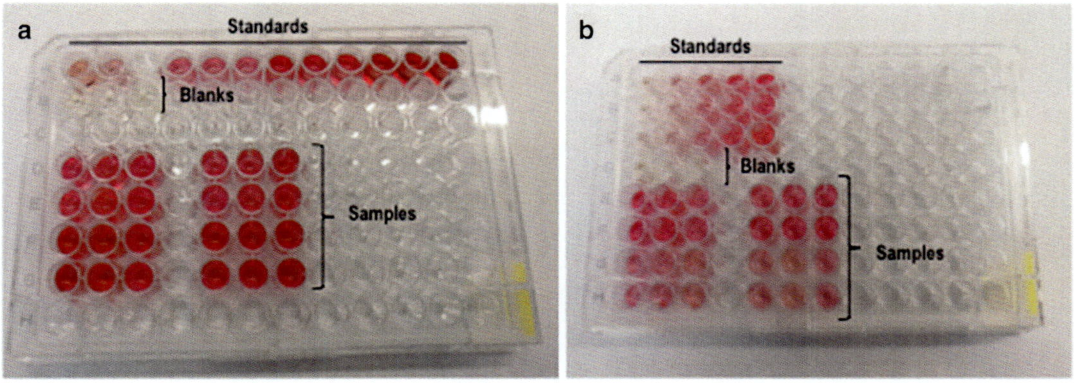

Fig. 5 Example of microplates for analysis. (**a**) Example of microplate for analysis in which the absorbance at 555 nm of the samples and standards is not comprised between 0.1 and 0.8, hence being unreliable for quantification. 0.5 M acetic acid solution was used as blank. (**b**) Example of microplate for analysis in which the absorbance at 555 nm of the samples and standards is comprised between 0.1 and 0.8, therefore being within the accurate range for quantification. 0.5 M acetic acid solution was used as blank

concentration step should be carried out (see manufacturer's protocol), or hydroxyproline assay should be conducted.

17. For hard tissues, it might be necessary to proceed to a second acid-pepsin extraction to completely recover all collagen. In order to do so, remove the supernatant from the first extraction and store it at −20 °C. Then proceed to an equal second extraction, and in the end mix the supernatants from both extractions and store them at −20 °C.
18. Do not allow the membranes to dry out once wet, and if you are not using the membranes, immediately leave fluid on the membrane until the device is used.
19. Wash the retentate with the same initial volume of sample added. Do not allow the filtrate liquid to touch the ultrafiltration membrane. If necessary, remove the ultrafiltration filter without inverting it, quickly discard the filtrate liquid, and reinsert the filter into the micro-tube.

Acknowledgments

This work forms part of the Teagasc Walsh Fellowship (Grant Award No. Ref: 2014045) and the ReValueProtein Research Project (Grant Award No. 11/F/043) supported by the Department of Agriculture, Food and the Marine (DAFM) under the National Development Plan 2007–2013 funded by the Irish Government. This work has also been supported from the Health Research Board, Health Research Awards Programme, under the grant agreement number HRA_POR/2011/84 and the Science Foundation Ireland and the European Regional Development Fund (Grant Agreement Number: 13/RC/2073).

References

1. Zeugolis DI, Paul RG, Attenburrow G (2009) Extruded collagen fibres for tissue-engineering applications: influence of collagen concentration and NaCl amount. J Biomater Sci Polym Ed 20(2):219–234. doi:10.1163/156856209X404505
2. Perez-Puyana V, Romero A, Guerrero A (2016) Influence of collagen concentration and glutaraldehyde on collagen-based scaffold properties. J Biomed Mater Res A 104(6):1462–1468. doi:10.1002/jbm.a.35671
3. Satyam A, Kumar P, Fan X et al (2014) Macromolecular crowding meets tissue engineering by self-assembly: a paradigm shift in regenerative medicine. Adv Mater 26(19):3024–3034. doi:10.1002/adma.201304428
4. Satyam A, Kumar P, Cigognini D et al (2016) Low, but not too low, oxygen tension and macromolecular crowding accelerate extracellular matrix deposition in human dermal fibroblast culture. Acta Biomater 44:221–231. doi:10.1016/j.actbio.2016.08.008
5. Li Y, Qi Y, Kim MS et al (2008) Increased renal collagen cross-linking and lipid accumulation in nephropathy of Zucker diabetic fatty rats. Diabetes Metab Res Rev 24(6):498–506. doi:10.1002/dmrr.874
6. Wang Z, Chesler NC (2012) Role of collagen content and cross-linking in large pulmonary arterial stiffening after chronic hypoxia. Biomech Model Mechanobiol 11(1-2):279–289. doi:10.1007/s10237-011-0309-z
7. Bhogal RK, Stoica CM, McGaha TL et al (2005) Molecular aspects of regulation of collagen gene expression in fibrosis. J Clin Immunol 25(6):592–603. doi:10.1007/s10875-005-7827-3
8. Thoua NM, Derrett-Smith EC, Khan K et al (2012) Gut fibrosis with altered colonic contractility in a mouse model of scleroderma. Rheumatology (Oxford) 51(11):1989–1998. doi:10.1093/rheumatology/kes191
9. Neuman RE, Logan MA (1950) The determination of hydroxyproline. J Biol Chem 184(1):299–306
10. Woessner JF, Jr. (1961) The determination of hydroxyproline in tissue and protein samples containing small proportions of this imino acid. Arch Biochem Biophys 93:440-447. doi:10.1016/0003-9861(61)90291-0
11. Zeugolis DI, Paul RG, Attenburrow G (2008) Factors influencing the properties of reconstituted collagen fibers prior to self-assembly: animal species and collagen extraction method. J Biomed Mater Res A 86(4):892–904. doi:10.1002/jbm.a.31694
12. Zeugolis DI, Li B, Lareu RR et al (2008) Collagen solubility testing, a quality assurance step for reproducible electro-spun nano-fibre fabrication. A technical note. J Biomater Sci Polym Ed 19(10):1307–1317. doi:10.1163/156856208786052344
13. Kumar P, Satyam A, Cigognini D et al (2016) Low oxygen tension and macromolecular crowding accelerate extracellular matrix deposition in human corneal fibroblast culture. J Tissue Eng Regen Med. doi:10.1002/term.2283
14. Cigognini D, Gaspar D, Kumar P et al (2016) Macromolecular crowding meets oxygen tension in human mesenchymal stem cell culture – a step closer to physiologically relevant in vitro organogenesis. Sci Rep 6:30746. doi:10.1038/srep30746
15. Yurovsky VV (2003) Tumor necrosis factor-related apoptosis-inducing ligand enhances collagen production by human lung fibroblasts. Am J Respir Cell Mol Biol 28(2):225–231. doi:10.1165/rcmb.2002-0140OC
16. Wilda H, Gough JE (2006) In vitro studies of annulus fibrosus disc cell attachment, differentiation and matrix production on PDLLA/45S5 Bioglass composite films. Biomaterials 27(30):5220–5229. doi:10.1016/j.biomaterials.2006.06.008
17. Junqueira LC, Bignolas G, Brentani RR (1979) Picrosirius staining plus polarization microscopy, a specific method for collagen detection in tissue sections. Histochem J 11(4):447–455. doi:10.1007/BF01002772
18. Rabau MY, Dayan D (1994) Polarization microscopy of picrosirius red stained sections: a useful method for qualitative evaluation of intestinal wall collagen. Histol Histopathol 9(3):525–528
19. Lareu RR, Zeugolis DI, Abu-Rub M et al (2010) Essential modification of the Sircol Collagen Assay for the accurate quantification of collagen content in complex protein solutions. Acta Biomater 6(8):3146–3151. doi:10.1016/j.actbio.2010.02.004

Chapter 23

Methods for the Assessment of Active Transforming Growth Factor-β in Cells and Tissues

Alison E. John, Joanne Porte, Gisli Jenkins, and Amanda L. Tatler

Abstract

The potent and pluripotent cytokine TGFβ has important roles in normal homeostasis and disease pathogenesis. Once released from cells, TGFβ exists in both latent and functionally active forms. Large amounts of latent TGFβ are secreted from cells and sequestered in extracellular matrix, only a small proportion of which is activated at any given time. Accurate assessment of TGFβ activity levels is an important measurement in biological research and requires methods distinct from measuring total levels of TGFβ expression as small changes in TGFβ activity levels could be masked by the large amounts of latent TGFβ available to be measured. In this chapter, we describe detailed experimental methods for assessing levels of active TGFβ in cells and tissues. This chapter includes methods for the assessment of TGFβ activity in cells in vitro, in ex vivo precision cut tissue, and in vivo.

Key words Transforming growth factor-β, Fibrosis, Remodeling, Integrins

1 Introduction

Transforming growth factor-β (TGFβ) is a ubiquitously expressed, pluripotent cytokine, which is fundamental to development, homeostasis, and repair and has been implicated in the pathogenesis of many diseases. It is potently pro-fibrotic, pro-angiogenic, anti-inflammatory, and immunosuppressive and can be either anti- or pro-tumorigenic. There are three mammalian isoforms, namely, TGFβ1, TGFβ2, and TGFβ3, with TGFβ1 being the most abundant form.

During posttranslational processing of TGFβ proteins, the pro-peptide is cleaved from the protein by the endopeptidase furin convertase [1]. All TGFβ isoforms are released from cells non-covalently associated with the pro-peptide, known as the latency-associated peptide (LAP), which renders the cytokine inactive (Fig. 1). This is known as the small latent complex. Once released, latent TGFβ interacts with the N-terminus of latent TGFβ binding proteins (LTBPs) forming the large latent complex, which binds to

Laure Rittié (ed.), *Fibrosis: Methods and Protocols*, Methods in Molecular Biology, vol. 1627,
DOI 10.1007/978-1-4939-7113-8_23, © Springer Science+Business Media LLC 2017

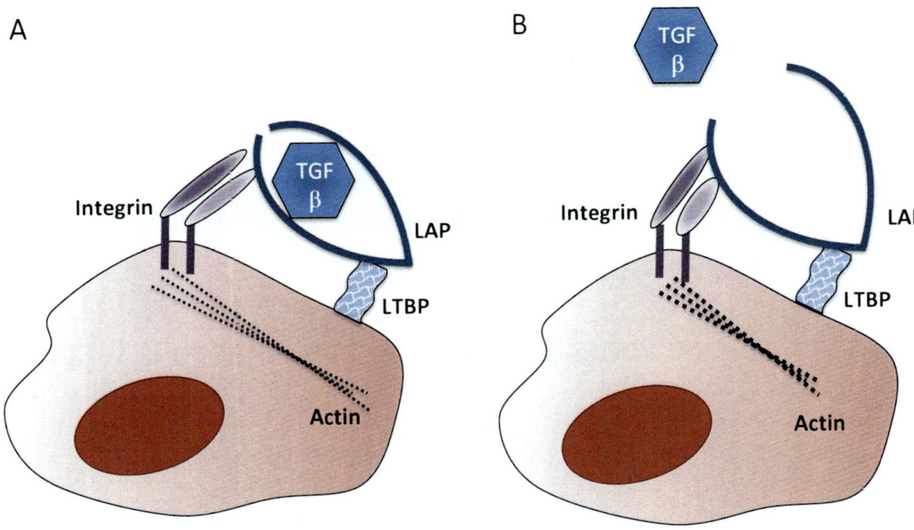

Fig. 1 Latent TGFβ activation. (**a**) TGFβ homodimers are released from cells non-covalently associated with latency-associated peptides (LAPs), which render the cytokine inactive. This is known as the small latent complex. LAP interacts with the N-terminus of latent TGFβ binding proteins (LTBPs), which serve to tether the small latent complex to proteins within the extracellular matrix, forming the large latent complex. Furthermore, LAP binds to cell surface integrins via an RGD integrin binding domain forming a direct link between the large latent complex and the actin cytoskeleton within the cell. (**b**) Reorganization of the actin cytoskeleton such as during cell contraction results in force generation. The force is transduced via the integrin to the LAP within the large latent complex. This causes a conformational change within LAP causing the release of active TGFβ from the large latent complex

proteins within the extracellular matrix (ECM) [2]. Cells sequester the large latent complex in their ECM. In this manner, cells surround themselves with large stores of latent TGFβ awaiting activation, and it is the activation of latent TGFβ that is the rate-limiting step in TGFβ bioavailability [3].

For TGFβ activation to occur, the interaction between TGFβ and LAP must be cleaved or structurally altered to allow the active TGFβ homodimer to bind to its receptor (Fig. 1). Several distinct mechanisms of TGFβ activation have been described. Physical measures such as extremes of temperature or pH have been shown to activate TGFβ, and proteases such as plasmin, MMP-14, and tryptase [4] can cleave the LAP from TGFβ. Additionally, the glycoprotein thrombospondin-1 [5] and certain cell surface integrins, including $\alpha_v\beta_6$, $\alpha_v\beta_5$, $\alpha_v\beta_3$, and $\alpha_v\beta_1$ [6–8], can activate TGFβ by inducing a conformational change within LAP. The primary mechanism of TGFβ activation employed in vivo during development appears to be integrin mediated since transgenic mice that cannot activate TGFβ via integrins recapitulate the phenotype of TGFβ1 null mice [9]. Furthermore, mice lacking α_v-containing integrins (a subunit common to all TGFβ-activating integrins) in myofibroblasts are protected from fibrosis in multiple organ systems [10], highlighting the importance of integrin-mediated TGFβ activation in fibrogenesis. Interestingly, integrin-mediated TGFβ activation may have a role in regulating expression of certain TGFβ-activating integrins, leading to a positive feedback loop that may be an important process in disease pathogenesis [11].

With the exception of $\alpha_v\beta_8$ integrins, integrin-mediated TGFβ activation involves mechanotransduction of intracellular force from the cell cytoskeleton to the latent TGFβ complex via the integrins on the cell surface (Fig. 1). Integrin-mediated TGFβ activation results in the release of free TGFβ molecules from the latent complex [12]. Once activated, the released TGFβ rapidly binds to its receptor on adjacent cells to initiate TGFβ signaling in a paracrine fashion. Furthermore, within a given tissue or cell type, the proportion of latent TGFβ which is activated in response to a stimulus is small [13, 14]; therefore, detection of released active TGFβ in biological fluids in vivo and supernatants in vitro can be problematic. To circumvent this issue, specific methods of measuring active TGFβ in vitro, ex vivo, and in vivo have been developed. It is crucial that suitable methods for measuring TGFβ activity levels are selected since many methods that determine overall expression levels of TGFβ do not account for the activation status of the cytokine. This chapter gives detailed methodologies to assess TGFβ activation in the lungs in vivo, in ex vivo precision cut lung slices and in cells in vitro. In vitro and ex vivo methods include transformed mink lung cell (TMLC) assay and phosphorylated SMAD2 (pSMAD 2) western blotting, while in vivo methods include pSMAD2 assays, using multiplex immunoassay, ELISA, or immunohistochemistry.

In the TMLC assay, mink lung epithelial cells transfected with an expression construct containing a truncated plasminogen-activator inhibitor-1 (PAI-1) promoter fused to the firefly luciferase gene are commonly used as a reporter cell for TGFβ activity [15]. These TMLCs were developed in 1994 and have become a gold standard in measuring TGFβ activity, being extensively utilized in research publications [6, 8, 13, 16–21]. The assay is one of the most sensitive and reliable methods of assessing TGFβ activity in vitro. TMLCs express luciferase in response to all three isoforms of TGFβ and exhibit no response to other inducers of PAI-1, including fibroblast growth factor and epidermal growth factor [15]. TMLCs can be used to measure active TGFβ released in fluids such as conditioned media from either cultured cells or precision cut lung slices. Furthermore, they can be cocultured with a cell type of interest to increase sensitivity when measuring integrin-mediated TGFβ activation, which rapidly binds to TGFβ receptors on nearby cells. For example, $\alpha_v\beta_6$-mediated TGFβ activation can be accurately assessed by coculturing TMLCs with mouse embryonic fibroblasts (MEF) that are stably transfected with the $\alpha_v\beta_6$ integrin (MEF-β_6) [19]. These cells can also be used to determine levels of total TGFβ (i.e., latent plus active) present in conditioned media samples by heating the sample to activate all TGFβ present. The use of a TGFβ1 standard curve acts as a positive control for the assay and allows for the quantification of TGFβ concentrations activated. For accuracy, tests are performed in triplicate.

Quantification of pSMAD2 using multiplex immunoassay assays and ELISAs allows the assessment of TGFβ activity in vivo by measuring the most proximal step of the TGFβ signaling cascade. Smad2 is phosphorylated by the TGFβ receptor when the active cytokine binds to it. The method using tissue can be applied to determine global TGFβ activity in any tissues; however, the method using bronchoalveolar lavage (BAL) cells is specifically used to detect TGFβ activation by lung epithelial cells. This method allows the measurement of TGFβ activation by alveolar epithelial cells in vivo using inflammatory cells, predominantly macrophages, present in the BAL fluid [14] (Fig. 2). The alveolar macrophages are in direct cell-cell contact with the epithelium, and the relative ease with which they can be isolated from in vivo lungs makes them an excellent in vivo reporter cell. TGFβ activated by epithelial cells binds to TGFβ receptors on the macrophage cell surface, resulting in the phosphorylation of SMAD2, which can be detected by multiplex immunoassay and/or ELISA.

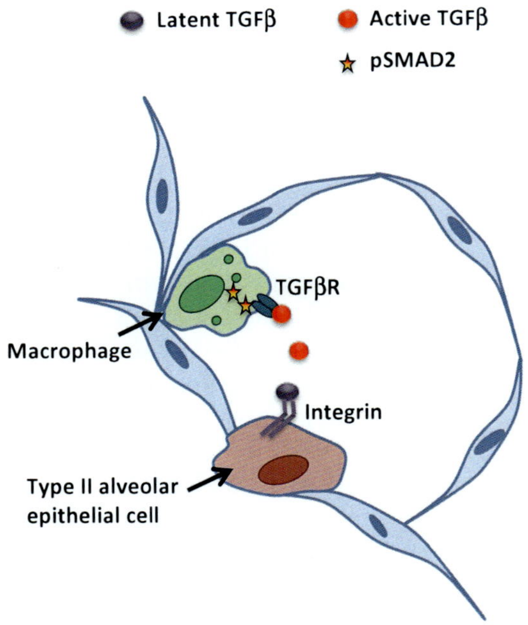

Fig. 2 Bronchoalveolar lavage cells as a reporter for active TGFβ. Alveolar macrophages line the alveolar spaces and lie in direct contact with the epithelial cells that comprise the alveoli. When TGFβ is activated by alveolar epithelial cells, the active cytokine binds to the TGFβ receptor on the cell surface of macrophages causing the phosphorylation of SMAD2. Alveolar macrophages can easily be removed from the lungs by bronchoalveolar lavage and phospho-SMAD2 (pSMAD2) levels determined

Lastly, utilizing immunohistochemistry to measure phospho-SMAD2 (pSMAD2) allows macroscopic visualization of TGFβ activity across an entire tissue. While this method is qualitative rather than quantitative, it can give valuable information about the cell types within a tissue that are responding to active TGFβ.

2 Materials

2.1 Transformed Mink Lung Cell (TMLC) Assay

1. TMLC culture medium: Dulbecco's Modified Eagle medium (DMEM) supplemented with 10% (v/v) fetal calf serum, 4 mM L-glutamine, and 250 μg/ml G418 antibiotic
2. Cell culture equipment and supplies (incubator, biosafety cabinet, cell culture dishes, pipettes, etc.).
3. Recombinant TGFβ.
4. Luciferase assay kit: most products contain cell lysis buffer, luciferase assay substrate, and luciferase assay buffer (we use the Luciferase Assay System from Promega).
5. White opaque plate.
6. Luminometer.

2.2 Phosphorylated Smad2 Western Blotting

1. Recombinant TGFβ.
2. Protein molecular weight marker (we use Rainbow molecular weight marker).
3. Polyacrylamide gel casting apparatus.
4. Electrophoresis apparatus.
5. Transfer apparatus.
6. Phosphate buffered saline (PBS).
7. Lysis buffer: 20 mM Tris–HCl, pH 7.4, 137 mM NaCl, 1% Triton X-100, 2 mM ethylenediaminetetraacetic acid (EDTA), 10% (w/v) glycerol, 25 mM β-glycerophosphate, 1 mM $NaVO_4$. Just prior to use, add protease inhibitor cocktail (we use P1860 from Sigma-Aldrich) and phosphatase inhibitor cocktail (we use #37492 from Active Motif).
8. Cell scraper.
9. SDS-PAGE gels can be purchased, pre-casted, or casted in advance with the following reagents:
   (a) Buffer 1: 1.5 M Tris–HCl, 0.4% SDS, pH 8.8.
   (b) Buffer 2: 0.5 M Tris–HCl, 0.4% SDS, pH 6.8.
   (c) 30% bis-acrylamide.
   (d) Distilled H_2O.
   (e) 10% (w/v) ammonium persulfate.
   (f) Tetramethylethylenediamine (TEMED).

10. Tris buffered saline (TBS) supplemented with Tween-20 (TBS-T): 25 mM Tris pH 7.4–7.6, 150 mM NaCl, 0.1% (v/v) Tween-20.
11. Blocking solution: 5% (v/v) non-fat milk diluted in TBS-T.
12. Laemmli buffer: 125 mM Tris–HCl, pH 6.8, 20% (v/v) glycerol, 2% (w/v) sodium dodecyl sulfate (SDS), 2 mg/ml bromophenol blue. Just before use, add 60 μl/ml β-mercaptoethanol.
13. Running buffer: 25 mM Tris, 190 mM glycine, 0.1% (w/v) SDS.
14. Transfer buffer: 25 mM Tris, 190 mM glycine, and 20% (v/v) methanol.
15. Polyvinylidene difluoride (PVDF) membrane.
16. Primary antibody anti-Phospho-Smad2 (we use and anti-Ser456/467, #3108 from Cell Signaling, diluted 1:1000 in blocking solution).
17. Secondary antibody conjugated to horseradish peroxidase (we use a goat anti-rabbit HRP #P0448 from Dako, diluted to 333 μg/ml with blocking solution).
18. Saran Wrap.
19. Dark room.
20. X-ray film cassette.
21. Tape.
22. Developing fluid.
23. Fixer solution.
24. Marker pen.
25. Electrogenerated chemiluminescence (ECL) western blotting detection liquid.
26. ECL Hyperfilm.

2.3 Measurement of pSMAD2 in Lung Tissue and Bronchoalveolar Lavage Cells

1. Pestle and mortar.
2. Liquid nitrogen.
3. Dry ice.
4. Cell lysis buffer: 20 mM Tris–HCl, pH 7.5, 150 mM NaCl, 1 mM EDTA, 1 mM EGTA, 1% (w/v) Triton X-100, 2.5 mM sodium pyrophosphate, 1 mM β-glycerophosphate, 1 mM Na_3VO, 1 μg/ml leupeptin. We use a 10X stock of this buffer (#9803 from Cell Signaling) and add a protease and phosphatase inhibitor cocktail before use (we use the Halt Protease and Phosphatase Inhibitor Cocktail from ThermoScientific).
5. Protein quantification kit (e.g., a bicinchoninic acid assay).
6. Multiplex immunoassay system and supplies. In this protocol, we will describe method using the Bio-Plex® system from Bio-Rad and the following supplies:

   (a) Milliplex TGFβ Signaling Magnetic Bead Panel 6-plex (Millipore #48-614MAG).
   (b) Handheld Magnetic Separation Block for 96-well plates (Millipore #40-285).
7. PathScan Total SMAD2 Sandwich ELISA Kit (Cell Signaling Technologies #7244C).
8. GST-SMAD2 standard (Sigma #SRP5131).

2.4 Measurement of pSMAD2 in Tissue by Immunohistochemistry

1. Formalin-fixed paraffin wax-embedded tissue.
2. Microtome.
3. Dehydrating station with xylene (two jars) and ethanol (100% (v/v, two jars), 70% (v/v, two jars), and water (two jars)).
4. PBS.
5. Citrate buffer: 10 mM citric acid, pH 6.0.
6. Microwave.
7. Peroxidase blocking solution: 3% (v/v) H_2O_2 in methanol.
8. Hydrophobic PAP pen.
9. Blocking solution: 5% (v/v) goat serum, 0.1% (w/v) bovine serum albumin in PBS.
10. Anti-pSMAD2 primary antibody (we use #3108 from Cell Signaling diluted 1:500 in blocking solution).
11. Goat anti-rabbit secondary antibody (most of them diluted to 5 μg/ml in PBS).
12. ABC reagent (we use the one from Vector): 5 ml PBS plus two drops reagent A and two drops reagent B. Allow to stand for 30 min prior to use.
13. 3′,3′-diaminobenzidine tetrahydrochloride (DAB).
14. Mayer's hematoxylin.
15. Depex mounting medium.

3 Methods

3.1 Transformed Mink Lung Cell (TMLC) Assay

3.1.1 Measurement of Global TGFβ Activity in Conditioned Medium

1. Maintain TMLCs in TMLC culture medium at 37 °C, 5% CO_2.
2. Trypsinize TMLCs, resuspend them in growth supplement-free DMEM, and count cells using a hemocytometer.
3. Seed the TMLC in a 96-well plate at a density of 1×10^5 cells/well, and allow them to adhere for 3 h at 37 °C, 5% CO_2.
4. Conditioned media from either in vitro cell experiments or ex vivo precision cut tissue experiments will be used as test samples (*see* **Note 1**).

5. Prepare a little more than 300 μl of each standard: dilute recombinant TGFβ to 250, 500, and 1000 ng/ml in growth supplement-free DMEM.
6. Aspirate and discard the TMLC medium from **step 3**, and add 100 μl of the test samples and TGFβ1 standards in triplicate to the plate.
7. Incubate the plate at 37 °C, 5% CO_2 for 16 h.
8. Remove the medium by aspiration.
9. Wash the wells with PBS and remove all liquid.
10. Add 50 μl of reporter lysis buffer per well to disrupt the cells (*see* **Note 2**).
11. Transfer the cell lysates to a white opaque plate.
12. Analyze using a luminometer: inject 100 μl of luciferase substrate into each well prior to the luminescence measurement.
13. Calculate TGFβ concentration in test samples based on the standard curve obtained from reading of standards run in parallel.

3.1.2 Measurement of Integrin-Mediated TGFβ Activation by TMLC Coculture Assay

1. Culture the experimental cell of interest in a 96-well plate until fully confluent.
2. Maintain TMLC cells in TMLC culture medium at 37 °C, 5% CO_2.
3. Switch the experimental cells' medium to supplement-free medium for 24 h to induce a growth arrest.
4. Trypsinize the TMLCs, count them using a hemocytometer, and resuspend them in growth supplement-free medium at a cell density of 0.5×10^6 cells/ml.
5. Aspirate the medium from the experimental cells, and seed TMLCs directly on top by adding 100 μl/well of the cell suspension prepared in **step 4**.
6. Prepare the test samples and standards: dilute test compounds in serum-free DMEM to the desired concentration. Prepare a TGFβ standard curve by diluting recombinant TGFβ1 in serum-free DMEM to 500, 1000, and 2000 ng/ml.
7. Add 100 μl of the test samples and TGFβ1 standards to the plate, in triplicate.
8. Incubate the plate at 37 °C, 5% CO_2 for 16 h.
9. Remove all media by aspiration and wash all wells with PBS, removing all liquids.
10. Add 50 μl of reporter lysis buffer per well to disrupt the cells (*see* **Note 2**).
11. Transfer cell lysates to a white opaque plate.

12. Analyze using a luminometer. Inject 100 μl of luciferase substrate into each well prior to the luminescence measurement.
13. Calculate TGFβ concentration in test samples based on the standard curve obtained from reading of standards run in parallel.

3.2 Measurement of pSMAD2 by Western Blotting

1. In vitro experiments on growth-arrested (i.e., cultured 24 h in serum-free medium) test cells are performed in duplicate in 12-well plates.
2. Stimulate two wells with 2 ng/ml of TGFβ1 as a positive control for the assay. Incubate the cells for 4 h at 37 °C, 5% CO_2.
3. Place the plates on ice, remove the culture medium, and wash the wells in ice-cold sterile PBS.
4. Add 50 μl of ice-cold lysis buffer to each well, ensuring that all cells are covered, and scrap the monolayer with a cell scraper.
5. Collect samples from each well pooling the samples from duplicate wells, thus giving a final volume of 100 μl per treatment.
6. Quantify the protein concentration of each sample using a protein assay kit. Calculate volume of samples required to yield 100 μg of proteins.
7. Set up a 10% polyacrylamide gel by either using purchased pre-casted gels (then proceed directly to **step** 7g) or by preparing gels according to the following steps:

   (a) Prepare a 10% polyacrylamide resolving gel by mixing 6.66 ml of 30% bis-acrylamide, 5.2 ml buffer 1, and 7.92 ml distilled H_2O. Add 200 μl of 10% ammonium persulfate and 50 μl of TEMED just prior to casting the gel.

   (b) Pour the resolving gel between the glass plates of the gel casting apparatus, leaving a 1.5 cm gap between the top level of the resolving gel and the top of the plates. Gently pipet 1 ml of water on top of the resolving gel to prevent gel from crusting.

   (c) Incubate at room temperature (RT) until the polyacrylamide resolving gel is set (*see* **Note 3**).

   (d) Pour out the water.

   (e) Prepare a polyacrylamide stacking gel by mixing 1.3 ml 30% bis-acrylamide, 2.5 ml buffer 2, and 6.1 ml distilled H_2O. Add 50 μl of 10% ammonium persulfate and 10 μl of TEMED just prior to casting the gel.

   (f) Pour the stacking gel onto the solidified resolving gel up to the top of the glass plates; insert a plastic comb to produce wells, and allow the gel to solidify at RT.

(g) Gently remove the comb.

(h) Insert the polyacrylamide gel into the electrophoresis tank, and add running buffer to the middle compartment and to the outside compartment of the tank.

8. Mix the corresponding volume of 100 μg of each protein lysate 1:3 (v/v) with Laemmli buffer in a microtube, and heat samples to 95 °C for 5 min.
9. Briefly centrifuge the microtubes, and pipet the samples into the wells of the polyacrylamide gel. Add 8 μl of molecular weight markers to one well of the gel from control.
10. Apply 150 mV across the gel for 90 min.
11. Cut a PVDF membrane, and filter paper to the polyacrylamide gel's dimensions.
12. Activate the PVDF membrane by soaking it in methanol for 30 s and then in tap water.
13. Soak the electrophoresed gel, PVDF membrane, and all sponges, and filter paper to be used in the transfer in transfer buffer for 2 min.
14. Lay the electrophoresed gel onto the PVDF membrane, and insert the assembly into the transfer apparatus sandwiched between filter paper and a sponge layer. Prior to closing the transfer cassette, gently run a roller over the "sandwich" to expel air bubbles, which can interfere with efficient transfer of the proteins to the PVDF membrane.
15. Place the transfer assembly into the transfer tank containing ice-cold transfer buffer, ensuring the terminals are loaded in the correct orientation (i.e., cathode to cathode) (*see* **Note 4**).
16. Insert an ice block into the tank (*see* **Note 5**), and apply 110 V through the transfer apparatus for 35 min.
17. Disassemble the transfer assembly, and incubate the membrane in blocking solution on a rocker for 1 h at RT.
18. Wash the membrane three times with TBS-T for 5 min each time.
19. Apply the primary antibody diluted in blocking solution to the membrane, and incubate overnight at 4 °C on a rocker.
20. Wash the membrane three times with TBS-T for 5 min each time.
21. Apply the secondary antibody diluted in blocking solution to the membrane, and incubate for 1 h on a rocker at RT.
22. Wash the membrane three times with TBS-T for 5 min each time.
23. Prepare the ECL detection reagent by mixing equal volumes of reagent 1 and reagent 2.

24. Blot excess liquid from the membrane, and apply the ECL reagent to the protein side of the membrane. Incubate for 45 s.
25. Blot ECL detection reagent from the membrane, and wrap the membrane in Saran Wrap, ensuring that no air bubble is trapped.
26. In a dark room, tape the wrapped membrane securely in to an X-ray film cassette, and lay a sheet of X-ray Hyperfilm on top of the membrane. Close the cassette.
27. Expose the film to the membrane for an appropriate time until a good signal is found (approximately 20–30 min) (*see* **Note 6**).
28. In the dark room, remove the film from the cassette, and place it in a tank of developing fluid (1:5 dilution in water) until bands appear.
29. Transfer the film to a tank of water for 3 min to wash and then to a tank of fixer solution (1:5 dilution in water) until the cloudy background of the film appears clear.
30. Wash the film in water and allow it to dry.
31. Lay the dry film over the membrane, and mark the presence of the molecular weight markers on the film with a marker pen.

3.3 Measurement of pSMAD2 in Lung Tissue and Bronchoalveolar Lavage Cells by Multiplex Immunoassay

3.3.1 Sample Preparation

1. To prepare lung tissue:
   (a) Freeze whole lung tissue, and ground to fine powder in a pestle and mortar under liquid nitrogen.
   (b) Aliquot into tubes pre-cooled on dry ice.
   (c) Lyse 100–300 mg of frozen lung powder by addition of 0.5 ml ice-cold cell lysis buffer, and incubate on ice for 30 min during which time samples are agitated using a vortex mixer intermittently for 1 min.
2. To prepare bronchoalveolar lavage (BAL) cells:
   (a) BAL cells are easily and quickly collected by performing a bronchial wash through injecting a saline solution into the lungs and collecting the fluid, which will contain cells on collection. Collect BAL cells into ice-cold PBS containing protease and phosphatase inhibitor cocktail, and count cells using a hemocytometer.
   (b) Pellet the BAL cells by centrifugation at 350 *g* for 10 min at 4 °C.
   (c) Carefully discard the supernatant (*see* **Note 7**).
   (d) Lyse BAL cell pellets (2.5–5 × 10^5 cells) by adding 30 μl of ice-cold cell lysis buffer, and incubate on ice for 30 min during which time samples are agitated using a vortex mixer intermittently for 1 min.

3.3.2 Generation of Protein Lysates

1. Freeze lysed samples for a minimum of 30 min at −80 °C to aid cell lysis.
2. Thaw samples on ice.
3. Clarify protein lysates by centrifugation at 10,000 *g* for 5 min at 4 °C.
4. Carefully transfer supernatants to fresh, pre-chilled tubes.
5. Assess protein levels using a protein quantification kit according to the manufacturer's protocol.
6. Equalize protein lysate concentrations to 2.5 mg/ml for lung tissue samples and 0.3 mg/ml for BAL cell samples by adding appropriate volumes of ice-cold cell lysis buffer.
7. Aliquot samples and store at −80 °C.

3.3.3 Analysis of pSMAD2 Using Multiplex Immunoassay

1. Perform the Milliplex TGFβ Signaling Magnetic Bead Panel 6-plex assay according to the manufacturer's instructions and using the black Greiner 96-well plates.
2. Prepare a 7-point standard curve by making 1:3 serial dilutions of the HepG2 control lysate (in Bio-Plex kit) in assay buffer. Standard curve concentrations are 200, 66.7, 22.2, 7.4, 2.5, 0.82, and 0 μg/ml.
3. Load 12.5 μl of each sample and standard into each well, and dilute 1:1 by adding 12.5 μl Milliplex TGFβ Signaling Assay buffer. Assay all samples in triplicate.
4. Collect data on the Bio-Plex reader, with samples acquired at high RP1 target, with 50 beads per region and a sample time of 60 s.
5. Fit standard curves to a 5-parameter plot with curves optimized after the run.

3.3.4 Analysis of Total SMAD2

1. Perform the PathScan Total SMAD2 Sandwich ELISA according to the manufacturer's instructions.
2. Both BAL cells and lung samples are assayed at a dilution determined to ensure they fall within the range of the standard curve (in our studies, about 1:20 lysate/diluent). Assay all samples and standards in triplicate.
3. Prepare a 7-point standard curve by making 1:3 serial dilution of GST-SMAD2 in ELISA sample diluent. For analysis of BAL cell SMAD2 levels, the highest standard concentration is 10 ng/ml. For lung samples, the highest standard concentration is 50 ng/ml.

3.4 Measurement of pSMAD2 in Tissue by Immunohistochemistry

1. Prepare 5 μm thick formalin-fixed paraffin wax-embedded tissue sections using a microtome (*see* **Note 8**). Cut an extra slide for negative control.
2. Bake slides at 60 °C for 1 h.

3. Remove the paraffin wax from the tissue sections by placing the slides in xylene for 5 min twice.
4. Remove the xylene from the dehydrated tissue by placing the sections in 100% ethanol for 5 min twice.
5. Rehydrate the tissue sections by first placing in 70% ethanol for 5 min twice and then placing them in distilled water for 5 min twice.
6. Bring citrate buffer to boiling point using a microwave.
7. Place the tissue sections in the boiling citrate buffer, and heat in a microwave for 20 min (*see* **Notes 9** and **10**).
8. Cool the slides to RT and wash them for 3 min in PBS twice.
9. Block the endogenous peroxidase activity by placing the slides in peroxidase blocking solution for 30 min at RT.
10. Wash the slides for 3 min in PBS twice.
11. Draw a circle around the tissue sections using a hydrophobic PAP pen.
12. Incubate the sections at RT for 30 min in blocking solution by pipetting blocking solution inside the hydrophobic pen circle.
13. Add 350 μl of primary antibody to the tissue sections, and incubate overnight at 4 °C in a humidified chamber. Incubate the extra slide cut in **step 1** in blocking solution only (this is the negative control for the immunohistochemistry procedure).
14. Wash all the slides for 3 min in PBS twice.
15. Apply 350 μl of secondary antibody to the tissue sections, and incubate for 30 min at RT.
16. Wash the slides for 3 min in PBS twice.
17. Add 350 μl of ABC reagent to the slides and incubate for 30 min at RT.
18. Wash the slides for 3 min in PBS twice.
19. Incubate the slides in DAB for 5 min at RT, and then place them immediately in PBS to halt color progression.
20. Place the tissue sections are placed in Mayer's hematoxylin for 1 min at RT to counterstain the cell nuclei blue.
21. Place slides in running tap water for 1 min to remove excess hematoxylin.
22. Place the counterstained slides in PBS for 1 min to aid the formation of the blue shade in cell nuclei.
23. Dehydrate the tissue sections by sequentially placing in 70% ethanol for 5 min twice and 100% ethanol for 5 min twice.
24. Place the slides in xylene for 5 min twice to clear the ethanol from the sections.

25. Apply two small drops of mounting medium directly onto the tissue, and gently place a glass coverslip on top. Remove any trapped bubbles by carefully pressing on the coverslip with forceps to push the bubbles out from under the coverslip.

4 Notes

1. Samples can be stored at −80 °C until the assay, when they should be thawed on ice. These samples are used neatly in the assay or can be heated to 100 °C for 5 min and then cooled prior to using in the assay to determine levels of total TGFβ (i.e., latent plus active) present [17].
2. Lysed plates can be stored at −80 °C until analysis.
3. To check if polyacrylamide resolving gel is set, gently tilt the gel casting apparatus sideways: if the gel is set, the water will collect in the corner, but the gel's upper level will not move and form a straight line.
4. The SDS-denatured proteins are charged negatively. Therefore, they will migrate toward the positive pole when current is applied. The PVDF membrane should then be placed between the gel and the positively charged electrode (i.e., the anode).
5. Where not available, the transfer tank can be stood in ice to ensure the transfer stays cool.
6. The appropriate time will need to be determined empirically as membrane exposure can be repeated.
7. Cell pellets can be frozen and stored at −80 °C or processed immediately.
8. Upon cutting, ensure sections are placed on the positively charged side of the glass slides.
9. This step, called antigen retrieval, is to unmask the pSMAD2 epitopes.
10. Care must be taken to ensure the tissue remains submerged in buffer.

References

1. Dubois CM, Laprise MH, Blanchette F et al (1995) Processing of transforming growth factor beta 1 precursor by human furin convertase. J Biol Chem 270(18):10618–10624. doi:10.1074/jbc.270.18.10618
2. Saharinen J, Taipale J, Keski-Oja J (1996) Association of the small latent transforming growth factor-beta with an eight cysteine repeat of its binding protein LTBP-1. EMBO J 15(2):245–253. doi:10.1074/jbc.271.47.29891
3. Annes JP, Munger JS, Rifkin DB (2003) Making sense of latent TGFbeta activation. J Cell Sci 116(Pt 2):217–224. doi:10.1242/jcs.00229
4. Tatler AL, Jenkins G (2012) TGF-beta activation and lung fibrosis. Proc Am Thorac Soc 9(3):130–136. doi:10.1513/pats.201201-003AW
5. Schultz-Cherry S, Murphy-Ullrich JE (1993) Thrombospondin causes activation of latent trans-

forming growth factor-beta secreted by endothelial cells by a novel mechanism. J Cell Biol 122(4):923–932. doi:10.1083/jcb.122.4.923

6. Jenkins RG, Su X, Su G et al (2006) Ligation of protease-activated receptor 1 enhances alpha(v) beta6 integrin-dependent TGF-beta activation and promotes acute lung injury. J Clin Invest 116(6):1606–1614. doi:10.1172/JCI27183
7. Wipff PJ, Rifkin DB, Meister JJ et al (2007) Myofibroblast contraction activates latent TGF- 1 from the extracellular matrix. J Cell Biol 179(6):1311–1323. doi:10.1083/jcb.200704042
8. Tatler AL, John AE, Jolly L et al (2011) Integrin alphavbeta5-mediated TGF-beta activation by airway smooth muscle cells in asthma. J Immunol 187(11):6094–6107. doi:10.4049/jimmunol.1003507
9. Yang Z, Mu Z, Dabovic B et al (2007) Absence of integrin-mediated TGFbeta1 activation in vivo recapitulates the phenotype of TGFbeta1-null mice. J Cell Biol 176(6):787–793. doi:10.1083/jcb.200611044
10. Henderson NC, Arnold TD, Katamura Y et al (2013) Targeting of alphav integrin identifies a core molecular pathway that regulates fibrosis in several organs. Nat Med 19(12):1617–1624. doi:10.1038/nm.3282
11. Tatler AL, Goodwin AT, Gbolahan O et al (2016) Amplification of TGFbeta Induced ITGB6 Gene Transcription May Promote Pulmonary Fibrosis. PLoS One 11(8):e0158047. doi:10.1371/journal.pone.0158047
12. Shi M, Zhu J, Wang R et al (2011) Latent TGF-beta structure and activation. Nature 474(7351):343–349. doi:10.1038/nature10152
13. Xu MY, Porte J, Knox AJ et al (2009) Lysophosphatidic Acid Induces {alpha}v{beta}6 Integrin-Mediated TGF-{beta} Activation via the LPA2 Receptor and the Small G Protein G{alpha}q. Am J Pathol 174(4):1264–1279. doi:10.2353/ajpath.2009.080160
14. John AE, Wilson MR, Habgood A et al (2016) Loss of epithelial Gq and G11 signaling inhibits its TGFbeta production but promotes IL-33-mediated macrophage polarization and emphysema. Sci Signal 9(451):ra104. doi:10.1126/scisignal.aad5568
15. Abe M, Harpel JG, Metz CN et al (1994) An assay for transforming growth factor-beta using cells transfected with a plasminogen activator inhibitor-1 promoter-luciferase construct. Anal Biochem 216(2):276–284. doi:10.1006/abio.1994.1042
16. Munger JS, Huang X, Kawakatsu H et al (1999) The integrin alpha v beta 6 binds and activates latent TGF beta 1: a mechanism for regulating pulmonary inflammation and fibrosis. Cell 96(3):319–328
17. Tatler AL, Porte J, Knox A et al (2008) Tryptase activates TGFbeta in human airway smooth muscle cells via direct proteolysis. Biochem Biophys Res Commun 370(2):239–242. doi:10.1016/j.bbrc.2008.03.064
18. Bedke N, Sammut D, Green B et al (2012) Transforming growth factor-beta promotes rhinovirus replication in bronchial epithelial cells by suppressing the innate immune response. PLoS One 7(9):e44580. doi:10.1371/journal.pone.0044580
19. Porte J, Jenkins G (2014) Assessment of the effect of potential antifibrotic compounds on total and alphaVbeta6 integrin-mediated TGF-beta activation. Pharmacol Res Perspect 2(4):e00030. doi:10.1002/prp2.30
20. Jolly L, Stavrou A, Vanderstoken G et al (2014) Influenza Promotes Collagen Deposition via alphavbeta6-integrin Mediated Transforming Growth Factor beta Activation. J Biol Chem. doi:10.1074/jbc.M114.582262
21. Tatler AL, Barnes J, Habgood A et al (2016) Caffeine inhibits TGFbeta activation in epithelial cells, interrupts fibroblast responses to TGFbeta, and reduces established fibrosis in ex vivo precision-cut lung slices. Thorax 71(6):565–567. doi:10.1136/thoraxjnl-2015-208215

Chapter 24

Visualizing In Vitro Type I Collagen Fibrillogenesis by Transmission Electron Microscopy

J. Robin Harris

Abstract

Techniques and protocols for the in vitro formation of collagen type I fibrils and the extensive biochemical variation of the fibrillogenesis conditions are presented. In all cases, the incubation and fibrillogenesis product can be readily monitored by transmission electron microscopic study of negatively stained specimens. Representative TEM data is presented and discussed within the context of the products of the fibrillogenesis protocols, from which the extensive biochemical and structural possibilities of this integrated approach can be appreciated.

Key words Collagen type I, Heterotrimer, Fibrillogenesis, Negative staining, Electron microscopy, D-Banded fibril, Tactoid, Segment long spacing (SLS) crystallite, ATP, Polyphosphate, Sulfonated diazo dye

1 Introduction

The formation in vitro of D-banded paracrystalline fibrils from type I collagen (D refers to the ~67 nm linear periodic distance), using acid-soluble solubilized collagen heterotrimers on transferring to a physiological saline solution, has long been established. Structurally these fibrils are essentially identical to those found in vivo. However, investigation of the detail of early heterotrimer association leading to fibril formation has been neglected until recent years. This applies to both in vitro fibril formation in physiological saline solutions and in other more experimental conditions (i.e., variation of ionic constituents, ionic strength, pH, time, and temperature), leading to similar, intermediate, or deviant fibrillar forms. With the present widespread use of collagen as a coating agent for cell culture and in the cosmetics industry, together with the expansion of biotechnological and biomedical applications of collagen and the understanding of bone mineralization, such investigations could well yield fundamental data of considerable importance. Thus, although biochemical manipulation of collagen fibrillogenesis in a controlled

Laure Rittié (ed.), *Fibrosis: Methods and Protocols*, Methods in Molecular Biology, vol. 1627,
DOI 10.1007/978-1-4939-7113-8_24, © Springer Science+Business Media LLC 2017

manner has been somewhat neglected, in this chapter a number of lines of investigation will be presented, some of which could well be expanded upon further in the future. Most significant within this context is the segment long spacing (SLS) crystallite form, created under mildly acidic conditions by adenosine triphosphate (ATP). This established SLS form consists of a lateral association of collagen heterotrimers, creating discrete ~300 nm long rodlike bundles with a markedly different banding pattern to that of the D-banded collagen fibril. Nevertheless, this SLS banding pattern correlates well with the widely accepted partial heterotrimer overlap and spacing model for the three-dimensional organization of rigid heterotrimers within the D-banded collagen fibril.

Although the methods presented here are devoted to collagen type I alone, it can be anticipated that other members of the collagen superfamily could be likewise investigated using biochemical manipulation, singly, in combination and with other extracellular matrix proteins. Collagen fibrils were one of the first biological samples to be studied in the 1950s by TEM. As a high-resolution X-ray structure of collagen fibrils has yet to emerge, despite much progress from synthetic collagen-like peptides, the transmission electron microscope (TEM) continues to make a major structural contribution alongside other biophysical techniques.

The author has successfully utilized TEM of negatively stained specimens for the study of numerous macromolecules, including collagen, for many years [1–3]. In the hands of others, atomic force microscopy (AFM) has also come into widespread usage for the study of collagen fibrils [4, 5], but in general the TEM possesses a superior macromolecular resolution, and negative staining provides the possibility of rapidly preparing multiple specimens for subsequent TEM study.

In this methodological chapter, protocols for the in vitro creation of collagen type I fibrillogenesis under a range of different conditions will be presented, along with representative TEM data from negatively stained specimens and referencing to relevant literature. Application of this approach to other members of the large family of collagen isoforms will not be included here, while not diminishing their likely future relevance.

The availability of a reliable source of purified material is essential for studies on collagen fibrillogenesis. Fortunately, several commercial companies (e.g., SERVA Electrophoresis, Sigma, BD Biosciences, EPC, IBIDI, GIBCO) produce an acid-soluble collagen type I product still containing the N- and C-terminal telopeptides, as well as a pepsin-treated product with the telopeptides removed. Synthetic collagen-like polymer polypeptides are also available (BIO/DATA Corporation). Alternatively, investigators can easily prepare acid-soluble collagen type I with all of the above characteristics, as detailed in Chapter 19 of this volume. The stability of purified acid-soluble collagen type I in 0.1% acetic acid (2–4 mg/ml) is excellent, facilitating 4 °C storage prior to aliquoting for laboratory use.

2 Materials

2.1 Biochemistry

1. Rat tail collagen type I (Collagen R 2.0 mg/ml sterile solution in 0.1% acetic acid, SERVA Electrophoresis) (*see* **Note 1**). Store in refrigerator.
2. Routine laboratory reagents can be purchased from Sigma-Aldrich or an alternative reliable supplier.
3. 1 M Tris–HCl pH 8.0 and 7.5 prepared by the careful addition of concentrated HCl, while adjusting the pH using a pH meter. Store at room temperature.
4. 100 mM glycine–HCl pH 2.5 buffer prepared by the addition of 1.0 M HCl while adjusting pH using a pH meter. Store at room temperature.
5. Glacial acetic acid (~17.5 M): prepare aqueous dilutions to required % (v/v) or molarity.
6. 100 mM phosphate buffer pH 7.5: prepared from sodium phosphate monobasic and dibasic by mixing correct proportions as indicated in a standard table, with final pH adjustment using a pH meter. Store in refrigerator.
7. 100 mM citrate–phosphate buffer pH 6.0: prepared from citric acid and dibasic sodium phosphate by mixing correct proportions as defined in a standard table, and check with a pH meter. Store in refrigerator.
8. 1.0 M sodium chloride aqueous solution. Store at room temperature.
9. 1X and 3X phosphate-buffered saline (PBS). Store in refrigerator.
10. 100 mM sodium tri(poly)phosphate. Store frozen as 100 μl aliquots.
11. 100 mM sodium ATP. Store frozen as 100 μl aliquots.
12. Diazo dyes: prepare 100 mM aqueous stock solutions of Congo red, Direct red 80 (Sirius red), Evans blue, and methyl blue, and store at room temperature.

2.2 Electron Microscopy

1. The number of small materials required for preparing negatively stained specimens is considerable and can be best appreciated by direct observation of the technique within an EM laboratory or by reference to published works [1, 6].
2. 2% uranyl acetate (w/v) (Agar Scientific (*see* **Note 2**)). Store at room temperature (*see* **Note 3**).

3. 2% ammonium molybdate (w/v) (Agar Scientific (*see* **Note 2**)) pH 6.9: adjust pH using 1.0 M NaOH under a pH meter. Store at room temperature.

3 Methods

3.1 Negative Staining

A detailed protocol for negative staining can be found in ref. [6]. Specimens are prepared on EM grids covered by a glow discharge-treated thin carbon support film, with adsorption of the collagen samples followed by distilled water washing, droplet negative staining, and rapid air-drying. It is desirable to study specimen grids in a TEM as rapidly as possible, particularly for grids negatively stained with ammonium molybdate. Specimen grids negatively stained with uranyl acetate have been found to be stable over many months.

3.2 Formation of D-Banded Collagen Type I Fibrils

Procedures for the formation of fibrils from purified collagen have been available for many years. Technical variations are numerous, but the procedure given below is based upon the use of buffered NaCl solutions (*see* **Note 4**); an established alternative using phosphate buffer alone is available [7]. The use of slow dialysis versus direct rapid dilution of the acetic acid solution of high-concentration collagen (2.0 mg/ml) into buffered saline has always to be considered. The procedure given below will, in the main, use direct dilution.

1. To a 2 ml polypropylene microcentrifuge tube, add 200 μl 1 M NaCl, followed by 20 μl 1 M Tris–HCl (pH 7.5) buffer.
2. Make the volume to 990 μl with deionized water followed by 10 μl of the collagen stock solution (*see* **Note 5**). Mix well by repeatedly inverting the tube, followed by incubation at room temperature for 24 h or longer (*see* **Notes 6** and 7).
3. Take aliquots for the preparation of negatively stained specimens and then store the tube at 4 °C.
4. Study the grids containing negatively stained specimens in an appropriate TEM and record digital images. D-banded spindle-shaped fibrils and multi-fibril fibers with aligned D-bands should be readily detected (Fig. 1 and Subheading 3.4).

3.3 Collagen Type I Fibrillogenesis Under Varying Experimental Conditions

The number of parameters that can be varied when performing collagen fibrillogenesis is considerable, e.g., protein concentration, ionic strength, NaCl concentration, buffer type and concentration, pH, time of incubation, temperature, etc. This biochemical approach was introduced by Harris and Reiber [2] and expanded upon by Harris et al. [3]. Two generalized protocols will be given below, within which the user can readily adjust the different parameters for collagen type I and other collagen isoforms, as desired.

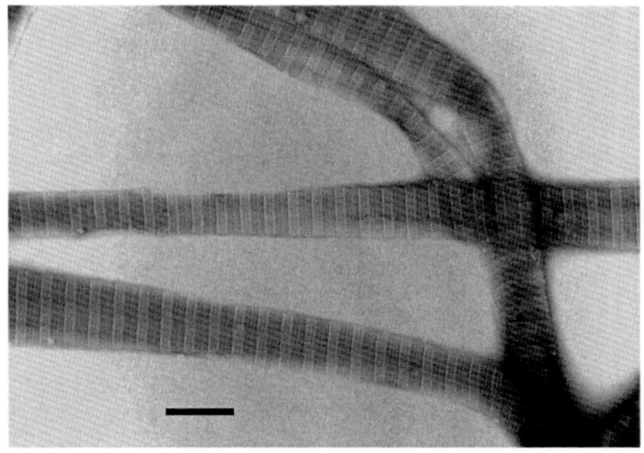

Fig. 1 Acetic acid-soluble collagen type I following pH adjustment to 7.0 with phosphate-buffered 150 mM NaCl and 24 h incubation. Mature D-banded collagen fibers are shown. Each mature D-banded fiber is composed of closely adhering transversely aligned spindle-shaped fibrils. Negatively stained with 2% uranyl acetate. The scale bar indicates 200 nm. From Harris and Reiber [2] with the permission of Elsevier Science

For multiple samples, the direct rapid addition of collagen to a 1 ml test volume is more convenient than dialysis of a diluted collagen sample against a large volume of buffered saline solution. However, when concentrating on the fibrillar end product rather than assembly intermediates, slow dialysis of a 1.0 mg/ml solution of the acid-soluble collagen against a large volume of buffer solution is also appropriate [2].

3.3.1 Formation of Collagen D-Banded Tactoid Fibers

Spindle-shaped collagen tactoid fibers containing an oblique packing of D-banded fibrils have been documented in the literature [8]. Their formation has also been encountered under different conditions when performing experimental fibrillogenesis with variation of NaCl and Tris–HCl concentration and pH [2].

1. To a short length of well-soaked dialysis tubing, add 100 μl of 1.0 mg/ml collagen solution and seal the two ends.
2. Dialyze 24 h against 500 or 1000 ml 150 mM NaCl, 10 mM citrate–phosphate buffer (pH 6.0).
3. Remove dialyzed sample from tubing and store at 4 °C.
4. Take 20 μl aliquots for the preparation of negatively stained EM specimens.
5. Study specimen grids in a TEM and record digital images (*see* Fig. 2 and Subheading 3.4).

3.3.2 Variation of NaCl Concentration During Collagen Fibrillogenesis

Increase of the NaCl concentration over the range 10–500 mM during fibrillogenesis provides information on the role of NaCl or Tris–HCl (more specifically the chloride anion) during collagen heterotrimer assembly into pre-fibrillar and fibrillar assemblies.

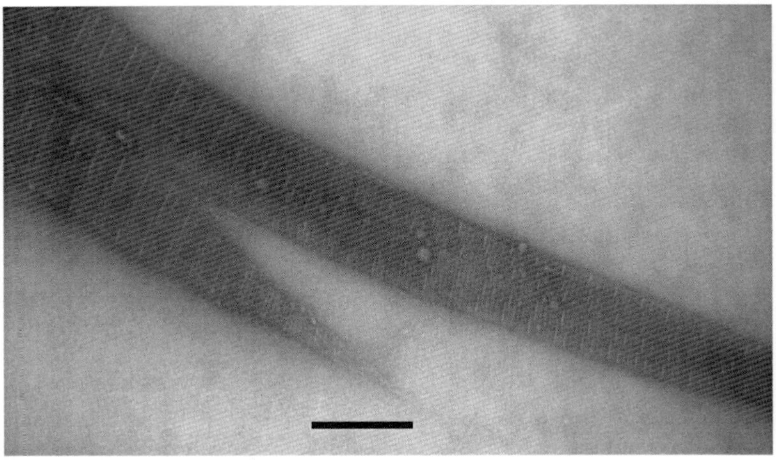

Fig. 2 Acetic acid-soluble collagen type I following adjustment of the pH to 6.0 with citrate–phosphate buffer in the presence of 150 mM NaCl. Deviant spindle-shaped D-banded collagen fiber tactites are shown, within which there is lateral misalignment of the D-banding between adjacent fibrils. Negatively stained with 2% uranyl acetate (cf. Figs. 3d, 5d, and 6). The scale bar indicates 200 nm. From Harris and Reiber [2] with the permission of Elsevier Science

In addition, variation of pH can be introduced, leading to numerous possibilities [3].

1. Set up series of 2 ml polypropylene microcentrifuge tubes containing 1 ml 10–500 mM NaCl in 10 or 20 mM phosphate buffer (pH 7.5).
2. To each tube add 10 μl 2.0 mg/ml collagen type I solution (final concentration 0.02 mg/ml), and rapidly mix by inversion.
3. Incubate the tubes at room temperature for 24 h.
4. Take 20 μl aliquots for the preparation of negatively stained specimens.
5. Study specimens in a TEM and record digital images. Representative data is shown in Fig. 3 (also *see* Subheading 3.4).

3.4 Collagen Type I Segment Long Spacing (SLS) Crystallite Formation

3.4.1 Collagen Type I SLS Crystallite Formation by ATP Treatment

As with D-banded collagen fibril formation in vitro, an established low-pH ATP procedure for producing the characteristic ~300 nm SLS crystallite (a rodlike parallel bundle of aligned heterotrimers) has been available for many years [9]. Similarly, it is of biochemical and structural interest to know the fibrillogenesis outcome following the use of a range of modified parameters when performing collagen-ATP treatment.

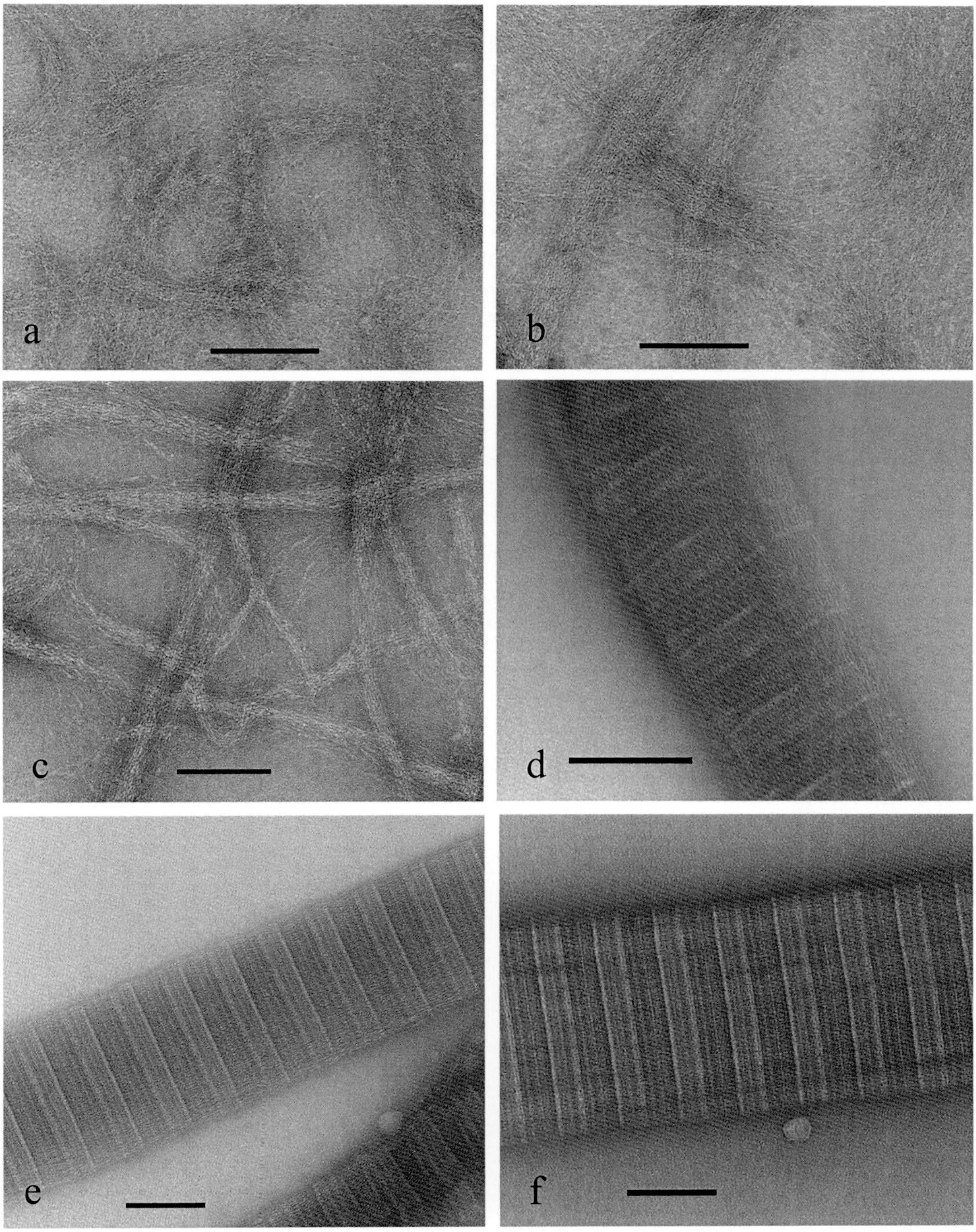

Fig. 3 Collagen type I fibrillogenesis in the presence of increasing concentrations of NaCl in 10 mM phosphate buffer, pH 7.0. (**a**, **b**) At low concentrations of NaCl (10 and 20 mM, respectively), initial aggregates show early indications of banding and form diffuse pre-fibrils. (**c**) In 50 mM NaCl, more compact pre-fibrils show a clearer indication of preliminary banding. (**d**) In 75 mM NaCl, faintly banded fibrils cluster into multi-fibril fibers that display a disordered diffuse D-banding, due to misaligned fibrils. Note the absence of free heterotrimers on the background, indicating efficient incorporation into fibrils. (**e**) In 100 mM NaCl, the characteristic ~67 nm collagen D-banding of tightly packed multi-fibril collagen fibers predominates. (**f**) In 500 mM NaCl, the clarity of the collagen D-banding and the intermediate banding is even more sharply pronounced, within well-formed compact multi-fibril collagen fibers. Negatively stained with 2% uranyl acetate. The scale bars indicate 100 nm. From Harris et al. [3] with the permission of Elsevier Science

Standard Treatment of Collagen with 1 mM ATP at Low pH

The low-pH treatment of collagen with ATP (a polyphosphate) to generate SLS crystallites is a remarkable and currently not fully exploited or explained phenomenon. Although the presence of collagen SLS crystallites in vivo is extremely rare, the fact that the initially flexible acetic acid-soluble collagen heterotrimer is transformed into a more rigid structure and able to aggregate as a series of N-/C-terminal aligned molecules must indicate specific/strong polyanion-binding properties. This in turn may relate to the likely chloride anion binding by collagen under physiological in vivo and in vitro conditions in the presence of an optimal NaCl concentration (*see* Subheading 3.2, **step 1**) to generate D-banded fibrils.

1. To a 2 ml polypropylene microcentrifuge tube, add 1 ml deionized water and 10 μl of 100 mM sodium ATP (check pH of 1 mM ATP, or alternative concentration, using narrow-range pH paper; pH 2.5–3.0 is desirable; if too close to neutral, add a small volume of 0.1% acetic acid or 100 mM glycine–HCl buffer pH 2.5).
2. Add 10 μl 2.0 mg/ml collagen type I solution in 0.1% acetic acid.
3. Incubate the solution for 2 h at room temperature (*see* **Note 8**).
4. Take 20 μl aliquots for the preparation of negatively stained specimens.
5. Study specimen grids in a TEM and record digital images. Representative SLS images are shown in Fig. 4 (also *see* Subheading 3.4 and **Note 9**).

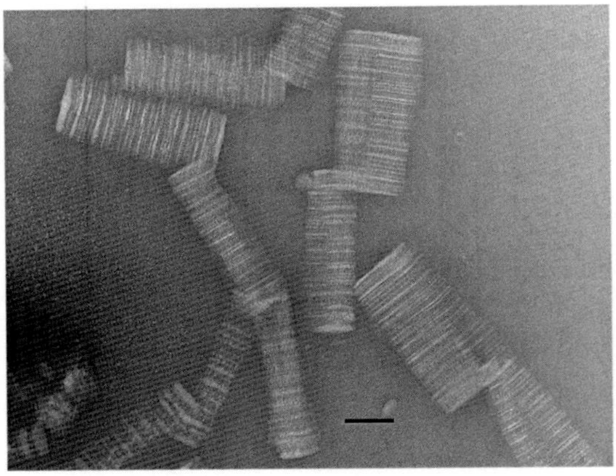

Fig. 4 Characteristic collagen type I 300 nm SLS banded crystallites formed in the presence of 1 mM ATP at low pH (pH 2.5–3.5). Each SLS crystallite is formed by the aggregation of a number of thinner SLS rods. Some misalignment is apparent (*top left*). Negatively stained with 2% uranyl acetate. The scale bar indicates 100 nm. From Harris and Lewis [14] with the permission of Elsevier Science

Collagen Treatment with ATP Under Varying pH Conditions

Apart from the variation of ATP concentration at low pH (pH 2.5), it is also of interest to show the different collagen aggregation states that are produced at progressively higher pH, e.g., in the presence of 1 mM ATP (up to pH 8.0).

1. Set up a series of 2 ml polypropylene microcentrifuge tubes containing 1 ml 1 mM ATP.
2. Adjust the pH of solution in each tube to give a pH range 2.5–7.5 by the addition of small volumes of 100 mM glycine–HCl (pH 2.5) or 100 mM Tris–HCl (pH 8.0). Check the pH by withdrawing a 2 μl aliquot and application to narrow-range pH paper.
3. Add 10 μl 2.0 mg/ml collagen type I in 0.1% acetic acid and mix. Recheck the pH and adjust as required.
4. Incubate for 24 h at room temperature.
5. Take 20 μl aliquots for the preparation of negatively stained specimens.
6. Study the specimen grids in a TEM and record digital images. Representative data is shown in Figs. 5 and 6, and *see* Subheading 3.4.

3.4.2 Collagen Type I SLS Crystallite Formation by Sulfonated Diazo Dye Treatment

Several sulfonated diazo dyes are known to histochemically stain collagen fibrils and amyloid fibrils within tissues, but little knowledge is available as to their reaction with in vitro-formed fibrils in solution. Using preformed collagen type I fibrils to investigate this situation, the unexpected formation of SLS-like aggregates has been detected in the presence of certain diazo dyes but only in the presence of a higher than usual NaCl concentration. The dyes Direct red (Sirius red) and Evans blue apparently dissociate collagen fibers into SLS structures, whereas Congo red and methyl blue split collagen fibers into individual fibrils (*see* **Note 10**).

1. Prepare collagen type I D-banded fibrils/fibers in 500 mM NaCl 20 mM Tris–HCl buffer (pH 7.5) as in Subheading 3.1 (*see* **Note 11**).
2. Using a 0.1 ml aliquot of the collagen fibril solution, add 10 μl 1.0 mM Direct red or Evans blue (diluted from stock solution with deionized water), and mix by repeated inversion.
3. Incubate tubes overnight at room temperature, and then take 20 μl aliquots for the preparation of negatively stained specimens (*see* **Note 12**).
4. Study specimen grids in a TEM and record digital images (Fig. 7). The presence of sheetlike SLS aggregates, composed of a number of aligned ~17 nm banded SLS rods, ~300 nm in length (cf. [10]), should be readily detected for comparison with the ATP and sodium tri(poly)phosphate-induced collagen type I SLS crystallites (Fig. 8).

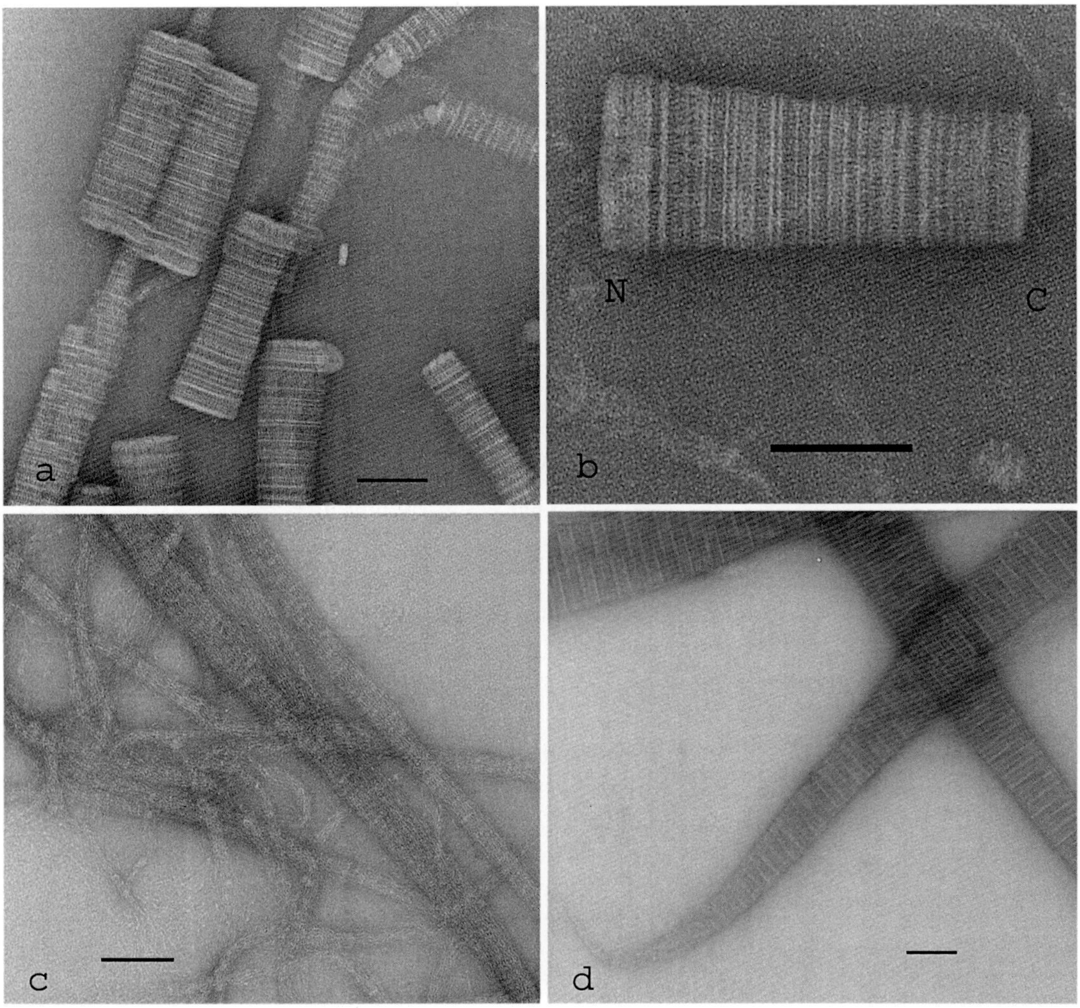

Fig. 5 Collagen type I interaction with 1 mM ATP at increasing pH, with incubation for 24 h at 22 °C. (**a**) At low pH (pH 2.5), characteristic 300 nm SLS crystallites readily form, with a tendency to link together as a network. (**b**) Higher-magnification image of a single SLS crystallite, with the heterotrimer C- and N-terminal orientation indicated (following Kobayashi et al. [13]). Note the well-defined asymmetric banding pattern along the SLS crystallite, with respect to heterotrimer orientation. (**c**) At pH 5.0, the collagen molecules aggregate in a more fibrillar manner, with the creation of loosely associated pre-fibrils and fibrils showing an indication of D-banding. (**d**) At pH 7.0, the collagen molecules associate to form ~67 nm D-banded fibrils that aggregate as spindle-shaped fiber structures, sometimes termed tactoids. Note that within these tactoids, the banding of individual D-banded fibrils tends to be longitudinally misaligned with respect to one another within the fiber bundle, unlike typical D-banded collagen fibers (cf. Figs. 2d and 6). All images are negatively stained with 2% (w/v) uranyl acetate. The scale bars indicate 100 nm. From Harris and Lewis [14] with the permission of Elsevier Science

3.5 Technical Comments and Discussion of the Collagen Negative Stain TEM Data

From the above series of closely related protocols, it will be readily appreciated that a large number of technical variations can readily be introduced around any one set of conditions or treatments. This can lead to a large number of TEM specimens and the

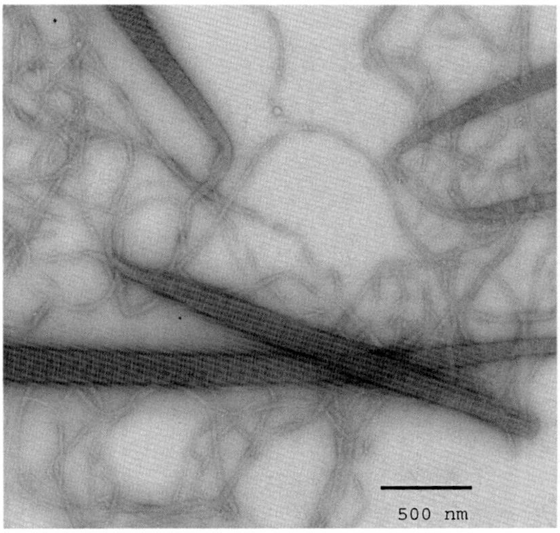

Fig. 6 Collagen type I treated with 1 mM ATP at pH 7.0 for 24 h (as in Fig. 5d), shown at lower-magnification D-banded tactoid fibers, surrounded by unincorporated pre-fibrillar aggregates. Negatively stained with 2% (w/v) uranyl acetate

accumulation of many images. It is only by assessing the reproducibility of the data from any one set of biochemical conditions that the experimenter can place faith upon the validity of the TEM data produced. Nevertheless, the constant minor modification of such protocols, with accumulated experience, is the essence of experimental advancement, leading to new data.

An understanding of the limitations of negative stain TEM specimen preparation, particularly with respect to the stability of SLS structures, is important. In the future, it is likely that unstained frozen-hydrated collagen specimen will be produced from such fibrillogenesis experiments as presented above, but the limitation here may be the reduced number of specimen grids that can be conveniently studied by cryoEM compared to those that have been negatively stained, air-dried, and studied by TEM under ambient conditions. However, the more successful samples can be selected by negative staining and subsequently used for the preparation of a reduced number of cryo-specimens [1].

The ionic and pH conditions for preparing ~67 nm D-banded collagen fibrils and aligned multi-fibril fibers in vitro (Fig. 1) have been well defined and have provided material for numerous biological, biomedical, and biotechnological studies. The deviant tactoid fibers formed under less optimal conditions (Fig. 2) contain misaligned D-banded fibrils that impart oblique banding pattern to the multi-fibril fiber [2, 8]. Remarkably, similar tactoid forms can also be formed in the presence of 1 mM ATP at neutral pH (Figs. 5 and 6), underlying the greater collagen heterotrimer reactivity with the polyphosphate group, compared to the chloride anion under in vitro

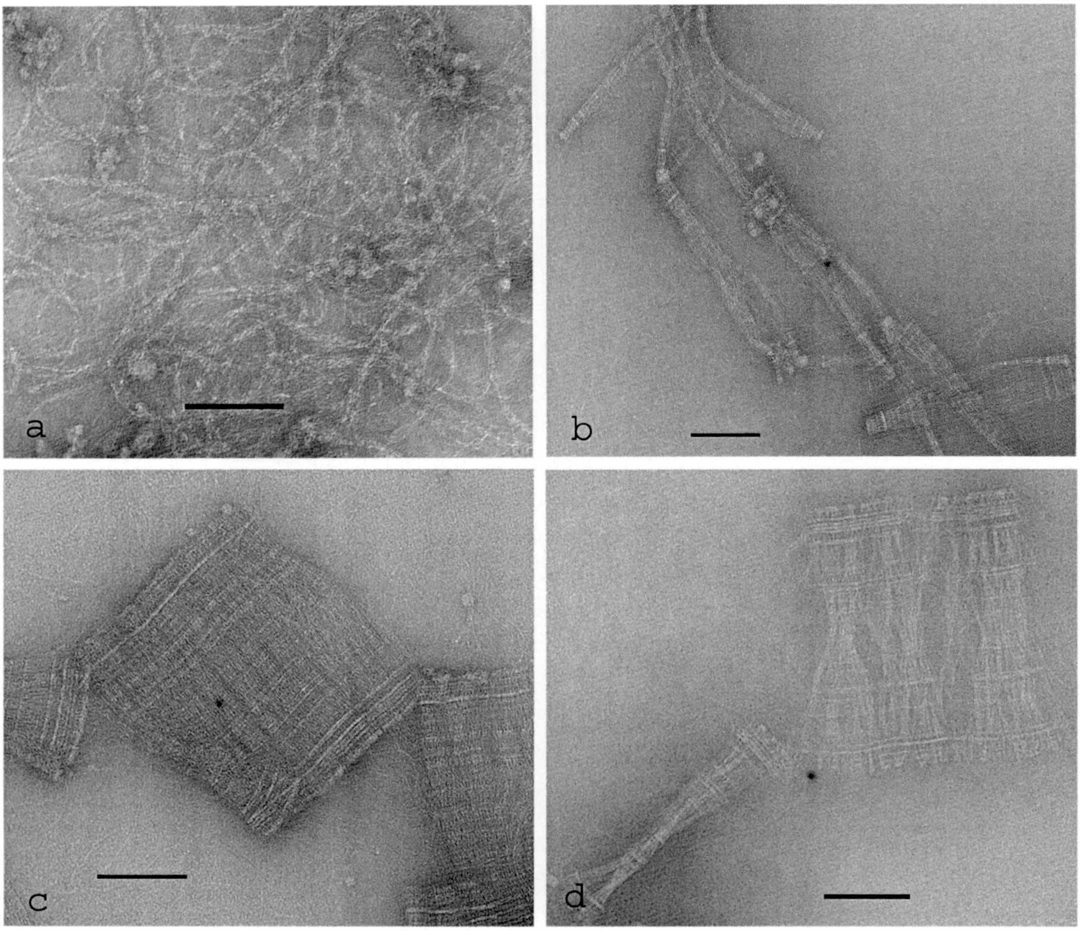

Fig. 7 Collagen type I interaction with the hexasulfonated diazo dye Direct red 80/Sirius red. (**a**) The addition of 0.1 mM Direct red 80 to collagen type I at pH 2.5 for 24 h induced the formation of a disordered fibrillar pigmented flocculate, with no indication of banding. (**b**) Preformed D-banded collagen fibrils in 500 mM NaCl, 20 mM Tris–HCl at pH 7.5 treated with 0.1 mM Direct red 80 for 15 min at 22 °C. The early stage of collagen aggregation into thin SLS-like bundles is shown. (**c**) Preformed D-banded collagen fibrils in 500 mM NaCl, 20 mM Tris–HCl at pH 7.5, treated with 0.1 mM Direct red 80 for 24 h at 22 °C. Sheetlike SLS structures are present, which appear to be aggregates of the thinner SLS rods shown in (**b**). (**d**) As for (**c**), but negatively stained with 5% (w/v) ammonium molybdate 0.1% trehalose (pH 7.0), showing splaying out of an SLS-like sheet in to individual bundles and also collagen heterotrimers. This suggests destabilization of the SLS structures due to a combination of the repeated water washing and ammonium molybdate negative staining of the specimen grid. Images (**a**–**c**) were negatively stained with 2% (w/v) uranyl acetate. The scale bars indicate 100 nm. From Harris and Lewis [14] with the permission of Elsevier Science

and in vivo physiological conditions, where a much higher molarity (e.g., 150 mM) is required. This is exemplified by performing collagen type I fibrillogenesis with progressively increasing NaCl concentrations at neutral pH as shown in Fig. 3. Here the progressive formation of pre-fibrillar aggregates, containing loosely adhering collagen heterotrimers (Fig. 3a–c), to faintly D-banded fibrils

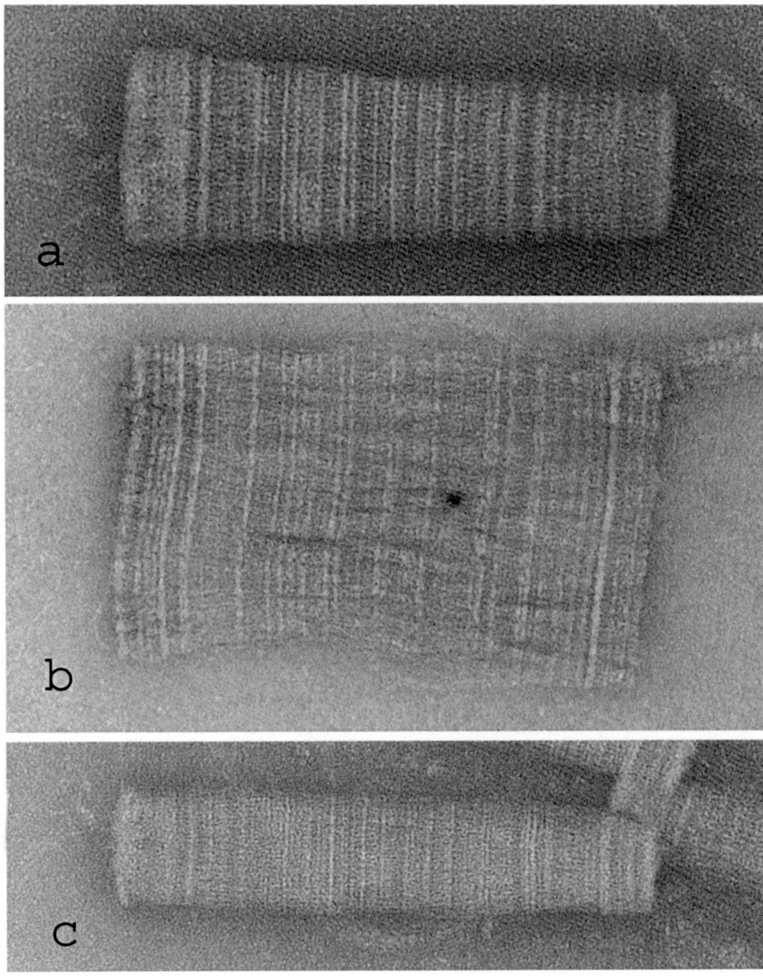

Fig. 8 A direct comparison of collagen type I SLS crystallites, formed (**a**) in the presence of 1 mM ATP, (**b**) 0.1 mM Direct red 80, and (**c**) 1.0 mM sodium tri(poly) phosphate (NaTP). The variation in the intensity of the SLS banding pattern is an indication of the different molecular mass contribution of these discretely bound collagen heterotrimer-linking reagents, within the banded SLS structures. All images negatively stained with 2% (w/v) uranyl acetate. The SLS length is ~300 nm. From Harris and Lewis [14] with the permission of Elsevier Science

(Fig. 3d) and clearly D-banded fibrils and fibers at higher NaCl concentrations (Fig. 3e, f) within which the more tightly associated heterotrimers create the main 67 nm D-banding together with the clear sequence of intermediate bands, all due to the linear partial overlap and spacing pattern of the heterotrimers and their superimposition within the individual fibrils (*see* **Note 13**).

The collagen type I segment long spacing (SLS) crystallite is an alternative experimentally induced aggregate or fibrillogenesis form, within which a number of collagen heterotrimers are all aligned side by side as 300 nm compact rodlike structures.

Although defined in the 1950s, this aggregation state has not been fully analyzed in structural terms using the more highly purified collagen products currently available and might yet be of some significance for the final understanding of the anion-binding properties of collagen and the formation of the D-banded fibril. In Fig. 4, typical 1 mM ATP-induced SLS crystallites formed at low pH are shown, within which a discrete series of bands are apparent, due to the superimposition of bulky positively charged amino acid side chains within the heterotrimer, together with their bound ATP. Unexpectedly, an increase of the pH of the 1 mM ATP solution leads to more usual D-banded fibrils as neutral pH is approached (Fig. 5), as mentioned above. As with the saline-induced fibrillogenesis studies, variation of ATP concentration and time dependency, as well as the use of other polyphosphates, can yield information on intermediate SLS assembly forms. A wide range of sulfonated diazo dyes are known to bind to fibrillar collagen, but in solution under acidic conditions, only a disordered heterotrimer aggregate is produced (Fig. 7a). However, when D-banded fibrils or the collagen heterotrimer solution is treated in the presence of a high NaCl concentration at neutral pH (e.g., 500 mM or 3X PBS), sheetlike SLS crystallites are formed, clearly composed of a number of thin SLS rods (Fig. 7b, c). The SLS banding pattern shown here, due to the presence of bound Direct red 80 in this instance, correlates well with the SLS banding pattern of ATP and sodium tri(poly)phosphate-induced SLS, as shown in Fig. 8. The variation of banding intensity is a reflection of the varying mass of the three bound polyanionic reagents, together with some variation in SLS thickness. The thinner sheetlike SLS aggregates induced by Direct red 80 closely resemble those produced from pepsin-digested collagen type I in the presence of ATP, as shown by a number of authors.

Dissociation of these dye-induced or ATP-induced SLS structures readily occurs likely due to loss of bound dye or ATP, following water washing (to remove the NaCl and unbound dye during specimen preparation) prior to negative staining of the carbon-adsorbed protein. This is particularly apparent when ammonium molybdate is used as the negative stain (Fig. 7d), where the individual relatively straight/rigid collagen heterotrimers can be seen [14], unlike the flexuous soluble heterotrimers initially present in the 0.1% acetic acid solution [3]. Unlike the cationic negative stain uranyl acetate, anionic ammonium molybdate does not impart a rapid stabilizing effect on protein structure [11]. Prior stabilization of SLS structures with 0.1% (v/v) glutaraldehyde prevents procedurally induced dissociation during negative staining. Overall, the data presented emphasize the value of negative staining for the structural assessment of collagen fibrillogenesis and indeed for other fibrous proteins.

4 Notes

1. Although purified collagen type I from man and other species is available from several companies, the user should give attention to the extraction procedures employed. Acetic acid extraction will leave the collagen terminal telopeptides intact, whereas subsequent pepsin treatment will remove the telopeptides, known to be important for heterotrimer crosslinking and D-banded fibril formation. However, pepsin-digested collagen type I is able to form segment long spacing (SLS) structures.
2. Apart from Agar Scientific, there are a number of readily accessible suppliers worldwide for EM consumables, e.g., Ted Pella Inc., SPI Supplies, TAAB Laboratories and Equipment Ltd, and NanoSolutions Pte Ltd.
3. Do not seal tubes containing uranyl acetate solution with aluminum foil (which will decompose if contact occurs). Due to the low-level radioactivity of uranyl acetate, appropriate handling and disposal should be adopted.
4. The NaCl concentration used will generally be in the range 100–200 mM, and the pH can be controlled with 20 mM Tris–HCl or phosphate buffer (pH 7.5). Standard phosphate-buffered saline (PBS) solution can also be used.
5. The acetic acid concentration will now be reduced to 0.001% and buffered by the 20 mM Tris–HCl. The pH can be checked using narrow-range pH paper.
6. Incubation of the collagen solution can be done at varying temperatures. Fibril formation will be more rapid at higher temperatures, i.e., 37 °C. In general, avoid refrigeration and low room temperatures. Incubation for 24 h should enable most if not all the collagen heterotrimers to be incorporated into the fibrils.
7. As an alternative to rapid mixing, a 1.0 mg/ml collagen solution can be dialyzed for 24 h against a large volume (1:1000) of PBS or 200 mM NaCl, 20 mM Tris–HCl (pH 7.5). In general, the aim here is to achieve a high level of fibril formation rather than incomplete formation. The latter can more readily be addressed using alternative salt concentrations and pH (*see* Subheading 3.3.2)
8. A time-dependent study of SLS formation has revealed that they do indeed form extremely rapidly (fully formed SLS crystallites are present by 10 min, with little background protein). An ATP concentration range (e.g., 0.1–10.0 mM) can readily be performed, from which the intermediate assemblies underlying SLS formation can be defined (data not shown) [14].
9. Other nucleoside triphosphates and sodium tri(poly)phosphate are as effective as ATP for collagen SLS formation,

whereas a number of other phosphate compounds such as fructose 1,6-diphosphate and perdisulfuric acid are less effective [12].

10. It is significant that diazo dye treatment of the acetic acid solution of collagen heterotrimers at low pH does not produce SLS structures, as is the case with ATP; here a disordered fine fibrillar aggregate is produced (Fig. 7a), as also shown for Amaranth and Cibacron blue [10].

11. Alternatively, direct addition of 0.1 mM Direct red 80 or Evans blue to diluted acid-soluble collagen in 500 mM NaCl, 20 mM Tris–HCl (pH 7.5) or collagen in 3X PBS will also produce SLS aggregates. The use of lower ionic strength saline does not facilitate SLS formation.

12. Apparently the level of sulfonation of the diazo dye is critical for collagen fibril dissociation for SLS formation, as will be the dye concentration. Direct red possesses six sulfonic acid groups, Evans blue has four, and methyl blue has three and Congo red two. Other diazo dyes such as Amaranth, Cibacron blue, Coomassie blue, Ponceau S, and trypan blue have not yet been studied in the system presented.

13. The reader will readily appreciate the fact that the range of possibilities for varying the fibrillogenesis conditions for collagen type I alone is quite enormous. If extended to the fibrillogenesis of other members of the collagen superfamily, proteolytic fragments, gene products, and synthetic collagen-like peptides and to their interaction with extracellular matrix proteins, the biochemical manipulation presented here could have future value.

Acknowledgments

This and related work was performed by the author as a scientific staff member in the laboratories of the Institute of Zoology, University of Mainz, Germany, with the support of Professor Juergen Markl, and also in retirement using equipment in EM Research Services at Newcastle University, UK, with the support of Professor Richard J. Lewis, Institute of Cellular and Molecular Biosciences.

References

1. Harris JR, Royal Microscopical S (1997) Negative staining and cryoelectron microscopy: the thin film techniques. BIOS Scientific Publishers in association with the Royal Microscopical Society, Oxford, UK

2. Harris JR, Reiber A (2007) Influence of saline and pH on collagen type I fibrillogenesis in vitro: fibril polymorphism and colloidal gold labelling. Micron 38(5):513–521. doi:10.1016/j.micron.2006.07.026

3. Harris JR, Soliakov A, Lewis RJ (2013) In vitro fibrillogenesis of collagen type I in varying ionic and pH conditions. Micron 49:60–68. doi:10.1016/j.micron.2013.03.004
4. Loo RW, Goh JB, Cheng CC et al (2012) In vitro synthesis of native, fibrous long spacing and segmental long spacing collagen. J Vis Exp 67:e4417. doi:10.3791/4417
5. Fang M, Holl MM (2013) Variation in type I collagen fibril nanomorphology: the significance and origin. Bonekey Rep 2:394. doi:10.1038/bonekey.2013.128
6. Harris JR, De Carlo S (2014) Negative staining and cryo-negative staining: applications in biology and medicine. In: Kuo J (ed) Electron microscopy: methods and protocols. Humana, Totowa, NJ, pp 215–258. doi:10.1007/978-1-62703-776-1_11
7. Holmes DF, Kadler KE (2006) Collagen fibril assembly in vitro. In: Harris JR, Graham JM, Rickwood D (eds) Cell biology protocols. John Wiley & Sons, Chichester, pp 375–378
8. Bruns RR (1976) Supramolecular structure of polymorphic collagen fibrils. J Cell Biol 68(3):521–538
9. Gross J, Highberger JH, Schmitt FO (1954) Collagen structures considered as states of aggregation of a kinetic unit. The tropocollagen particle. Proc Natl Acad Sci U S A 40(8):679–688
10. Paige MF, Goh MC (2001) Ultrastructure and assembly of segmental long spacing collagen studied by atomic force microscopy. Micron 32(3):355–361. doi:10.1016/S0968-4328(00)00038-X
11. Zhao FQ, Craig R (2003) Capturing time-resolved changes in molecular structure by negative staining. J Struct Biol 141(1):43–52. doi:10.1016/S1047-8477(02)00546-4
12. Bowden JK, Chapman JA, Wynn CH (1968) Precipitation of collagen in the segmented long-spacing form by various organic and inorganic compounds. Biochim Biophys Acta 154(1):190–195
13. Kobayashi K, Ito T, Hoshino T (1985) Electron microscopic demonstration of acid-labile, 4D-staggered intermolecular association of collagen formed in vitro. Coll Relat Res 5(3):253–260
14. Harris JR, Lewis RJ (2016) The collagen type I segment long spacing (SLS) and fibrillar forms: formation by ATP and sulphonated diazo dyes. Micron 86:36–47

Chapter 25

Histological and Electron Microscope Staining for the Identification of Elastic Fiber Networks

Elaine C. Davis and Ling Li

Abstract

Elastic fibers are a major component of the extracellular matrix and are present in many tissues. Routine histology and standard electron microscopy procedures often do not allow for clear identification of elastic fibers making their organization and ultrastructure difficult to study. In this paper, we describe staining methods and procedures to enhance the contrast of elastin at both the light and electron microscope levels.

Key words Histology, Light microscopy, Electron microscopy, Elastin, Elastic fibers

1 Introduction

Elastic fibers are present in the extracellular matrix of many tissues, but are most prevalent in tissues that undergo repetitive stretch and recoil, such as the blood vessels, lung, and skin. Abnormal elastic fibers, as a result of genetic mutations in the elastin gene or genes of elastic fiber-related proteins or as a consequence of degradation, can lead to a number of diseases. For example, in the aorta, elastin is found in sheets or laminae, forming concentric layers in the media of the vessel interposed with smooth muscle cells [1]. Aberrant assembly of these laminae can result in the disruption of the normal architecture of the media resulting in an altered smooth muscle cell phenotype and aneurysm formation [2]. In the skin, abnormal and/or a reduced amount of elastic fibers can result in loose, inelastic skin; a condition called cutis laxa [3]. Similarly, loose and saggy skin is seen as one ages due to the progressive destruction of dermal elastic fibers as a result of sun exposure (UV damage). Finally, destruction of elastic fibers in the lung, such as seen in heavy smokers, can contribute to the development of emphysema and COPD [4].

To study the distribution, organization, and integrity of elastic fibers in tissues, routine histological stains, such as hematoxylin

Laure Rittié (ed.), *Fibrosis: Methods and Protocols*, Methods in Molecular Biology, vol. 1627, DOI 10.1007/978-1-4939-7113-8_25, © Springer Science+Business Media LLC 2017

and eosin or toluidine blue, are generally not effective at the light microscope level (except for the large elastic laminae in the aorta, which can be recognized with these stains). Delicate fibers, such as those found in the lung and skin, cannot be identified. Here, we describe a procedure that specifically stains elastic fibers black, making even the finest fibers stand out against a lightly stained background (Fig. 1). Since the elastic fibers are so clearly seen using this method, immunostaining is not necessary for detection of insoluble elastin fibers.

In our work, we have found that elastic fibers that appear normal at the light microscope level can actually be defective when observed at the electron microscope (EM) level. A clear demonstration of this can be seen in our work on the fibulin-5 knockout mouse [5]. Fibulin-5 is an elastic fiber-related protein that is necessary for elastic fiber assembly [6]. Like elastin, mutations in fibulin-5 cause cutis laxa, and the skin of the fibulin-5 knockout mouse is saggy and shows very few elastic fibers in the dermis [5, 6]. Surprisingly, short, normal appearing elastic fibers can be seen

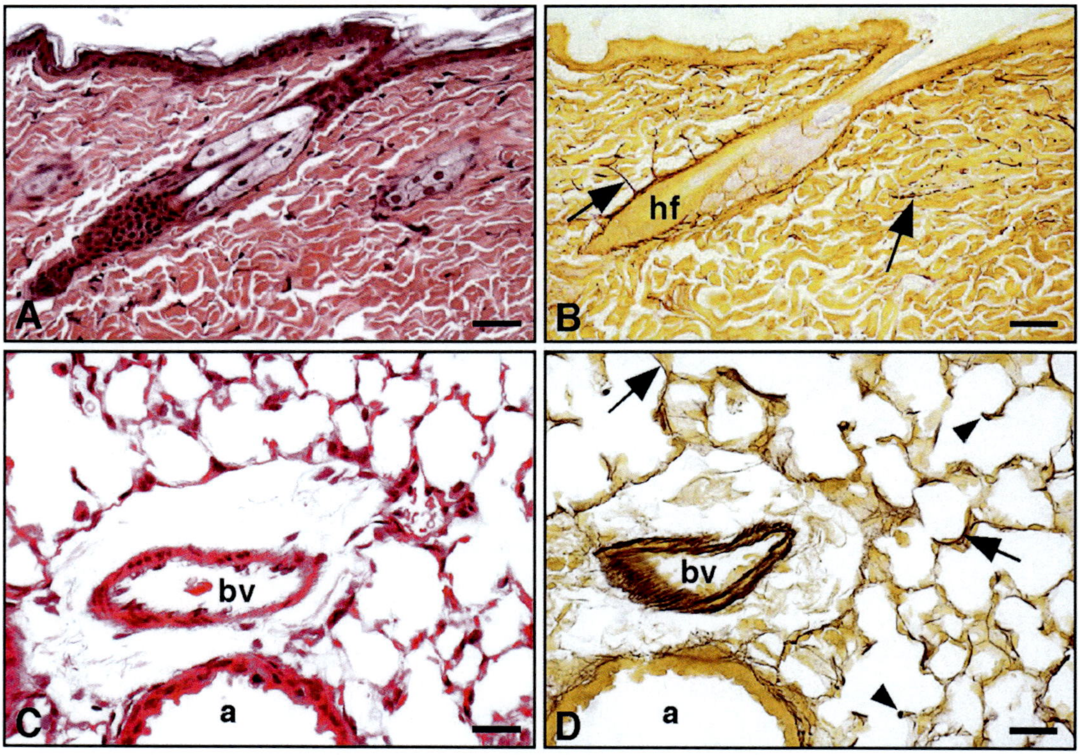

Fig. 1 Light microscope images of the skin (**a**, **b**) and lung (**c**, **d**). Serial sections were stained with either hematoxylin and eosin (**a**, **c**) or Hart's stain (**b**, **d**). In the hematoxylin and eosin-stained tissues, elastic fibers are not observed. In contrast, elastic fibers in the skin are evident around the hair follicles (hf) and in the dermis (*arrows*) of Hart's stained tissue. In the lung, the elastic fiber network is extensive, and delicate fibers can be seen in the alveolar walls (*arrows*), alveolar tips (*arrowheads*), media of blood vessels (bv) and subjacent to the epithelium in the airways (a). Bars = 500 μm

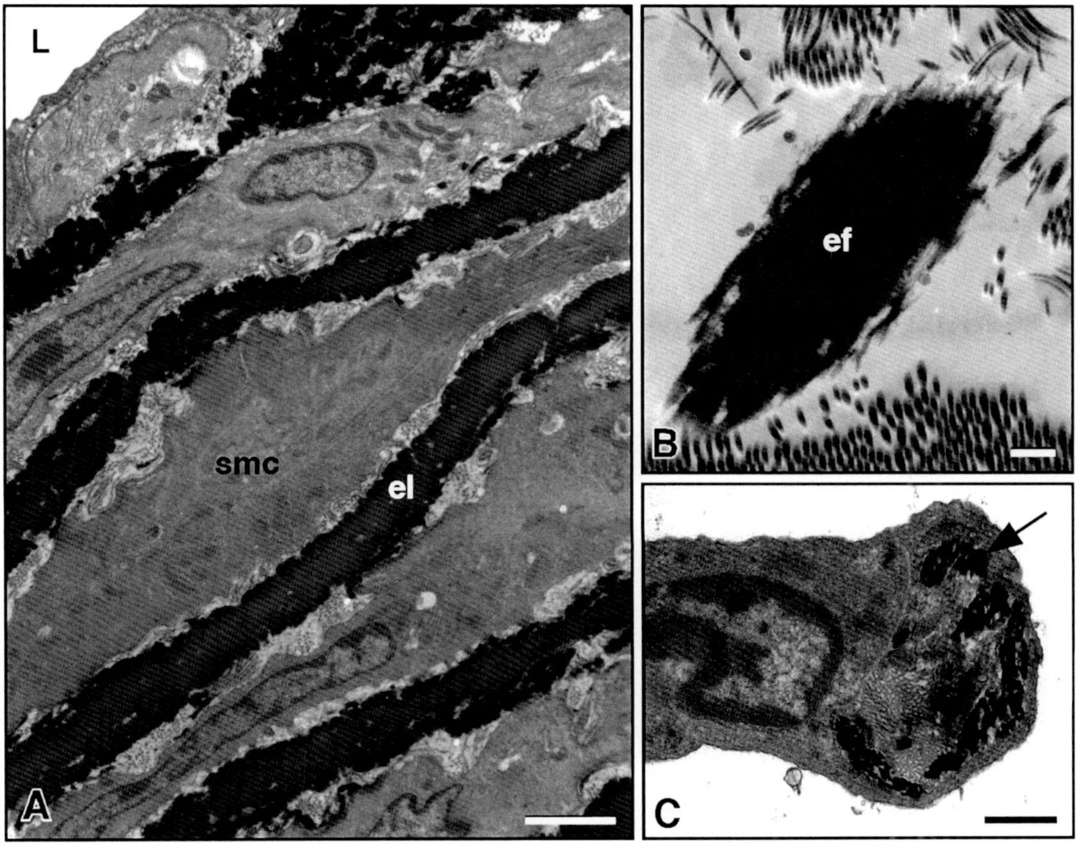

Fig. 2 Electron microscope images of elastin in mouse aorta (**a**), human skin (**b**), and the alveolar tip in mouse lung (**c**, *arrow*). *L* lumen, *smc* smooth muscle cell, *el* elastic lamina, *ef* elastic fiber. Bars = 2 μm (**a**), 500 nm (**b**), 1 μm (**c**)

around the hair follicles. Only with the power of EM were we able to discern that these elastic fibers were not normal, but instead consisted of small globules of elastin adjacent to a microfibrillar scaffold. These results were easy to demonstrate due to a procedure that we use to stain elastin black at the EM level (Fig. 2). This procedure is described here.

2 Materials

Most solutions are prepared fresh immediately before use. For EM, chemicals and reagents should be EM grade and purchased from suppliers of EM products.

2.1 Hart's Staining

1. Staining racks and dishes (*see* **Note 1**).
2. 65 °C oven.
3. Xylene or xylene alternative (we use CitriSolv Hybrid Solvent) (*see* **Note 2**).

4. Resorcin-fuchsin stock solution: We use F-379-1 from Rowley Biochemical. This stock solution can also be made from scratch as follows: Add 2 g basic fuchsin, 4 g resorcinol, and 200 ml deionized water (diH_2O) in a beaker. Mix and boil the solution for 1 min. Add 25 ml 29% (w/v) ferric chloride solution and boil for 1 min. Cool, filter, and leave precipitate on the filter paper until dry. Place precipitate in a beaker and add 200 ml 95% (v/v) ethanol. Heat carefully until the precipitate is fully dissolved. Discard the filter paper and add 4 ml HCl. Adjust solution to exactly 200 ml with 95% (v/v) ethanol. Filter and store at room temperature; stable for 1 year.
5. Hart's working solution: Mix 10 ml resorcin-fuchsin stock solution, 100 ml 70% (v/v) ethanol, and 2 ml 12.1 M HCl. Store at room temperature.
6. Metanil yellow solution: Mix 0.25 g metanil yellow, 100 ml diH_2O, and 0.25 ml of glacial acetic acid. Filter and store at room temperature.
7. Coverslips #1 thickness.
8. Organic mounting medium (we use Permount® from ThermoFisher).

2.2 Electron Microscopy

1. 6.5 ml polyethylene scintillation vials with snap caps.
2. 0.2 M sodium cacodylate buffer: Dissolve 4.28 g sodium cacodylate in ~80 ml diH_2O, bring pH to 7.4, and adjust volume to 100 ml. Store at 4 °C. This is a 2X stock solution.
3. Fixative: 3% glutaraldehyde in 0.1 M sodium cacodylate buffer. For 10 ml, mix 1.2 ml 25% (w/v) EM grade glutaraldehyde, 5 ml 0.2 M sodium cacodylate buffer, and 3.8 ml diH_2O. Make sufficient fixative for perfusion and tissue fixation (*see* **Note 3**).
4. 1% osmium tetroxide in 0.1 M sodium cacodylate buffer: Prepare in fume hood. Open a prescored ampoule containing 2 ml of 4% (w/v) osmium tetroxide. Using a long (9″) Pasteur pipette, transfer the osmium to a 15 ml conical tube. Add 2 ml diH2O and 4 ml of 0.2 M sodium cacodylate buffer. Cap and mix by inversion.
5. 2% tannic acid in 0.1 M cacodylate buffer and 2% uranyl acetate in diH_2O: Make these solutions fresh and filter before use (*see* **Notes 4** and **5**). Only about 1 ml is needed per sample.
6. Methanol.
7. Propylene oxide.
8. Epoxy resin Epon™ 812: Weigh directly into a 100 ml disposable beaker 23 g Epon 812, 14 g nadic methyl anhydride (NMA), and 13 g dodecenyl succinic anhydride (DDSA). Add 1 ml of the accelerator DMP-30 (use a 1 ml syringe with no

needle), and stir mixture with a wooden tongue depressor for at least 3 min in a fume hood.

9. Flat embedding molds.

3 Methods

Carry out all procedures at room temperature unless indicated otherwise. Chemicals that must be used in a fume hood are indicated. Detailed methods for the EM procedure and images of the mouse aortic wall using this method have been published [1].

3.1 Hart's Staining

1. Put the microscope slides with paraffin sections in a staining rack and place in a 65 °C oven for 30 min (*see* **Note 6**).
2. Let slides cool to room temperature and deparaffinize in three changes CitriSolv, followed by one change of CitriSolv/ethanol (1:1) for 5 min each, in a fume hood (*see* **Note 2**).
3. Rehydrate sections in a graded series of ethanol (100, 95, 70, 50%, tap water) for 5 min per solution.
4. Wipe off any excess water from around the sections and immerse the slides in Hart's working solution for 5–12 h (*see* **Note 7**).
5. Rinse slides gently in tap water for 45 s three times and wipe off the excess water from around the sections.
6. Place slides in metanil yellow solution for 1 min and 45 s (*see* **Note 8**).
7. Rinse slides gently in tap water for three times 1 min and wipe off the excess water from around the sections.
8. Dehydrate sections in a graded series of ethanol to CitriSolv as follows: 95% ethanol for 1 min, 100% ethanol for 1 min, CitriSolv/ethanol (1:1) for 3 min, and pure CitriSolv for 10 min.
9. Mount a coverslip over the section(s) with organic mounting medium.

3.2 Electron Microscopy

1. Cut tissues into 1.0 mm^3 pieces and place in fixative. Incubate for 4 h at 4 °C on a rotator (*see* **Note 9**).
2. Wash tissues four times 10 min in 0.1 M sodium cacodylate buffer at 4 °C on a rotator (*see* **Note 10**).
3. Postfixation: Incubate tissues in 1% osmium tetroxide in 0.1 M sodium cacodylate buffer for 1 h at 4 °C on a tissue rotator (*see* **Note 11**).
4. Wash tissues four times 10 min in 0.1 M sodium cacodylate buffer at 4 °C on a rotator (*see* **Note 10**).

5. Perform first en bloc staining: Incubate tissues in 2% tannic acid in 0.1 M sodium cacodylate buffer for 1 h at 4 °C on a tissue rotator [7].
6. Wash tissues four times 10 min in diH_2O at 4 °C on a rotator (*see* **Note 12**).
7. Perform second en bloc staining: Incubate tissues in 2% uranyl acetate in diH_2O for 1 h at 4 °C on a tissue rotator in the dark (*see* **Note 13**).
8. Wash tissues for 10 min in diH_2O at room temperature on a rotator (*see* **Note 14**).
9. Dehydrate tissues in a graded series of methanol (10, 25, 40, 55, 70, 85, 90, 95%, and twice in 100%) on a tissue rotator at room temperature for approximately 8 min each (*see* **Note 15**).
10. Incubate tissues in two changes of 100% propylene oxide on a tissue rotator at room temperature for approximately 8 min each (*see* **Note 16**).
11. Infiltrate the tissues with propylene oxide/Epon ratios on a tissue rotator at room temperature as follows: 3:1 for 1 h, 1:1 for at least 2 h, and 1:3 overnight (*see* **Note 17**).
12. The next day, make a fresh batch of Epon. Remove the 1:3 propylene oxide/Epon solution using a Pasteur pipette, and add a small amount of fresh Epon to each vial. Leave vials in the fume hood with the caps off for 4–6 h (*see* **Note 18**).
13. Embed the tissues in flat embedding molds with the tissue pieces oriented as desired in the tapered end. Polymerize the Epon blocks in an oven at 65 °C for 2–3 days (*see* **Note 19**).
14. Sectioning of the Epon blocks is routine and generally done in a core facility (*see* **Note 20**).
15. For the best contrast, sections should be placed on Formvar-coated grids and counterstained according to the method of Franc and colleagues [8], also described in [1].

4 Notes

1. It is best to have a series of dishes so that the slides, in the staining rack, can be moved from one solution to the next. Solutions can be used more than once.
2. CitriSolv Hybrid Solvent is a safer alternative to xylene and does not ship/store as flammable.
3. We use 50–100 ml for perfusion, depending on the number of animals, and 2 ml per sample for subsequent fixation.

4. Do not use aluminum foil for the sealing of uranyl acetate solutions as the foil decomposes upon contact with uranyl acetate (eventually contaminating the solution).
5. Uranyl acetate is made from depleted uranium, meaning it contains traces of radioactive isotopes. Please handle and discard according to local regulatory guidelines.
6. Paraffin section should be 5 μm in thickness and mounted on positively charged glass slides.
7. Hart's working solution can be reused many times. Longer incubation times are needed if the working solution is newly prepared. To save on the amount of stain needed, Coplin jars can be used.
8. Incubation time in metanil yellow can be adjusted for desired result. If the staining is too yellow, small elastic fibers may be masked. The sections can just be covered with the stain, rather than using a staining dish.
9. For mouse tissues, we fix by cardiac perfusion. Blood is first cleared using normal saline until the liver has paled. The solution is then switched to 3% glutaraldehyde in 0.1 M sodium cacodylate buffer (pH 7.4), and the animal is perfused for 3–5 min. A good indication that the fixation is working is that the muscles should twitch and the tail should move. Tissues are then dissected from the animal, cut into small pieces, and placed in fresh fixative. We generally prepare six or eight pieces per tissue and use 6.5 ml polyethylene scintillation vials with snap caps for processing.
10. Tissues can be washed and then left overnight at 4 °C on a tissue rotator in a fresh change of buffer.
11. Osmium tetroxide (OsO_4) is highly poisonous even at low exposure levels and must be prepared and used in the fume hood. Once the vials are capped, they can be moved to a rotator in the refrigerator. Prepare the smallest amount of solution necessary. We prepare it fresh and use about 1 ml per tissue sample. Waste 2% osmium solution should be mixed 1-part osmium to 2-parts corn oil. Store waste in the fume hood in a disposable container with a tight lid, such as a 50 ml conical for small amounts or a used plastic 1 liter tissue culture medium bottle for larger amounts. Notify waste management for disposal/pickup procedures.
12. Longer washes or more washes can be carried out if the tissue pieces are a bit large. The wash solution should be clear.
13. Uranyl acetate must be kept in the dark as much as possible since it is photoreductive and will precipitate.
14. Only one wash is needed because the excess uranyl acetate will be removed during the subsequent dehydration steps.

15. Tissue can be left in 70% methanol overnight or longer. This is a good stopping point. We generally use three overnight stopping points: (a) in the wash after fixation, (b) in the wash after osmium, and (c) in 70% methanol during dehydration.
16. Propylene oxide is very toxic and highly volatile. Open the bottle in the fume hood and use as little as possible, about 1 ml per sample is enough. Place waste in a disposable plastic container (such as a 50 ml beaker) and leave in the fume hood. The solution will evaporate very quickly.
17. Prepare propylene oxide/Epon solutions immediately before use. Use a 50 ml disposable beaker. Pour a small volume of Epon in the beaker and add the appropriate amount of propylene oxide. The two solutions won't mix until stirred so you can eyeball it. Stir very well for several minutes using a wooden tongue depressor. Tape or parafilm the caps in place for the overnight incubation to ensure they don't pop off.
18. This final step is to infiltrate the tissue pieces with pure Epon and evaporate any remaining propylene oxide. It may help to very gently nudge the pieces up into the Epon so they are not stuck on the bottom of the vial. We use wooden plain-tipped applicator sticks. Try not to touch the tissues because they are very fragile; just move the solution around the pieces and draw them up into the Epon.
19. Labels should be included in the blocks. We use small strips of paper with the block information printed on them (Arial 5-point works well). The strips are placed in the bottom of each well before filling with Epon. An example of a label could be 27-wt-S1, representing experiment 27, wild-type animal, skin sample, block number 1.
20. We routinely have the core cut several 0.5 μm "semi-thin" sections from each EM block and place them on a microscope slide. The slides are then put on a slide warmer or hot plate at the lowest setting to dry. Once dry, the sections are covered with a few drops of toluidine blue (with the heat source still on) for 1–2 min depending on the darkness of staining you would like to achieve. After gently rinsing in water, the sections can be dried and mounted with Permount. Large elastic fibers or laminae show up well with this staining method. The sections also provide an overview of what will be on the EM grid and can serve as a reference for further trimming of the block, if necessary.

Acknowledgments

This work was supported by NSERC grant 355710 and funding from the Faculty of Medicine, McGill University to E.C.D.

References

1. Davis EC (1993) Smooth muscle cell to elastic lamina connections in developing mouse aorta. Role in aortic medial organization. Lab Invest 68(1):89–99
2. Huang J, Davis EC, Chapman SL et al (2010) Fibulin-4 deficiency results in ascending aortic aneurysms: a potential link between abnormal smooth muscle cell phenotype and aneurysm progression. Circ Res 106(3):583–592. doi:10.1161/CIRCRESAHA.109.207852
3. Urban Z, Davis EC (2014) Cutis laxa: intersection of elastic fiber biogenesis, TGFbeta signaling, the secretory pathway and metabolism. Matrix Biol 33:16–22. doi:10.1016/j.matbio.2013.07.006
4. Black PN, Ching PS, Beaumont B et al (2008) Changes in elastic fibres in the small airways and alveoli in COPD. Eur Respir J 31(5):998–1004. doi:10.1183/09031936.00017207
5. Choi J, Bergdahl A, Zheng Q et al (2009) Analysis of dermal elastic fibers in the absence of fibulin-5 reveals potential roles for fibulin-5 in elastic fiber assembly. Matrix Biol 28(4):211–220. doi:10.1016/j.matbio.2009.03.004
6. Yanagisawa H, Davis EC, Starcher BC et al (2002) Fibulin-5 is an elastin-binding protein essential for elastic fibre development in vivo. Nature 415(6868):168–171. doi:10.1038/415168a
7. Wagner RC (1976) The effect of tannic acid on electron images of capillary endothelial cell membranes. J Ultrastruct Res 57(2):132–139. doi:10.1016/S0022-5320(76)80103-7
8. Franc S, Garrone R, Bosch A et al (1984) A routine method for contrasting elastin at the ultrastructural level. J Histochem Cytochem 32(2):251–258. doi:10.1177/32.2.6198356

Chapter 26

Method for Picrosirius Red-Polarization Detection of Collagen Fibers in Tissue Sections

Laure Rittié

Abstract

The extracellular matrix is critical in guiding cell behavior in normal and pathologic tissues, particularly in cancers and fibrosis. Highlighting the organization (or disorganization) of a collagen-containing matrix can be very useful for understanding or grading pathophysiological conditions. The picrosirius red stain (also called "Sirius red" stain) is one of the best understood histochemical techniques able to selectively highlight collagen networks. Relatively inexpensive, the technique relies on the birefringent properties of collagen molecules. While the picrosirius red stain alone does not selectively bind collagen network, it becomes more specific than the other common collagen stains when combined with polarized light detection. This is why the selective histochemical procedure for collagen detection should be called the picrosirius-polarization method. In this chapter, we will provide essential explanation and detailed protocols and tips to allow collagen researchers not only to better understand how this staining technique works but also to easily apply this technique to their collagen-related research.

Key words Collagen, Sirius red, Polarization, Orientation, Birefringence

1 Introduction

Fibrillar collagens make up to 6% of the human body and are incorporated in many organs and tissues including the heart, skin, bones, ligaments, and tendons. Fibrillar collagens are the main components of the extracellular matrix. The extracellular matrix is increasingly regarded as critical in guiding cell behavior in normal and pathologic tissues, particularly in cancers and fibrosis. Highlighting the organization (or disorganization) of a collagen-containing matrix may be very useful for understanding or grading pathophysiological conditions.

Various histological or histochemical methods have been developed to visualize collagen fibers within tissues. The most common collagen-staining methods are the Masson trichrome, van Gieson, Herovici, or Sirius red stains. Although Masson, van Gieson, and Herovici stains' interpretation is usually relatively

Laure Rittié (ed.), *Fibrosis: Methods and Protocols*, Methods in Molecular Biology, vol. 1627,
DOI 10.1007/978-1-4939-7113-8_26, © Springer Science+Business Media LLC 2017

straightforward (each color corresponding to a particular component of the extracellular matrix), they rely on the reaction of a mixture of dyes with proteins with mechanisms of action that remain mostly unclear. Thus, dyes' selectivity toward different components of the extracellular matrix remains uncertain. For example, Herovici proposed a polychromic technique to distinguish collagen I and III networks, staining them in red and blue, respectively. In this case, however, the selectivity of the stain was shown to depend on the competitiveness of the two acidic dyes, as opposed to histochemical reactions per se, as each dye stains the entire collagen network when used separately [1]. This makes the reaction extremely condition-dependent and hard to interpret without reasonable doubt.

The picrosirius red stain (also called "Sirius red" stain) is one of the best understood histochemical techniques. It relies on the birefringent properties of collagen. Albeit much more specific than the other common collagen stains, the picrosirius red stain may seem difficult to interpret for biologists not familiar with the details of the physical concepts of birefringence and its detection. In this chapter, we will provide essential details that will allow collagen researchers to better understand how this staining technique works.

Many optical materials such as glass are optically isotropic. This means they reflect light equally in all directions. However, not all biological materials interact with light in an isotropic manner. Anisotropic materials interact with light in a manner that is dependent upon the orientation of the molecule, relative to the incident light. Fibrillar collagens, with their typical rod-like shape and asymmetrical axis, are highly anisotropic. When light hits an anisotropic material, it is refracted into two rays traveling at different speed and with vibration directions oriented at 90° to one another. This phenomenon is called "double" or "bi"-refraction. Birefringence is a measure of the difference in refractive index between the two refracted rays (Fig. 1).

Picrosirius red is an elongated birefringent molecule (Fig. 2). In tissues, picrosirius red binds to a variety of molecules, not just collagens. When bound to collagen, however, it orients parallel to the collagen fibrils, thereby greatly enhancing their natural birefringence [2]. Thus, the complex fibrillar collagen/Sirius red is much more birefringent than complexes made of Sirius red and other proteins. Sirius red-bound fibrillar collagens can then be detected under polarized light, where they appear bright and in sharp contrast with the rest of the tissue that remains dark/black (Fig. 3) (*see* **Notes 1** and **2**). Thus, the selective histochemical procedure for collagen detection should be called the picrosirius-polarization (PSR-POL) method. Collagen types I, II, and III all bind to Sirius red at an average of 126 molecules of dye per collagen molecule [3]. The C1q component of the complement, which contains a collagenous domain that can bind a wide variety of

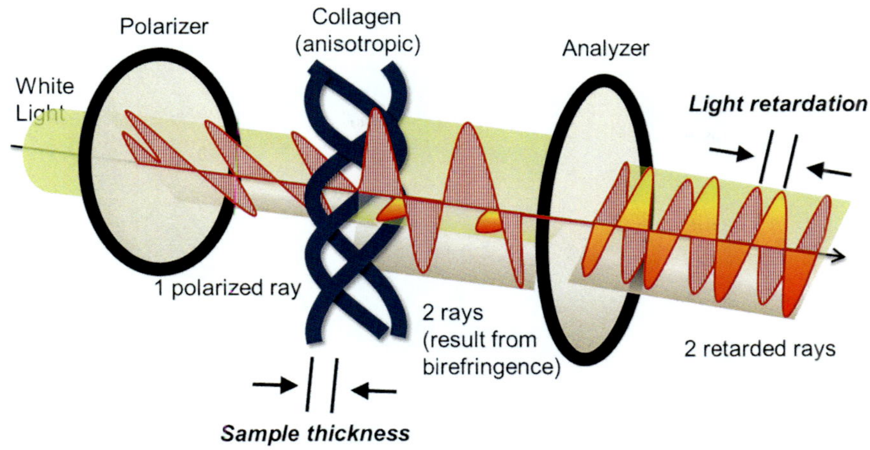

Fig. 1 Basic principle of birefringence and its detection through crossed polarizers. To detect birefringence, white light from the microscope illuminator (*path is left to right*) is polarized before interacting with the sample. Upon crossing collagen molecules (anisotropic), the polarized light is refracted and divided into two separate rays. The two rays of light initially vibrate perpendicular to each other, until an analyzer (often a quarter-wave plate) "flips" one ray so that it becomes parallel to the other ray to allow its detection. The relative retardation of one ray with respect to the other is indicated by an equation (thickness multiplied by refractive index difference) and governs intensity of detection. Because refractive index difference is constant for a given material (i.e., collagen fibers), the intensity of detection is thus directly proportional to the thickness of the material (fibers within the tissue if tissue sections are kept at a constant thickness)

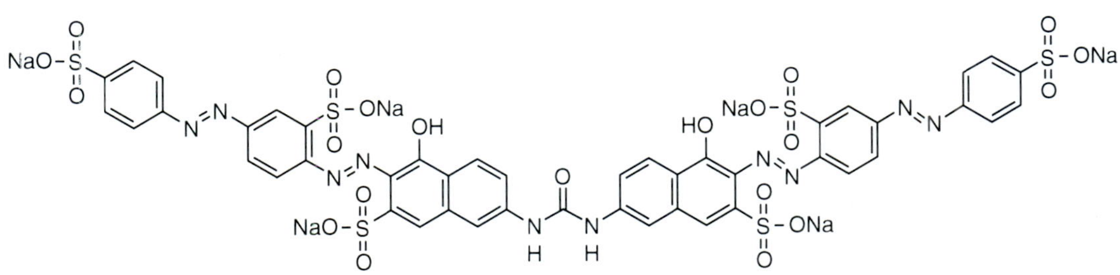

Fig. 2 Sirius red's molecular formula. Sirius red (Direct Red 80 or Sirius red F3B, C.I. number = 35780) is an elongated molecule that contains six salt-forming -SO_3H sulfonic groups that interact with the basic groups aligned on the elongated collagen molecule (auxochromic interactions) and four -N = N- azo structures that act as chromophores

polyanions [4, 5], is the only known non-collagenous protein that increases birefringence with Sirius red [3].

Three anatomical structures have been reported to interfere with PSR-POL: keratohyaline granules of cornified epithelia (i.e., stratum corneum of the skin), mucus-producing cells of the intestine, and the heart of fishes [2]. The exact mechanism of this interaction is unclear. PSR-POL appears to be selective for collagen in all other structures studied so far. In the case of the skin, the presence of the epidermis between the stratum corneum and the collagen-containing dermis allows clear discrimination between the two structures, and this interference is typically not an issue (Fig. 4).

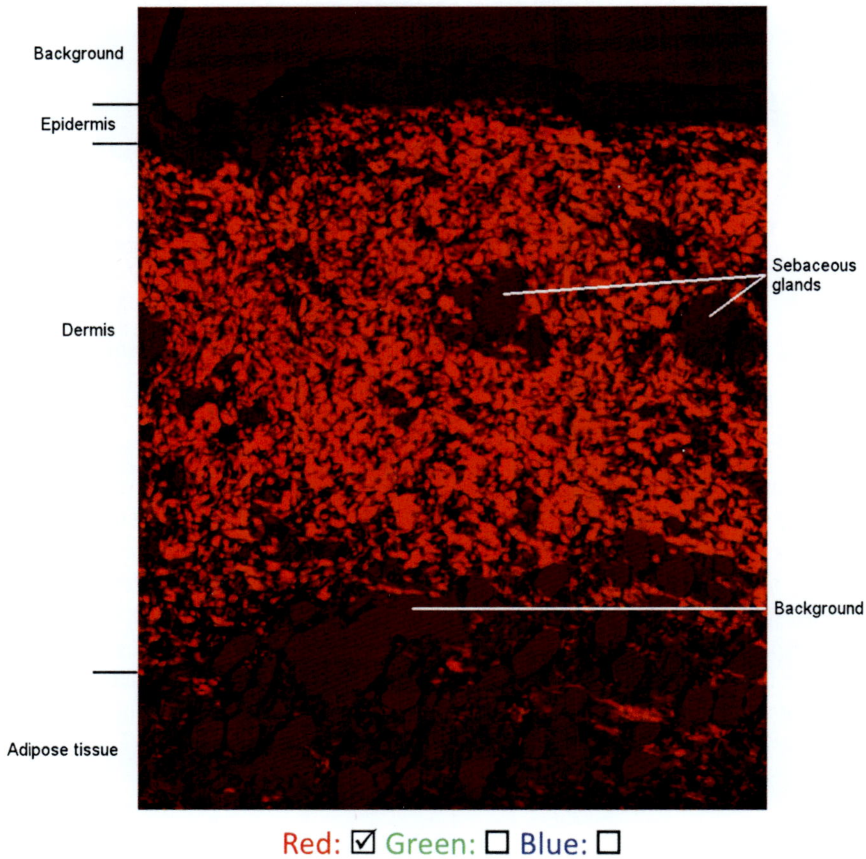

Fig. 3 Rat abdominal skin revealed by picrosirius red-polarization (PSR-POL). Sirius red-bound fibrillar collagens can be detected under polarized light, where they appear *bright red*, and in sharp contrast with the rest of the tissue that remains *dark* or *black*. Structures devoid of collagen (e.g., sebaceous glands, epidermis) appear similar to background. Some collagen fibers appear completely *black*: they are the ones for which polarization is extinct due to their orientation relative to the polarizer (an inherent characteristic of linear polarization, used here)

Picrosirius red is typically detected with a bright-field excitation (i.e., white light), although utilizing a fluorescent light setting with Sirius red has also been reported [6]. Utilizing a regular bright-field microscope to image a Sirius red-stained tissue will not be suitable for identifying collagen because, as explained above, the picrosirius red dye binds all proteins in the tissue. Without polarization, Sirius red-stained tissue appears pink-red, and all areas are stained, including epithelial structures that do not contain collagen proteins (Fig. 5a, b). Observing the same tissue with a polarized light not only allows clear identification of collagen networks (Fig. 5c–d) but also allows semiquantitative appreciation of potential collagen alterations that are not readily evident without polarization (Fig. 5, compare b and d). Thus, PSR-POL is a very useful method for studying collagen networks. This method is relatively easy too.

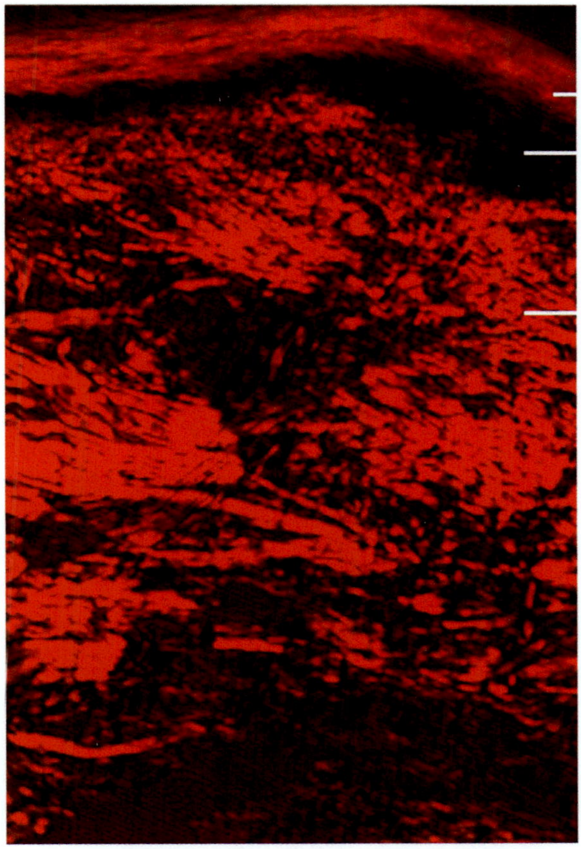

Fig. 4 Example of an anatomical structure known to interfere with picrosirius red-polarization (PSR-POL). In forearm human skin, the keratohyaline granules of the cornified layers make the stratum corneum of the skin virtually as bright as the collagen network itself. The epidermis between the two structures is an anatomical marker that is typically used to differentiate the stratum corneum and collagen network

PSR-POL was shown to correlate well with another highly specific collagen-imaging method, i.e., second harmonic generation (SHG) imaging [8] (also *see* Chap. 27 for protocols and tips on SHG imaging). Importantly, however, PSR-POL detects higher fiber counts, alignment, length, straightness, and width compared with SHG imaging [8] and can be used at lower magnification. Thus, because of its relatively inexpensive cost, PSR-POL may provide sufficient information in a conventional laboratory for certain types of collagen quantification [8].

Microscope equipment that allows PSR-POL detection may vary. Figure 6 depicts a typical microscope setting for PSR-POL collagen detection that we use in our laboratory. It involves inserting a polarizer between the bright light source and the sample and an analyzer between the sample and the detector (i.e., eyepiece or digital camera). This device utilizes the linearly polarized light

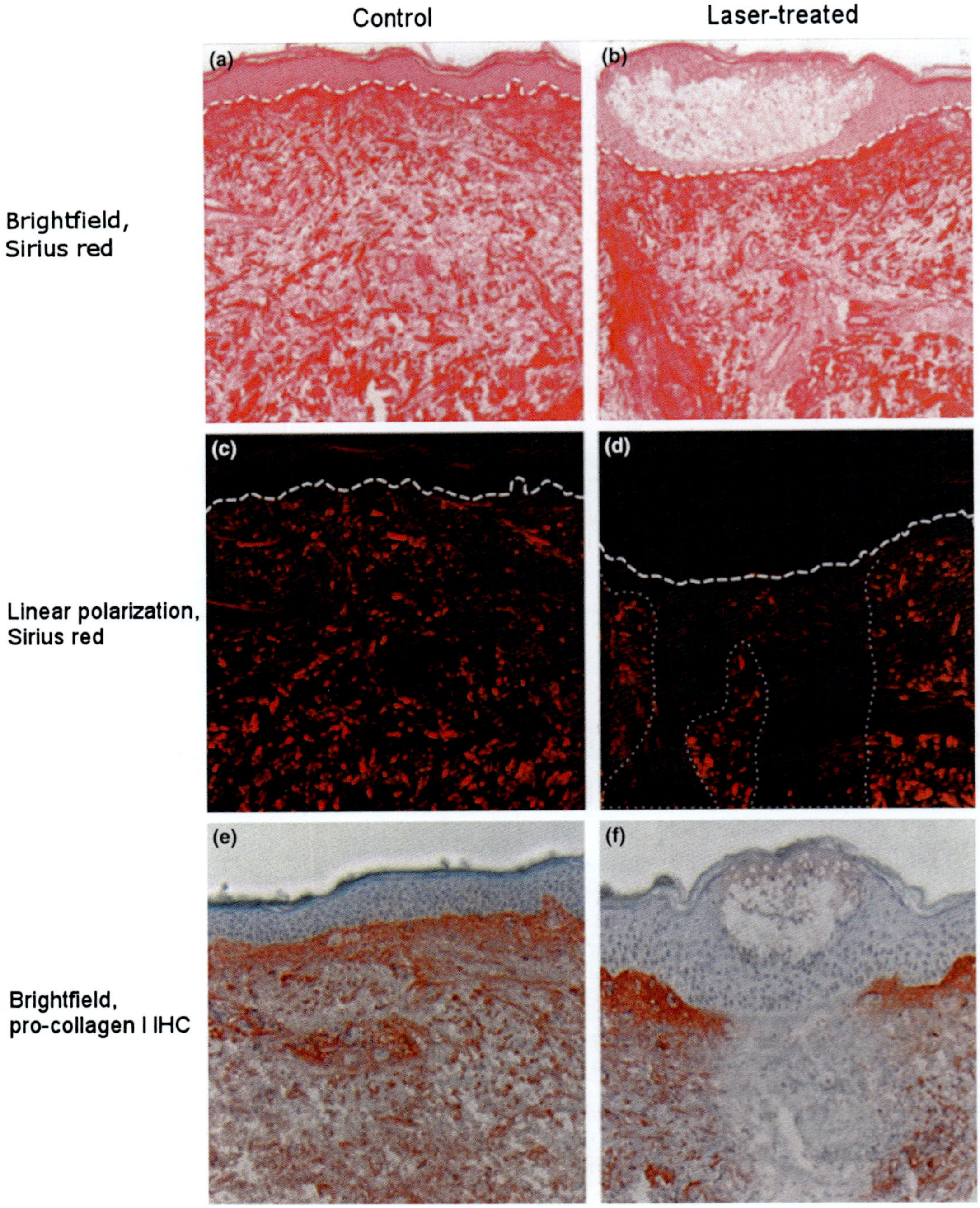

Fig. 5 Picrosirius red stain must be combined to polarized light detection to show collagen specificity. Photodamaged forearm skin, untreated (**a**, **c**, **e**) or 24 h after in vivo treatment with fractional photothermolysis (**b**, **d**, **f**), as described in [7]. (**a**, **b**) Sirius red staining viewed by bright-field microscopy without polarization: Sirius red is not specific of collagen in these conditions and all tissues appear *pink-red*. (**c**, **d**) Sirius red staining viewed by bright-field microscopy with linear polarization: Sirius red-bound fibrillar collagens appear *bright red* and in sharp contrast with the rest of the tissue that remains *black*. Altered collagen fibrils in the dermis (demarcated by *dotted lines*) are also apparent. Heavy *dashed line* indicates dermal-epidermal junction. (**e**, **f**) Procollagen I immunohistochemistry image of a consecutive section is shown for comparison and reveals areas of reduced staining in the papillary dermis of treated skin. Reproduced from [7] with permission

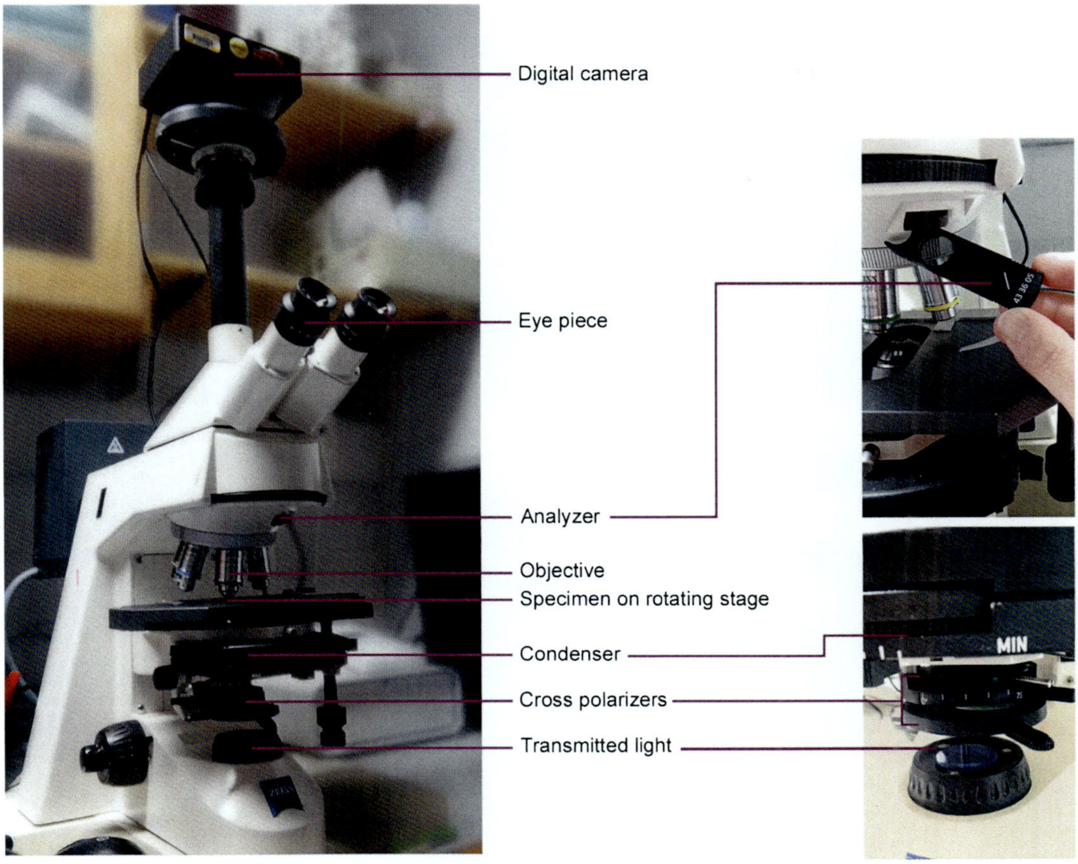

Fig. 6 Typical microscope setting for PSR-POL detection. *Left*, from bottom to top: the illuminator produces a white light that successively passes through cross polarizers, a condenser, the specimen, the objective, and the analyzer (quarter-wave plate) before being detected either by the observer through the eyepiece or by a digital camera. This path corresponds to the path shown in Fig. 1. *Right*: close-up of the illuminator and crossed polarizers (*bottom*) and of the analyzer (*top*). The optional *blue* filter that covers the illuminator for conventional imaging should be removed for PSR-POL imaging. The crossed polarizers are mounted on a holder of the microscope and can be rotated to orient the extinction areas (Maltese cross) to produce the best results for a particular sample (all images of a batch should be imaged with the polarizers positioned at the same angle). The analyzer slides into the slot that normally hosts the UV safety shield on this particular microscope

described in Fig. 1. It is important to note that linearly polarized devices have an inherent reduced intensity of light that occurs in the vicinity of each ±45° and ±135° angle relative to the transmission axis of the polarizer. This phenomenon of extinction creates an artefactual "Maltese cross" shadow of detection. This has not been a problem for us since we typically image skin, a tissue that can easily be oriented in a consistent direction relative to the polarizer using the epidermis as reference. Other tissues such as bones or liver cannot be that easily oriented, and the presence of a Maltese cross can greatly affect detection accuracy (Fig. 7). To circumvent this obstacle, one can potentially image the same sample twice, precisely

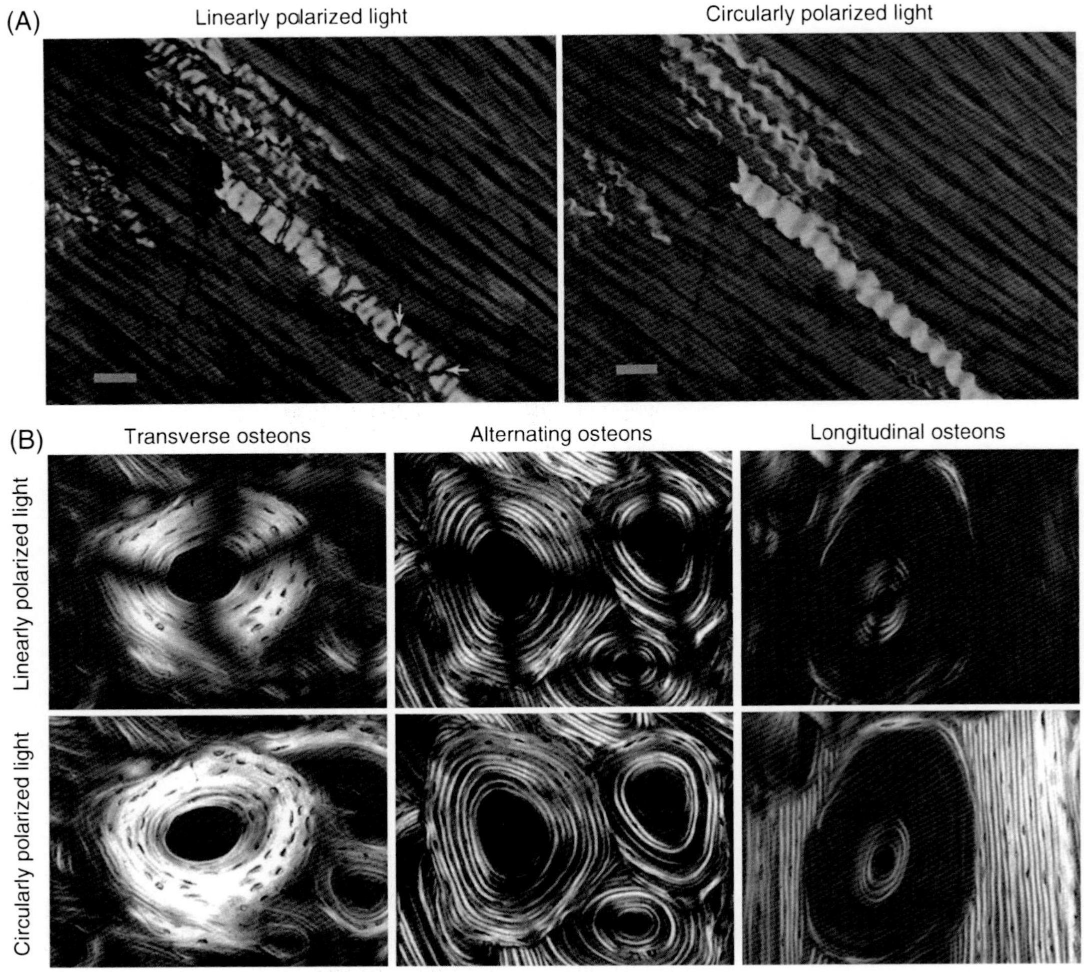

Fig. 7 Comparison of picrosirius red images obtained with linear vs. circular polarization. (**a**) Rat myocardium sections stained with picrosirius red. Highly birefringent collagen fibers appear *bright*. *Left*: Tissue viewed with linearly polarized light; *arrows* indicate portions of the collagen fibers that appear dark because they are aligned parallel to the transmission axis of one of the polarizing filters. *Right*: Same field viewed with circularly polarized light; all of the collagen fibers appear bright, and extinction zones have disappeared. *Scale bars*, 25 μm. Reproduced from [9] with permission. (**b**) *Left*: Transverse (*right*), alternating (*middle*), and longitudinal (*right*) osteons contain lamellae composed of collagen fibers that are transverse, alternating, and longitudinal to the osteon axis, respectively. Artefactual extinction in the form of a Maltese cross is seen in linearly polarized light images (*top row*) but not in circularly polarized light images (*bottom row*). Images are from human (*bright and alternating*) and spider monkey (*longitudinal osteons*) femurs, respectively. Frames, 475 μm wide. Reproduced from [10] with permission

rotating the sample by 45° angle between images and performing a post-processing maximum projection on realigned images. However, collagen fibers are frequently wavy or even crimped; it is thus very likely that some fibers will display some dark zones no matter how the microscope stage is rotated (*see* Fig. 7a). Alternatively, and most preferably, the use of circularly polarized light eliminates the Maltese cross [9–11]. Circularly polarized light systems have an arrangement of filters that allows refracted light emerging from a birefringent specimen in all 360° of arc to be polarized along the transmission axis of the analyzer. A direct comparison of linearly and circularly polarized light system is depicted in Fig. 7.

Important elements of the detection system are the detector and detector settings. Images shown in Figs. 3, 4, and 5c, d were detected on a digital camera that was set to record only the red channel. This setting is great to reveal bright red collagen fibers against a dark/black background. The drawback is that the background appears similar between areas without tissue and areas with tissue devoid of collagen (Fig. 3, compare areas labeled background with sebaceous glands). To circumvent this and visualize anatomical references that may be useful for result interpretation or specimen orientation, the experimenter has two options possible: she/he can take successive pictures with and without polarization, as shown in Fig. 5. This method is totally acceptable but very cumbersome because it entails placing/removing polarizers and changing illuminator power settings between images and thus can be prone to manipulator error. A second option involves changing the detector settings to record the red, green, and blue (RGB) channels all at once (instead of red only) (Fig. 8). The RGB image can be very useful because background and collagen-devoid anatomical structures then become distinct. Such strategy is thus preferable for qualitative approaches. However, it makes quantitative approaches trickier because, as seen in Fig. 8, some collagen fibers appear in various colors, including orange, yellow, and green. It was proposed that, when viewed under crossed polarizers, birefringence intensity indicates the degree of alignment of the fibers and the hue of birefringence indicates either the direction of collagen fiber alignment or distinct patterns of physical aggregation [12, 13]. Thus, while it might be fairly easy to visually appreciate a difference in hue between two specimens, interpretation might not be straightforward. Quantifications of RGB images need to be approached accordingly, with great caution and abundant controls and validation steps (*see* **Note 3**).

2 Materials

1. Coplin jars.
2. 2% (w/v) paraformaldehyde solution in phosphate buffer saline (PBS) (*see* **Note 4**).
3. For formalin-fixed paraffin-embedded (FFPE) tissue sections:
   (a) Xylene or equivalent.
   (b) Absolute ethanol.
   (c) Deionized or distilled water (diH_2O).

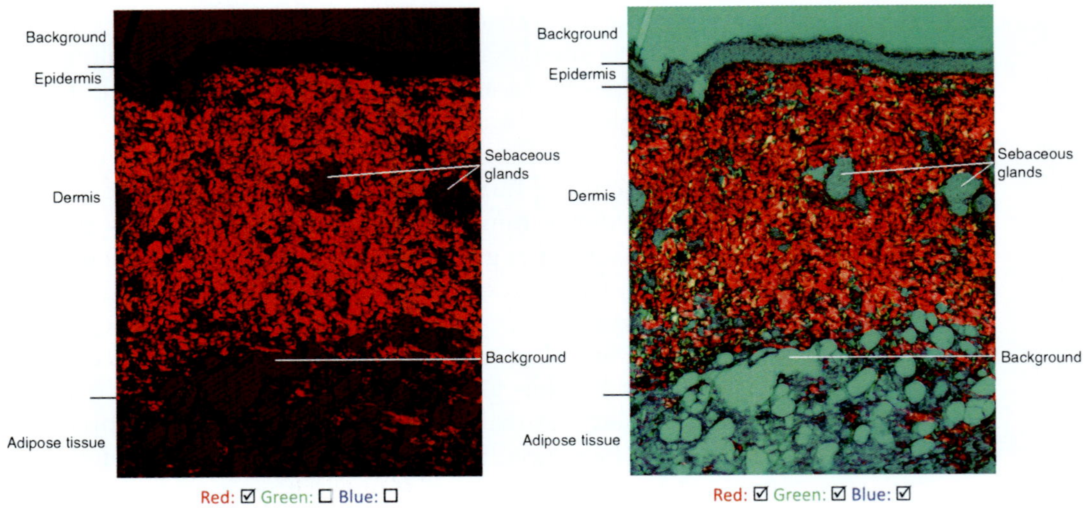

Fig. 8 Effects of detector settings on PSR-POL images. The two images depict the same forearm skin sample stained with picrosirius red. Both images were generated with bright-field microscopy with linear polarization. The image on the left was taken with the digital camera set to record only the red channel, while the image on the right was taken with the digital camera set to record the three color channels (*red, green, and blue, RGB*). Recording the three color channels makes the background without tissue appear teal, while histological details (e.g., cell membranes and nuclei) are visible in the epithelial tissue devoid of collagen (in *blue/purple* hues, see epidermis and sebaceous glands). Also note that some collagen fibers have various colors, while others are still *black* (the extinction phenomenon still occurs)

4. Sirius red working solution: prepare 1 l of saturated picric acid (i.e., 1.3% (w/v) picric acid solution in diH_2O; also called 2,4,6-trinitrophenol), add 1 mg Sirius red F3B (also called Direct red 80, color index: C.I. 35782), and stir. The final concentration of Sirius red is 0.1% (w/v). Store at room temperature for several months (*see* **Note 5**).
5. Wash solution: add 5 ml glacial acetic acid (i.e., ~18 M) to 995 ml diH_2O. Store at room temperature.
6. Rehydration station: place eight Coplin jars containing xylene (2 jars), 100% ethanol (2 jars), 95% ethanol (1 jar), 90% ethanol (1 jar), 70% ethanol (1 jar), and diH_2O (1 jar) in a fume hood.
7. Organic mounting medium such as Permount® or Cytoseal®, Pasteur pipettes with latex bulbs and coverslips (*see* **Note 6**).

3 Methods

1. For frozen tissue sections, proceed to **step #2**. For FFPE tissue sections, skip to **step #5**.
2. Thaw frozen tissue sections (7–20 μm thick) at room temperature by leaving them on the bench for 5–10 min.

3. Fix thawed tissue sections by immersing slides in 2% paraformaldehyde for 20 min at room temperature.
4. Rinse three times in diH_2O. Skip to **step #6**.
5. Dewax FFPE tissue sections in three rinses of xylene (ten dips or 2–3 min incubation each), three rinses of absolute ethanol (ten dips or 2–3 min incubation each), and three rinses in diH_2O (*see* **Note 7**).
6. Stain in Sirius red working solution for 1 h (*see* **Note 8**).
7. Remove excess staining by washing twice with wash solution (ten dips or 2–3 min each).
8. Dehydrate slides by immersing them through a series of increasing alcohol concentrations: Transfer slides sequentially to diH_2O, 70%, 90%, 95%, and 100% (v/v) ethanol (ten dips or 2–3 min incubation each). Rinse slides to a second 100% ethanol solution to ensure that all water is removed.
9. Replace ethanol with xylene by immersing slides in two successive xylene solutions.
10. Mount slides with organic mounting medium and coverslips (*see* **Note 9**).
11. Observe stained tissue with polarized light microscope.

4 Notes

1. It is critical to understand that the picrosirius red stain alone is not selective for collagen detection but must be combined to polarized light detection.
2. Because the birefringence displayed by Sirius red-bound collagen is due to collagen's molecular arrangement, the PSR-POL method can also be used to study pathological conditions in which molecular disorganization (e.g., collagen degradation) occurs. It is expected that collagen molecular disorganization will result in alterations of birefringence patterns compared to healthy tissue.
3. The reader is reminded that one workaround would be to record the RGB image for qualitative assessment and later extract the red channel (with software tools such as ImageJ or GIMP) for quantification.
4. Paraformaldehyde is toxic and should be handled in a fume hood and with personal protection equipment according to local safety policies. We highly recommend purchasing an already made solution (16% (w/v) or lower) and dilute it to 2% (w/v) with PBS. Alternatively, heat ~800 ml PBS at 60 °C on a hot plate with a magnetic stirrer. Add 20 g paraformaldehyde powder and stir until dissolution (~30 min). When dis-

solution is complete, turn off the heat and let the solution cool down with agitation maintained several hours to overnight. Adjust volume to 1 l with PBS and 0.22 μm filter the solution for storage. Use within 3 months.

5. There are many Sirius red dyes available. Make sure you purchase the right dye, corresponding to the unique color index.
6. Most commercial microscope objectives are designed to be used with a cover glass that has a standard thickness of 0.17 mm (i.e., #1.5 thickness) and a refractive index of 1.515. The amount of mounting medium to be used should be determined empirically and should be the lowest amount that allows covering the entire coverslipped area once cured (all mounting media tend to shrink upon drying). Adding too much mounting medium will increase the volume between the slide and cover glass, and therefore, if the sample is adhered on the slide, increase the minimal possible distance between the objective and sample. If this distance is too large, it will prevent high magnification observation (the objective can't get close enough of the sample that remains blurry).
7. If you are considering using immunohistochemistry in parallel with picrosirius red staining, please keep in mind that antigen retrieval methods cause collagen fibers to shrink. This makes IHC/Sirius red staining combination on FFPE tissue challenging. A detailed method for simultaneous detection of antigen and Sirius red in FFPE tissues has been proposed [14]. We have not tested it.
8. One hour incubation has been shown to achieve optimal staining. Staining intensity does not increase with longer times. Shorter times however should be avoided as the staining tends to fade with mounting and with time.
9. Do not let the tissue dry after the second xylene change. Instead, leave slides in xylene and mount slides one by one. Tissue may stay in xylene for a relatively prolonged period of time. When mounting, keeping a thin film of xylene on the slide will help disperse the mounting medium and coverslipping will be easier. Allow excess xylene to evaporate and leave slides in the fume hood until mounting medium dries (~1 h).

References

1. Levame M, Meyer F (1986) Le Picropolychrome de Herovici: application à l'identification des collagènes de types I et III. [Herovici's picropolychromium. Application to the identification of type I and III collagens]. Pathol Biol 35(8):1183–1188
2. Junqueira LC, Bignolas G, Brentani RR (1979) Picrosirius staining plus polarization microscopy, a specific method for collagen detection in tissue sections. Histochem J 11(4):447–455. doi:10.1007/BF01002772
3. Junquiera LC, Junqueira LC, Brentani RR (1979) A simple and sensitive method for the quantitative estimation of collagen. Anal Biochem 94(1):96–99. doi:10.1016/0003-2697(79)90795-4

4. Muller-Eberhard HJ (1975) Complement. Annu Rev Biochem 44:697–724. doi:10.1146/annurev.bi.44.070175.003405
5. Acton S, Resnick D, Freeman M et al (1993) The collagenous domains of macrophage scavenger receptors and complement component C1q mediate their similar, but not identical, binding specificities for polyanionic ligands. J Biol Chem 268(5):3530–3537
6. Vogel B, Siebert H, Hofmann U et al (2015) Determination of collagen content within picrosirius red stained paraffin-embedded tissue sections using fluorescence microscopy. MethodsX 2:124–134. doi:10.1016/j.mex.2015.02.007
7. Orringer JS, Rittié L, Baker D et al (2010) Molecular mechanisms of nonablative fractionated laser resurfacing. Br J Dermatol 163(4):757–768. doi:10.1111/j.1365-2133.2010.09998.x
8. Drifka CR, Loeffler AG, Mathewson K et al (2016) Comparison of picrosirius red staining with second harmonic generation imaging for the quantification of clinically relevant collagen fiber features in histopathology samples. J Histochem Cytochem 64(9):519–529. doi:10.1369/0022155416659249
9. Whittaker P, Kloner RA, Boughner DR et al (1994) Quantitative assessment of myocardial collagen with picrosirius red staining and circularly polarized light. Basic Res Cardiol 89(5):397–410. doi:10.1007/BF00788278
10. Bromage TG, Goldman HM, McFarlin SC et al (2003) Circularly polarized light standards for investigations of collagen fiber orientation in bone. Anat Rec B New Anat 274(1):157–168. doi:10.1002/ar.b.10031
11. Rich L, Whittaker P (2005) Collagen and picrosirius red staining: a polarized light assessment of fibrillar hue and spatial distribution. Braz J Morphol Sci 22(2):97–104
12. Borges LF, Gutierrez PS, Marana HR et al (2007) Picrosirius-polarization staining method as an efficient histopathological tool for collagenolysis detection in vesical prolapse lesions. Micron 38(6):580–583. doi:10.1016/j.micron.2006.10.005
13. Nerurkar NL, Baker BM, Sen S et al (2009) Nanofibrous biologic laminates replicate the form and function of the annulus fibrosus. Nat Mater 8(12):986–992. doi:10.1038/nmat2558
14. Gadd VL (2014) Combining immunodetection with histochemical techniques: the effect of heat-induced antigen retrieval on picro-Sirius red staining. J Histochem Cytochem 62(12):902–906. doi:10.1369/0022155414553667

Chapter 27

Probing Collagen Organization: Practical Guide for Second-Harmonic Generation (SHG) Imaging

Riccardo Cicchi and Francesco S. Pavone

Abstract

Second-harmonic generation (SHG) microscopy is a powerful microscopy technique for imaging collagen and other biological molecules using a label-free approach. SHG microscopy offers the advantages of a nonlinear imaging modality together with those ones of a coherent technique. These features make SHG microscopy the ideal tool for imaging collagen at high resolution and for characterizing its organization at various hierarchical levels. Considering that collagen organization plays a crucial role in fibrosis and in its development, it would be beneficial for the researcher working in the field of fibrosis to have a manual listing crucial points to be considered when imaging collagen using SHG microscopy. This chapter provides an answer to this demand with state-of-the-art protocols, methods, and laboratory tips related to SHG microscopy. We also discuss advantages and limitations of the use of SHG for studying fibrosis.

Key words SHG microscopy, Collagen, Polarization scanning, Forward backward, Detection, Numerical aperture, Ti:sapphire laser

1 Introduction

Since their first implementations, more than a quarter of century ago, nonlinear optical (NLO) microscopy techniques are considered a powerful imaging tool for both biological and biomedical applications [1–3]. In the last two decades, NLO microscopy techniques were successfully employed in several research fields, from single molecule biophysics, through cell biology, up to tissue imaging and biomedical diagnostics. NLO microscopy offers several advantages compared to single-photon-based techniques, especially for tissue imaging. They enable label-free deep optical sectioning capabilities even inside optically turbid samples [4, 5]. Compared to linear imaging techniques, NLO processes are characterized by increased penetration depth capability [6–8], better spatial resolution [9, 10], and more efficient excitation capability [11–13]. In fact, the use of near-infrared (NIR) wavelengths offers the advantage of a reduced scattering with respect to linear techniques when

Laure Rittié (ed.), *Fibrosis: Methods and Protocols*, Methods in Molecular Biology, vol. 1627,
DOI 10.1007/978-1-4939-7113-8_27, © Springer Science+Business Media LLC 2017

exciting transition located in the blue-ultraviolet spectral range and hence a deeper penetration inside optically turbid samples as biological tissues [6, 14]. In addition, the spatial resolution achievable is comparable to confocal microscopy, but without undesirable out-of-focus photoeffects. Further, scattered photons unable to reach the focal volume do not contribute to the excitation with the result of avoiding detrimental effects on the spatial resolution when imaging deep into a highly scattering medium.

Among NLO imaging techniques, an extremely powerful modality for imaging collagen in biological tissues is represented by second-harmonic generation (SHG) microscopy [1, 2]. SHG microscopy can provide background-free morphological information by revealing the distribution of anisotropic biological structures with large hyperpolarizability [15, 16], such as collagen [17, 18], muscle [19–23], or microtubules [24]. SHG is a nonlinear second-order optical process occurring in non-centrosymmetric systems with a large hyperpolarizability. This condition, satisfied at the molecular level by the presence of electron-donor and electron-acceptor moieties connected by a π-conjugated system, is necessary but not sufficient for generating a detectable SHG signal. In fact, the additional condition of having a structural anisotropy of the molecular emitters at the focal volume scale needs to be matched. Both conditions are satisfied in anisotropic biological molecules such as collagen, making SHG microscopy an ideal tool for imaging collagen, as demonstrated by the applications in various collagen-rich tissues, such as the cornea [25–27], tendon [28, 29], and arteries [30, 31]. The coherent nature of the optical process at the basis of SHG microscopy allows not only to image collagen but also to probe its organization at various scale levels. In particular, SHG microscopy has been already largely used for selectively investigating collagen fiber orientation and their structural changes in human dermis [32–37] (Fig. 1), keloid [37–39], thermally treated samples [27, 29, 40–42], and also tumor microenvironments [43–49] (quantitative methods described in Chap. 28). The possibility to characterize collagen organization makes SHG microscopy an ideal tool for studying and diagnosing connective tissues in altered physiological conditions, as demonstrated by studies conducted on muscles [50], bones [51, 52], and cartilages [53, 54].

Considering that collagen I is one of the most efficient SHG molecular emitter, together with the fact that it plays a crucial role in the development of fibrosis, it is easy to understand that SHG microscope represents a privileged microscopic tool for studying and diagnosing connective tissues in general and fibrosis in particular. In fact, SHG microscopy have been already successfully employed for imaging and characterizing fibrosis in various biological tissues, including cutaneous scar tissue [34], renal tissue [55, 56], lung tissue [57], and liver [58, 59]. However, a commercial microscope exclusively dedicated to SHG imaging is still lacking. Very often, SHG microscopes used in laboratory research are

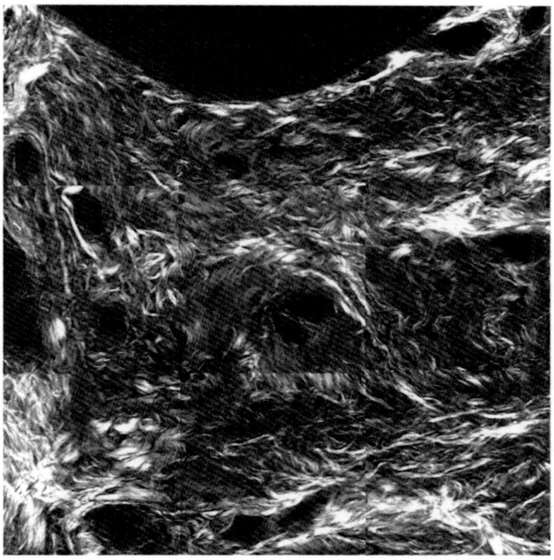

Fig. 1 SHG image of a collagen network within the human dermis, acquired from an ex vivo skin sample using 840 nm as excitation wavelength. Field of view: 1.2 mm

adapted from commercial (confocal or multiphoton) microscopes. However, for some applications, ex novo design or adaptation from an existing laser scanning confocal/multiphoton microscope is required to fit the technical specifications of the experiments to be performed. Several technical and experimental aspects have to be considered. This chapter aims to provide a practical guide to the researchers who want to adapt their confocal/multiphoton microscope to perform SHG microscopy.

2 Materials

2.1 Excitation and Scanning System

This section describes one of the most important parts of a laser microscope: the laser scanning system. Starting from basic principles, we then focus our attention on the different elements constituting the scanning system.

2.1.1 Laser Source

SHG is a second-order optical process characterized by a low transition probability, so that an extremely high spatial and temporal density of photons is required in the focal volume in order to excite such a process and to detect a non-negligible signal. The high photon density is realized spatially by using high-numerical aperture (NA) objective lens (as it will be explained in Subheading 2.1) and temporally by using femtosecond-pulsed laser sources.

1. The most common source in SHG imaging is the Ti:sapphire oscillator. Typically, it emits pulses of a duration in the 80–200 fs range, with a repetition rate generally between 50 and

100 MHz. The output is tunable in the 700–1000 nm spectral range, corresponding to the range in which biological molecules have a significant cross section for SHG. All these features make Ti:sapphire the ideal laser source for an SHG microscope. The cost is quite high (typically in the 100k Euro range).

2. Another femtosecond-pulsed option is represented by the Cr:forsterite laser. This source emits pulses comparable to those of the Ti:sapphire in terms of width and repetition rate, but in the wavelength range 1150–1300 nm. Even if at these wavelengths the SHG cross section of biological molecules is reduced, the Cr:forsterite provides an efficient source not only for second- but also for third-harmonic generation microscopy [60–62]. The cost is approximately half of the Ti:sapphire's.
3. An alternative cheaper option is represented by femtosecond-pulsed fiber lasers. These compact and robust lasers provide a pulsed emission comparable with that of the Ti:sapphire in terms of pulse width and repetition rate, but they cannot be tuned. Their cost is in the order of 20–30 kEuro and their maximum power is in the order of W.

2.1.2 Optical Scheme for Laser Scanning

In wide-field microscopy, the entire specimen is immersed in a uniform bath of light, and the image is acquired in one shot onto a camera equipped with a charge-coupled device (CCD) detector, whereas in laser scanning microscopy, the sample illumination scheme is totally different. Scanning is achieved by illuminating the specimen point by point with a focused laser beam that is moved across the sample and by collecting the SHG signal point by point onto a high-sensitivity single-point detector. The basic optical principles used for performing such scanning are illustrated in Fig. 2.

Figure 2a shows a collimated laser beam in two configurations: parallel to the optical axis and tilted. When parallel to the optical axis, the beam is focused in a point geometrically defined by the intersection of the optical axis with the focal plane. When tilted at an angle α, the focal point is located within the focal plane at a distance d from the optical axis, related to the tilting angle α and to the focal length of the lens f by the following equation:

$$d = f \tan\alpha \tag{1}$$

For small tilting angles, Eq. 1 becomes

$$d = f\alpha \tag{2}$$

Beam tilting required for scanning is obtained by means of a scanning head (see the following section), optically relayed to the objective lens by a telescope (Fig. 2b). The telescope re-conjugates the scanning system with the objective back aperture, so that the laser beam is kept centered on the back aperture during scanning. In addition, the telescope magnifies the laser beam diameter in

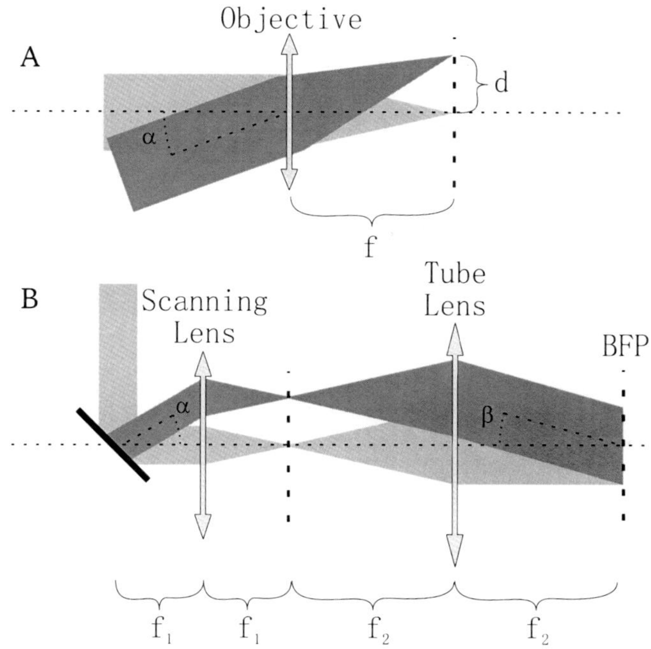

Fig. 2 Basics of laser beam scanning. (**a**) Working principle of an objective lens with focal length (f). (**b**) Schematic path of a beam propagating through a typical telescopic system composed of two lenses with focal lengths f_1 and f_2, respectively. BFP indicates the back focal plane of the objective lens, corresponding to the input diaphragm of the objective itself. *Double arrow*: thin lens. *Thick dark line*: mirror. *Thin dashed line*: optical axis. *Light gray*: laser beam aligned with the optical axis. *Dark gray*: laser beam tilted with respect to the optical axis. *Thick dashed lines*: conjugate optical planes. *BFP* back focal plane

order to fill the objective back aperture and take full advantage of the numerical aperture (NA) offered by the objective lens (*see* Subheading 2.2). In particular, the magnification (M) obtained corresponds to:

$$M = \frac{f_2}{f_1} \tag{3}$$

Finally, the telescope de-multiplies (by a factor equal to the magnification) the angle spanned by the laser beam during scanning (α), enhancing the scanning sensitivity in the objective focal plane, so that the angle spanned by the beam in the focal plane (β) is equal to:

$$\beta = \frac{1}{M}\alpha \tag{4}$$

This process allows enhancing the scanning sensitivity in the focal plane.

2.1.3 Scanning Head

The scanning head provides the beam tilting required for laser scanning. This is generally achieved by using galvanometric mirrors (galvo-mirrors), acousto-optic deflectors (AODs), or polygonal rotating mirrors as scanners. A brief description of the most common scanning heads is provided below.

1. The most common scanning head consists of a couple of small mirrors mounted onto two galvanometer-based scanners. The galvanometers are made by a magnet and a current-driven coil that allows tilting the mirror at an angle proportional to the current in the coil. They are very often equipped with a position sensor and a closed-loop servo system. They offer good precision and high-resolution scanning. Typically, the scan rate is several microseconds per pixel. Faster acquisition speed can be obtained by using resonant scanners.
2. When scanning with nonresonant galvanometers, the scanning speed has an upper limit in order to avoid extreme acceleration and deceleration of the scanner when inverting scanning directions. This limitation is circumvented by driving the faster scanner with a resonant sinusoidal waveform. In fact, a sinusoid can be used at very high scan rates without having extremely high accelerations. Obviously, the pixel clock has to be modified according to the scanner speed. In fact, the image pixels are scanned at the highest speed in the image center, with the speed decreasing when moving to the image edges. Scanning is then restricted to the portion of the oscillation where the velocity of the scanner is almost linear in order to avoid problems related with speed nonlinearity.
3. A valid alternative, if extremely high scanning speeds are required, consists of instruments equipped with AODs. AODs take advantage of ultrasonic waves, generated by a piezoelectric transducer, to generate within a crystal pressure waves that can diffract or deflect incident laser light (Bragg diffraction). The deflection angle depends on the frequency of the acoustic wave, and it can be controlled by properly driving the transducer. These devices benefit from having few moving mechanical parts and negligible inertia, allowing fast speed as well as random access scanning. The main disadvantage is due to the dispersive properties of these devices, which are suited only for monochromatic light.
4. Another potential solution able to reach extremely high scanning speed consists in substituting the faster galvanometer scanner with a polygonal mirror scanner. The polygonal scanning mirror is a prism with polygonal basis having mirrors placed onto the external faces. A laser beam hitting on the external face of a rotating polygonal mirror translates into a beam deflection with a sawtooth profile, useful for scanning the specimen with a raster waveform.

2.2 Objective Lens

The objective lens is the crucial part of a microscope, since it determines the spatial resolution achievable. In wide-field microscopy, the spatial resolution achievable is limited by the diffraction. In an SHG microscope, the spatial resolution corresponds to the size of the excitation volume, which is generally smaller than the diffraction limit. In addition to the spatial resolution achievable, various specifications have to be taken into account when choosing an objective lens.

1. *Numerical aperture (NA)*: the NA of the excitation objective should be not less than 0.5, as a general rule, to ensure sufficient photon spatial density in the focus for nonlinear excitation. Objective lenses with high NA are generally preferable because both spatial resolution and signal-to-noise ratio increase with NA. On the other hand, high NA corresponds in general to a high magnification and a small field of view. In addition, high-NA objectives can introduce spurious effects when working with polarization.
2. *Objective transmission*: the spectral range for the excitation is normally located in the NIR range (typically 700–1000 nm). An objective lens with good transmission in this range allows having better excitation efficiency. On the other hand, if the same objective is used also for detection, it is preferable to have high transmission in the visible range, since SHG signal is spectrally located in the 350–500 nm range. As a rule, it is better to maximize collection efficiency rather than excitation efficiency, since the amount of laser power available is generally much higher than the maximum power sustainable by the specimen.
3. *Working distance (WD)*: the WD generally imposes a limit on the imaging depth within a specimen, since high-NA objectives commonly have worked in the 100–200 μm range. Hence, the working distance of the objective should be chosen according to the sample to be investigated. On the other hand, long WDs generally correspond to low NAs, so that a trade-off between WD and NA should be considered according to the required optical performances and to the sample to be imaged.
4. *Back aperture*: the size of the objective back aperture has to be chosen carefully according to the size of the laser beam. In fact, it is very important that the excitation beam slightly overfills the objective back aperture in order to take advantage of all of the available NA of the objective and maximize the spatial resolution. Figure 3 summarizes the effects that occur on laser power and beam waist size in the optical configuration of overfilling (Fig. 3a), perfect filling (Fig. 3b), and underfilling (Fig. 3c). In particular, the perfect filling (Fig. 3b) maximizes the laser power transmitted by the objective while maintaining small beam waist (high spatial resolution). The large overfilling

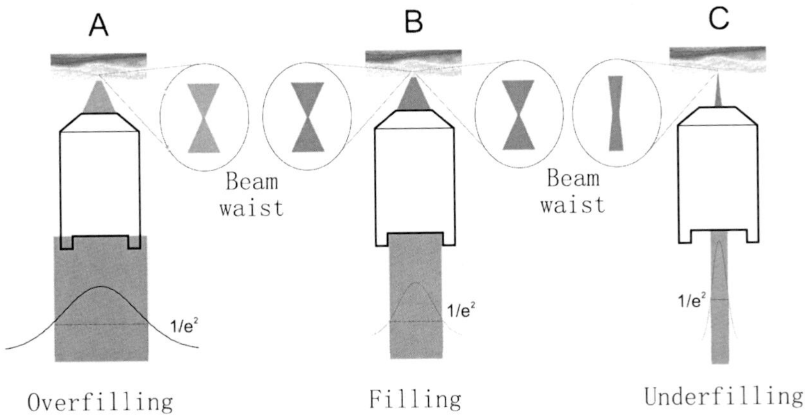

Fig. 3 Working principle of an objective lens that focuses a collimated laser beam with different beam size, as compared to the entrance diaphragm of the objective. (**a**) Overfilling: low power transmission and high spatial resolution. (**b**) Perfect filling: good power transmission and high spatial resolution. (**c**) Underfilling: maximum power transmission and low spatial resolution. $1/e^2$ represents the distance from the optical axis at which the beam intensity is reduced by a factor of e^2 with respect to the axial intensity. For a Gaussian beam, this corresponds to a distance HWHM (half width at half maximum) of the Gaussian intensity profile

in Fig. 2a allows maintaining a small beam waist (high spatial resolution) but with a reduced laser power. The underfilling condition (Fig. 3c) maintains high power transmission at the price of a large beam waist (low resolution).

2.3 Detection System

This section describes the detection system. In particular, various types of detector suitable for SHG microscopy will be described, highlighting advantages and drawbacks of each detector type and leaving the treatment of detection schemes (i.e., forward detection, backward detection) and filtering to the following section (*see* Subheadings 3.2–3.4).

1. *Photomultiplier tubes (PMTs)*: The most commonly used detector type in SHG microscopy is without doubt the PMT. A PMT consists in a vacuum device equipped with a light-sensitive photocathode, a number of dynodes (used as amplifying stages), and an anode for delivering the output signal. The photoelectrons emitted by the cathode are accelerated and amplified in each dynode by an electric field. The overall gain is in the range of 106–108. A large variety of photocathode and dynode geometries have been developed. Basically, the sensitivity and the spectral response in a PMT depend on the photocathode material, whereas the dynode geometry and electric field affect the gain and the temporal response.
2. *Avalanche photodiodes (APDs)*: An APD is a normal photodiode, electrically driven with a voltage close to or slightly above the breakdown voltage. With this approach, when a photon hits the sensitive area and generates an electron-hole pair, the pair is

accelerated creating an avalanche that can be detected as a current pulse. APDs have a very high quantum efficiency in the green spectral range (up to 0.7), but it drops quickly when moving to shorter wavelengths.

3. *Micro-channel plates (MCPs)*: An MCP is a particular type of photomultiplier. The working principle is similar to the conventional PMT, with the only difference that the amplification is achieved in a conductive channel instead of in a multiple dynode stage. MCPs are the fastest detectors in terms of temporal response. The sensitivity is comparable to PMTs and the achievable gain is slightly higher.
4. *Hybrid detectors*: Hybrid detectors consist of a recent technology in which the sensitive element is a photocathode, as in PMTs, and the dynode stage for amplification is substituted by an APD. Basically, they are comparable with PMTs in terms of sensitive area and quantum efficiency, but the output pulse is in general shorter. This allows having higher count rates and faster temporal response. They are particularly indicated for applications in which temporal resolution is important such in fluorescence lifetime measurements.

The crucial features to be taken into account when choosing a detector for SHG microscopy are the sensitivity, the achievable gain level, and the size of the sensitive area. Regarding the sensitivity, it is important to choose the detector with the highest sensitivity at the detection wavelength. This allows maximizing the signal-to-noise ratio for a certain acquisition time, or equivalently minimizing the acquisition time for a certain signal-to-noise ratio. The achievable gain level is not so crucial, and it should be chosen according to the post-amplification gain in the electronic chain. An extremely crucial feature is represented by the size of the sensitive area. As a general rule, the choice between these features has to be done depending on whether the optical detection of SHG is performed in descanned or in non-descanned mode. In descanned mode, the position stability of the focused SHG light within the detector allows using detectors with a very small sensitive area and high quantum efficiency, such as an APD. On the other hand, in non-descanned mode, it is necessary to use a detector with larger sensitive area, such as a PMT. Hence, the choice of the detector is free for the descanned mode, whereas a PMT is mandatory in non-descanned mode. The size of the sensitive area should be chosen according to the size of the scanned area. The size of the scanned area depends in turn on the magnification obtained with the objective and the focusing optics. A too small sensitive area can cause a limited field of view as well as a bright central region and darker sides in the images. In practice, the descanned mode allows using detectors with higher quantum efficiency (such as APDs), at the price of a detector position far away from the objective lens, corresponding to a lower signal collected. The non-descanned mode allows placing the detector closer to the objective lens, at the price of using a detector with lower quantum efficiency. As a general rule, the non-descanned mode is preferable for SHG microscopy when imaging deep into a highly scattering sample and when performing forward detection. In fact, descanning in forward detection is impractical because a second scanning system driven synchronously is required.

3 Methods

3.1 Laser Power Adjustment

Commercial femtosecond-pulsed laser sources commonly used for SHG microscopy, such as the Ti:sapphire laser, provide an optical power output much higher than that one required for safely imaging biological samples. In addition, very often they do not offer a power regulation system, so that the beam needs to be attenuated before entering the imaging system. Adjustable attenuation can be obtained by using a neutral density filter ring with variable optical density: the power on the specimen can be controlled by rotating the filter, manually or with a motorized mount for a control from remote. This solution might be problematic with extremely high peak power sources, because the filter coating could be damaged. An alternative approach is based on polarization and uses polarization optics. Laser output beam is normally linearly polarized, so that a rotatable half-wave plate (for rotating polarization), used in combination with a polarizing beam splitter cube, can represent a variable attenuator. In fact, the optical power transmitted through the polarization beam splitter cube depends on the rotation angle of the half-wave plate. The half-wave plate can be rotated manually or with a motorized rotational mount for a remote control. All these optical elements have to be chosen for sustaining the high peak intensity of femtosecond pulses, with particular attention devoted to the beam splitter cube.

3.2 Forward Detection

SHG is a coherent process preserving both energy and momentum. Therefore, a prominent amount of the emitted signal has the same direction as the exciting wave vector. More in detail, in almost all the biological specimen, SHG light has a spatial emission pattern with two lobes oriented at a certain angle with respect to the optical axis. The angle depends on the phase anomaly in the focus, on the NA of the exciting objective lens, and on the orientation of the molecular emitters with respect to the optical axis. Hence, considering that most of the SHG signal generated in a biological specimen is forward scattered, it is easy to understand that the most popular detection geometry used in SHG microscopy is forward-scattering detection.

Various features have to be taken into account when choosing the collection condenser for forward detection of SHG. Below, we list some important points to consider.

1. In principle, the ideal optical geometry is obtained using a collection objective with the same NA of the excitation objective (preferably the same as the excitation objective).
2. The use of a collection condenser with lower NA than the excitation objective causes a substantial loss of collected photons.
3. As a general rule for the implementation, it is preferable that the NA of the collection condenser is slightly higher than that of the excitation objective. In this way, losses due to an unavoidable misalignment of the confocality during experiments (for example in axial scanning) are prevented.
4. The condenser should have optimal transmittance for SHG light without considering the transmittance in the NIR.
5. Even if condensers with high NA are in principle preferable because of a better photon collection efficiency, high NA generally corresponds to a short WD. The WD of the condenser, on the other hand, is a crucial parameter to be considered, since it limits the maximum thickness of the specimen that can be imaged. A trade-off between WD and NA should be considered.

3.3 Backward Detection

Although the prominent amount of SHG signal is scattered in forward direction, backward detection is possible as well in an SHG microscope, especially in specific conditions as listed below.

1. There is a non-negligible amount of SHG signal emitted in the backward direction, so that imaging can be performed with epi- (i.e., backward) detection. However, the amount of SHG backward-emitted is generally much lower than the forward emission [12, 63].
2. When imaging massive specimens or living specimens, forward detection is intrinsically prevented by the specimen thickness, and only backward detection is possible. However, with this kind of samples, the signal collected in backward direction is strongly enhanced by multiple scattering events that cause the forward-emitted SHG light to be back-scattered within the backward collection cone. The amount of backscattered signal generated by multiple scattering is generally in the range from 5 to 20% of the forward-emitted signal.
3. When using backward detection modality, the excitation/collection objective should have optimal transmittance for both excitation and SHG light. If it is not possible to satisfy both conditions, optimizing the transmittance in the SHG spectral range is preferable since the laser power available is generally redundant for imaging.

3.4 Combined Forward–Backward Detection

As described in the previous sections, forward or backward detection should be chosen according to the characteristics of the specimen to be examined. Independently from the sample and from the experimental setup, the optimal configuration for the detection consists in detecting both forward- and backward-scattered SHG light by means of two separated objective lenses and two separated detectors. The advantages connected with this approach are listed below.

1. Enhancement of the detected signal (and of the signal-to-noise ratio) because the second objective used for collection enlarges the collection cone.
2. From the theoretical formulation of SHG, it is possible to derive that the ratio between forward-emitted and backward-emitted SHG (F/B SHG ratio) depends on the angle between the hyperpolarizability and the optical axis. Hence, by measuring the ratio between forward- and backward-scattered SHG light, it is possible to estimate the mean orientation of the emitters contained in the focal volume with respect to the optical axis. This information is very useful for characterizing a specimen emitting SHG, because it provides information related to molecular structural organization [64, 65].

4 Polarization and Polarization Scanning

4.1 Polarization Scanning of the Exciting Beam

An important feature to be considered in imaging applications involving SHG is represented by the polarization of the exciting beam. In fact, the SHG intensity in the far field depends on the mutual orientation between the molecular hyperpolarizability and the direction of oscillation of the driving electric field. Considering this feature, it is easy to understand that the use of an exciting beam having circular polarization on the sample is recommended in order to avoid artefacts in the image. In fact, to use a circular polarization for exciting the sample makes the generated SHG signal independent on the direction of molecular hyperpolarizability. This is a fundamental feature for acquiring SHG images that are independent from the polarization of the exciting beam. On the other hand, the capability to vary the polarization of the incident beam in a controlled manner can open the possibility to extract structural molecular information from the imaged specimen. In fact, the use of a polarization scanning approach allows measuring the distribution of SHG molecular emitters within the focal volume, which is in turn related to the molecular structural morphology of the specimen. This kind of measurements is commonly performed through the acquisition of multiple images in correspondence of multiple orientations of the polarization of the incident laser beam. This approach produces a polarization SHG image, where a polarization profile is embedded in each pixel. The polarization profile has a behavior that depends on the molecular orientation of the emitters within the focal volume. A proper fitting procedure, with a function calculated from the SHG theory, allows extracting the morphological parameters that describe the structural organization of the specimen with a spatial resolution of a single pixel.

The optical equipment to be used for polarization scanning could be implemented in a commercial microscope without dramatic difficulties. However, it is important to insert the optical components in a section where the laser is collimated and as close as possible to the objective lens. The optical components required for performing polarization scanning on an SHG microscope are listed below and have to be inserted in the path in the same order than listing. In particular, these are a first polarizer, a quarter-wave plate, and a second rotating polarizer (Fig. 4).

1. The first polarizer is used for making the polarization linear. Even if the laser output is normally linearly polarized, beam traveling through several optics has a detrimental effect on the polarization.
2. The quarter-wave plate is inserted in the optical path immediately after the first polarizer. The quarter-wave plate needs to be properly oriented in order to have a circularly polarized beam as output.
3. The rotating polarizer serves for scanning the sample with a linear rotating polarization. Rotation is normally ensured by mounting the polarizer on a rotating motorized opto-mechanical mount.

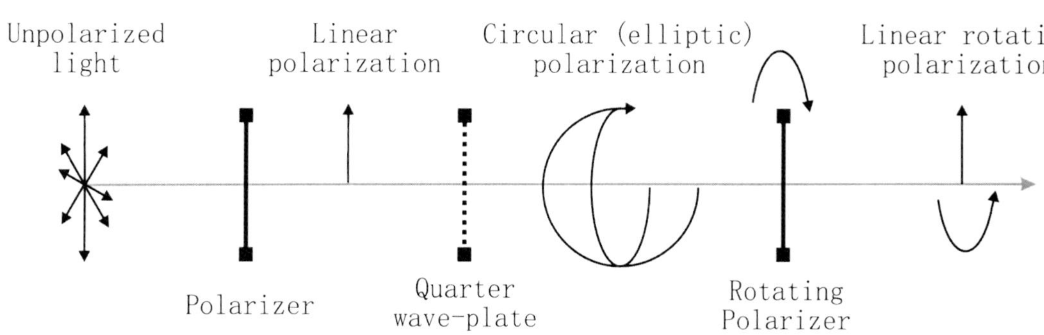

Fig. 4 Schematic sketch of a polarization scanning equipment to be used in an SHG microscope. The input non-polarized light (most general case) is made linearly polarized by means of a first polarizer. Then, the quarter-wave plate makes the polarization circular. A second rotating polarizer allows making a linearly rotating polarization. Entering the last polarizer with circular polarization allows maintaining a constant laser power during polarization scanning. If a dichroic mirror (not shown in the sketch) introduces ellipticity in the polarization, the quarter-wave plate needs to be rotated at a certain angle in order to compensate the phase retardation introduced by the dichroic mirror and have a circular polarization in front of the rotating polarizer

It should be noted that the light beam entering the rotating polarizer must have a perfect circular polarization in order to avoid intensity fluctuations of the beam during polarization scanning. This can be obtained by rotating the quarter-wave plate at an angle that allows compensating for the polarization ellipticity introduced in the beam by other optical components, especially the dichroic mirror used for decoupling SHG light from the laser path. In fact, the dielectric coating on the dichroic mirror has a detrimental effect on the polarization, making it elliptical. In this case, the quarter wave-plate needs to be properly rotated for introducing a compensating effect, so that the beam is polarized with circular polarization at the entrance of the rotating polarizer.

4.2 Filtering

The choice of proper optical filters is another crucial step for selecting an SHG microscope. Optical filtering is commonly obtained in an SHG microscope by means of three different optical elements: a dichroic mirror, a short-pass blocking filter, and a narrow band-pass filter. Practical rules to be followed when choosing and placing optical filters are reported below for each of the optical elements listed above.

1. The dichroic mirror is for decoupling SHG light from the laser path. It should be placed as close as possible to both the collection objective and the detector in order to minimize signal losses. The cutoff wavelength should be chosen in a spectral range comprised between the excitation and the SHG wavelength.
2. The short-pass filter is for blocking spurious contamination of the excitation light in the detection path. It has to be placed in the detection path, independently from the detection scheme (forward or backward). The optical density at the laser emission wavelength should be at least 6–7, in order to avoid the unwanted detection of NIR photons. On the other hand, the filter transmission within the SHG spectral range should be as high as possible (generally more than 90%).
3. The narrow band-pass filter is for exclusively detecting SHG photons, thus preventing the detection of fluorescence light. The central wavelength of the band-pass should be half the SHG wavelength. The spectral width of the filter is chosen depending on the spectral broadening of excitation laser pulses. For a Ti:sapphire laser, a dielectric band-pass filter with 20 nm FWHM is a good choice.

Acknowledgments

We acknowledge funding from the Italian Ministry for Education, University and Research in the framework of the Flagship Project NANOMAX, from Tuscany Region and EU FP7 BiophotonicsPlus projects "LITE" (Laser Imaging of The Eye) and "LighTPatcH" (Led Technology in Photo Haemostasis), from the European Union Seventh Framework Programme (FP7/2007–2013) under grant agreement number 284464 and number 604102 (Human Brain Project), from the Italian Ministry of Health (GR-2011-02349626), from Fondazione Pisa, and from Ente Cassa di Risparmio di Firenze. Part of this work was performed in the frame of the Proof of Concept Studies for the ESFRI research infrastructure project Euro-BioImaging at the PCS facility LENS.

References

1. Sheppard CJR, Gannaway J, Kompfner R et al (1977) The scanning harmonic optical microscope. IEEE J Quantum Electron 13E:100D. doi:10.1109/JQE.1977.1069615
2. Gannaway JN, Sheppard CJR (1978) Second-harmonic imaging in the scanning optical microscope. Opt Quant Electron 10(5):435–439. doi:10.1007/bf00620308
3. Denk W, Strickler JH, Webb WW (1990) Two-photon laser scanning fluorescence microscopy. Science 248(4951):73–76. doi:10.1126/science.2321027
4. Dunn AK, Wallace VP, Coleno M et al (2000) Influence of optical properties on two-photon fluorescence imaging in turbid samples. Appl Opt 39(7):1194–1201. doi:10.1364/AO.39.001194
5. Helmchen F, Denk W (2005) Deep tissue two-photon microscopy. Nat Methods 2(12):932–940. doi:10.1038/nmeth818
6. Gu M, Gan XS, Kisteman A et al (2000) Comparison of penetration depth between two-photon excitation and single-photon excitation in imaging through turbid tissue media. Appl Phys Lett 77(10):1551–1553. doi:10.1063/1.1308059
7. Oheim M, Beaurepaire E, Chaigneau E et al (2001) Two-photon microscopy in brain tissue: parameters influencing the imaging depth. J Neurosci Methods 111(1):29–37. doi:10.1016/S0165-0270(01)00438-1
8. Beaurepaire E, Oheim M, Mertz J (2001) Ultra-deep two-photon fluorescence excitation in turbid media. Opt Commun 188(1–4):25–29. doi:10.1016/S0030-4018(00)01156-1
9. Sheppard CJR, Gu M (1990) Image formation in two-photon fluorescence microscopy. Optik 86(3):104–110
10. Nakamura O (1999) Fundamental of two-photon microscopy. Microsc Res Tech 47(3):165–171. doi:10.1002/(SICI)1097-0029(19991101)47:3<165::AID-JEMT2>3.0.CO;2-D
11. Xu C, Zipfel W, Shear JB et al (1996) Multiphoton fluorescence excitation: new spectral windows for biological nonlinear microscopy. Proc Natl Acad Sci U S A 93(20):10763–10768. doi:10.1073/pnas.93.20.10763
12. Zipfel WR, Williams RM, Christie R et al (2003) Live tissue intrinsic emission microscopy using multiphoton-excited native fluorescence and second harmonic generation. Proc Natl Acad Sci U S A 100(12):7075–7080. doi:10.1073/pnas.0832308100
13. Zipfel WR, Williams RM, Webb WW (2003) Nonlinear magic: multiphoton microscopy in the biosciences. Nat Biotechnol 21(11):1369–1377. doi:10.1038/nbt899
14. Centonze VE, White JG (1998) Multiphoton excitation provides optical sections from deeper within scattering specimens than confocal imaging. Biophys J 75(4):2015–2024. doi:10.1016/S0006-3495(98)77643-X
15. Fine S, Hansen WP (1971) Optical second harmonic generation in biological systems. Appl Opt 10(10):2350–2353. doi:10.1364/AO.10.002350
16. Mohler W, Millard AC, Campagnola PJ (2003) Second harmonic generation imaging of endogenous structural proteins. Methods 29(1):97–109. doi:10.1016/S1046-2023(02)00292-X
17. Roth S, Freund I (1979) Second-harmonic generation in collagen. J Chem Phys 70(4):1637–1643. doi:10.1063/1.437677
18. Freund I, Deutsch M, Sprecher A (1986) Connective tissue polarity. Optical second-harmonic microscopy, crossed-beam summation, and small-angle scattering in rat-tail tendon. Biophys J 50(4):693–712. doi:10.1016/S0006-3495(86)83510-X
19. Boulesteix T, Beaurepaire E, Sauviat MP et al (2004) Second-harmonic microscopy of unstained living cardiac myocytes: measurements of sarcomere length with 20-nm accuracy. Opt Lett 29(17):2031–2033. doi:10.1364/OL.29.002031

20. Both M, Vogel M, Friedrich O et al (2004) Second harmonic imaging of intrinsic signals in muscle fibers in situ. J Biomed Opt 9(5):882–892. doi:10.1117/1.1783354
21. Plotnikov SV, Millard AC, Campagnola PJ et al (2006) Characterization of the myosin-based source for second-harmonic generation from muscle sarcomeres. Biophys J 90(2):693–703. doi:10.1529/biophysj.105.071555
22. Llewellyn ME, Barretto RP, Delp SL et al (2008) Minimally invasive high-speed imaging of sarcomere contractile dynamics in mice and humans. Nature 454(7205):784–788. doi:10.1038/nature07104
23. Nucciotti V, Stringari C, Sacconi L et al (2010) Probing myosin structural conformation in vivo by second-harmonic generation microscopy. Proc Natl Acad Sci U S A 107(17):7763–7768. doi:10.1073/pnas.0914782107
24. Dombeck DA, Kasischke KA, Vishwasrao HD et al (2003) Uniform polarity microtubule assemblies imaged in native brain tissue by second-harmonic generation microscopy. Proc Natl Acad Sci U S A 100(12):7081–7086. doi:10.1073/pnas.0731953100
25. Yeh AT, Nassif N, Zoumi A et al (2002) Selective corneal imaging using combined second-harmonic generation and two-photon excited fluorescence. Opt Lett 27(23):2082–2084. doi:10.1364/OL.27.002082
26. Han M, Giese G, Bille J (2005) Second harmonic generation imaging of collagen fibrils in cornea and sclera. Opt Express 13(15):5791–5797. doi:10.1364/OPEX.13.005791
27. Matteini P, Ratto F, Rossi F et al (2009) Photothermally-induced disordered patterns of corneal collagen revealed by SHG imaging. Opt Express 17(6):4868–4878. doi:10.1364/OE.17.004868
28. Stoller P, Kim BM, Rubenchik AM et al (2002) Polarization-dependent optical second-harmonic imaging of a rat-tail tendon. J Biomed Opt 7(2):205–214. doi:10.1117/1.1431967
29. Theodossiou T, Rapti GS, Hovhannisyan V et al (2002) Thermally induced irreversible conformational changes in collagen probed by optical second harmonic generation and laser-induced fluorescence. Lasers Med Sci 17(1):34–41. doi:10.1007/s101030200007
30. Zoumi A, Lu X, Kassab GS et al (2004) Imaging coronary artery microstructure using second-harmonic and two-photon fluorescence microscopy. Biophys J 87(4):2778–2786. doi:10.1529/biophysj.104.042887
31. Cicchi R, Matthaus C, Meyer T et al (2014) Characterization of collagen and cholesterol deposition in atherosclerotic arterial tissue using non-linear microscopy. J Biophotonics 7(1–2):135–143. doi:10.1002/jbio.201300055
32. Stoller P, Reiser KM, Celliers PM et al (2002) Polarization-modulated second harmonic generation in collagen. Biophys J 82(6):3330–3342. doi:10.1016/S0006-3495(02)75673-7
33. Yasui T, Tohno Y, Araki T (2004) Characterization of collagen orientation in human dermis by two-dimensional second-harmonic-generation polarimetry. J Biomed Opt 9(2):259–264. doi:10.1117/1.1644116
34. Cicchi R, Sestini S, De Giorgi V et al (2008) Nonlinear laser imaging of skin lesions. J Biophotonics 1(1):62–73. doi:10.1002/jbio.200710003
35. Su PJ, Chen WL, Hong JB et al (2009) Discrimination of collagen in normal and pathological skin dermis through second-order susceptibility microscopy. Opt Express 17(13):11161–11171. doi:10.1364/OE.17.011161
36. Pena AM, Fagot D, Olive C et al (2010) Multiphoton microscopy of engineered dermal substitutes: assessment of 3-D collagen matrix remodeling induced by fibroblast contraction. J Biomed Opt 15(5):056018. doi:10.1117/1.3503411
37. Cicchi R, Kapsokalyvas D, De Giorgi V et al (2010) Scoring of collagen organization in healthy and diseased human dermis by multiphoton microscopy. J Biophotonics 3(1–2):34–43. doi:10.1002/jbio.200910062
38. Medyukhina A, Vogler N, Latka I et al (2011) Automated classification of healthy and keloidal collagen patterns based on processing of SHG images of human skin. J Biophotonics 4(9):627–636. doi:10.1002/jbio.201100028
39. Chen J, Zhuo S, Jiang X et al (2011) Multiphoton microscopy study of the morphological and quantity changes of collagen and elastic fiber components in keloid disease. J Biomed Opt 16(5):051305. doi:10.1117/1.3569617
40. Lin SJ, Hsiao CY, Sun Y et al (2005) Monitoring the thermally induced structural transitions of collagen by use of second-harmonic generation microscopy. Opt Lett 30(6):622–624. doi:10.1364/OL.30.000622
41. Lo W, Chang YL, Liu JS et al (2009) Multimodal, multiphoton microscopy and image correlation analysis for characterizing corneal thermal damage. J Biomed Opt 14(5):054003. doi:10.1117/1.3213602
42. Matteini P, Cicchi R, Ratto F et al (2012) Thermal transitions of fibrillar collagen unveiled by second-harmonic generation microscopy of corneal stroma. Biophys

J 103(6):1179–1187. doi:10.1016/j.bpj.2012.07.055

43. Guo Y, Savage HE, Liu F et al (1999) Subsurface tumor progression investigated by noninvasive optical second harmonic tomography. Proc Natl Acad Sci U S A 96(19):10854–10856. doi:10.1073/pnas.96.19.10854
44. Brown E, McKee T, diTomaso E et al (2003) Dynamic imaging of collagen and its modulation in tumors in vivo using second-harmonic generation. Nat Med 9(6):796–800. doi:10.1038/nm879
45. Provenzano PP, Eliceiri KW, Campbell JM et al (2006) Collagen reorganization at the tumor-stromal interface facilitates local invasion. BMC Med 4(1):38. doi:10.1186/1741-7015-4-38
46. Lin SJ, Jee SH, Kuo CJ et al (2006) Discrimination of basal cell carcinoma from normal dermal stroma by quantitative multiphoton imaging. Opt Lett 31(18):2756–2758. doi:10.1364/OL.31.002756
47. Han X, Burke RM, Zettel ML et al (2008) Second harmonic properties of tumor collagen: determining the structural relationship between reactive stroma and healthy stroma. Opt Express 16(3):1846–1859. doi:10.1364/OE.16.001846
48. Nadiarnykh O, LaComb RB, Brewer MA et al (2010) Alterations of the extracellular matrix in ovarian cancer studied by second harmonic generation imaging microscopy. BMC Cancer 10:94. doi:10.1186/1471-2407-10-94
49. Raja AM, Xu S, Sun W et al (2010) Pulse-modulated second harmonic imaging microscope quantitatively demonstrates marked increase of collagen in tumor after chemotherapy. J Biomed Opt 15(5):056016. doi:10.1117/1.3497565
50. Plotnikov SV, Kenny AM, Walsh SJ et al (2008) Measurement of muscle disease by quantitative second-harmonic generation imaging. J Biomed Opt 13(4):044018. doi:10.1117/1.2967536
51. Nadiarnykh O, Plotnikov S, Mohler WA et al (2007) Second harmonic generation imaging microscopy studies of osteogenesis imperfecta. J Biomed Opt 12(5):051805. doi:10.1117/1.2799538
52. Lacomb R, Nadiarnykh O, Campagnola PJ (2008) Quantitative second harmonic generation imaging of the diseased state osteogenesis imperfecta: experiment and simulation. Biophys J 94(11):4504–4514. doi:10.1529/biophysj.107.114405
53. Reiser KM, Bratton C, Yankelevich DR et al (2007) Quantitative analysis of structural disorder in intervertebral disks using second harmonic generation imaging: comparison with morphometric analysis. J Biomed Opt 12(6):064019. doi:10.1117/1.2812631
54. Tiwari N, Chabra S, Mehdi S et al (2010) Imaging of normal and pathologic joint synovium using nonlinear optical microscopy as a potential diagnostic tool. J Biomed Opt 15(5):056001. doi:10.1117/1.3484262
55. Strupler M, Pena AM, Hernest M et al (2007) Second harmonic imaging and scoring of collagen in fibrotic tissues. Opt Express 15(7):4054–4065. doi:10.1364/OE.15.004054
56. Strupler M, Hernest M, Fligny C et al (2008) Second harmonic microscopy to quantify renal interstitial fibrosis and arterial remodeling. J Biomed Opt 13(5):054041. doi:10.1117/1.2981830
57. Pena AM, Fabre A, Debarre D et al (2007) Three-dimensional investigation and scoring of extracellular matrix remodeling during lung fibrosis using multiphoton microscopy. Microsc Res Tech 70(2):162–170. doi:10.1002/jemt.20400
58. Gailhouste L, Le Grand Y, Odin C et al (2010) Fibrillar collagen scoring by second harmonic microscopy: a new tool in the assessment of liver fibrosis. J Hepatol 52(3):398–406. doi:10.1016/j.jhep.2009.12.009
59. Guilbert T, Odin C, Le Grand Y et al (2010) A robust collagen scoring method for human liver fibrosis by second harmonic microscopy. Opt Express 18(25):25794–25807. doi:10.1364/OE.18.025794
60. Barad Y, Eisenberg H, Horowitz M et al (1997) Nonlinear scanning laser microscopy by third harmonic generation. Appl Phys Lett 70:922–924. doi:10.1063/1.118442
61. Oron D, Yelin D, Tal E et al (2004) Depth-resolved structural imaging by third-harmonic generation microscopy. J Struct Biol 147(1):3–11. doi:10.1016/S1047-8477(03)00125-4
62. Debarre D, Supatto W, Pena AM et al (2006) Imaging lipid bodies in cells and tissues using third-harmonic generation microscopy. Nat Methods 3(1):47–53. doi:10.1038/nmeth813
63. Mertz J, Moreaux L (2001) Second-harmonic generation by focused excitation of inhomogeneously distributed scatterers. Opt Commun 196:325–330. doi:10.1016/S0030-4018(01)01403-1
64. Vanzi F, Sacconi L, Cicchi R et al (2012) Protein conformation and molecular order probed by second-harmonic-generation microscopy. J Biomed Opt 17(6):060901. doi:10.1117/1.JBO.17.6.060901
65. Cicchi R, Vogler N, Kapsokalyvas D et al (2013) From molecular structure to tissue architecture: collagen organization probed by SHG microscopy. J Biophotonics 6(2):129–142. doi:10.1002/jbio.201200092

Part IV

Optical and Computational Methods

Chapter 28

Methods for Quantifying Fibrillar Collagen Alignment

Yuming Liu, Adib Keikhosravi, Guneet S. Mehta, Cole R. Drifka, and Kevin W. Eliceiri

Abstract

Recent evidence has implicated collagen, particularly fibrillar collagen, in a number of diseases ranging from osteogenesis imperfecta and asthma to breast and ovarian cancer. A key property of collagen that has been correlated with disease has been the alignment of collagen fibers. Collagen can be visualized using a variety of imaging techniques including second-harmonic generation (SHG) microscopy, polarized light microscopy, and staining with dyes or antibodies. However, there exists a great need to easily and robustly quantify images from these modalities for individual fibers in specified regions of interest and with respect to relevant boundaries. Most currently available computational tools rely on calculation of pixel-wise orientation or global window-wise orientation that do not directly calculate or give visible fiber-wise information and do not provide relative orientation against boundaries. We describe and detail how to use a freely available, open-source MATLAB software framework that includes two separate but linked packages "CurveAlign" and "CT-FIRE" that can address this need by either directly extracting individual fibers using an improved fiber tracking algorithm or directly finding optimal representation of fiber edges using the curvelet transform. This curvelet-based framework allows the user to measure fiber alignment on a global, region of interest, and fiber basis. Additionally, users can measure fiber angle relative to manually or automatically segmented boundaries. This tool does not require prior experience of programming or image processing and can handle multiple files, enabling efficient quantification of collagen organization from biological datasets.

Key words Fibrillar collagen, Collagen quantification, Collagen alignment, Collagen organization, Curvelet transform, Fiber tracking, Second-harmonic generation microscopy, Tumor-associated collagen signatures, Cancer imaging, Extracellular matrix

1 Introduction

Fibrillar collagens are one of the prominent extracellular matrix components. Studies have shown that specific changes in collagen alignment play an important role in contributing to the mechanical properties of tissues [1–4] and are associated with disease progression as shown in breast [5–7] and pancreatic [8–10] cancers.

Authors Yuming Liu and Adib Keikhosravi contributed equally to this work.

Laure Rittié (ed.), *Fibrosis: Methods and Protocols*, Methods in Molecular Biology, vol. 1627, DOI 10.1007/978-1-4939-7113-8_28, © Springer Science+Business Media LLC 2017

Image analysis methods suitable for quantifying fibrillar collagen alignment and orientation are generally based on the intensity derivatives [11–16] or intensity variation [17], Fourier transform [18–22] or Hough transform [23, 24] or directional filters [25–27], or fiber tracking algorithm [28–31]. Derivative-based methods can usually yield pixel-wise orientation and require additional steps to detect fiber edges. The filter or transform-based methods can usually only yield global measurements for a window with a given size and would be time-consuming to yield pixel-wise orientation. Fiber tracking algorithms use fiber propagation criteria based on, for example, local fiber center location and orientation to form individual fibers and are usually computationally demanding and have been challenged in extracting complex fiber networks.

Given the importance of fiber alignment and the need for transparency on how it is being quantified, an emphasis of the collagen research community has been to develop open-source approaches rather than closed-source proprietary tools. Besides being freely available with fewer barriers to use and adaption, open-source tools allow for one to examine the algorithms being used to assure the best results and also allow programmers to adapt or reuse code in their specific workflows. Also, software licenses of most open-source scientific programming efforts are commercially friendly opening up opportunities for adaptation by commercial imaging tools.

Currently freely available open-source software tools for collagen alignment quantification include the ImageJ [32] plug-ins "FibrilTool" [15] and "Orientation J" [13, 33], the MATLAB (MathWorks, Natick, MA, USA) stand-alone applications "CytoSpectre" [34, 35], "CurveAlign" [25, 31, 36], and "CT-FIRE" [37, 38]. FibrilTool is based on the first derivative and borrows the concept of local nematic tensor as applied in the field of liquid crystal physics. It calculates the main orientation and alignment of the fibers within the region of interest (ROI) by using the average local nematic tensors over an ROI. This tool needs manual involvement to evaluate the results and to choose ROIs that are suitable for analysis. Hence, it can be time-consuming for high-throughput processing. Orientation J uses the first derivative and a Gaussian weighting function to construct a structure tensor commonly used in the field of image processing. It calculates the orientation and anisotropy information for each pixel and has additional steps to identify pixels belonging to a fiber and assign a weight to elongated structures for orientation calculation. This tool involves manual operation to annotate the ROI and is convenient for processing a single image or an image stack, but it is not trivial to process a large number of images. CytoSpectre uses Fourier transform-based spectrum analysis to extract the orientation and its anisotropy within a specified window. It does not require additional pre- or post-processing steps, is highly robust to background noise, and can be easily used for processing multiple images. However, this tool can only provide global information rather than the localized fiber measurements.

Here, we describe the latest version of CurveAlign (CurveAlign 4.0), which provides a powerful and comprehensive platform for quantifying fibrillar collagen on a global, ROI, and fiber basis. The development of this program was driven by our active work in characterizing the role of collagen organization in disease [4–10, 31, 38–45]. This software platform uses two fiber analysis methods, CT-FIRE [38] and curvelets fiber representation (CFR) [25]. While these analysis methods can be downloaded and used as separate tools, we will here refer to the "CurveAlign" platform where CurveAlign can be run in both the CT-FIRE and CFR modes. CT-FIRE first uses the curvelet transform (CT) [46] to de-noise the image and enhance the fiber edges and then uses a fiber tracking algorithm (FIRE) [29] to form individual fiber networks, which includes major steps of fiber boundary detection, fiber center point identification, fiber extension from the center points, short fiber removal, and fiber network creation. While CFR does not extract individual fibers, it uses the curvelets in CT to directly represent the edges of fiber segments since curvelets have high-resolution information about their scale, location, and orientation and can optimally represent the local curve-like shapes. In contrast to other comparable methods, CFR does not need to add additional steps to detect fiber edges as in many pixel-wise approaches or to assume that spatial frequency of pixel intensity change can represent the fiber distribution as in the Fourier transform-based approach. In addition, measuring relative angle of the collagen fibers with respect to a boundary of interest, such as the tumor-stroma interface [5], is an important image analysis capability but is not available in the tools briefly mentioned above except for CurveAlign. Specifically, alignment can be calculated as angle relative to manually drawn boundaries or boundaries segmented through computational means [31]. Moreover, since fiber-wise orientation is calculated, CurveAlign also calculates alignment related to each fiber or fiber segments besides the alignment for a full image and an ROI. That is, each fiber or fiber segment has features related to alignment of specified surrounding rectangular regions (called box alignment) or nearest number of fibers (named nearest alignment) as described in detail in our previous publication [31].

CurveAlign capabilities have been successfully applied to numerous studies of collagen alignment. For example, the CT-FIRE module has been used to quantify fiber alignment in SHG images acquired from human pancreatic histology tissues. This enabled Drifka and colleagues to determine that stromal collagen alignment is significantly higher in pancreatic cancer compared to normal and chronic pancreatitis tissue [9]. Moreover, it was discovered that the degree of collagen alignment in pancreatic

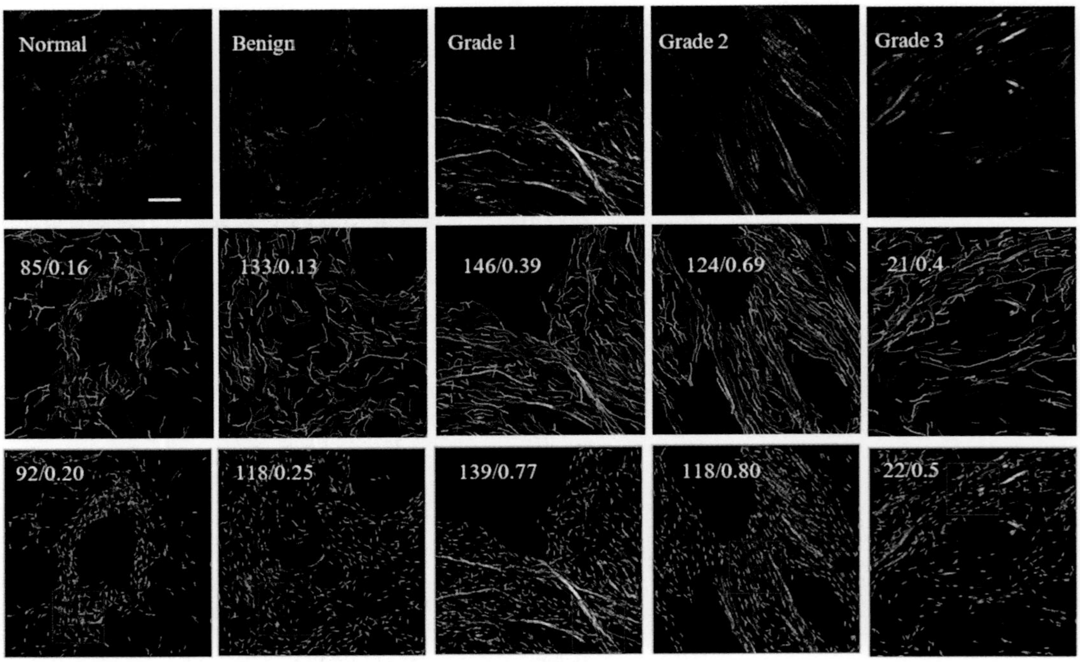

Fig. 1 An example of using CT-FIRE mode without the boundary mode of CurveAlign for both full image and ROI analyses in pancreatic tissue. The *top row* shows the SHG image from different types of pancreatic tissue. The *middle row* shows the CT-FIRE extracted fibers highlighted by different colored lines for the purpose of contrast, which are overlaid upon the SHG image. The *bottom row* is the "Overlay" image generated by CurveAlign showing the location (*red dots*) and orientation (*green lines*) of the extracted fibers as well as the annotated ROI overlaid upon the SHG image. The quantification of the full image and the representative ROI are displayed in the format of "mean orientation/alignment" at the top left corner of the *middle row* and *bottom row*, respectively. Both full image-based and ROI-based quantifications show that collagen fibers are more aligned in malignant ducts (Grade 1–3) than in normal and benign ducts. Default parameters were used here. Image size is 1024 x 1024 pixels, and ROI size is 256 x 256 pixels. The scale bar at the top left column indicates 50 μm, and all images are shown at the same scale

tumors correlates with patient survival [10]. A demonstration of CurveAlign in CT-FIRE mode, without a boundary for both a full image and ROI-based analysis, in pancreatic tissue [9] is shown in Fig. 1. CurveAlign has also been used in breast cancer research: for example, in CFR mode to quantify collagen alignment in breast cancer tissue where it indicated significantly less aligned fibers after treatment of a tumor [47]. It was also used in an in vitro study of breast carcinoma cells in 3D culture to show how the angle of fibers with respect to the boundaries formed by groups of cells differs under varying culture conditions and pharmacological perturbations [44]. In CT-FIRE mode, it was used to automatically quantify both the angle with respect to a boundary and localized fiber-based relative alignments, which are important factors in human breast carcinoma prognosis [31]. A demonstration of using

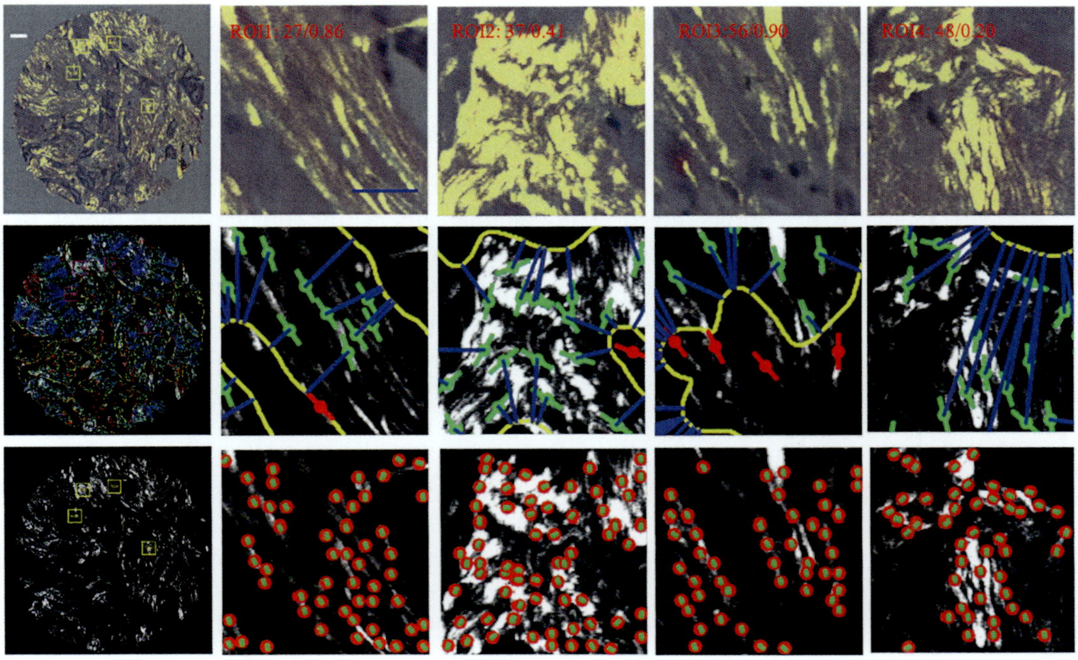

Fig. 2 An example of using CurveAlign to quantify relative angle and ROI-based alignment on breast cancer tissue microarray. The first column shows the SHG image (*in yellow*) overlaid on the bright-field H&E image with four rectangular ROI annotations (*in yellow*) (*top*), the orientations and locations of extracted fibers using CT-FIRE mode (*in green color*) with four ROI annotations (*in magenta*) overlaid on the SHG image (*in gray*) (*middle*), and four rectangular ROI annotations (*in yellow*) overlaid on the SHG image (*in gray*) (*bottom*), respectively. The remaining four columns from *left* to *right* show the cropped images of the four ROIs, where for the ones in the top row, ROI name as well as its mean relative angle and ROI-based alignment in the format of "ROI name: mean relative angle/ROI alignment." In the middle row, the *blue line* is used to associate the center of fiber extracted by CT-FIRE with the corresponding boundary locations, and the *red line* shows the fibers located either beyond the distance range or within the boundary. In the bottom row, the locations and orientations of fiber segments analyzed by CFR mode were indicated by *red dots* and *green lines*. From the figure, we can see that fibers in ROI 1 and ROI 3 are both well aligned, but there are more fibers in ROI 3 that are more perpendicularly aligned with respect to the tumor boundary. The boundary creation parameter is the same as in Fig. 6, i.e., pixel per micron ratio was set to 2; fiber extraction in CT-FIRE used default settings; the distance parameter was set to 250 pixels; the fraction of kept curvelets is set to 0.06. The image size is 2048 x 2048 pixels, and the sizes of ROI are identically set to 128 x 128 pixels. The scale bar for the full size image at the first column of the first row indicates 100 μm, scale bar for the ROI image at the second column of the first row indicates 25 μm, and all images either full size images or ROIs are shown at the same scale

both CT-FIRE mode and CFR mode for quantification of relative angle and ROI-based alignment is shown in Fig. 2.

There are three kinds of alignments calculated in CurveAlign: (1) alignment with respect to the horizontal named "angle" or "orientation," ranging from 0 to 180°; (2) alignment with respect to a boundary named "relative angle" or "relative orientation," ranging from 0 to 90°; and (3) alignment of fibers with respect to each other named "alignment coefficient," ranging from 0 to 1. In CurveAlign, to calculate the alignment coefficient, the angle is first multiplied by 2 to map to the orientation range of [0-2π], and then the alignment coefficient is calculated as the normalized vector sum of orientation vectors or mean resultant vector length in circular statistics. The alignment coefficient ranges from 0 to 1, with 1 indicating perfectly aligned fibers, and smaller values representing more randomly distributed fibers. To be noted, the alignment coefficient indicates the dispersity of the fiber orientations and has been defined in different ways or terms, such as anisotropy index [21] based on eigenvalues of a second rank tensor, coherence [13] based on structure tensor eigenvalues, anisotropy based on circular variance [15] in circular statistics, or mean vector length [12, 31] in circular statistics (as in CurveAlign). Hereafter, the name "alignment" will be used to simplify the term of "alignment coefficient" unless stated otherwise.

The schematic workflow for quantifying collagen alignment in a single image with CurveAlign is shown in Fig. 3. The details of each step will be described in Subheading 3.1. The graphical user interface (GUI) of CurveAlign is modular, and some functions were implemented in different modules, which are separate from but can be called from the main GUI. To process multiple images in a batch mode, if needed, the CT-FIRE (CTF), boundary creation, and ROI manager modules can be used to prepare the required CTF output file, boundary mask file, or ROI annotation file in advance, respectively. Once all the required files associated with each image are provided, one can simply follow the same procedure as that for a single image analysis to run the quantification for all of the images. Output can be in the form of overlaid images of the extracted fibers or curvelets on the original image, table of summary statistics, heatmap showing the alignment or relative angle distribution, Excel files of the fiber alignment coefficient and angles, as well as others. Post-processing module can combine output of CurveAlign to show combined summary statistics of the quantified fiber features including collagen fiber alignment and orientation.

2 Materials

2.1 Images

Collagen is typically imaged using SHG microscopy, polarized light microscopy, or dyes and stains in conjunction with bright-field or fluorescence microscopy [48–54]. CurveAlign can analyze any image file readable by MATLAB regardless of the imaging modality used to collect it. As SHG imaging is a label-free modality offering optical sectioning and high specificity and resolution, it has become a popular fibrillar collagen imaging method (*see* Chap. 27 for protocols and tips). Our group and others have widely used SHG microscopy to investigate collagen in a variety of tissue types

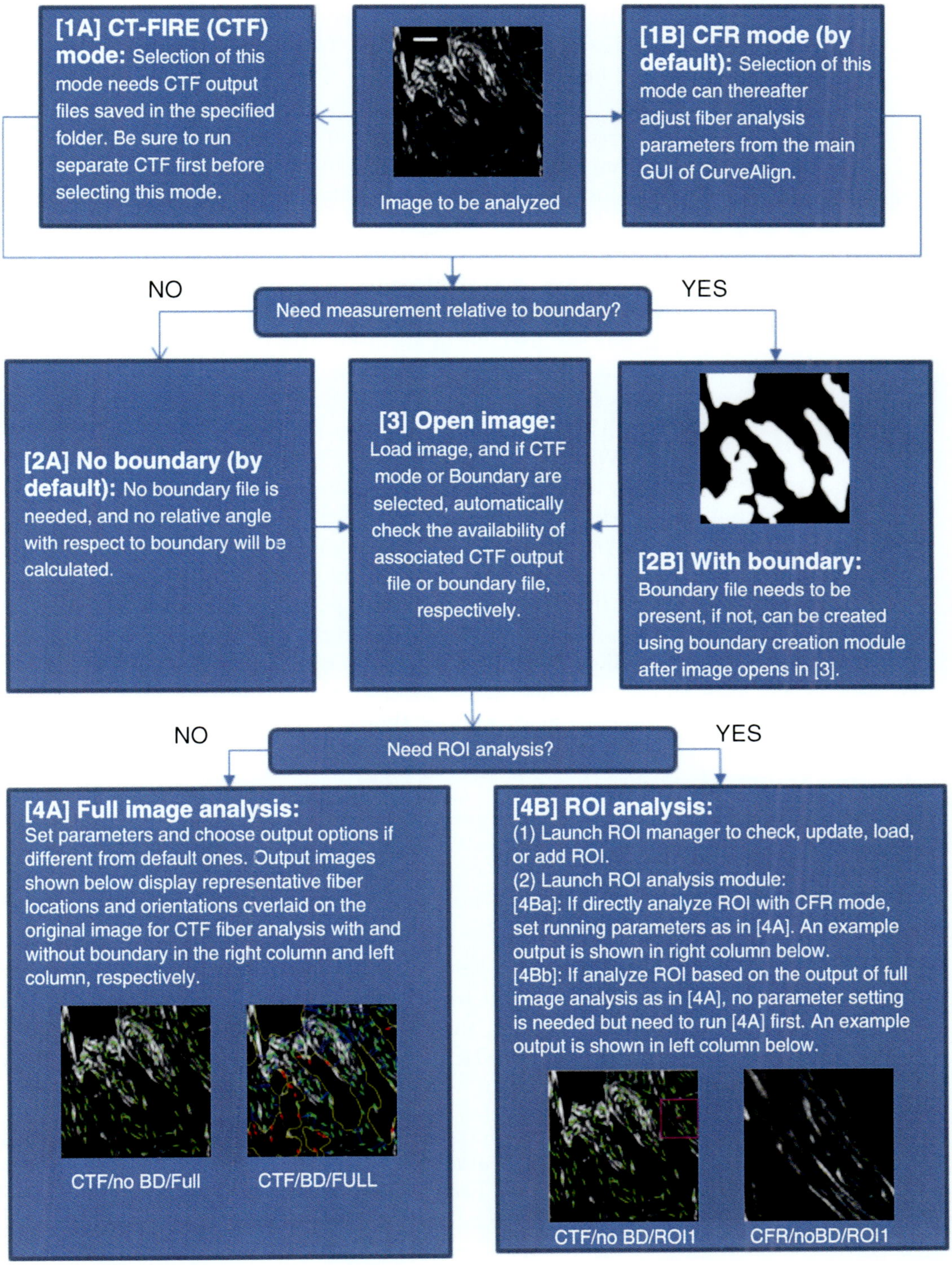

Fig. 3 Schematic workflow of quantifying collagen alignment using CurveAlign for a single image. For the images in step 4, the fiber location and orientation were highlighted by *red dots* and *green lines*, respectively; the *red lines* indicate the fibers are out of the interested region. For [4B], there are two types of ROI analysis, type 1 ([4Ba]) can directly run CFR mode on the annotated ROI, but type 2 [4Bb] needs to run a full image analysis first either in CFR mode or in CT-FIRE mode. CTF, CT-FIRE; CFR, curvelets fiber representation; BD, with boundary; no BD, without boundary; FULL, full image analysis; and ROI, ROI analysis. The scale bar shown in the image at the *top middle column* indicates 50 μm, and all images are shown at the same scale

including human breast cancer tissue [38] and human pancreatic cancer tissue [9]. Data from these two studies in .tif file format will be used here for a demonstration.

2.2 Software

Download the MATLAB Runtime Compiler (MCR) and the CurveAlign software from [36] and follow the detailed requirements and installation instructions from the above web page. A user guide is also available for download: it provides detailed information for installation and operation.

Both stand-alone and source-code versions are freely available. The stand-alone version does not require a full MATLAB installation, but the user needs to install the freely available MATLAB MCR package (download link available at [36]). As CurveAlign requires significant memory use especially for big image processing or parallel computing, we only provide stand-alone applications for 64-bit Windows or Mac systems. These programs can be run on Unix as well but require code compilation for this operating system including Linux. The source-code version requires a full MATLAB installation including toolboxes of Signal Processing, Image Processing, Statistics Analysis, and Parallel Computing.

For the stand-alone version, open the software by double clicking (in Windows system) or right-clicking (in Mac) on the CurveAlign icon. This will launch the main GUI shown in Fig. 4a. Figure 4b shows the GUI for CT-FIRE individual analysis that can be launched by clicking on the "CT-FIRE" button (labeled as 6 in Fig. 4a).

3 Methods

3.1 Collagen Fiber Analysis with CurveAlign

1. Download and install MATLAB MCR and CurveAlign (*see* Subheading 2.2).
2. *Fiber analysis mode selection* (step 1 of Fig. 3): Select the fiber analysis method from the drop-down menu (labeled as 1 in Fig. 4a) among the following four options from CFR mode (CT) and CT-FIRE mode (segments, fibers, and endpoints) (*see* **Notes 1–3**):
   (a) *CT*: The curvelet transform is performed on the image(s), and each curvelet corresponds to an observation in the feature list. Each curvelet has a unique angle and position. In this case, no individual fiber is extracted and the curvelets that indicate the representative locations and directions of fiber segments are calculated as shown in Fig. 5a.
   (b) *CT-FIRE segments*: The output from CT-FIRE as illustrated in Fig. 5b is used as the input, providing information about the fibers in the image. Each fiber is represented

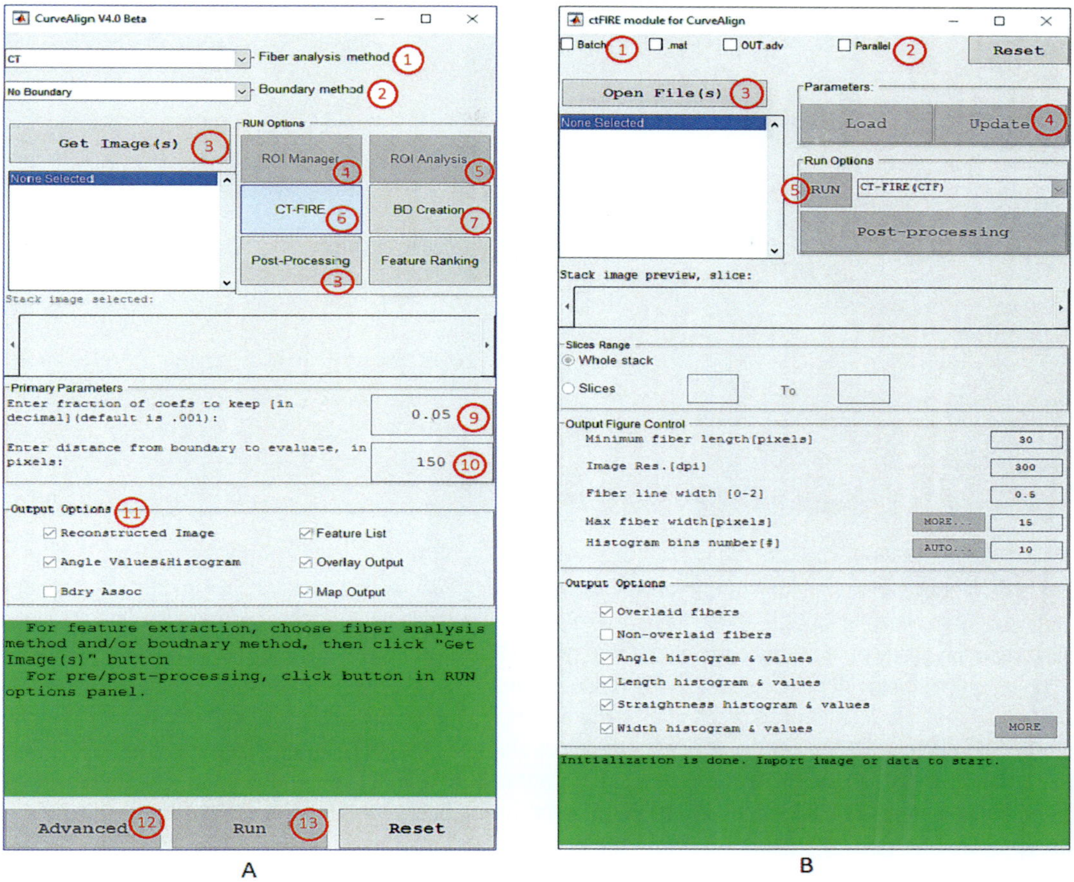

Fig. 4 Graphical user interface of CurveAlign (**a**) and CT-FIRE (**b**)

as segments with individual orientations and locations, and each fiber segment in the CT-FIRE output file corresponds to an observation in the CurveAlign feature set. Each segment has equal length (set at 5 pixels by default) and has a unique angle and position.

(c) *CT-FIRE fibers:* The output from CT-FIRE as illustrated in Fig. 5b is used as the input, providing information about the fibers in the image. Each fiber center point in the CT-FIRE output file corresponds to an observation in the feature set. Each center point has a unique angle corresponding to the average angle of the fiber. The position is the midpoint between the fiber endpoints by default.

(d) *CT-FIRE fiber endpoints:* The output from CT-FIRE as illustrated in Fig. 5b is used as the input, providing information about the fibers in the image. Each fiber endpoint in the CT-FIRE output file corresponds to an observation in the feature set. Each endpoint has a unique angle and position. The angle corresponds to the angle of the entire fiber.

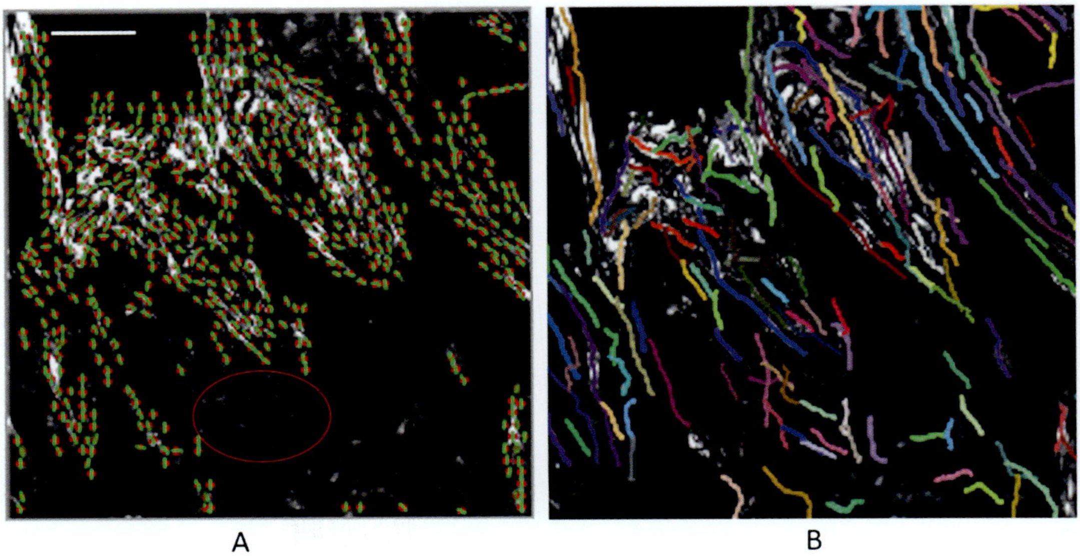

Fig. 5 Two fiber analysis modes in CurveAlign: (**a**) representative curvelets used in CFR mode; (**b**) extracted individual fibers used in CT-FIRE. This image of a relatively low-resolution portion of a breast tissue microarray illustrates the ability of the CurveAlign platform to extract fibers even when the fibers are relatively low signal to noise ratio but also demonstrates the difference between the two modes in fiber extraction. In (**a**), the *red dots* show the fiber location and green lines show the orientation. In (**b**), extracted fibers are displayed in different colored lines. CFR mode (**a**) indicates the most prominent fibers but does not provide individual fiber extraction as in CT-FIRE mode (**b**), which instead provides the information for entire fibers. CFR mode missed some fibers in the region annotated in *red ellipse* in (**a**) where fibers have relative lower intensity values. For the fiber analysis here, all parameters were kept as default ones except that, in CFR mode, the fraction of kept curvelet was set to 0.06. The image size is 512 pixels x 512 pixels. The scale bar at the *upper left* corner of (**a**) indicates 50 μm, and all images are shown at the same scale

3. *Determine boundary conditions* (step 2 of Fig. 3): Select the boundary processing mode from drop-down menu (labeled as 2 in Fig. 4a) among the following options: No Boundary, CSV Boundary, and TIFF Boundary (*see* **Notes 4** and **5**). For calculations of fiber angles with respect to a boundary, a corresponding boundary file for each image or each stack has to be provided. The user can follow the instructions on the screen to manually or automatically annotate either a "CSV" (comma-separated values format based, x-y coordinates) boundary file or a "TIFF" boundary file. The boundary files created in CurveAlign will be saved according to the file directory and file naming conventions described below.

(a) *CSV boundaries*: Previously stored boundary files can be used that contain the x-y positions of points along the boundary. CSV boundary files can also be manually annotated in later steps. CSV files must adhere to the following naming convention if they are defined outside CurveAlign: If the image is named "TACS-3a.jpg," the CSV file must be named "boundary for TACS-3a.jpg.csv." The boundary file must be in a sub-directory named "CA_Boundary."

(b) *TIFF boundaries* allow for identifying whether a fiber is inside an ROI. Mask files are used to indicate where region boundaries are located. The mask files should be 8-bit image files where the inside of ROIs is given a value of 255 or 1 and outside a value of 0. Mask files must be registered with the collagen image files and therefore have the same dimensions as the image files. TIFF boundary files must adhere to the following naming convention if they are defined outside CurveAlign. If the image is named "1B–a5.tif," the TIFF boundary file must be named "mask for 1B–a5.tif.tif." The boundary file must be presented in a sub-directory named "CA_Boundary". Boundary creation module can be launched by clicking on the "BD Creation" button labeled as 7 in Fig. 4a. An example of automatic TIFF boundary creation is shown in Fig. 6.

4. *Load image(s) or data file(s)* (step 3 of Fig. 3): Click on "Get Image(s)" button (labeled as 3 in Fig. 4a) and browse to an image. Images may be single or stacks. If needed, select multiple images in the dialog using the technique appropriate for your operating system (e.g., in Windows, hold CTRL while selecting multiple files).
5. *Annotate the ROIs* (step 4B of Fig. 3) by clicking on the "ROI Manager" button (labeled as 4 in Fig. 4a). Two new windows ("ROI Manager" and "CurveAlign ROI analysis output table") will open. Options to delineate and annotate different shapes of ROI as shown in Fig. 7b are provided in the drop-down menu of the "ROI Manager" window (Fig. 7a) and include rectangle, polygon, ellipse, freehand drawing arbitrary shapes, or specified rectangle. To create an ROI, select the desired shape in the drop-down menu, draw the shape directly on the image with a drag-and-drop mouse gesture, and click on "Save ROI(s)" (or press the "s" key). The newly created ROI then becomes listed on the left column of the ROI window with the default name ROI1, ROI2, etc. (Fig. 7a). ROIs can be renamed, deleted, combined with other ROIs, and saved into or loaded from a ".mat" file, mask image file, or ".txt" file. After drawing and saving an ROI, press the "d" key to continue to draw ROIs, or drag the previous ROI to a new position to create a new ROI. If original image name is "ImageName.tif," ROI file is named "ImageName_ROIs.mat" and saved in a subfolder of the image's directory named "ROI_management" (*see* **Note 6**).

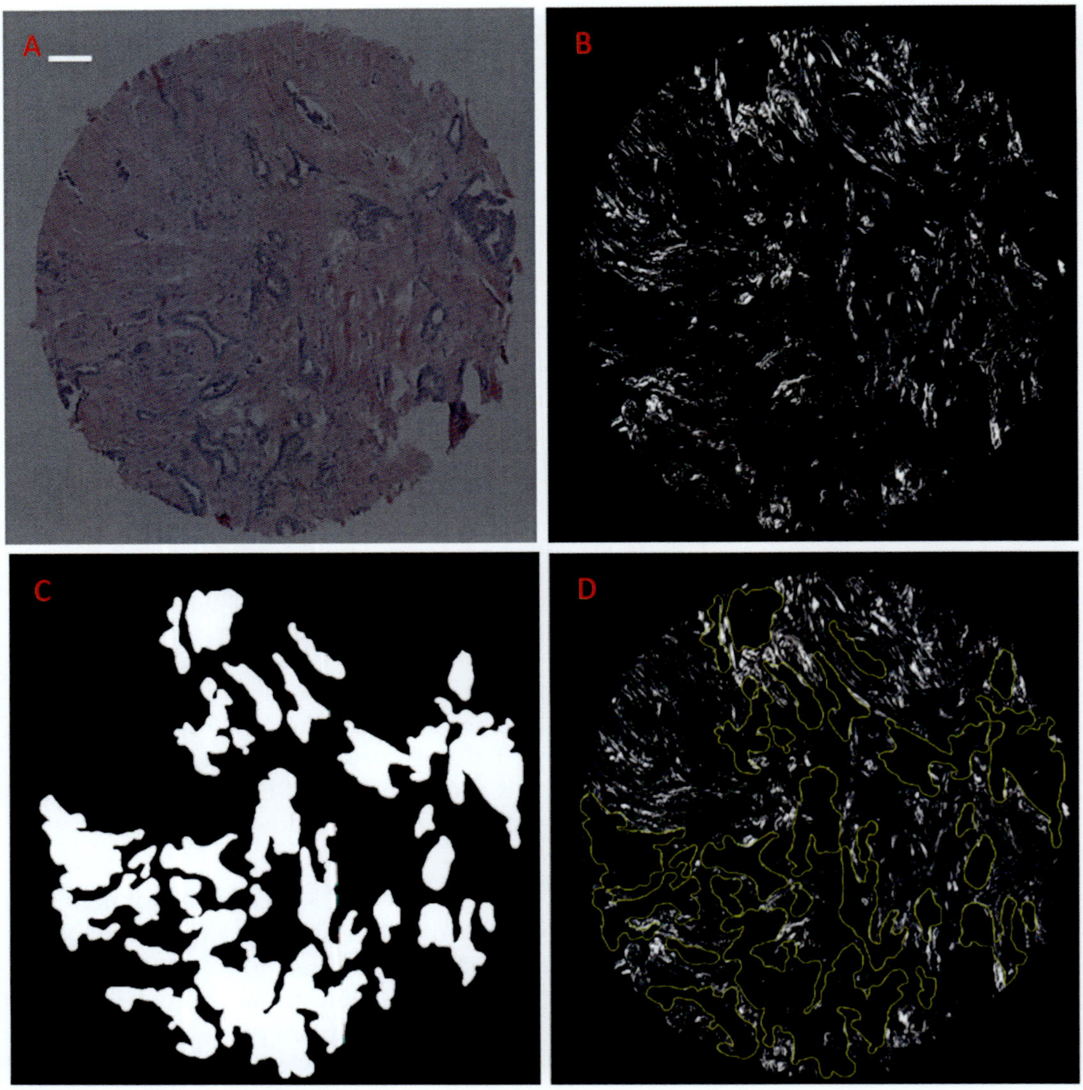

Fig. 6 Automatic tumor boundary creation for a breast cancer TMA core. The bright-field H&E image (**a**) is co-registered with the SHG image (**b**), and the boundary mask image (**c**) is created from segmentation of the H&E image. The boundaries were detected and overlaid on the SHG image (**d**). The only necessary parameter to be input for the segmentation is the pixel per micron ratio of the image (set to 2 in this image). The scale bar at the *upper left* corner of (**a**) indicates 100 μm, and all images are shown at the same scale

6. *Set running parameters* in the CurveAlign main window (steps 4A and 4B of Fig. 3):

(a) If fiber extraction mode "CT" is selected, enter the "fraction of coefs to keep" (labeled as 9 in Fig. 4a) to use the fraction of the largest coefficients of CT for curvelets calculation.

(b) When calculating the angle of fibers with respect to a boundary (relative angle), the user can spatially restrict the area over which fibers are analyzed. To define this radius from

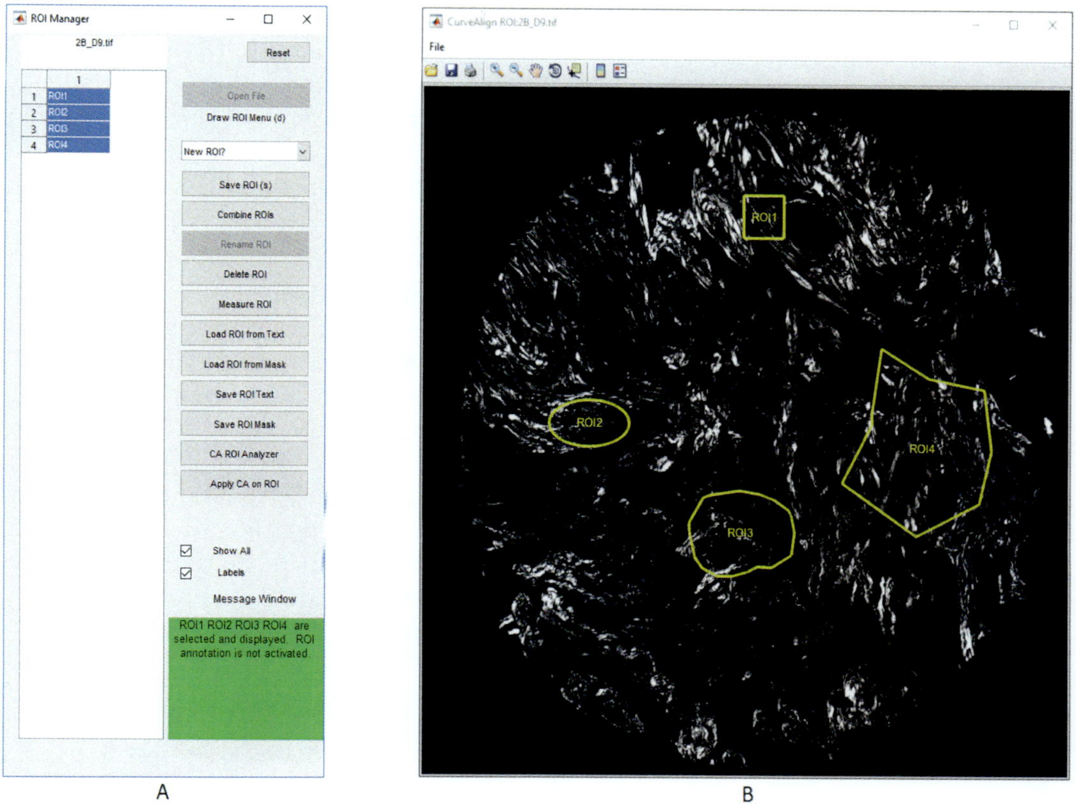

Fig. 7 Screenshot of the ROI manager being used to annotate different shapes of ROIs. (**a**) ROI manager user interface; and (**b**) ROI output figure

the boundary line, enter the distance in pixels (labeled as 10 in Fig. 4a).

(c) Select the desired outputs using the check boxes at the bottom of the main window in Fig. 4a (labeled as 11).

7. *Run the program and explore the results* (step 4 of Fig. 3): For full image analysis, click on the "Run" button labeled as 13 at the bottom of Fig. 4a. The progress information is displayed in a window highlighted in green color at the bottom of Fig. 4a, and the output data and images will open and will be automatically saved in a subfolder called "CA_Out" in the directory of the original image(s). For ROI image analysis, click on the "ROI analysis" button (labeled as 5 on Fig. 4a). It will prompt a window to select the ROI analysis mode (*see* **Notes 7** and **8**).
8. Post-processing: This module is used to combine the output of different images in the same folder. In the main window, click on "Post-Processing" (labeled as 8 on Fig. 4) to launch the post-processing module. In the "post-processing CA features"

window, click on the "Get CA output folder" button to select the output folder for the processed images. Click on the "OK" button to have the combined output results. Among the Post-Processing Options, the default is to combine "mean of all features" of each image; another useful option is "Combine feature files" to combine the features of all the fibers in the processed images.

9. The outputs of CurveAlign can be displayed in images, tables, and histograms and are mainly saved in the subfolders of "CA_Out," "CA_ROI," and "CA_Boundary" in the format of mask image file, overlaid image, heatmap image, ".CSV" file, ".mat" file, and excel file. A demonstration of some typical outputs is shown in Fig. 8.

3.2 Analysis Time Estimates

The estimated time scale for running each step on an image with size of 1024 × 1024 pixels with moderate fiber density is shown below. These times are estimates and depend on the size of the file, the particular CurveAlign features deployed, the central processing unit (CPU) type, and the amount of random-access memory (or RAM) a user has available.

- CurveAlign CRF mode for fiber representation: a few seconds
- CurveAlign CT-FIRE mode for fiber extraction: ~100 s
- CurveAlign boundary analysis: tens of seconds

3.3 Anticipated Results

We conducted tests on computer-generated artificial fibers, different types of SHG images, and polarized light microscope images. By comparing the orientation and alignment calculated by CurveAlign to real values generated by computer program, manually measured values by a panel of experts, or the values computed by Orientation J under certain conditions, we found that, in most cases, CurveAlign yields statistically reliable results that have a good correlation to results yielded from other approaches (comparison not shown here).

3.4 Advantages and Limitations

The main advantages of the CurveAlign software platform include: (1) Its capability to directly track or represent fibers or fiber segments and make the fiber tracking results visible to the user. This trait is particularly useful to provide direct fiber-wise alignment analysis. (2) It allows relative orientation measurements against boundaries that can be manually or automatically created by the tool itself. (3) It is a comprehensive platform that can meet different needs of collagen quantification for images, stacks, and ROIs and is suitable for high-throughput collagen analysis.

Meanwhile, there have been some limitations or challenges for each of the two fiber analysis modes CT-FIRE and CFR. While the CT-FIRE mode can provide the most complete information for each individual fiber and can be applied to most images with large heterogeneities in terms of contrast and noise level, there are three

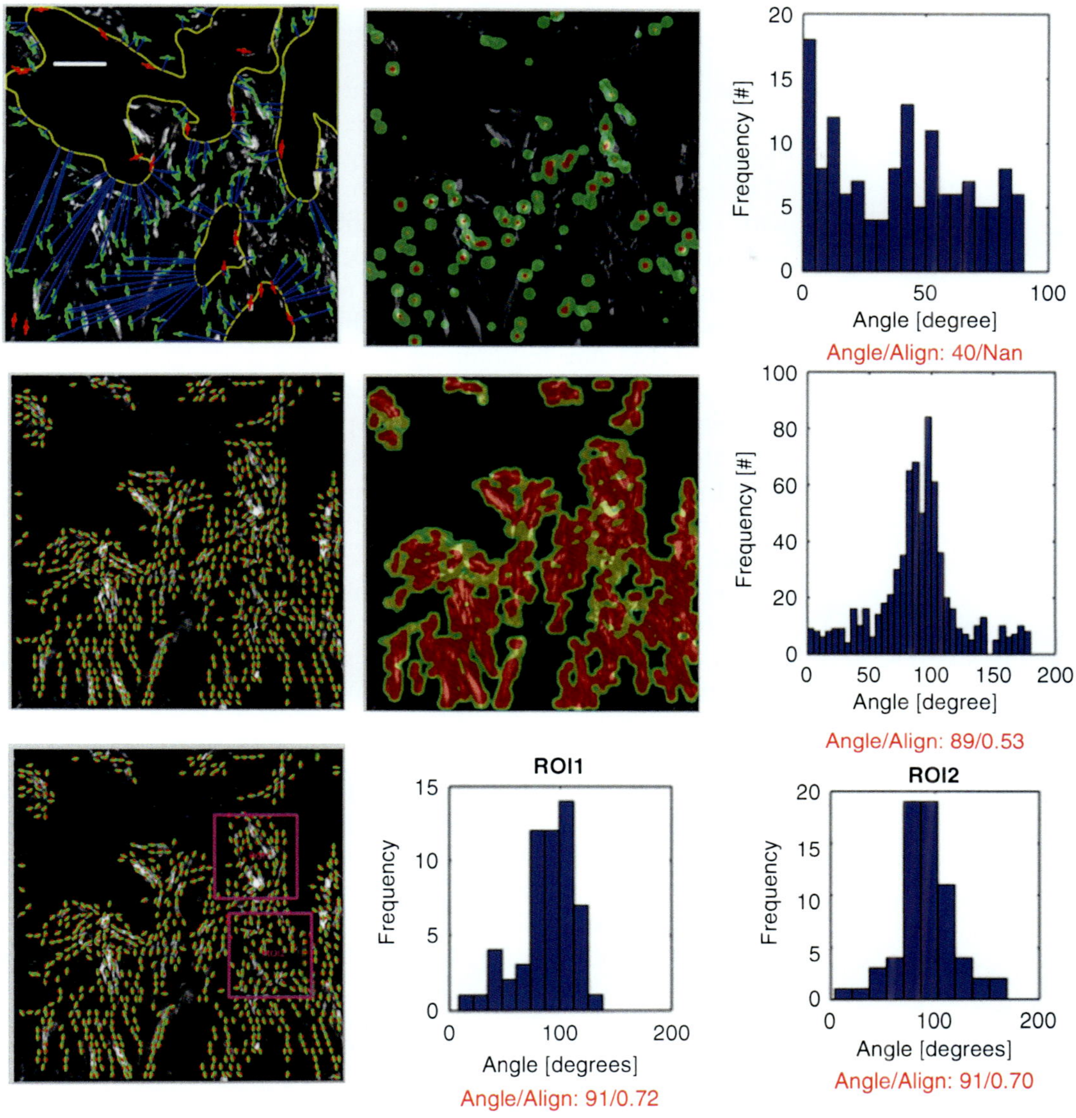

Fig. 8 Demonstration of typical outputs of CurveAlign: (1) The *top row* shows the relative angle (with respect to a boundary) using fibers extracted in CT-FIRE mode, the *left column* of this row shows that the *blue line* is used to associate the center of the fiber extracted by CT-FIRE with the corresponding boundary location, and the *red line* is used to show the fibers located either beyond the distance range or within the boundary; the heatmap at the *middle column* uses *red color* to indicate larger relative angles, and the histogram at the *right column* shows the distribution of the relative angle of fibers within the range of 0 to 90°; (2) the *middle row* shows the angle (with respect to the horizontal) measurement with CFR mode, and the *left column* of this row uses a *red dot* to indicate the center of fiber segments and a *green line* to indicate the fiber orientation at that point; the heatmap at the *middle column* uses *red color* to indicate well aligned fiber regions, and the histogram at the *right column* shows the distribution of the angles within the range of 0 to 180°; and (3) the *bottom row* shows ROI analysis based on the result from the CFR results shown in the *middle row*. Two magenta rectangular ROIs are annotated on the SHG image at the first column of this row, the histograms of angles within these two ROIs are displayed at the *middle* and *right columns*. Both the mean angle and alignment coefficient are listed below each histogram except that alignment is not calculated based on the relative angle data. The boundaries were cropped from the mask image shown in Fig. 6; fiber extraction in CT-FIRE used default settings; the distance parameter was set to 250 pixels; the fraction of kept curvelets is set to 0.06, the image size is 512 x 512 pixels, and the sizes of ROI are identically set to 128 x 128 pixels. The scale bar at the *upper left* corner of the *top row* indicates 50 μm, and all images are shown at the same scale

major challenges for the CT-FIRE mode: (1) The software has difficulty to extract an intact fiber (especially those having curvy shapes and varying intensities along their length) from a dense fiber network. The tracking of such a long curvy fiber may end up with a few fiber segments along the fiber propagation direction. In order to overcome this issue, the local pixel-wise orientation and anisotropy information (that can be readily calculated as described in other approaches [11–16]) can be combined to form a fiber. Alternatively, other techniques [28] such as those based on energy minimization along the fiber extension can be adapted to the current fiber extracting algorithm. In practice, if the orientation of individual fibers is not of interest, this issue is not actually a problem. In CurveAlign, the CT-FIRE segment mode can be selected as the fiber analysis method, which theoretically would yield comparable results to other applicable methods. (2) If fiber thicknesses vary a lot in an image, either the thinnest or the thickest fibers have to be compromised to some extent since only fibers whose thicknesses are within a fixed searching range can be accessed in the current fiber propagation algorithm. The fiber tracking strategy algorithm can be adapted to consider fiber thickness at different scales by adding fiber edge or ridge detection with automatic scale selection [55]. (3) The fiber tracking algorithm is computationally demanding, and it may take a much longer time than most derivative- or transform-based tools. The speed issue will need to be properly addressed before the program can perform real-time image processing or analysis of very large images (e.g., 10,000 × 10,000 pixels). Options include simplifying the fiber tracking algorithm to make it faster and combining ROI analysis (by automatically dividing image to smaller tilts) and parallel computing. These options will be investigated in future versions of the software. Of note, we have enabled parallel computing in CT-FIRE mode. Although this addition cannot reduce the processing time for each image, it allows the computer to process multiple images simultaneously depending on how many CPU cores in the computer are available for running CurveAlign, allowing for more rapid batch analysis of many images.

The CFR mode can directly find optimal representation of fiber edges using curvelets without any additional edge detection algorithms (that might be needed for derivative- or transform-based methods). The CFR mode operates at a similar time scale to derivative- or transform-based methods, which means it runs much faster than fiber tracking algorithms like CT-FIRE. However, in the current version of CT-FIRE (version 2.0), there are two major limitations. (1) It cannot be applied to images with a large variation in contrast. The program tends to bias toward fibers with highest intensities. A practical solution is using the ROI manager to annotate regions with even contrast for analysis and check the overlay results to make sure the extracted fiber edge matches the visual inspection. (2) It only uses the curvelets in one scale to characterize fiber edges and may not be able to faithfully represent all the fibers at different scales of thickness. In the current tool, we can set the scale relative to a specific thickness and set different group radius to group curvelets belonging to the same fiber, which can partially resolve this issue. A future solution would be to develop a strategy to combine the fiber information at different scales or do automatic scale selection [12] when calculating local curvelets orientation.

3.5 Troubleshooting and Practical Tips

Parallel computing techniques can be used for the CT-FIRE mode, which can save significant fiber extraction time for a batch of images. In some situations (e.g., for images with acceptable contrast), the CFR mode is equivalent to "CT-FIRE segments" option.

3.5.1 Adjust Parameters in CFR Mode

Some advanced settings can be selected by clicking on the "Advanced" button (labeled as 12 in Fig. 4a) and make changes to corresponding values, including:

1. The radius of grouping the curvelets, which is largely determined by the range of fiber thickness. The larger the grouping radius, the fewer curvelets can be displayed.
2. Scale: the default scale to be analyzed in CT-FIRE mode is the second finest scale. However, depending on the primary thickness the fiber and the image size, the scale can be set to a coarser scale, like the third finest scale, the fourth finest scale, etc.
3. Control of the alignment or relative angle heatmap. There are three related parameters, i.e., heatmap standard deviation filter for the no-boundary case, heatmap square max filter size, and heatmap Gaussian disc filter sigma. To do an accurate quantitative comparison of the heatmap, e.g., counting the number of pixels of different colors, those three parameters have to be set constant between analyses.

3.5.2 Adjust Parameters in CT-FIRE Mode

The primary parameters to be adjusted are the background intensity (named "thresh_im2" in the parameter setting window) and the searching radius (named "s_xlinkbox" in the parameter setting window) to find the center line of a fiber. The background threshold is associated with the noise level: the larger the threshold, the less collagen information remains. The searching radius is associated with the range of fiber thicknesses: the larger the value, the fewer of the smaller fibers information can be extracted. There are other parameters that can be used to find the optimal fiber extraction or representation. However, their effects on the final assessment of the alignment are minor and in most cases are negligible.

3.5.3 Using Boundaries

The automatic boundary creation is based on corresponding hematoxylin and eosin (H&E)-stained slide data (and not the primary

SHG data) to best visualize the tumor boundary (Fig. 6). This gives the best result to calculate the angle of collagen fibers with respect to a tumor boundary (relative angle). The current version is optimized for H&E-stained human breast samples (with the corresponding SHG) but can be used for other epithelial cancers. The automatic boundary creation is needed to have a map of tumor locations, which includes image color enhancement, color segmentation, finding nuclei and grouping them, and removing unwanted regions. Due to having two steps of color enhancement in this algorithm, it should be robust for variations in stain hue or imaging systems. To improve the accuracy of the segmentation, a white balancing as a pre-processing step sometimes can help.

The segmentation process requires the bright-field H&E image be registered to the SHG image in the beginning. The registration algorithm includes several steps: first, enhancing the colors using decorrelation stretch [49]; second, extracting the collagen-like structure from the bright-field image by color separation; and third, registering the image from step two to the SHG image using an iterative algorithm at different scales. As a rule of thumb, for the best results from the registration algorithm, the fields of view of the two images shouldn't differ by more than 10%, and the SHG signal intensity shouldn't be too weak.

When boundaries are used as part of the analysis, CurveAlign computes up to two relative angles per observation. The first is the nearest point angle and the second is the intersection point angle. The nearest point angle is the relative angle between the observation point and the tangent angle of the region boundary at the point nearest to the observation point. The intersection point angle is the relative angle between the observation point and the intersection point of the fiber, interpolated out a user-defined distance, and a boundary. For most applications in breast cancer, for example, nearest point angle is the preferred one.

3.5.4 Additional Tips

For the alignment quantification, in particular for fiber-based or ROI-based ones, the number of fiber or fiber segments should be larger than ten to yield a statistically robust measurement. Although the alignment coefficient and mean of orientations or angles are the main metrics used for quantifying fibrillar collagen alignment, CurveAlign also outputs other orientation-related metrics such as the variance, standard deviation, median, skewness, Kurtosis, etc. to characterize the distribution or dispersion of collagen fiber orientations. These provide additional useful information for some potential applications.

Visual inspection of the output images, which includes extracted fibers or curvelets overlaid on the original image, enables the user to assess the results for any image without the need for comparing against a ground truth. In addition, we can compare the statistics change by adjusting the primary parameters mentioned above. In many cases we tested, the alignment or orientation did not have significant change if the visual inspection is properly conducted.

3.6 Future Directions

For the current version of the CurveAlign platform (which includes software versions CurveAlign 4.0 and CT-FIRE 2.0), there are several improvements that we would like to make, many of them already mentioned above. Much of future development will be focused on usability, particularly in making it easier to run each mode and to be more modular. This will entail combining the functionality of CurveAlign and CT-FIRE more than it currently is, ideally into one common program. We also need to continue to improve the speed and performance of analysis. This will include exploring the better use of parallelization and possible deployment of graphics processing units. We also have plans to improve the image processing capabilities of CurveAlign by linking it to our Bio-Formats [56] and ImageJ efforts [32, 57, 58] . This need for image processing will also address a biological need to better track cells and tumor changes with the collagen alignment. This type of cell and fiber analysis can be used with machine learning approaches such as the WEKA toolkit in ImageJ [59]. We also are actively using and developing the CurveAlign platform to quantitate other properties of collagen organization such as length, width, straightness, and density. Another future development based on biological imaging need is adding support for three-dimensional quantitation of collagen. To date, the majority of the reported collagen analysis studies are of 2D sections out of 3D image stacks. As imaging work continues to characterize the role of collagen, there are likely to be studies that characterize collagen in 3D, including changes in collagen fiber between focal planes. We plan on adding true 3D support to our platform to accommodate such analysis. Additional feature requests can be made by any user at the CurveAlign website.

4 Notes

1. CFR mode is usually applicable to images without a large variation in contrast. Options in CT-FIRE mode are applicable to situations where individual fibers are most concerned and can be used to analyze images of any contrast. Importantly, the accuracy of the CT-FIRE mode is influenced by the complexity of fiber networks and not as efficient as the CFR mode (also *see* Subheading 3.5). CFR mode can be used to screen images with any type of collagen network.
2. There are default parameters for both CFR mode and CT-FIRE mode. Although most of those parameters are suitable for

many images, optimal parameters can be set according to the image contrast, image size, fiber thickness distribution, and collagen density distribution as discussed in Subheading 3.5.

3. For CFR mode, the fraction of coefficient to keep (labeled as 9 in Fig. 4a) is usually the only parameter to be adjusted to represent the most prominent fibers. In general, the smaller the image size is, the larger this parameter is. For CT-FIRE mode, the .mat file generated by CT-FIRE must be in the subfolder "ctFIREout" of the original image. To launch the CT-FIRE module as shown in Fig. 4b, click the CT-FIRE button (labeled as 6 in Fig. 4a). After clicking on "Open File(s)" button (labeled as 3 in Fig. 4b) to load image, click the "Update" button (labeled as 4 in Fig. 4b) to confirm or update default parameters. Some practical tips to adjust the parameters can be seen in Subheading 3.5. Click on "RUN" button (labeled as 5 in Fig. 4b) to run CT-FIRE fiber extraction, and the progress information will be displayed in both the information window highlighted in green color at the bottom of Fig. 4b and in the command window. To run CT-FIRE on multiple images, first check on the "Batch" box (labeled as 1 in Fig. 4b), and optionally, check on the "Parallel" box (labeled as 2 in Fig. 4b) to enable parallel computing.
4. No boundaries: Fibers will be compared to each other, but not to a boundary.
5. CSV boundary is an open boundary and is only used for CT mode, and only one boundary can be defined in this boundary condition. Alternatively, the TIFF boundary condition can contain one or more boundaries and can replace the CSV boundary if it is carefully annotated and thus is a preferred option for most applications.
6. If ROI analysis is desired, after images are loaded, click on the "ROI manager" button (4 in Fig. 4a) to launch ROI manager window (Fig. 7a) to define an ROI for each image, update a previously defined ROI, or load ROI files defined in other tools (such as Fiji or ImageJ) in the format of mask image file or ".txt" file.
7. If the full image has already been analyzed by either CT-FIRE mode or CFR mode, choosing "ROI post-processing" will extract the features from the processed output. (CT-FIRE mode only supports ROI post-processing in the current version).
8. If the full image has not been analyzed, CurveAlign can be applied to the specified ROI for analysis in CFR mode. If the ROI is of rectangular shape, which is the most commonly used shape, we recommend choosing the option "CA on cropped rectangular ROI." For all other shapes, choose the option "CA

on mask with ROI of any shape." As described in Subheading 3.5, full image analysis in CFR mode tends to be biased toward fibers with higher intensity. ROI analysis in CFR mode can focus fiber alignment analysis on a smaller region with improved fiber representation.

Acknowledgments

We thank many users and contributors to CT-FIRE and CurveAlign over the years including Rob Nowak, Carolyn Pehlke, Jeremy Bredfeldt, Matt Conklin, Paolo Provenzano, Patricia Keely, and Jayne Squirrell. This work was supported by NIH grants R01CA179556 and U54DK104310 to K.W.E.

References

1. Lanir Y (1983) Constitutive equations for fibrous connective tissues. J Biomech 16(1):1–12. doi:10.1016/0021-9290(83)90041-6
2. Martin RB, Lau ST, Mathews PV et al (1996) Collagen fiber organization is related to mechanical properties and remodeling in equine bone. A comparison of two methods. J Biomech 29(12):1515–1521. doi:10.1016/S0021-9290(96)80002-9
3. Chen C-H, Cheng C-H (1996) Effective elastic moduli of misoriented short-fiber composites. Int J Solids Struct 33(17):2519–2539. doi:10.1016/0020-7683(95)00160-3
4. Tian L, Wang Z, Liu Y et al (2016) Validation of an arterial constitutive model accounting for collagen content and crosslinking. Acta Biomater 31:276–287. doi:10.1016/j.actbio.2015.11.058
5. Provenzano PP, Eliceiri KW, Campbell JM et al (2006) Collagen reorganization at the tumor-stromal interface facilitates local invasion. BMC Med 4(1):38. doi:10.1186/1741-7015-4-38
6. Conklin MW, Eickhoff JC, Riching KM et al (2011) Aligned collagen is a prognostic signature for survival in human breast carcinoma. Am J Pathol 178(3):1221–1232. doi:10.1016/j.ajpath.2010.11.076
7. Keikhosravi A, Bredfeldt JS, Sagar AK et al (2014) Second-harmonic generation imaging of cancer. Methods Cell Biol 123:531–546. doi:10.1016/B978-0-12-420138-5.00028-8
8. Drifka CR, Eliceiri KW, Weber SM et al (2013) A bioengineered heterotypic stroma-cancer microenvironment model to study pancreatic ductal adenocarcinoma. Lab Chip 13(19):3965–3975. doi:10.1039/c3lc50487e
9. Drifka CR, Tod J, Loeffler AG et al (2015) Periductal stromal collagen topology of pancreatic ductal adenocarcinoma differs from that of normal and chronic pancreatitis. Mod Pathol 28(11):1470–1480. doi:10.1038/modpathol.2015.97
10. Drifka CR, Loeffler AG, Mathewson K et al (2016) Highly aligned stromal collagen is a negative prognostic factor following pancreatic ductal adenocarcinoma resection. Oncotarget 7(46):76197–76213. doi:10.18632/oncotarget.12772
11. Meijering E, Jacob M, Sarria JC et al (2004) Design and validation of a tool for neurite tracing and analysis in fluorescence microscopy images. Cytometry A 58(2):167–176. doi:10.1002/cyto.a.20022
12. Rubbens MP, Driessen-Mol A, Boerboom RA et al (2009) Quantification of the temporal evolution of collagen orientation in mechanically conditioned engineered cardiovascular tissues. Ann Biomed Eng 37(7):1263–1272. doi:10.1007/s10439-009-9698-x
13. Rezakhaniha R, Agianniotis A, Schrauwen JT et al (2012) Experimental investigation of collagen waviness and orientation in the arterial adventitia using confocal laser scanning microscopy. Biomech Model Mechanobiol 11(3–4):461–473. doi:10.1007/s10237-011-0325-z
14. Kabir MM, Inavalli VV, Lau TY et al (2013) Application of quantitative second-harmonic generation microscopy to dynamic conditions. Biomed Opt Express 4(11):2546–2554. doi:10.1364/BOE.4.002546

15. Boudaoud A, Burian A, Borowska-Wykret D et al (2014) FibrilTool, an ImageJ plug-in to quantify fibrillar structures in raw microscopy images. Nat Protoc 9(2):457–463. doi:10.1038/nprot.2014.024
16. Sun M, Bloom AB, Zaman MH (2015) Rapid quantification of 3D collagen fiber alignment and fiber intersection correlations with high sensitivity. PLoS One 10(7):e0131814. doi:10.1371/journal.pone.0131814
17. Quinn KP, Georgakoudi I (2013) Rapid quantification of pixel-wise fiber orientation data in micrographs. J Biomed Opt 18(4):046003. doi:10.1117/1.JBO.18.4.046003
18. Chaudhuri S, Nguyen H, Rangayyan RM et al (1987) A Fourier domain directional filtering method for analysis of collagen alignment in ligaments. IEEE Trans Biomed Eng 34(7):509–518. doi:10.1109/TBME.1987.325980
19. Pourdeyhimi B, Dent R, Davis H (1997) Measuring fiber orientation in nonwovens part III: fourier transform. Text Res J 67(2):143–151. doi:10.1177/004051759706700211
20. Marquez JP (2006) Fourier analysis and automated measurement of cell and fiber angular orientation distributions. Int J Solids Struct 43(21):6413–6423. doi:10.1016/j.ijsolstr.2005.11.003
21. Sander EA, Barocas VH (2009) Comparison of 2D fiber network orientation measurement methods. J Biomed Mater Res A 88(2):322–331. doi:10.1002/jbm.a.31847
22. Sivaguru M, Durgam S, Ambekar R et al (2010) Quantitative analysis of collagen fiber organization in injured tendons using Fourier transform-second harmonic generation imaging. Opt Express 18(24):24983–24993. doi:10.1364/OE.18.024983
23. Pourdeyhimi B, Kim HS (2002) Measuring fiber orientation in nonwovens: the hough transform. Text Res J 72(9):803–809. doi:10.1177/004051750207200909
24. Bayan C, Levitt JM, Miller E et al (2009) Fully automated, quantitative, noninvasive assessment of collagen fiber content and organization in thick collagen gels. J Appl Phys 105(10):102042. doi:10.1063/1.3116626
25. Schneider CA, Pehlke CA, Tilbury K et al (2013) Quantitative approaches for studying the role of collagen in breast cancer invasion and progression. In: Pavone FS, Campagnola PJ (eds) Second harmonic generation imaging. Taylor & Francis, Boca Raton, FL, pp 373–390
26. Wen BL, Brewer MA, Nadiarnykh O et al (2014) Texture analysis applied to second harmonic generation image data for ovarian cancer classification. J Biomed Opt 19(9):096007. doi:10.1117/1.JBO.19.9.096007
27. Puspoki Z, Storath M, Sage D et al (2016) Transforms and operators for directional bioimage analysis: a survey. Adv Anat Embryol Cell Biol 219:69–93. doi:10.1007/978-3-319-28549-8_3
28. Mori S, van Zijl PC (2002) Fiber tracking: principles and strategies - a technical review. NMR Biomed 15(7–8):468–480. doi:10.1002/nbm.781
29. Stein AM, Vader DA, Jawerth LM et al (2008) An algorithm for extracting the network geometry of three-dimensional collagen gels. J Microsc 232(3):463–475. doi:10.1111/j.1365-2818.2008.02141.x
30. Jacques E, Buytaert J, Wells DM et al (2013) MicroFilament Analyzer, an image analysis tool for quantifying fibrillar orientation, reveals changes in microtubule organization during gravitropism. Plant J 74(6):1045–1058. doi:10.1111/tpj.12174
31. Bredfeldt JS, Liu Y, Conklin MW et al (2014) Automated quantification of aligned collagen for human breast carcinoma prognosis. J Pathol Inform 5(1):28. doi:10.4103/2153-3539.139707
32. Schneider CA, Rasband WS, Eliceiri KW (2012) NIH Image to ImageJ: 25 years of image analysis. Nat Methods 9(7):671–675. doi:10.1038/nmeth.2089
33. BIG > OrientationJ. http://bigwww.epfl.ch/demo/orientation/#soft. Accessed 23 Nov 2016
34. CytoSpectre: Spectral analysis of microscopy images. http://www.tut.fi/cytospectre/. Accessed 23 Nov 2016
35. Kartasalo K, Polonen RP, Ojala M et al (2015) CytoSpectre: a tool for spectral analysis of oriented structures on cellular and subcellular levels. BMC Bioinformatics 16:344. doi:10.1186/s12859-015-0782-y
36. CurveAlign | LOCI. http://loci.wisc.edu/software/curvealign. Accessed 26 Nov 2016
37. CT-FIRE | LOCI. http://loci.wisc.edu/software/ctfire. Accessed 26 Nov 2016
38. Bredfeldt JS, Liu Y, Pehlke CA et al (2014) Computational segmentation of collagen fibers from second-harmonic generation images of breast cancer. J Biomed Opt 19(1):16007. doi:10.1117/1.JBO.19.1.016007
39. Provenzano PP, Eliceiri KW, Yan L et al (2008) Nonlinear optical imaging of cellular processes in breast cancer. Microsc Microanal 14(6):532–548. doi:10.1017/S1431927608080884
40. Ajeti V, Nadiarnykh O, Ponik SM et al (2011) Structural changes in mixed Col I/Col V collagen gels probed by SHG microscopy: implications for probing stromal alterations in

human breast cancer. Biomed Opt Express 2(8):2307–2316. doi:10.1364/BOE.2.002307

41. Barcus CE, Keely PJ, Eliceiri KW et al (2013) Stiff collagen matrices increase tumorigenic prolactin signaling in breast cancer cells. J Biol Chem 288(18):12722–12732. doi:10.1074/jbc.M112.447631
42. Riching KM, Cox BL, Salick MR et al (2014) 3D collagen alignment limits protrusions to enhance breast cancer cell persistence. Biophys J 107(11):2546–2558. doi:10.1016/j.bpj.2014.10.035
43. Bauman TM, Nicholson TM, Abler LL et al (2014) Characterization of fibrillar collagens and extracellular matrix of glandular benign prostatic hyperplasia nodules. PLoS One 9(10):e109102. doi:10.1371/journal.pone.0109102
44. Barcus CE, Holt EC, Keely PJ et al (2015) Dense collagen-I matrices enhance pro-tumorigenic estrogen-prolactin crosstalk in MCF-7 and T47D breast cancer cells. PLoS One 10(1):e0116891. doi:10.1371/journal.pone.0116891
45. Corsa CA, Brenot A, Grither WR et al (2016) The action of discoidin domain receptor 2 in basal tumor cells and stromal cancer-associated fibroblasts is critical for breast cancer metastasis. Cell Rep 15(11):2510–2523. doi:10.1016/j.celrep.2016.05.033
46. Candes E, Demanet L, Donoho D et al (2006) Fast discrete curvelet transforms. Multiscale Model Simul 5(3):861–899. doi:10.1137/05064182X
47. Walsh AJ, Cook RS, Lee JH et al (2015) Collagen density and alignment in responsive and resistant trastuzumab-treated breast cancer xenografts. J Biomed Opt 20(2):26004. doi:10.1117/1.JBO.20.2.026004
48. Junqueira LC, Bignolas G, Brentani RR (1979) Picrosirius staining plus polarization microscopy, a specific method for collagen detection in tissue sections. Histochem J 11(4):447–455. doi:10.1007/BF01002772
49. Gillespie AR, Kahle AB, Walker RE (1986) Color enhancement of highly correlated images. I. Decorrelation and HSI contrast stretches. Remote Sens Environ 20(3):209–235. doi:10.1016/0034-4257(86)90044-1
50. Campagnola PJ, Wei MD, Lewis A et al (1999) High-resolution nonlinear optical imaging of live cells by second harmonic generation. Biophys J 77(6):3341–3349. doi:10.1016/S0006-3495(99)77165-1
51. Campagnola PJ, Millard AC, Terasaki M et al (2002) Three-dimensional high-resolution second-harmonic generation imaging of endogenous structural proteins in biological tissues. Biophys J 82(1 Pt 1):493–508. doi:10.1016/S0006-3495(02)75414-3
52. Ayala G, Tuxhorn JA, Wheeler TM et al (2003) Reactive stroma as a predictor of biochemical-free recurrence in prostate cancer. Clin Cancer Res 9(13):4792–4801
53. Allon I, Vered M, Buchner A et al (2006) Stromal differences in salivary gland tumors of a common histopathogenesis but with different biological behavior: a study with picrosirius red and polarizing microscopy. Acta Histochem 108(4):259–264. doi:10.1016/j.acthis.2006.05.007
54. Arun Gopinathan P, Kokila G, Jyothi M et al (2015) Study of collagen birefringence in different grades of oral squamous cell carcinoma using picrosirius red and polarized light microscopy. Scientifica (Cairo) 2015:802980. doi:10.1155/2015/802980
55. Lindeberg T (1998) Edge detection and ridge detection with automatic scale selection. Int J Comput Vision 30(2):117–156. doi:10.1023/A:1008097225773
56. Linkert M, Rueden CT, Allan C et al (2010) Metadata matters: access to image data in the real world. J Cell Biol 189(5):777–782. doi:10.1083/jcb.201004104
57. Schindelin J, Arganda-Carreras I, Frise E et al (2012) Fiji: an open-source platform for biological-image analysis. Nat Methods 9(7):676–682. doi:10.1038/nmeth.2019
58. Schindelin J, Rueden CT, Hiner MC et al (2015) The ImageJ ecosystem: an open platform for biomedical image analysis. Mol Reprod Dev 82(7–8):518–529. doi:10.1002/mrd.22489
59. Arganda-Carreras I, Kaynig V, Eliceiri KW et al (2016) Trainable weka segmentation: a machine learning tool for microscopy pixel classification. J Bioinformatics. submitted

Chapter 29

Exploring the Nano-Surface of Collagenous and Other Fibrotic Tissues with AFM

Andreas Stylianou, Vasiliki Gkretsi, Costas S. Patrickios, and Triantafyllos Stylianopoulos

Abstract

Atomic force microscope (AFM) is a powerful and invaluable tool for imaging and probing the mechanical properties of biological samples at the nanometric scale. The importance of nano-scale characterization and nanomechanics of soft biological tissues is becoming widely appreciated, and AFM offers unique advantages in this direction. In this chapter, we describe the procedure to collect data sets (imaging and mechanical properties measurement) of collagen gels and tumor tissues. We provide step-by-step instructions throughout the procedure, from sample preparation to cantilever calibration, data acquisition, analysis, and visualization, using two commercial AFM systems (PicoPlus and Cypher ES) and software that accompanied the AFM systems and/or are freeware available (WSxM, AtomicJ). Our protocols are written specifically for these two systems and the mentioned software; however, most of the general concepts can be readily translated to other AFM systems and software.

Key words Connective tissues, Stiffness, Force spectroscopy, Force maps, Mechanobiology, Young's modulus, Elasticity, Cancer

1 Introduction

Atomic force microscope (AFM) belongs to the scanning probe microscopy (SPM) family of techniques, and since its invention in 1986 [1], it has rapidly become a popular method for high-resolution imaging and studying the mechanical properties of a wide range of samples, including biological ones [2, 3]. An AFM system records the interactions between the AFM tip (which is mounted on a cantilever) and the sample and uses the obtained information to form 3D images (Fig. 1). Simultaneously to the high-resolution and nondestructive imaging of the surfaces, the cantilever-tip assembly can act as a force sensor [4], offering quantitative information of the mechanical properties of the sample [5–9]. AFM can operate both in air and liquid conditions [10] without special treatment of the specimen [11]. The unique features of AFM and especially its

Laure Rittié (ed.), *Fibrosis: Methods and Protocols*, Methods in Molecular Biology, vol. 1627, DOI 10.1007/978-1-4939-7113-8_29,

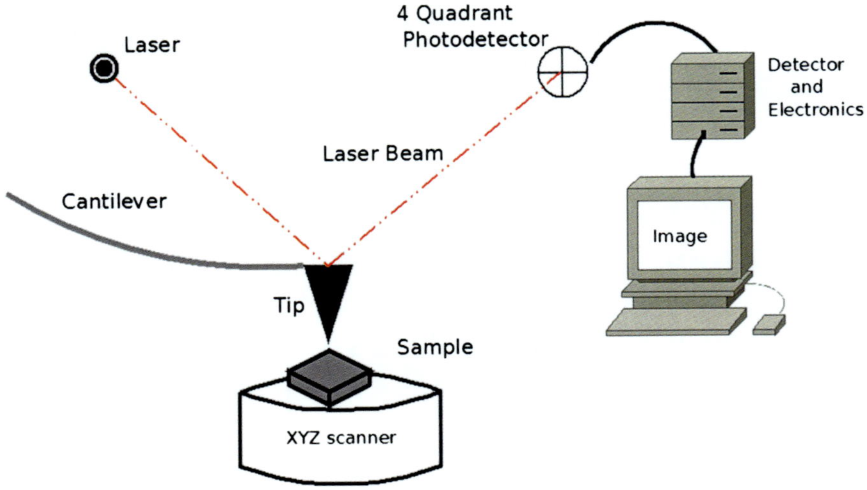

Fig. 1 Atomic force microscopy general components. A typical AFM apparatus consists of a cantilever, a sharp tip, a laser source, an XYZ scanner, a photodetector, a detector with the electronics, and a computer for the acquisition of the image. The tip scans the surface of the specimen by coming in physical contact with it. In order to control the x, y, and z position of the sample (or the position of the probe depending of the AFM system), piezoelectric actuators are typically used. The laser beam is reflected off the cantilever to the four-quadrant photodetector. Consequently, the photodetector can monitor the tip-surface forces through the vertical and lateral deflection of the probe. This information is transferred to the system detectors, electronics, and computer for the formation of the AFM images or the mechanical property analysis

potential to provide mechanical characterization of biological samples (e.g., Young's or elastic modulus, which is a measure of stiffness of an elastic material) offer new possibilities for characterization of soft biological tissues, cancerous tissues, and biopsies [12–14].

The investigation of the structure of collagenous and other fibrotic tissues is possible nowadays by means of various optical (e.g., fluorescence, second harmonic generation (SHG) spectroscopy, etc.) or electron (e.g., scanning electron microscope (SEM), transmission electron microscopy (TEM)) microscopy techniques. Although these techniques can access very precisely the structure of the specimen, they lack the ability to provide characterization of the mechanical properties and are unable to perform in physiological conditions. Among the several sophisticated instruments that can investigate the mechanical properties of biological samples (including properties of living samples, such as cells), AFM is probably the most readily accessible one. In the case of collagen-rich tissues, the AFM can be used to investigate collagen structures at different length scales, from collagen molecules to separate fibers under physiological conditions without destroying their native structure [15].

In this chapter we describe the protocols for AFM imaging and mechanical characterization of collagenous and other fibrotic tissues. We used pure collagen gels since they are controllable in vitro models and can mimic real tissue. By altering different parameters during sample preparation, it is possible to control and predetermine structural characteristics of the gels, such as the organization and stiffness of the collagen network, as well as to modify their structure according to different physiological or pathological conditions. Furthermore, inexperienced AFM users can start from this kind of samples so as to become familiar with AFM procedures, before investigating real tissues. Here, we provide step-by-step instructions throughout the procedure, from sample preparation to cantilever calibration, data acquisition, analysis, and visualization, using two commercial AFM systems, the PicoPlus (currently known as 5500 Atomic Force Microscope, Keysight Technologies) and the Cypher ES (Asylum Research, Oxford Instruments), and software that accompanies the AFM systems and/or freeware available (WSxM, AtomicJ). Although the procedures and protocols that are presented in this chapter are written specifically for the abovementioned AFM systems, they can easily be modified for other commercial available AFM systems and appropriate software. Throughout the chapter, we include advice and troubleshooting tips based on our own experience with these procedures and measurements.

We will provide protocols to perform AFM imaging in tapping or contact mode and in air or liquid environments. In tapping mode (also known as intermittent contact mode or AC mode), the cantilever is driven to oscillate to its resonance frequency, and the tip touches the sample surface only for a short time (it "taps" the surface). Tapping mode is widely used for biological samples as it overcomes issues related to friction, adhesion, electrostatic forces, and other difficulties that are more intense in contact mode. Contact mode is the most common in AFM, being the first mode that was developed. In contact mode, the AFM tip is in full contact with the specimen's surface. Contact mode can be more destructive than tapping mode, but this depends on how soft the sample is and what forces are being applied. Contact mode is preferred for combining imaging with mechanical property characterization, while in liquid conditions the use of tapping mode is preferred, since the oscillations created by the latter in the liquid environment can compromise the measurement. In constant force contact mode (the most common kind of contact mode, where a constant force is applied to the sample while scanning its surface), a feedback loop maintains a constant deflection of the tip based on the specified setpoint voltage. The error signal is the difference between the setpoint and the actual cantilever deflection. It is measured in volts by the photodetector and is read as the deflection. For each pixel, the system will record and plot the error signal (the difference in volts between the surface-induced deflection and the setpoint) as the deflection image (in volts). The correction signal (the voltage that the feedback loop applies to the z-piezo to maintain the deflection at the setpoint) is scaled by the piezo sensitivity (nm/V) and plotted as topography (in nanometers). As the tip passes over regions of varying friction, it will twist in the scan direction as well as deflect in the vertical axis. The detector then senses changes in the cantilever's twisting motion and prints it as the lateral deflection (Friction) signal, which is plotted as the Friction or Lateral image (in volts). Changes in lateral force on the tip can be caused either by changes in frictional properties across the sample or by variations in topography. The Friction signal will therefore be a convolution of these two components. Comparing the friction and topography images helps to differentiate the impact of topography versus friction.

PicoPlus is an older microscope than Cypher ES. Many of the procedures that can be performed automatically with new AFM systems need to be performed manually with this older system. Consequently, we added protocols to help readers that have access to this kind of microscopes.

For AFM image analysis, we describe the open access freeware software WSxM (5.0, develop 8) [16]. We selected this software because it is freely available and supports image processing of AFM images of many different commercially available microscopes. Although the AFM systems are accompanied by relevant software that enables the processing of the images, in many cases you may prefer to use this software (or other software such as Gwyddion [17]) so as to analyze and present images from different AFM systems with the same software. The described procedure presents only a very small portion of the functions that are available, and it can be used as a first-step guide.

In the next section, we describe a procedure for recording topographical characteristics and Young's modulus maps by using the so-called "force volume mode." Force volume mode can be considered to be an extension of AFM force spectroscopy, where the cantilever-tip assembly acts as a force sensor [18] and provides several methods for characterizing and measuring mechanical properties of the specimen surface [4]. Volume spectroscopy combines AFM imaging and force spectroscopy [4]. The strength of the interaction between the AFM tip and the sample is measured in defined areas and not only in individual points. In particular, the tip is periodically indented into the sample, and the mechanical property characterization is achieved through the study of the deformation of the cantilever as a function of the indented depth. After acquiring force-distance curves in all the areas of interest by nano-indenting each point separately, advanced calculations (either with plugins, home-based built-in algorithms, freeware, or commercially available software) are used to calculate mechanical properties like stiffness (e.g., material Young's modulus). In volume spectroscopy, a standard topography image is collected, and a specific procedure is performed to collect data that can provide parameters for calculating the mechanical properties of the sample and allow the formation of a map of the material's properties (e.g., a Young's modulus map). The final recorded data set in volume spectroscopy contains not only the three-dimensional image but also force spectroscopy data for all the user-selected points in the image [4]. These procedures can be conducted in liquid and at ambient temperatures, which permits direct measurement of living cells and tissues [19]. The procedure described in Subheading 3.5 covers general guidelines for calibrating the probes and volume spectroscopy in contact mode.

Finally, we will outline a procedure/protocol for analyzing the data that were obtained with volume spectroscopy to extract valuable information and form two-dimensional Young's modulus maps of the sample. All described data processing will be accomplished with the open-source software AtomicJ [20], but other freeware (e.g., WSxM [16], OpenFovea [21], Gwyddion [17]) or commercial software (e.g., SPIP™-Image Metrology) can also be used. Some researchers prefer to write their algorithms to analyze force-distance curves using software that can support nonlinear least-squares fitting (e.g., MATLAB® [22]); some software that accompany AFM systems can support this kind of analysis.

2 Materials

2.1 Sample Preparation

2.1.1 Collagen Gels

1. High concentration collagen (we use a 10 mg/ml rat tail collagen solution by Corning 354249).
2. Minimal Essential Medium (MEM) (10X): premixed, sterile. After dilution to 1X, store at 4 °C and keep sterile.
3. Human insulin solution (we use one from Sigma-Aldrich).
4. diH_2O.
5. 1 M NaOH.
6. Phosphate-buffered saline (PBS).
7. Cell culturing tubes and Petri dishes.
8. Cell incubator.

2.1.2 Tumor Tissue

1. Frozen tissue/tumor. For AFM analysis the tumor tissue can be studied either after harvesting or following cryopreservation. We typically use frozen tumors from mice, which were embedded in OCT in a disposable plastic base mold and frozen at -80 °C.
2. Optimal cutting temperature (OCT) compound.
3. Plastic base molds.
4. Cryostat and microtome blades.

2.2 Atomic Force Microscopy

1. AFM system. We employ two commercially available AFM systems, the PicoPlus AFM system from Molecular Imaging/ Agilent Technologies (now known as the 5500 AFM from Keysight Technologies) and the Cypher ES Environmental AFM from Asylum Research, Oxford Instruments (Fig. 2). The PicoPlus is an old-fashioned microscope, and the user has to develop many of the methods manually, while the Cypher has many automated features and advanced methodologies (*see* **Note 1**).
2. AFM probes. The selection of the appropriate probe in many cases is of crucial importance for AFM characterization. Firstly, the user should select an appropriate probe depending on the mode (contact or tapping mode) that will be used. Also, in some cases, the selection of the cantilever may rely on whether the imaging is performed in air or liquid. Furthermore, depending on the sample's stiffness and whether imaging or mechanical property characterization or a combination of the two is planned, cantilevers should be selected according to their spring constant (*see* **Note 2**). The different probes we use in our protocols are described in Table 1.
3. Circular cover glasses 13 mm, 1.0 thickness (*see* **Note 3**) or positively charged microscope slides.
4. AFM specimen discs 15 mm.
5. Double-sided adhesive tape.
6. Tweezers and screwdrivers.
7. Software: they are described in Subheading 3 with their respective analysis methods.

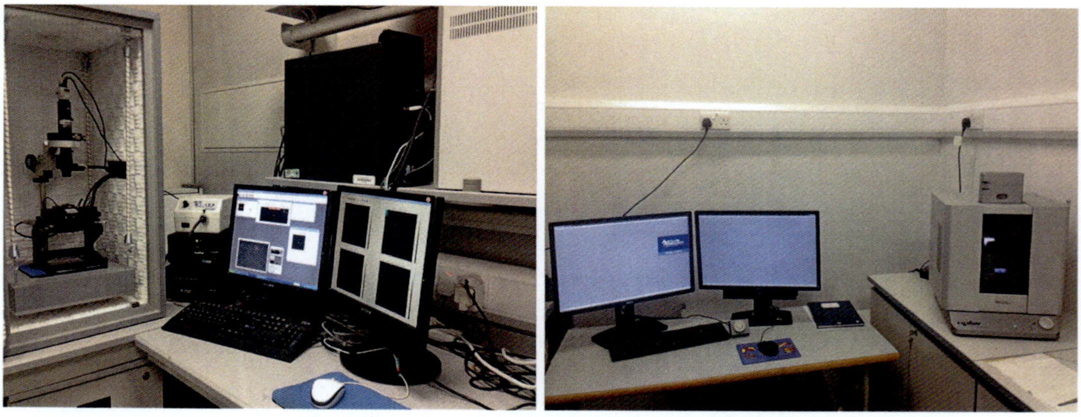

Fig. 2 The two AFM systems employed for our analysis. (*Left*) A PicoPlus molecular imaging and (*Right*) a Cypher ES AFM system

Table 1
Properties of AFM probes employed

		AFM probes						
		Cantilever				Tip		
Model	Application	Material	Shape	Resonance frequency (kHz)	Spring constant (N/m)	Material	Shape	Radius
SICON Applied nanostructures	Contact mode (in liquid)	Silicon	Rectangular	0.02–0.89	15 (5–25)	Silicon	Pyramidal	6 nm
AC160TS-R3 Olympus	AC MODE (AIR)	Silicon	Rectangular	300 (200–400)	26 (11–54)	Silicon	3-sided	9 nm
ACT applied nanostructures	AC MODE	Silicon	Rectangular	200–400	37 (25–75)	Silicon	Pyramidal	6 nm
PNP-TR NanoWorld Cantilever 1 Cantilever 2	Contact mode air/liquid Material property characterization	Silicon nitride	Triangular	67 17	0.32 0.08	Silicon nitride	Pyramidal	<10 nm
CP-PNP-BSG-A-5 Cantilever 1 Cantilever 2	Colloid probe	Silicon nitride	Triangular	67 17	0.32 0.08	Silicon nitride	Pyramidal	5 μm, <10 nm

3 Methods

3.1 Collagen Gel Preparation

The method below is a modification of previously published protocols [23] (*see* **Note 4**).

1. Set up workspace in sterile hood with an appropriate workflow.
2. Prepare the collagen mixture by mixing the following reagents, in this particular order, in a cell culturing tube: 10% 10X MEM, 1% (v/v) insulin, diH_2O, and collagen. The volume of collagen is calculated so that it will get the desired final collagen concentration (e.g., 0.5 mg/ml). The volume of diH_2O is calculated as to get 100% of the final volume.
3. Mix solution gently by inverting several times.
4. Adjust pH to 7.4 by adding 1 M NaOH. Mix solution gently by inverting several times. Follow the neutralization reaction by looking at the color of the solution that must become red. If the color is not changed, add more NaOH.
5. Add 200 μl of the neutralized collagen solution on a glass cover slip. Carefully cover the entire surface of the cover slip with collagen solution, and avoid creating bubbles.
6. Place the sample in a Petri dish, and allow to incubate at 37 °C (i.e., in a cell incubator) for at least 30 min.
7. Remove samples from the incubator, and carefully affix each cover slip to an AFM specimen disc with double-sided adhesive tape.
8. Let the samples air-dry at room temperature.

3.2 Tumor Tissue Preparation

1. Section the frozen tissue blocks with microtome blades on a cryostat. Generally, ~5 μm sections are used for AFM imaging purposes [24] and ~20 μm for AFM mechanical property characterization [25, 26].
2. Mount tissue sections on ~13 mm circular coverslips or positively charged microscope slides.
3. Allow tissue cryo-sections to thaw at room temperature.
4. Wash with distilled water to remove excess OCT.
5. Air-dry the sections.
6. Mount the samples on the AFM metal specimen discs using double-sided adhesive tape.

3.3 AFM Imaging with the Cypher ES

Protocols used with the Cypher ES were derived from information contained in the instrument's manuals [27–29].

3.3.1 Tapping Mode Imaging in Air

1. Power up the system:
   (a) Turn on the Cypher ES SPM.
   (b) Turn on the computer and start the relevant software (Asylum Research, Igor Pro 6.37, with the shortcut).
   (c) Click "yes" on the software prompt asking if you would like to home the engage motors.
   (d) On the "Mode Master" window, click on the "Standard" window, and then from the "Standard Modes" window select "Template."
2. Load the cantilever and the sample:
   (a) Rotate clockwise the "Engage Control Knob" on the Cypher, and hold until the cantilever holder is far from the sample.
   (b) Lift the door latch, open the enclosure door, unlock the scanner, and pull the scanner forward.
   (c) Release the cantilever holder, remove it, and set it aside.
   (d) Prepare cantilever mounting workspace (tweezers, screwdriver, box of cantilevers) (*see* **Note 5**).
   (e) Load cantilever: loosen the cantilever clip with the screwdriver, and remove the old cantilever if necessary. Grab a new cantilever with tweezers, slide the new cantilever under the clip, and secure it with the screwdriver (*see* **Note 6**).
   (f) Place the sample: use tweezers to place new sample on sample stage (*see* **Note 7**). We will exemplify below a collagen gel and a section from a tumor.
   (g) Place cantilever holder back in its place and secure it.
   (h) Slide scanner back to its position and close enclosure door.
3. Motor cantilever toward sample: place your eyes at the same level as the cantilever and sample so you can clearly see the gap between the two. Slowly turn the "Engage Control Knob" on the AFM enclosure counterclockwise to lower the cantilever holder. Close the gap between tip and sample to within 1 mm (*see* **Note 8**).
4. Focus on tip and align the laser:
   (a) In the lower left corner of the "Video" window from the menu bar, set the Zoom at 1.0.
   (b) At the bottom of the "Video" window, set the illumination bar to approximately one third of its full level.
   (c) Select the "Engage Panel" window (Fig. 3, left), and click on "Focus On Tip." This will move the objectives to the last known tip focus (which was set from the previous use of the system). Consequently, the focus will not be perfect (the cantilever may even not be visible at all). If you cannot see the cantilever case, use the four arrows at the top left

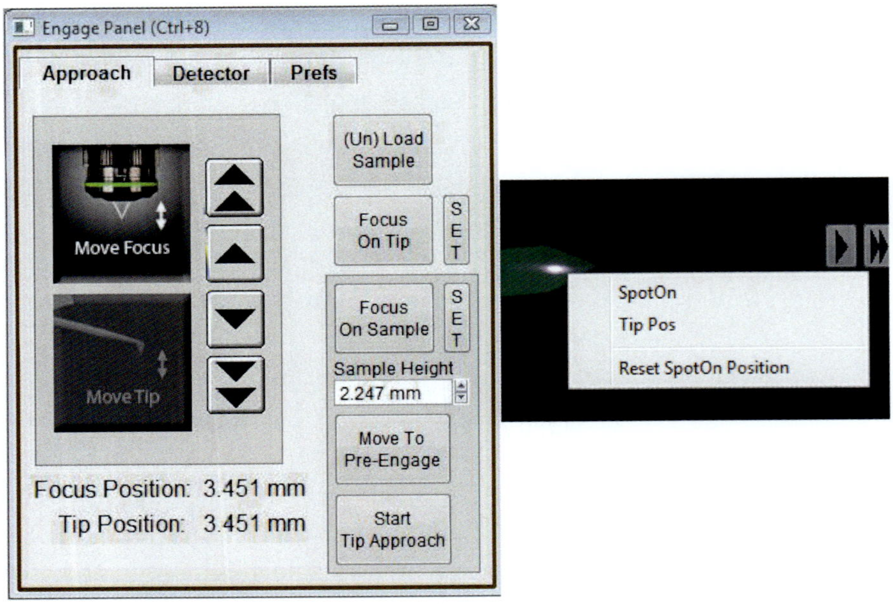

Fig. 3 Focus on tip and align the laser. (*Left*) The "Engage Panel" and (*Right*) the laser alignment procedure for the Cypher ES microscope

of the "Video" window to locate the cantilever in the image. If you do not manage to find the cantilever, it probably means that the cantilever chip is located off the side of the field of view. You will then need to move the cantilever to a more appropriate place on the cantilever holder.

(d) When you manage to locate the cantilever, fine-tune the focus: on the "Engage Panel" window, click on "Move Focus," and use the arrow buttons to focus the cantilever. Click on the "SET" button next to the "Focus On Tip" button to validate.

(e) Center the laser on the cantilever: right-click on the center of the cantilever, and select the "Spot On" option (Fig. 3, right). The laser spot is now visible on the cantilever where you clicked. If needed, set the spot position again.

5. Focus the sample: select the "Engage Panel" window, and use the arrows to motor the microscope objective down toward the sample until it comes in focus and locates the sample surface optically. Once in focus, hit the "SET" button next to the "Focus On Sample" button (*see* **Note 9**).

6. Tune the tip:

   (a) On the "Engage Panel" window, click on "Move to Pre-engage." Motors automatically bring the tip to 50 μm distance from the surface.

   (b) Adjust the spot position of the laser to near the end of the cantilever as described in **step 4e**.

(c) Center the laser on the photo detector by clicking on the red button at the center of the video window motion controls. This zeroes the "Deflection Signal."

(d) In the "Main" tab of the "Master Panel," select the "AC Mode" from the "Imaging Mode" pulldown menu.

(e) On the "Master Panel," select the "Tune" tab. Set the parameters as follows: "Auto Tune Low" to 50 kHz, "Auto Tune High" to 400 kHz, "Target Amplitude" to 1 V, and "Target Percent" to -5%.

(f) Click on "Auto Tune." A graph will pop up with the tune result. The resonance curve should peak around 300 kHz for the used cantilever (Fig. 4).

7. Engage the cantilever on the sample:

(a) On the "Master Panel" window (Fig. 5), select the "Main" tab. Set the set scan parameters (Scan Size, 20 μm; Scan Rate, 1 Hz (*see* **Note 10**); Scan points, 256 or 532; Point value, 600 mV; Gain, 30).

(b) On the "Engage Panel" window, click on "Start Tip Approach." When the system is ready, select the "Sum and Deflection Panel" window and click on "Engage."

8. Start the imaging and parameter tuning:

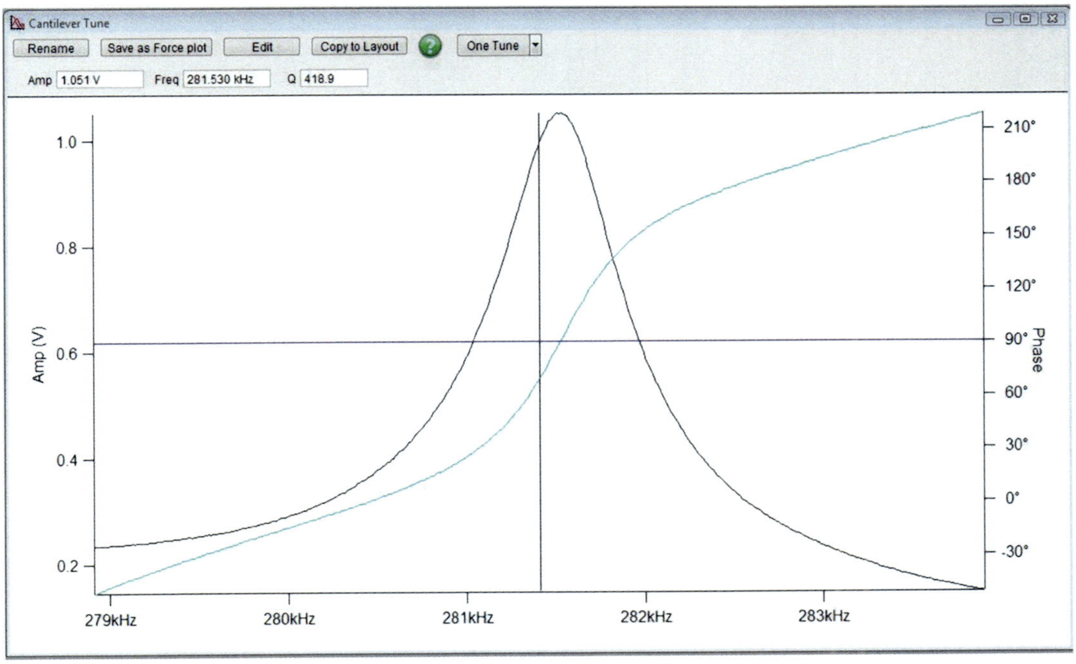

Fig. 4 Cantilever tune graph. The graph is the tuning result of an AC160TS-R3 probe with the "Target Percent" set to −5%

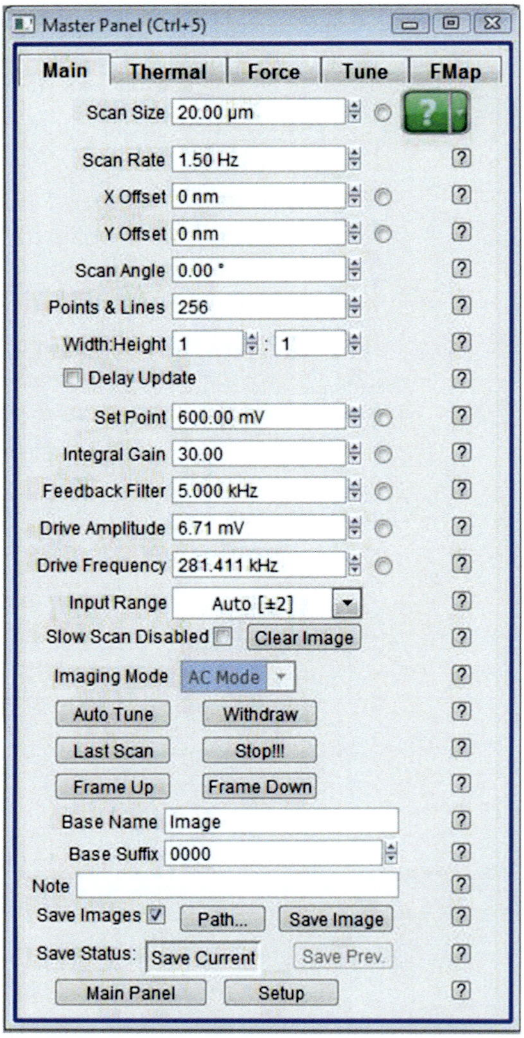

Fig. 5 The "Master Panel" of Cypher ES

(a) Select the "Master Panel" window. On the "Main" tab, click on "Frame Up" or "Frame Down," and imaging procedure will begin.

(b) Look at the "Scope Trace" below the image. This graph represents the most recent line of the image. Blue indicates the "Trace" (which is the tip moving from left to right), and red indicates the "Retrace" (which is the tip returning from right to left). Adjust "Setpoint," "Gain," and "Scan Speed" to get Trace and Retrace to overlap.

(c) After each scan images are automatically saved. Figure 6 depicts two taping mode images from collagen gel and a tumor section, respectively, that were obtained with this protocol.

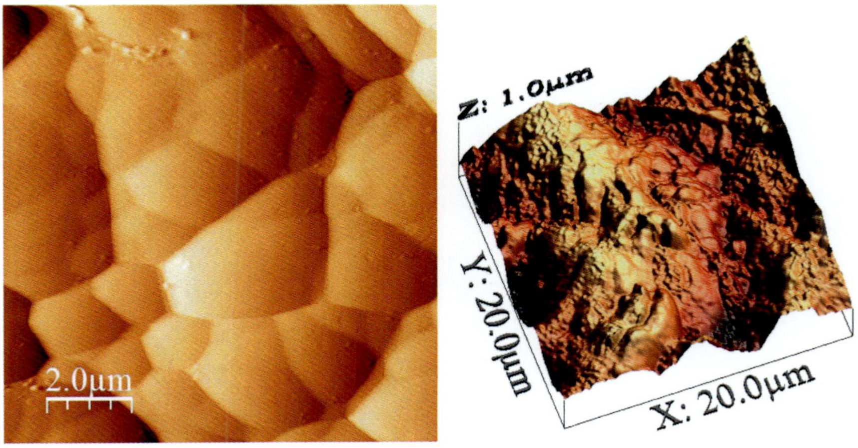

Fig. 6 AFM images in tapping mode in air with Cypher ES. (*Left*) Topography AFM image of a collagen I gel (0.5 mg/ml) and (*Right*) 3D topography image of a tumor section

3.3.2 Contact Mode Imaging in Air

1. **Step 6d** is replaced by: In the "Main" tab of the "Master Panel," select the "Contact Mode" from the "Imaging Mode" pulldown menu.
2. You do not need to tune the cantilever, so omit the "tune tip" procedure (**steps 6e** and **6f**). Instead, zero the deflection and pick a setpoint that is greater than 0, typically 0.5–1 V.
3. When in contact mode, the system can also provide deflection and lateral force images. In deflection the system uses the error signal of the feedback loop that is used to maintain the user setpoint deflection. In lateral force the system monitors the cantilever torsion (twisting) when scanning at 90° by comparing the amount of signal in the left and right halves of the four-quadrant photodiode. That is why the scan angle in the "Master Panel" should be set at 90° for lateral force microscopy.

Figure 7 depicts two contact mode images of a collagen gel (deflection and lateral force images, respectively), which were obtained with this protocol.

3.4 AFM Imaging with the PicoPlus

3.4.1 AFM Contact Mode Imaging in Liquid

In PicoPlus, contact mode imaging can be completed with any of the multipurpose scanners, using almost any AFM probe and nose assembly. Contact mode tips, however, are designed specifically for this application, with lower resonance frequency and softer cantilevers. Protocols used with the PicoPlus were derived from information contained in the instrument's manual [18]:

1. Power up the system:
   (a) Turn on all PicoPlus AFM parts (head electronic box (HEB), laser, camera), boot up the computer, and start the relevant software (PicoView) (*see* **Note 11**).

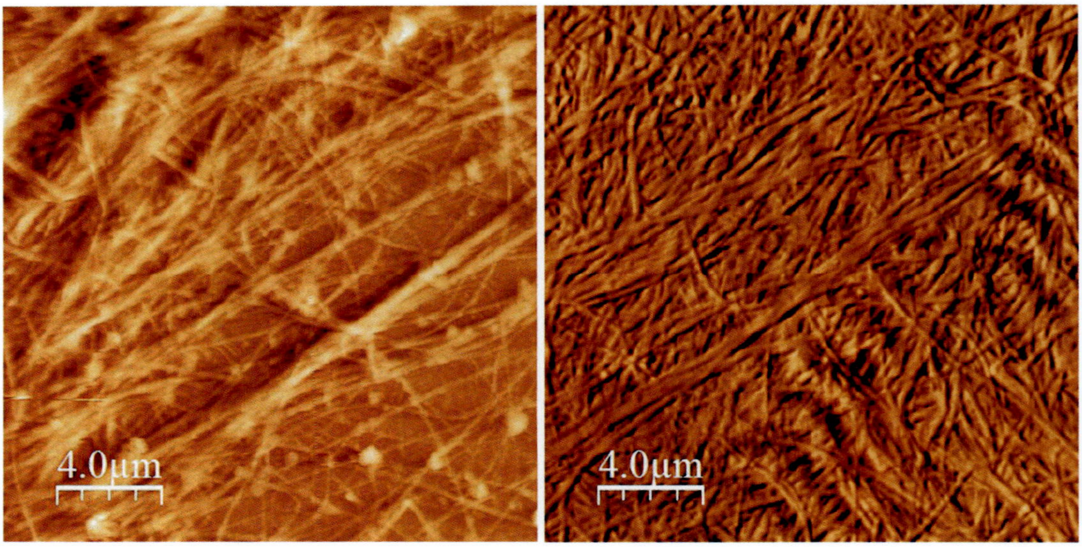

Fig. 7 AFM images in contact mode in air with Cypher ES. (*Left*) Deflection and (*Right*) lateral force microscopy AFM image of collagen I gel (0.5 mg/ml)

(b) Click on "Controls" and then on "Camera View" to open the "Camera View video" window (*see* **Note 12**).

(c) In the PicoView software, in the menu "Mode," select "Contact."

2. Load the cantilever and sample:

(a) Insert the nose assembly into the scanner.

(b) Insert a probe into the nose assembly (e.g., SICON or PNP-TR).

(c) Place the scanner in the microscope and connect its cables.

3. Find the cantilever in your microscope view (*see* **Note 13**):

(a) Align the laser on the cantilever with the laser alignment knobs that are located on the top of the scanner.

(b) Insert and align the detector. In the PicoView software, find the "Laser Alignment" window (this window will open automatically when you launch the software). If it is not open, you can open it by clicking on the "Laser Alignment" toolbar icon. Use the knobs on the detector to move the laser spot in the center of the four quadrants. For Contact Mode, the laser spot should be just below the dotted line (Fig. 8).

(c) Prepare the sample and mount the sample plate. Since we present the contact mode imaging in liquid, you will need the "Liquid Cell" that accompanies your system. The liquid cell enables in situ AFM imaging and characterization under liquid conditions that are more realistic when imaging

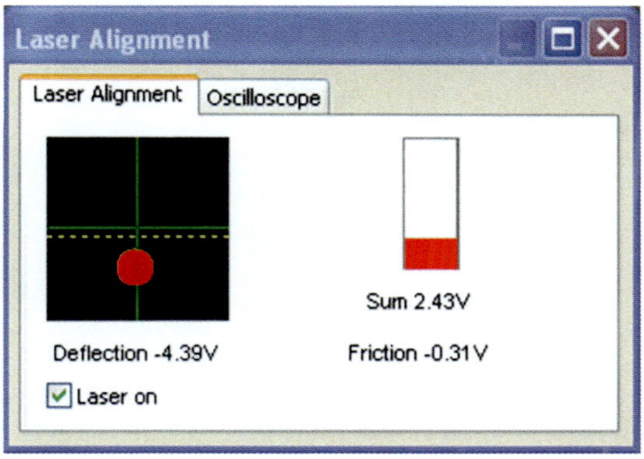

Fig. 8 Laser alignment window for contact mode. The red spot in the window demonstrates the deflection of the laser beam on the photo detector. In contact mode in the PicoPlus, the spot should be in the center of the vertical line and just below the *dotted line*

biological samples. Mount the liquid cell on the sample plate and insert the sample (e.g., collagen gel on a cover glass).

(d) Add some PBS into the liquid cell. Be careful so as not to overspill: use enough liquid to submerge the sample but not so much that the liquid rises to the top of the cell. This will prevent spillage when the scanner moves into the cell.

(e) Mount carefully the sample plate with the liquid cell on the AFM system.

4. Motor cantilever toward sample:

(a) Place your eyes at the level of the cantilever and the liquid cell with the sample, so that you can clearly see the gap between the two. Press the "Close" switch on the head electronic box (HEB) to raise the sample until the tip is immerged into the liquid (close to the sample surface but not touching the sample) (*see* **Note 14**).

(b) Now you will need to realign the photodetector due to the change in the laser location caused by the liquid. First, remove the photodetector and readjust its position. Then use the knobs of the detector to move the laser spot to the appropriate location.

(c) Locate the area of interest on the sample by manually moving the X/Y stage control micrometers while watching the video window (*see* **Note 15**).

5. Engage the cantilever on the sample:

(a) "Approach" the sample bringing the tip in contact with the surface. To ensure that the contact will be gentle, verify that the setpoint voltage is set appropriately: note the "Deflection" reading on the HEB front panel or in the

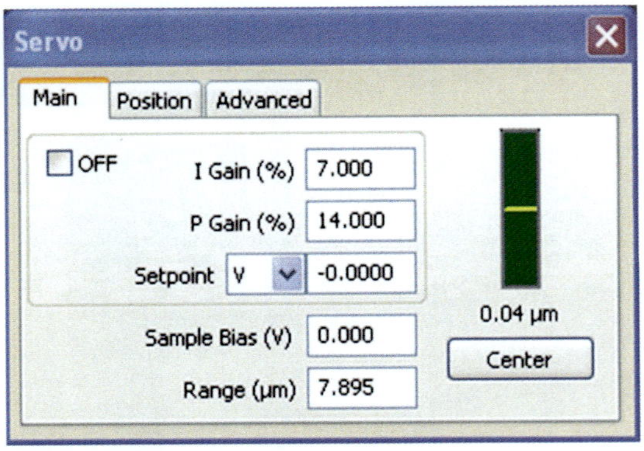

Fig. 9 Servo window showing setpoint voltage and Gains for the PicoPlus AFM system

PicoView's Laser Alignment window (both will display the same value). This is the current cantilever deflection, stated in volts. In the PicoView's Servo window, enter a setpoint value slightly more positive than the current deflection reading. This sets the deflection that the feedback loop will achieve and maintain.

(b) In the "Servo" window, make sure that the "I Gain" and "P Gain" (thereafter we will call these as "Gains") are set to 10%. These gains dictate how quickly the system will react to changes in tip deflection in order to maintain constant force. Ten percent is a good starting value (during imaging, you will reset the gains for better image quality; for collagen based samples, 7% and 14% work very well; Fig. 9).

(c) Click on the "Approach" icon in the PicoView's toolbar. The system will raise the sample until the deflection reaches the setpoint value.

6. Start the imaging and parameter tuning:

   (a) In the "Scan" and "Motor" window, select the "Scan" tab.

   (b) Enter a scan "Speed" stated in lines/second (ln/s). A typical starting value is 1–2 ln/s.

   (c) Select a resolution from the list (256 is a good starting value; for final images we recommend a 512 resolution).

   (d) In the "Realtime Images" window, display Topography, Deflection and Friction. Click on the "+" icon of the window to add a buffer. To set what each buffer will display, right-click inside the buffer frame, and select the "Input Signal" from the list. The list will vary depending on the imaging mode.

   (e) In the "Scan" and "Motor" windows, click on the "Down" blue arrow to initiate a scan starting at the top of the grid. Click on the "Up" blue arrow to initiate a scan from the bottom up. The image maps will begin to be rendered in the "Realtime Images" window.

(f) During imaging, adjust the "Setpoint" and Gains to achieve the better possible image depending on the use of cantilever and the sample.

3.4.2 AFM Tapping Mode Imaging in Air

The procedure is similar to the one described for tapping mode in Subheading 3.4.1, with the following exceptions:

1. For **step 1c**, in the menu "Mode," select "ACAFM" (Fig. 10).
2. For **step 2b**, choose appropriate probe (here we use the ACT probe).
3. For **step 5**, before engaging the tip, tune the tip:
   (a) Choose "AC Mode Tune" from the "Controls," or click on the "AC Mode Tune" icon (Fig. 11) to open the "AC Tune" window (Fig. 12).
   (b) On the "Auto" tab of the "AC Tune" window, set the following parameters: Start (kHz), 50; End (kHz), 500; Peak Amplitude (V), 5; and Off Peak (kHz), -0.10 (Fig. 12).
   (c) Click on "Auto Tune": this will bring up the Cantilever Tune Graph (Fig. 13).
   (d) In the "Servo" window, set "I Gain (%)" to 1 and "P Gain (%)" to 20 (Fig. 14), and make approach by clicking on the "Approach" icon in the PicoView's toolbar.

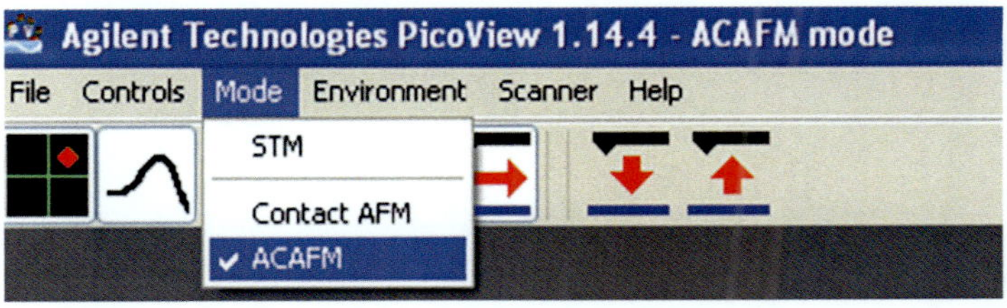

Fig. 10 Opening the "AC Tune" window in the PicoView software

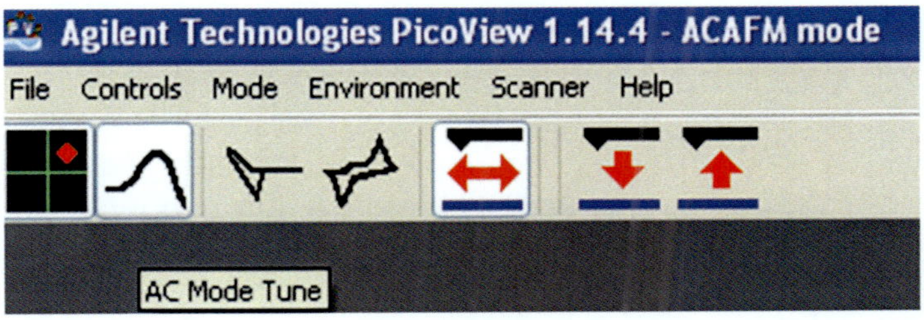

Fig. 11 AC Tune window and the set parameters in the "Auto" panel

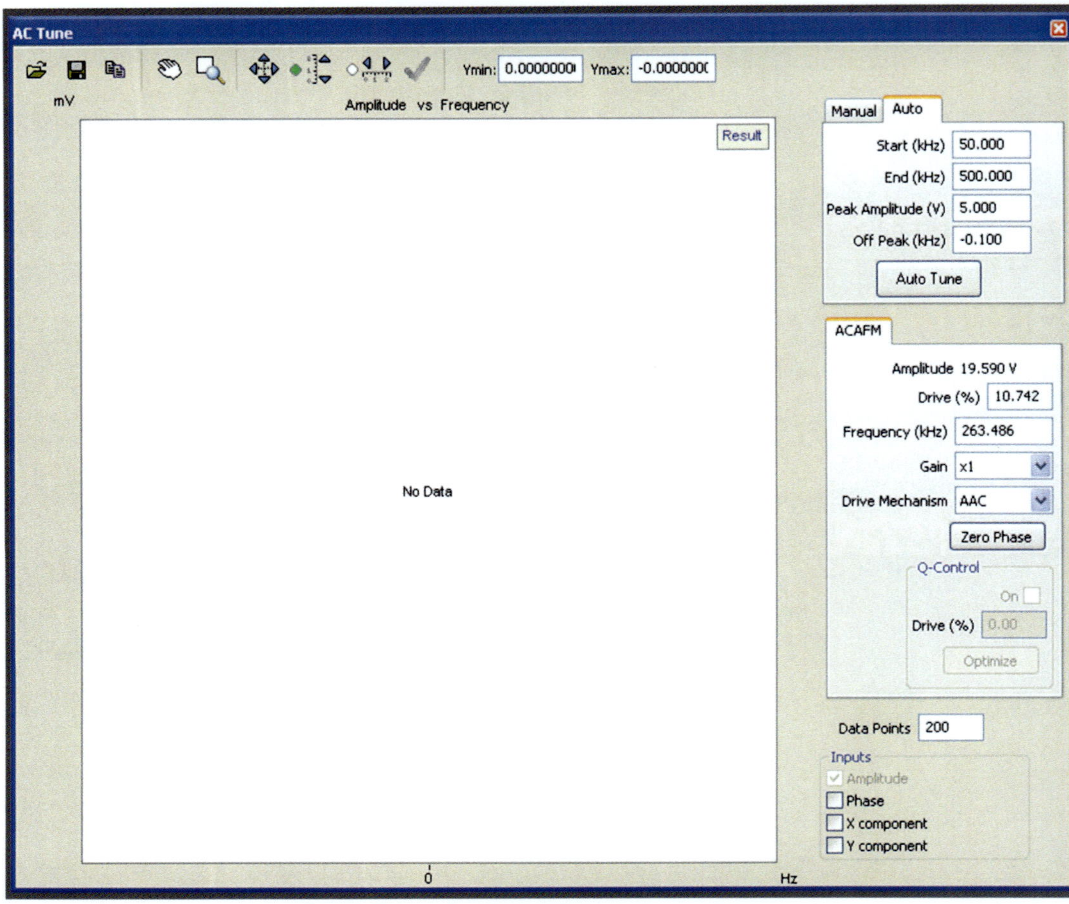

Fig. 12 Cantilever tune graph. The graph is the tuning results of an ACT probe with the "Off Peak" set to –0.1 kHz. The "Frequency" value was found to be 263.429 kHz as it can be seen in the "ACAFM" tap (the manufacturer gives a range of values from 200 to 400 kHz)

3.4.3 Analysis of AFM Images with the Open Access WSxM Software

1. Open the WSxM software.
2. A software message "SPM System not found" will pop. Click on "OK."
3. In the "File" menu, click on "Open." In the "File Type," set "All Files (*.*)," and select the file/image in the folder you want to analyze (Fig. 15, top).
4. The software will show the following message: "This file contains multiple data. What do you want?" (Fig. 15, bottom). Select the "Extract & Load" option. This will create a subfolder with the images and will also load the images in the software.
5. Upon loading the file, a number of different images will open (Fig. 16). In this example, we opened a file as it was saved in Cypher ES in tapping mode. Four images opened representing the Height, Amplitude, Phase, and ZSensor image.

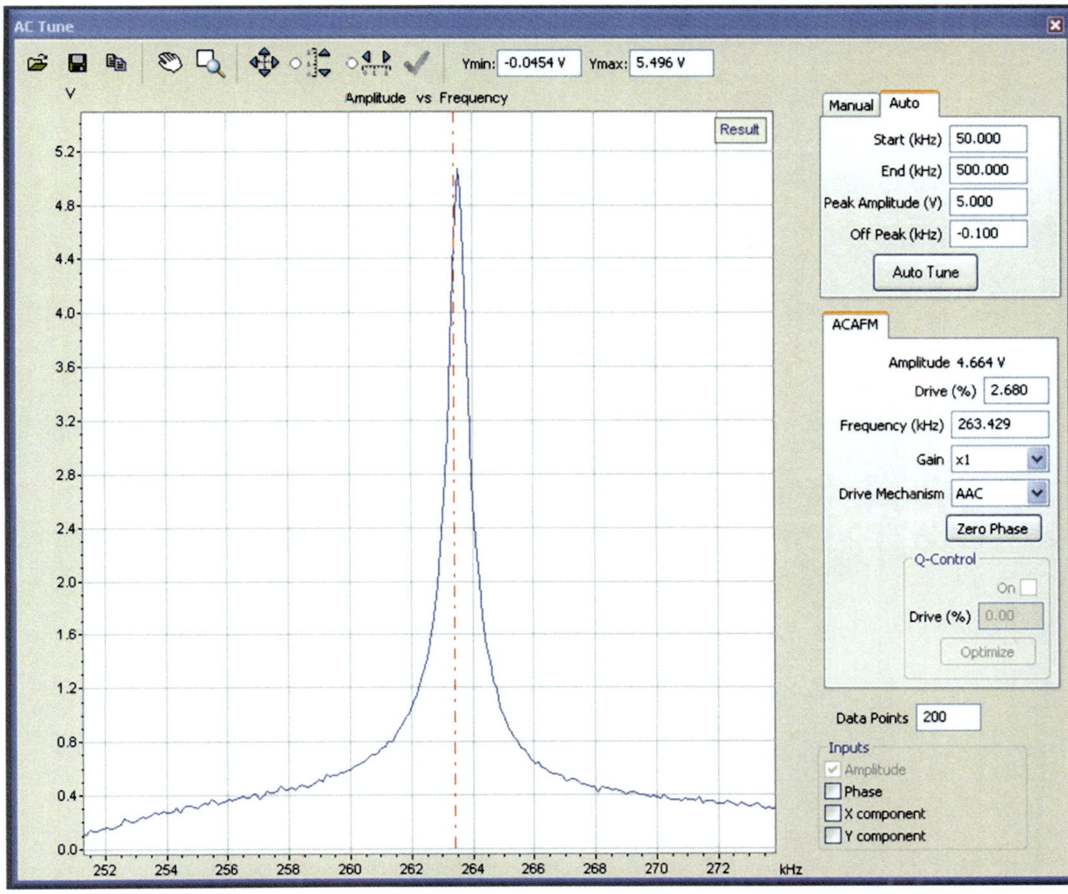

Fig. 13 The parameters in the "Servo" window just before the approach

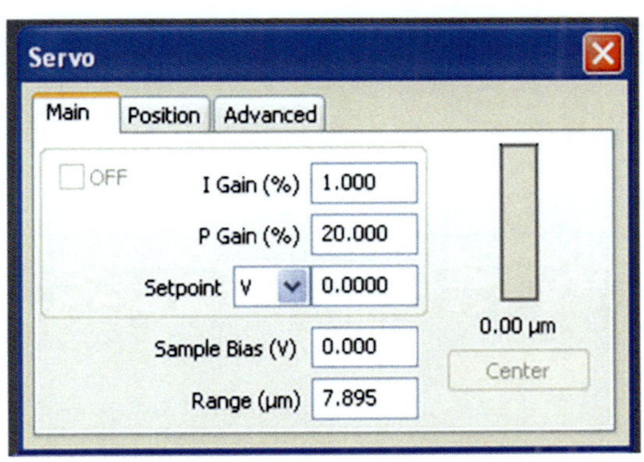

Fig. 14 Selection of AC AFM (tapping mode) in the PicoView software

6. Select the first image (Height) by clicking on the image. Height image is the most frequently used type of image in AFM. Also, when you want to measure distances or height values, it would be better to use this kind of image (as opposed

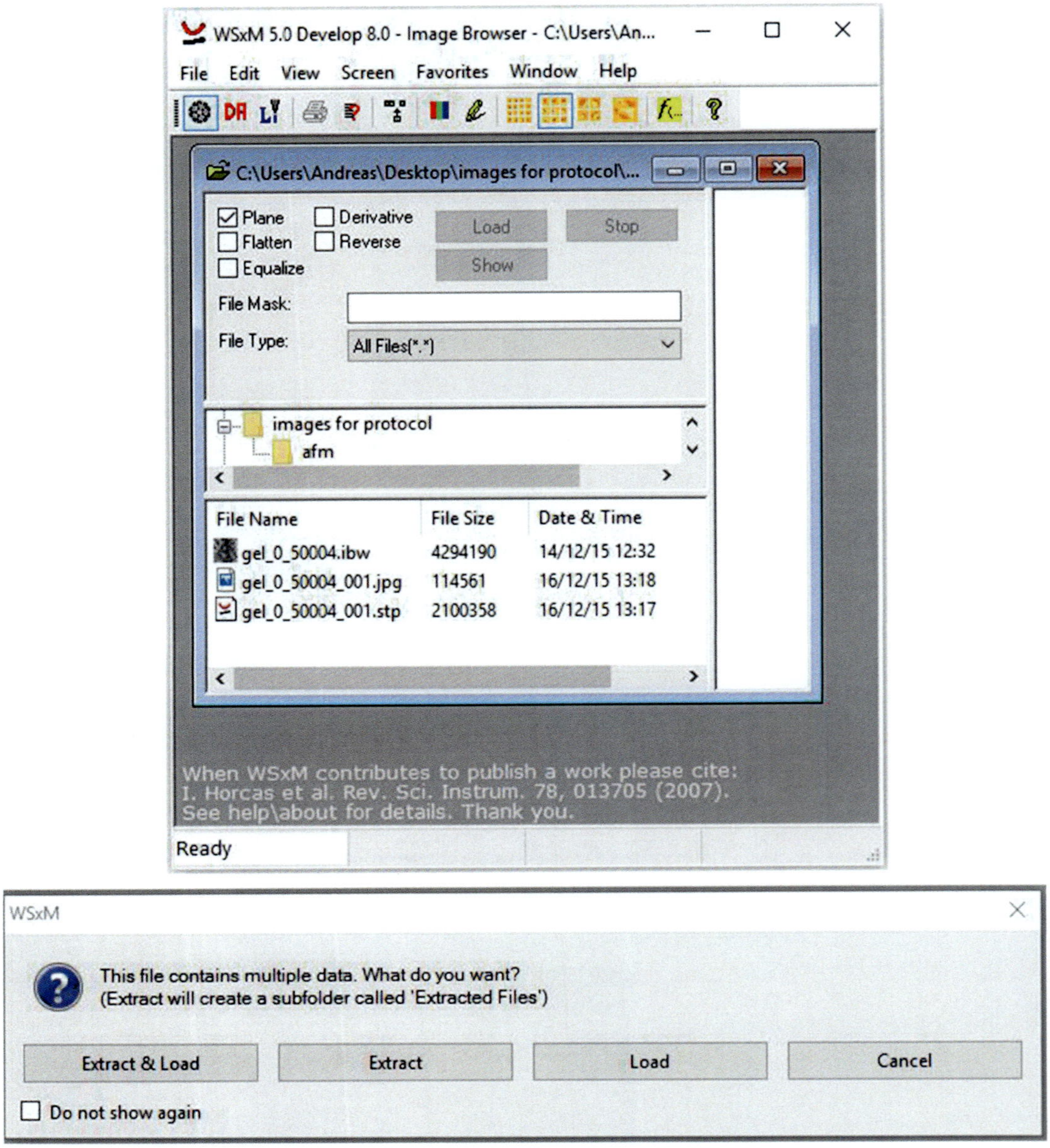

Fig. 15 WSxM software screenshots during the procedure of loading an image

to the Amplitude or Phase images) because it represents some of the surface features better.

7. In the "Screen" menu, click on "Palette settings." From the Pallet settings window, adjust the "Brightness" and "Contrast" to highlight the surface features you want to focus on.
8. In the "Display" menu, click on "Show Scale Bar" to add a scale bar on the image.
9. In the "Process" menu, click on "Profile." Drag a line on the figure, and a height profile of the line will appear (Fig. 17, top).

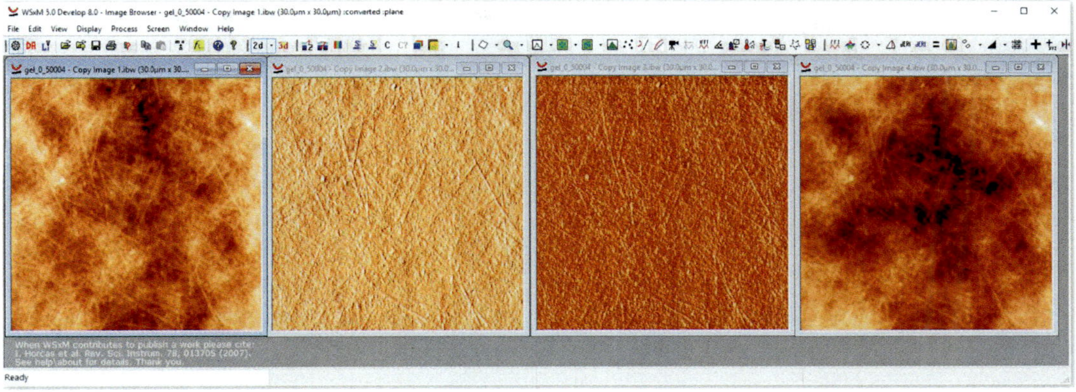

Fig. 16 Screenshot from WSxM software when a file from tapping mode imaging (Cypher ES) is loaded

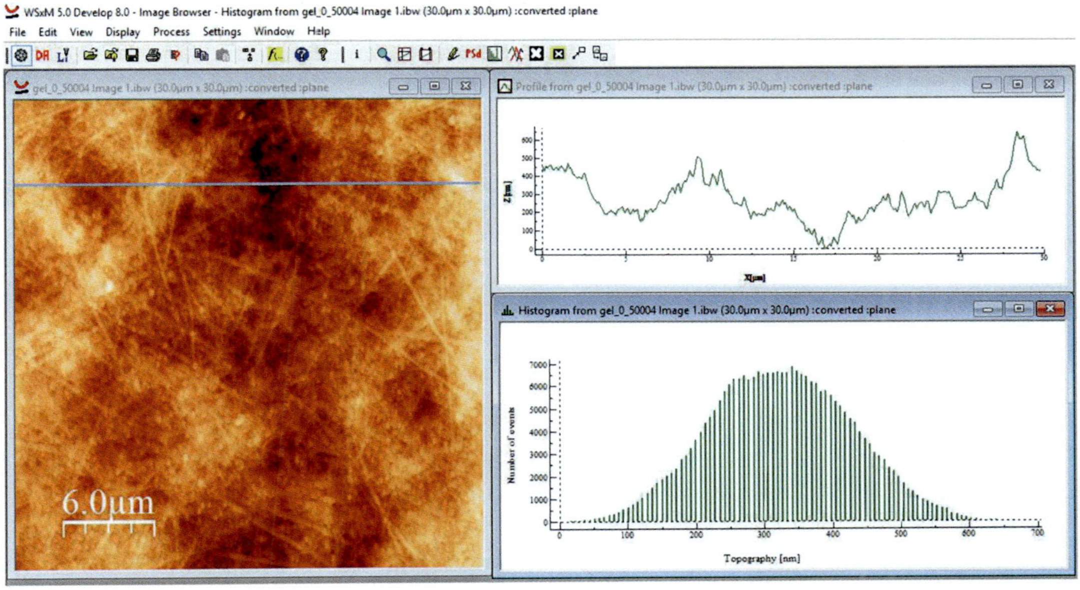

Fig. 17 Screenshot from WSxM software when a tapping mode was analyzed. (*Left*) Topography image of a collagen gel. (*Right Top*) Line profile of the line on the topography image. (*Right Bottom*) Histogram of the topography image

10. In the "Process" menu, click on "Roughness Analysis." The "Roughness Analysis" window will present a number of different values, including RMS Roughness, Roughness Average, and Average height. Write down the values you need and click on "OK." A "Histogram" of the surface will appear (Fig. 17, bottom right).
11. In order to save any of these figures as a .jpg image, click on the figure, go to the "File" menu, and select "Save as." Set the type as "JPEG FILES (*.jpg)," select the folder you want to save it in, type a name for your file, and click "Save."

3.5 AFM Mechanical Property Characterization

The following general guidelines should be carefully considered for calibrating the probes and volume spectroscopy in contact mode.

3.5.1 Calibration of Probes: General Principles

Each manufacturer provides a spring constant value (or a range of values) for its probes, but the actual spring constant can vary significantly from the estimated value [19]. Due to this uncertainty about the actual spring constant, the user should calibrate each cantilever that is used in quantitative mechanical property measurements [30]. Various methods for measuring cantilever spring constants are available in the literature [22].

In order to measure the mechanical properties of the sample, the sample is indented by the tip. Then the cantilever deflection is measured as a function of tip's z position [19]. Consequently, by using Hooke's law, the indentation force can be calculated. The indentation procedure provides force vs. indentation curves that can be used to extract the elastic modulus of the sample by fitting the curves to standard models, such as the Hertz model [19, 31]. Consequently, an important step in AFM force measurements is the calibration of the probe parameters that is required for accurate quantitative measurements. In particular, three parameters must be calculated, and two calibration procedures ("sensitivity calibration" and "spring constant calibration") should be performed. As previously mentioned, the force F between the tip and the specimen can be provided through Hooke's law in relation to the cantilever's deflection. In particular, in the case of AFM [4],

$$F = k.\alpha.V$$

where k is the cantilever's spring constant (cantilever's bending stiffness), α is the deflection sensitivity (that converts cantilever's deflection from volts to nanometers), and V is the measured cantilever's deflection (in volts). These three entities, k, α, and V, are the main entities that the AFM determines in force spectroscopy [4]. The deflection V is measured directly with the system's position-sensitive split photodiode detector, while the sensitivity calibration and the spring constant calibration should be performed in order to determine the α and k, respectively (*see* below).

3.5.2 Sensitivity Calibration

Sensitivity calibration (nm cantilever deflection per volt signal of the laser detection system) is straightforward [30]. It is important to acquire a force vs. distance curve on a clean, hard surface (like mica or glass). Then, the deflection sensitivity α is determined from this force vs. distance curve by simply positioning two cursors on its contact part [4].

3.5.3 Spring Constant Calibration

Spring constant calibration (N/m = nN/nm, nanonewtons force from the cantilever per nm of vertical deflection) is the most complicated part of the calibration [30]. Although the manufacturer provides the spring constant k, the provided value can be quite gross; 300% deviation from the stated estimate is not unusual [4]. That is why an accurate measurement of the spring constant is required. Several different methods have been developed (calculation from dimensions, dimensions plus frequency and/or quality factor (Q), added mass, reference cantilever, thermal noise analysis), with the thermal noise analysis becoming the main standard for AFM experiments. Furthermore, new and novel contactless and one-step procedure methods, like GetReal™, are emerging, providing new capabilities and eliminating some of the old procedure limitations (more below).

3.6 AFM Mechanical Property Characterization with Cypher ES

3.6.1 Spring Constant Calibration

The most common method is the "thermal tune" method. In this method, the system determines the natural resonant frequency of the cantilever by appropriate fitting [27]. More specifically, the thermal tune measures the thermal fluctuations of the cantilever as a function of time and fits the resonance peak (which is normally selected by the user) to a Lorentzian curve so as to calculate the cantilever spring constant [19]. The thermal tuning procedure should be performed in air with a clean, dry cantilever and the "deflection sensitivity" on a material that is very stiff compared to the cantilever, such as mica, glass, and tissue culture dish [19]. The following procedure is for the Cypher ES. Determination of the spring constant *k* is done by firstly calculating the deflection sensitivity (called InvOLS—inverse optical lever sensitivity—in Cypher ES) and secondly by determining the cantilever's resonant frequency with the thermal method.

1. Follow **steps 1–4e** detailed in Subheading 3.3.1 "Tapping Mode Imaging in Air." Use the appropriate probe for your experiment (here we use an AC160TS-R3, Olympus), and for the sample, use a freshly cleaved mica.
2. Perform a deflection sensitivity calibration:
   (a) Perform force curve: engage on the surface in contact mode. Set the trigger channel to DflV (deflection) and set the absolute trigger to 1 V. Take a force plot by clicking the "Single Force" button.
   (b) Find InvOLS: right-click on the contact region of the curve, and select "Calculate InvOLS" to calculate the InvOLS.
   (c) Perform line fit: on the "Cal" tab of the "Force" tab on the "Master" panel, select "Defl InvOLS" from the "Set Sensitivity" pulldown menu. A fit will be performed and the InvOLS will be updated.
3. Perform a thermal tune:

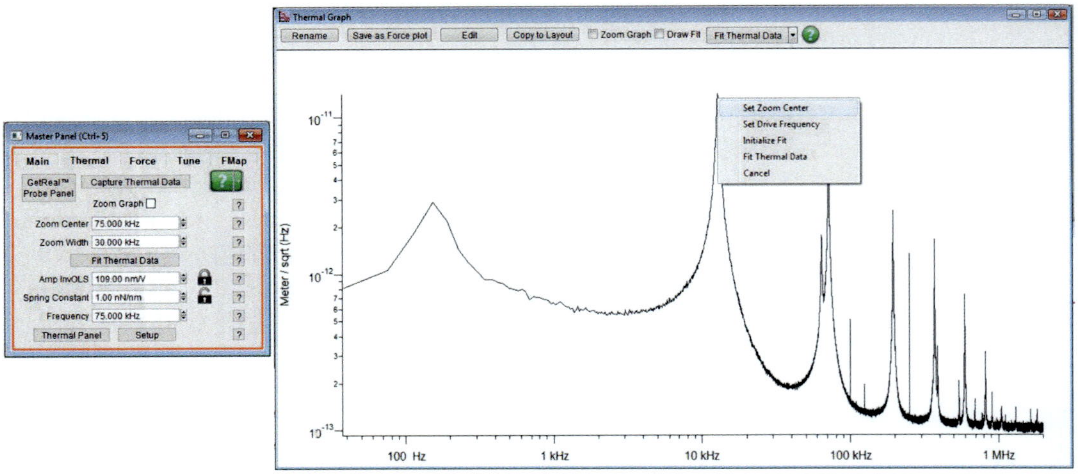

Fig. 18 Capturing thermal data. (*Left*) The "Thermal" tap of the "Master Panel" and (*Right*) a thermal graph

(a) Go to the "Thermal" tab which is located in the "Master Panel" (Fig. 18, left).

(b) Click on "Capture Thermal Data" and a spectrum will appear (Fig. 18, right). From the graph you can see that the baseline is mostly noise, but a sharp line/peak will be present. This peak is the probe resonant frequency. For the used probe, it should be around the frequency that is provided by the manufacturer. Click the "Stop" button to terminate the collection of the power spectra.

4. Thermal fitting for the spring constant:

(a) Select the peak, and zoom into the area by left mouse dragging around the higher peak (arrow in Fig. 18, right).

(b) Right-click to open the contextual menu and select the "Set Zoom Center" option.

(c) Click on "Fit Thermal" and a blue curve will appear (Fig. 19).

(d) Go to the "Master Panel," select the "Force" panel, and click on the "Cal." tab. Check the spring constant value (a new value will appear when the procedure has finished). If the procedure was performed appropriately, the *k* value will be in the range that is provided by the manufacturer.

3.6.2 Automated Calibration

In our work we prefer to use the GetReal™ function which is an automated probe calibration feature provided exclusively by Asylum Research (for Cypher™ and MFP-3D™ families of AFMs). This feature makes calibration very simple and easy, and, more importantly, with this technique there is no risk to damage or contaminate the tip during the calibration procedure, since the tip

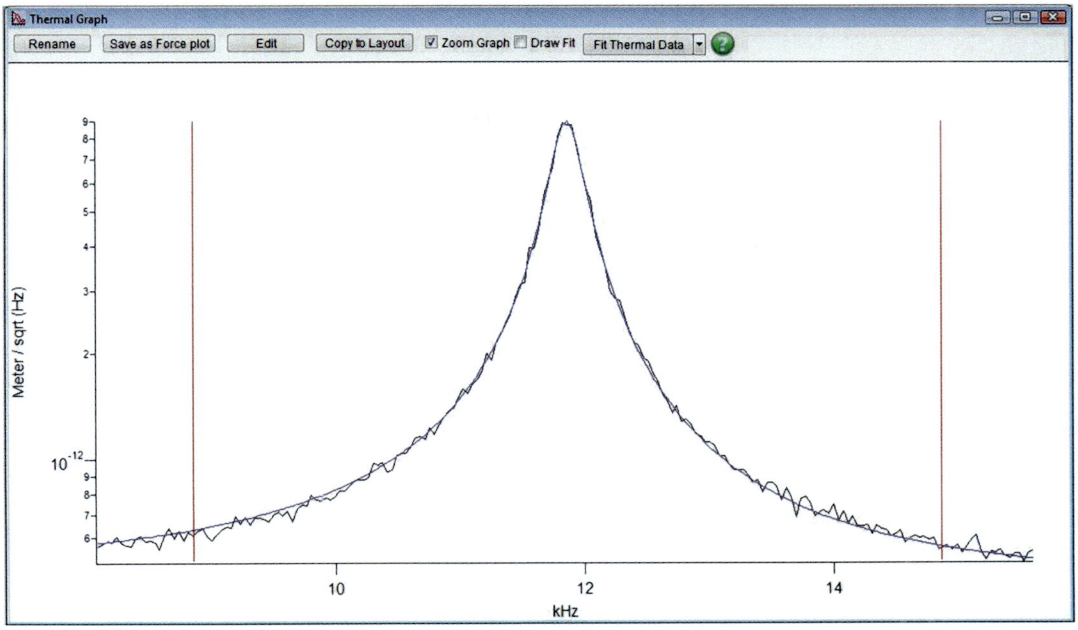

Fig. 19 A thermal graph after fitting the graph

never touches any surface. The GetReal function is based on the well-known spring constant calibration methods, the thermal noise [32] and Sader's method [33]. With this one-step calibration procedure, the inverse optical lever sensitivity (InvOLS) and spring constant (k) are both calibrated by just selecting the probe or probe characteristics.

1. Align the laser and the photodetector signal as it was presented in the previous sections for the Cypher ES (*see* Subheading 3.3.1 "Tapping Mode Imaging in Air").
2. Select "Thermal" tab on the "Master Panel" (Fig. 20, top).
3. Click on "GetReal™ Probe Panel" and the "Probe Panel" opens. Select the cantilever you are using (AC160TC in this example) (*see* **Note 16**).
4. Then click on "GetReal™ Calibration" and the calibration procedure will start. The rest of the calibration is completely automated.
5. Select the "Master Panel" window, select the "Force" tab, and click on "Cal." tab. During the procedure, a red circle will appear next to the "Defl InvOLS" and "Spring Constant" values (Fig. 20, bottom). When the procedure is finished, a green circle will appear next to the values, and the values will change with the calculated ones (*see* **Note 17**).

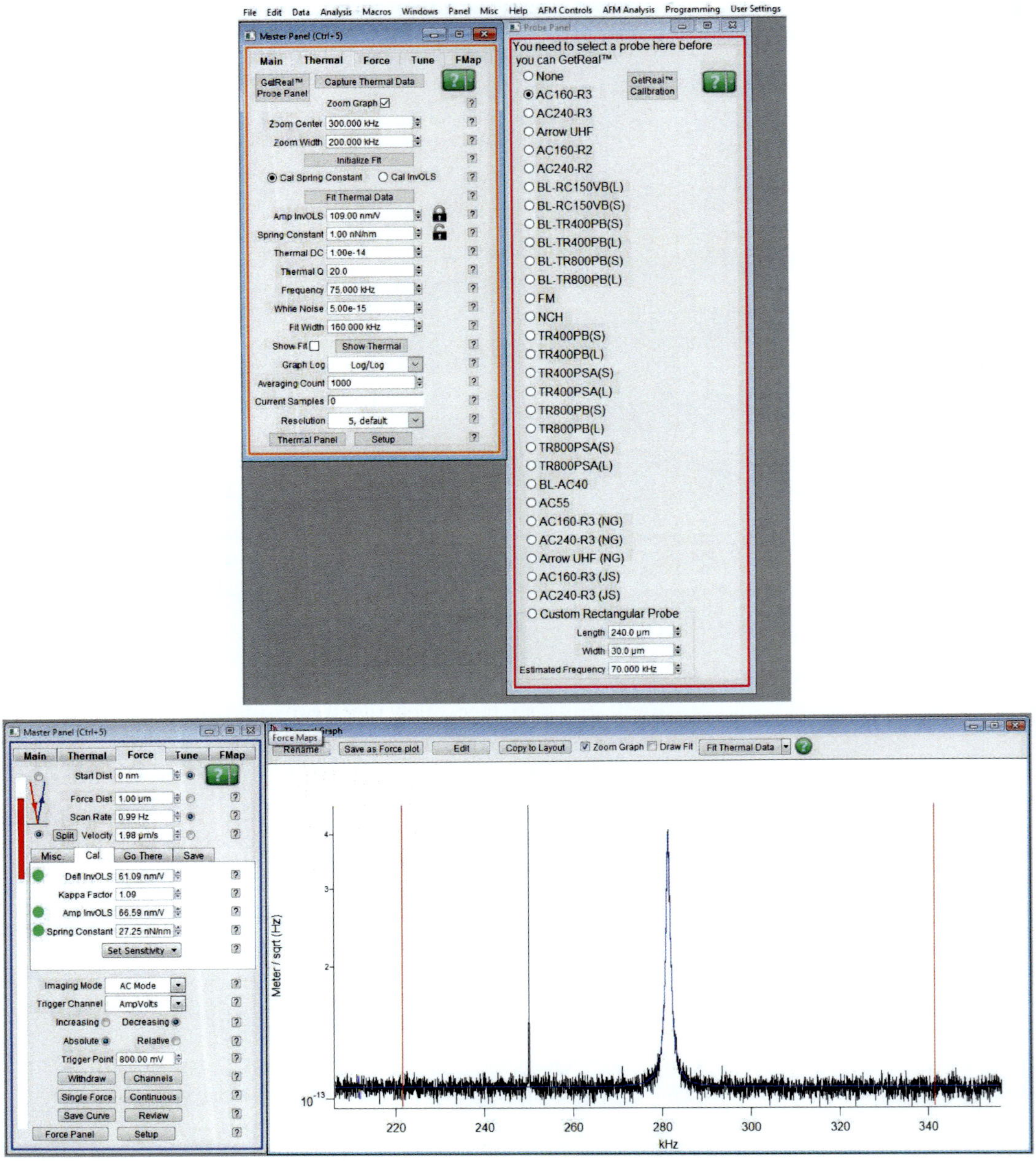

Fig. 20 GetReal calibration procedure. (*Top*) Probe Panel and (*Bottom*) Cal. Panel and Thermal Graph

3.6.3 Acquisition of Mechanical Property Data from Collagen Gels and Tumor Tissue

In this section we present the methodology to collect mechanical properties, especially the formation of force maps data with the Cypher ES. Force mapping is when force curves are acquired in an XY raster pattern to construct an image of mechanical properties of the sample (e.g., Young's modulus). With the Cypher ES, only adhesion and height maps can be displayed in real time, but off-line procedures can be performed to create other maps.

1. Prepare your system for contact mode imaging as described in Subheading 3.3.2 "Contact Mode Imaging in Air." Use an appropriate contact mode probe.

2. Proceed to a probe calibration procedure (*see* Subheading 3.6.1 "Spring Constant Calibration" and Subheading 3.6.2 "Automated Calibration") to determine the spring constant k and the deflection sensitivity of your probe. With the Cypher ES, the easiest way is to use the GetReal function.
3. Engage your probe to the area of interest. If you wish you may acquire an image of the selected area or you can continue directly to the force mapping.
4. In the "FMap" tab of the "Master Panel," define the scan size, the velocity, and the number of points and lines. Be careful, high values of the numbers of points and lines mean longer time to acquire your image.
5. Click on "Do Scan" to begin Force Map Acquisition.
6. The data can be used after the procedure to get Young's modulus maps (*see* Subheading 3.8 "Generation of Young's Modulus Maps with the Open Access AtomicJ Software").

3.7 AFM Mechanical Property Characterization with PicoPlus

3.7.1 Spring Constant Calibration

1. Perform a deflection sensitivity calibration:
   (a) Prepare your system for contact mode imaging as described in Subheading 3.4.1 "AFM Contact Mode Imaging in Liquid"). The calibration procedure should be first performed in air and then in liquid if necessary. Use the probe you want to calibrate (here we used PNP-TR, NanoWorld) and freshly cleaved mica as a sample (*see* **Note 18**).
   (b) The deflection sensitivity "Deflection Sens." parameter is found in the "Advanced" tab in the "Spectroscopy" window.
   (c) In the Servo dialog box, set the following parameters, set Gains at 8% and "Setpoint" to 0 V, and maximize the "Range" (to maximize the value, enter a very large number (e.g., 999), and the PicoView will adjust to the maximum value for the scanner). For our system the maximum value is 7.89 μm).
   (d) Select an area of interest. For calibration, select a clean area of mica surface (if the mica was cleaved appropriately, the entire surface is fresh, clean, and flat).
   (e) Approach the tip by clicking on "Approach" (*see* **Note 19**).
   (f) Open the spectroscopy function by clicking on the "Spectroscopy" toolbar icon. Ensure the plot type is set to "Force vs Distance."
   (g) Select the spectroscopy "Basic" tab, and set the "Sweeps" to 1, the "Duration" to 1, and the "Data Points" to 200.
   (h) Maximize the "Start," and minimize the "End" values by entering a very large number (e.g., 999) and a large negative number (e.g., −999), respectively. The PicoView will adjust to the maximum value for the scanner.

(i) Turn On the "Toggle Auto Full Scale" on the top of the screen.

(j) On the "Basic" panel of the spectroscopy window, click on the play button (►). The scanner will take a force vs. distance curve. If needed, adjust the "Start"/"End" parameters.

(k) In the plot window, right-click on the curve to add a "Ruler" to the linear part of the plot (in this part, the tip is in hard contact with the sample). Set the end points to cover a large proportion of this linear part of the curve.

(l) Right-click on the ruler and select "Deflection Sensitivity." The deflection sensitivity is now automatically set. You can check the value from the "Deflection Sens." in the "Advanced" tab in the "Spectroscopy" window.

(m) The units for the Y-axis can now be changed by clicking on the title of the curve "Force (V) vs. Distance" and selecting nm to display "Force (nm) vs. Distance."

2. Perform a thermal tune: for the PicoPlus AFM microscope, the thermal tuning can be performed with the "Thermal K Calibration," but not all the microscopes support this function since it is optional [22].

(a) Withdraw the tip from the sample surface by clicking on "Withdraw" at the top of the main window.

(b) Select the "Advanced" tab of the "Spectroscopy" window, and click on "Thermal K" to open the "Thermal K" plot window.

(c) Set the Acquisition time to 1 sec and Averages to 10.

(d) Click on "Plot" and a plot will be displayed.

(e) Click and drag the red and green circles to define the frequency range in which the resonance frequency should be found.

(f) Click on "Compute."

(g) Click on "Compute" several times until the provided force constant value is stable.

(h) Click on "Apply" in the "Thermal K" window. The thermal tune is done.

3.7.2 Acquisition of Mechanical Property Data from Collagen Gels and Tumor Tissue

1. Prepare your system for contact mode imaging as described in Subheading 3.4 "AFM Imaging with the PicoPlus." Use the probe you want to calibrate (here we used PNP-TR, NanoWorld).

2. Proceed to a probe calibration procedure (*see* Subheading 3.6.1 "Spring Constant Calibration") to determine the spring constant *k* and the deflection sensitivity of your probe. Since we will perform a force volume spectroscopy of collagen gel under liquid, perform a sensitivity calibration under liquid. We suggest the following:

(a) Use the "Thermal K" to acquire the value of spring constant k.

(b) Mount the previously selected tip in the cantilever holder of the PicoPlus AFM, and mount a freshly cleaved mica sample with the liquid cell filled with PBS (for the liquid cell, *see* Subheading 3.4.1 "AFM Contact Mode Imaging in Liquid").

(c) Perform a sensitivity calibration under PBS on freshly cleaved mica (*see* Subheading 3.6.1 "Spring Constant Calibration").

(d) Select the "Advanced" tab of the "Spectroscopy" window, and check the new value of "Deflection sens.," which corresponds to the measurement performed in PBS.

(e) In the same tab, set the value for the spring constant *k* as obtained from "Thermal K" (or from the manufacturer if you do not need accurate measurement).

(f) In the "Spectroscopy" window, change the values in the title to be "Force (nN) vs Distance."

3. Change the sample and mount a collagen gel in PBS.
4. Choose an area of interest and perform a contact mode imaging in PBS.
5. Move to an area on which you want to acquire force volume spectroscopy.
6. Proceed to the force scanning procedure:

(a) In the Servo dialog box, set the following parameters: set Gains as needed for the sample. Here we suggest starting with 10 and 10%. In our samples we get good results for setting the gains at 13 and 7%, respectively. Set the Setpoint to 0 V. Maximize the "Range" by entering a very large number (e.g., 999). Open the spectroscopy function by clicking on the "Spectroscopy" toolbar icon. Ensure the plot type is set to "Force vs Distance."

(b) Select the Spectroscopy Basic tab, and set the Sweeps to 1, the Duration to 1, and the Data Points to 200. Maximize the Start and minimize the End values by entering a very large number (e.g., 999) and a large negative number (e.g., -999), respectively.

(c) Select the "Basic" tab on the "Spectroscopy" window, and click on the "play" icon (►) to take a force vs. distance curve.

(d) After the initial sweep is completed, fine-tune the force-distance parameters by adjusting the sweep range as needed using the Start/End parameters in the "Setup" tab. We suggest you take at least one force-distance curve for each area you want to perform force volume spectroscopy on, in order to obtain good force-distance curves.

(e) Save successive force measurements after each force curve: select the "Spectroscopy" window; in the "File" menu, select "Set filename." In the "Save As" dialog box, enter a filename for the data set. Click on "Save." Alternatively, turn on auto-save by selecting "Auto Save" in the "File" menu.

7. Perform volume spectroscopy:

   (a) Select the "Volume" tab in the "Spectroscopy" window to display the topographic image. The transparency of the image can be adjusted by clicking on the image and rolling the mouse wheel.

   (b) Specify the resolution by selecting a volume from the pull-down menu.

   (c) Turn on the Toggle Auto Full Scale.

   (d) Save successive force measurements by having files saved automatically after each force curve (*see* **step 8e**).

   (e) Begin to take force measurements. Start the sweep of the selected area by clicking on "Scan Up" or "Scan Down."

8. Save your data by selecting "Save as" in the "File" menu.

9. Withdraw the AFM tip.

3.8 Generation of Young's Modulus Maps with the Open Access AtomicJ Software

1. Open the data processing software AtomicJ (*see* **Note 20**).
2. Click on the "Gear" icon "Process force curve and maps" to open the "Processing assistant" window (Fig. 21, left).
3. Click on "Add," and select the file with force volume data that you wish to analyze. Then click on "Next" to process all the curves that are stored in the selected file.

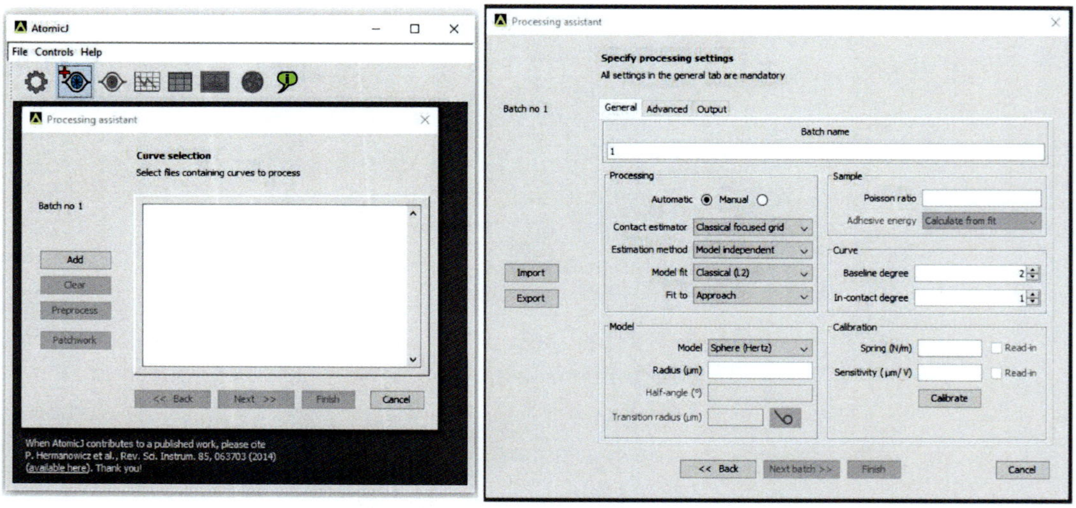

Fig. 21 Snapshots from AtomicJ. (*Left*) The "Processing assistant" window and (*Right*) the "General" panel of the "Processing assistant" window

4. Another "Processing Assistant" window will open (Fig. 21, right). In the "General" tab, enter the appropriate parameters (*see* **Note 21**).
   (a) Model: "Sphere (Hertz)" (*see* **Note 22**).
   (b) Radius (μm), "0.01" (provided by the probe manufacturer).
   (c) Poisson ratio, "0.3." (This parameter depends on your sample. For pure collagen samples, a value of 0.3 is usually used, while for cells a value of 0.5 is more appropriate. For tissues, use 0.5.)
   (d) Spring (N/m), "0.32." (This depends on the used tip. You can use the value that is provided by the manufacturer or, more appropriately, the value obtained via the spring constant calibration that you performed for this specific probe.)
   (e) Sensitivity (μm/V), "0.102" (you can find this value from the sensitivity calibration procedure that you performed for this specific probe; *see* **Note 23**).
5. Click on "Finish" and two windows will open, the "Graphical results" and the "Maps." In the "Maps" window you will find the following tabs (with the relevant maps or images): Young's modulus, transition indentation, transition force, contact position, contact force, deformation, adhesion force, topography trace, and deflection trace.
6. In the "Young's Modulus" tab (on which we focused in this chapter), Young's modulus values of the sample are represented in each square as values and as a pseudo-color (the matching of each color to the values is represented in the bar in the right side of the map; you can change it by double-clicking on the bar) (*see* **Note 24**).
7. Double-click on each square of Young's modulus map to open the corresponding curve. If a value appears out of range or not as expected, you can open the corresponding curve and check if the fitting is appropriate. Adjust the fitting by using the provided tools that you can find in the right side of the "Graphical results" window.
8. Finally, a useful feature is the formation of histograms. On the right side of the "Maps" window, click on "Draw Histogram," and the "Histogram Assistant" will appear. Select "Young's Modulus" and click "Next." In the next panel in the "Method" tab, select "Square Root" (you can select any other method among the provided ones), and check the "Add Fit" box and click finish.
9. Keep in mind that AtomicJ can provide many more information, images, maps, and charts. Check the user's manual for more details.

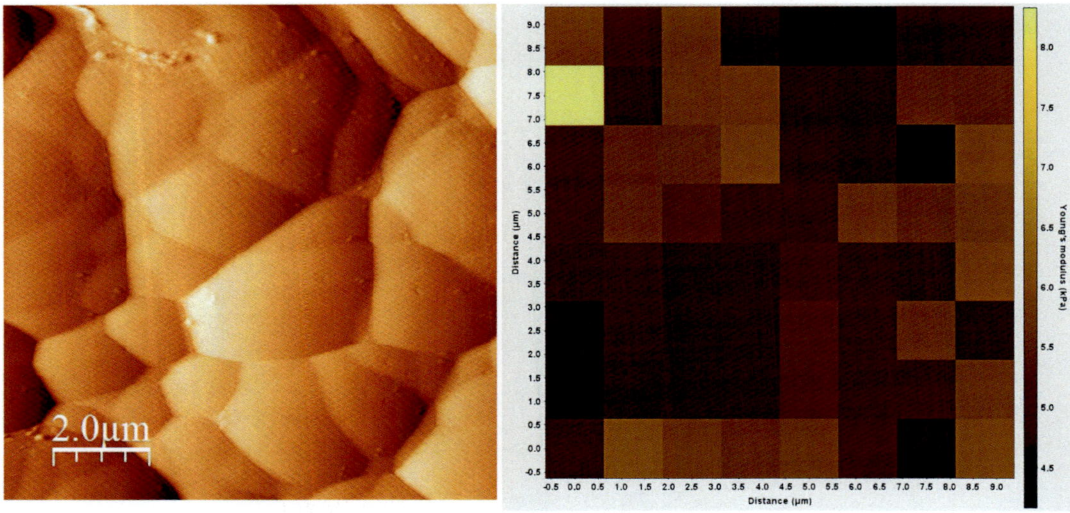

Fig. 22 Tissue with colloid AFM probe. (*Left*) Deflection AFM image and (*Right*) Young's modulus map of a tissue section with colloid AFM probe (contact mode, PicoPlus and AtomicJ)

3.9 AFM Characterization of Mechanical Properties of Tumor Tissue with Colloidal Probes (PicoPlus and AtomicJ)

1. Prepare your system for contact mode imaging. Use the probe you want to calibrate (here we used CP-PNP-BSG, sQube, with sphere diameter of 5 µm) (*see* **Note 25**).
2. Proceed to a probe calibration procedure (*see* Subheading 3.7 "AFM Mechanical Property Characterization with the PicoPlus" in mica in air.
3. Change the sample and mount a 20 µm-thick tissue section.
4. Choose an area of interest, and perform a contact mode imaging (since you have a colloidal probe, you will not get the resolution of that sharp AFM tips offer; Fig. 22, left).
5. Proceed to the force scanning procedure and volume spectroscopy (*see* Subheading 3.7.2 "Acquisition of Mechanical Property Data from Collagen Gels and Tumor Tissue" **steps 8** and **9**).
6. Take a series of force volume data and ensure you save your data.
7. Withdraw the AFM tip.
8. Analyze your data with AtomicJ. Use the Hertz model, your calibration values, and a value of 5 µm for tip diameter. Form Young's modulus maps (Fig. 22, right).

4 Notes

1. We elected to describe two AFM systems to help inexperienced AFM users to obtain as much information as possible since the available commercial systems are numerous and with quite

different characteristics. Of course, all protocols described here can be performed using just one AFM system and can be adjusted to any other commercially available AFM system with small modifications. Note that there are also biologically oriented AFM systems (commercially available or homebuilt) that combine the AFM technology with an inverted microscope. In this case, the user can simultaneously take advantage of both optical microscopy and AFM techniques [14].

2. New silicon nitride cantilevers should be used. The selection of the probe should be made very carefully since the tip and cantilever characteristics influence the final imaging result and the quantitative measurements [30]. For instance, for biological samples, soft rectangular or triangular cantilevers are preferred in ordered to prevent sample damage. In the case of collagen, which is quite stiff, stiffer cantilevers can be used. For high-resolution imaging, sharpened tips are a better choice, while for mechanical property characterization, it might be better to select tips with a large radius of curvature. Also, spherical tips, usually colloidal probes, are a good choice for measuring mechanical properties in biological samples, since the geometry is well defined. This permits the estimations of the elastic modulus with higher accuracy, while the possible puncture of the sample by the sharp tips is minimized [19].
3. Usually for AFM studies, mica discs are used. However, we tried to form our gels on glass cover slips and investigated them with AFM, and the results were satisfactory. Glass cover slips are cheaper and optically clear, characteristics that are useful when planning to make multiple experiments, and the samples are used as substrates for culturing cells.
4. Be careful with the selection of the original collagen solution. Not all the commercially available collagens are appropriate for collagen gels. *See* Chapter 15 for more information on the topic.
5. Different cantilevers can be used. We prefer the AC160TS cantilever for tapping mode.
6. When trying to pick up a cantilever, carefully hold the cantilever box with the other hand. Also, some users find it useful to first lay the chip down on a nonsticky surface and re-grip it before continuing. You can push or pull the cantilever into place so as to put the tip approximately in the center. You may nudge the cantilever chip from the side to align it, but *do not* nudge the end of the chip, as that could damage the cantilever.
7. In your first experiments, you may use a calibration grating (e.g., Asylum Research calibration grating sample, part # 900.237) as a sample to check that your methodology is correct.

8. You must be very careful because if you crash the cantilever holder on the sample surface, you may cause serious damage to your system components. If you are unsure about how far the tip is from the surface, leave the tip at a safe height (i.e., when you can see a clear gap between tip and surface). It will just take more time to approach the probe to the sample later in the procedure.
9. If you are not sure that you focused appropriately on the sample surface, use the arrows on the video window to move your sample. If the features are moving, the focus was probably correct. Also, if you did not manually move the tip close enough, you will never get a focused image of the sample. In this case move manually the tip to the surface so as to minimize the gap between the tip and the surface. Then try to focus again on the tip and on the sample. When you set the focus appropriately, check your system by clicking to the "Focus On Sample" and "Focus On Tip" so as to go back and forth between tip and sample.
10. For pure collagen samples (like gels or thin films), we have noticed that 1 Hz is a good starting point. After some scans and when you find an area of interest, you can set the scan rate to a smaller value, e.g., 0.5 Hz, to get your final image. In our experiments, smaller scan rates produce better images.
11. We recommend to always turn on the computer after turning on the AFM parts. If you first turn on the computer, you may face some issues related to miscommunication between the different components of the system.
12. For older software versions, you may have to open a second software (e.g., "PVR PLUS," KWorld) to view the camera.
13. In cases that you cannot *see* your cantilever very well with your microscope, you may use a flashlight under your probe.
14. Raise the sample slowly and carefully to avoid collision with the tip. Hard contact between the tip and the sample can damage either or both.
15. If your sample has tall features or steps, you may need to raise the scanner slightly to avoid contacting features as you move the stage. When imaging under liquid, it might be difficult to locate the area of interest. One way to solve this issue, if your sample can remain in dry conditions, is to first locate the area of interest in the dry sample and then use the liquid cell to add the liquid.
16. The GetReal function is compatible with a wide range of probe models, including those with rectangular, arrow-shaped, and V-shaped cantilevers. In addition, the "Custom Rectangular Probe" selection allows the user to calibrate any rectangular probe by using the length, width, and frequency provided by the probe manufacturer.

17. Although GetReal is a function of Asylum microscopes, if you have access to any of these microscopes, you can use this function to calibrate your probes and then use the probes and the calibration measurements on other microscopes.
18. Mica is the most widely used AFM substrate due to its flat surface, wide availability, and low cost. Mica consists of a series of thin, flat crystalline layers that can easily be split apart ("cleaved") [11]. You can cleave a mica disc or sheet by inserting a pin or a razor blade at its edge or by using an adhesive tape so as to remove a couple of the top layers. In our research, we prefer to use adhesive tapes, because using a blade may remove a larger number of layers and/or damage the surface. After cleaving the mica, its surface is fresh without having been exposed to the atmosphere, and it is anatomically flat [11]. That is why mica is used when one wants to achieve molecular resolution or to calibrate a probe on a hard, clean surface.
19. Here we suggest you to make a quick scan and acquire a contact mode of your mica surface to ensure that it is clean, devoid of contamination, and that you did not scratch the surface. If your area is not appropriate, click on "Withdraw" to move to another area of interest, approach the tip, and take image.
20. AtomicJ is licensed under the terms of the GNU General Public License. The software and its manual can be downloaded for free at SourceForge (http://sourceforge.net/projects/jrobust). AtomicJ is available in two versions, for 64-bit Windows (with Java 7 Runtime Environment) and for Windows, Linux, and Mac OS (with the platform-independent distribution).
21. You can use the "Advanced" panel if your final results are not appropriate. In this panel you can crop the parts of the curves that are out of limits. If your data acquisition was performed appropriately, you may not need to use this function.
22. Although the Hertz model is the most widely used, it includes many assumptions (like that the material is isotropic, linearly elastic, and infinitely deep) which are not the case for biological material. There are also several modifications to the Hertz model [34–37] that take into account these limits, but Hertz is still the basic model. Of course the software offers other models too, and you may use any other model from the provided one that may be more appropriate for your sample. As a first step, we suggest to use the Hertz model, which is the most established model.
23. If you didn't keep the value you can use the "Calibrate" procedure. Click the "Calibrate" button to recalculate the sensitivity by using the relevant file which contains the curve for a force-curve cycle with this probe on a hard material, such as mica.

24. If you want to remove the values and keep only the color representations, right-click on the image and select the "Live chart style." In the "Series" window, select the "Label" tab and uncheck the "Value labels."
25. Here we use colloidal probes. In the so-called colloidal probe technique, single colloids are attached to AFM cantilevers. This technique is appropriate for force measurements since the well-known geometry of the sphere in the cantilever enables better performance of the fitting models (like the Hertz model).

Acknowledgment

This work was supported by the European Commission through a Horizon 2020, Marie Skłodowska-Curie Individual Fellowship (MSCA-IF-2014-658769-MYO-DESMOPLASIA). The Cypher ES atomic force microscope was purchased through an infrastructure research grant (project IPE/NEKYP /0311/27) co-funded by the European Regional Development Fund and the Republic of Cyprus through Cyprus Research Promotion Foundation.

References

1. Binnig G, Quate CF, Gerber C (1986) Atomic force microscope. Phys Rev Lett 56(9):930–933. doi:10.1103/PhysRevLett.56.930
2. Gadegaard N (2006) Atomic force microscopy in biology: technology and techniques. Biotech Histochem 81(2-3):87–97. doi:10.1080/10520290600783143
3. Stylianou A, Yova D, Alexandratou E (2013) Nanotopography of collagen thin films in correlation with fibroblast response. J Nanophoton 7(1):073590. doi:10.1117/1.JNP.7.073590
4. Han WS, Serry FM Force spectroscopy with the atomic force microscope-application note. Agilent Technologies. doi:10.1371/journal.pone.0148974
5. Xia B, Miao Q, Chao J et al (2008) Charge transfer on porous silicon membranes studied by current-sensing atomic force microscopy. Chin Chem Lett 19(2):199–202. doi:10.1016/j.cclet.2007.12.003
6. Stylianou A, Politopoulos K, Yova D (2011) Atomic force microscopy imaging of the nanoscale assembly of type i collagen on controlled polystyrene particles surfaces. In: 5th European conference of the international federation for medical and biological engineering, pp 1058–1061. doi:10.1007/978-3-642-23508-5_275
7. Stylianou A, Yova D, Politopoulos K (2012) Atomic force microscopy quantitative and qualitative nanoscale characterization of collagen thin films. In: 5th international conference on emerging technologies in non-destructive testing, NDT, pp 415–420. doi:10.1201/b11837-75
8. Kontomaris SV, Stylianou A, Yova D et al (2012) Mechanical properties of collagen fibrils on thin films by Atomic Force Microscopy nanoindentation. In: 12th IEEE international conference on bioinformatics and bioengineering, BIBE, pp 608–613. doi:10.1109/bibe.2012.6399742
9. Stylianou A, Yova D (2013) Surface nanoscale imaging of collagen thin films by atomic force microscopy. Mater Sci Eng C 33(5):2947–2957. doi:10.1016/j.msec.2013.03.029
10. Allison DP, Mortensen NP, Sullivan CJ et al (2010) Atomic force microscopy of biological samples. Wiley Interdiscip Rev Nanomed Nanobiotechnol 2(6):618–634. doi:10.1002/wnan.104
11. Morris VJ, Kirby AR, Gunning AP (2008) Atomic force microscopy for biologists. Imperial College Press, London. doi:10.1142/P674
12. Lekka M, Gil D, Pogoda K et al (2012) Cancer cell detection in tissue sections using AFM. Arch Biochem Biophys 518(2):151–156. doi:10.1016/j.abb.2011.12.013

13. Gkretsi V, Stylianou A, Papageorgis P et al (2015) Remodeling components of the tumor microenvironment to enhance cancer therapy. Front Oncol 5:214. doi:10.3389/fonc.2015.00214
14. Stylianou A, Stylianopoulos T (2016) Atomic force microscopy probing of cancer cells and tumor microenvironment components. BioNanoScience 6(1):33–46. doi:10.1007/s12668-015-0187-4
15. Cisneros DA, Friedrichs J, Taubenberger A et al (2007) Creating ultrathin nanoscopic collagen matrices for biological and biotechnological applications. Small 3(6):956–963. doi:10.1002/smll.200600598
16. Horcas I, Fernández R, Gómez-Rodríguez JM et al (2007) WSXM: a software for scanning probe microscopy and a tool for nanotechnology. Rev Sci Instrum 78(1):013705. doi:10.1063/1.2432410
17. Nečas D, Klapetek P (2012) Gwyddion: an open-source software for SPM data analysis. Open Physics 10(1):181–188. doi:10.2478/s11534-011-0096-2
18. Keysight-Technologies (2014) Keysight 5500 Scanning Probe Microscope-User's Guide. http://nano.em.keysight.com/PDFs/5500%20User%20Guide%20Dec%202015%20REV%20H.pdf. Accessed 16 Oct 2016
19. Mackay JL, Kumar S (2013) Measuring the elastic properties of living cells with atomic force microscopy indentation. Methods Mol Biol (Clifton, NJ) 931:313–329. doi:10.1007/978-1-62703-056-4_15
20. Hermanowicz P, Sarna M, Burda K et al (2014) AtomicJ: an open source software for analysis of force curves. Rev Sci Instrum 85(6):063703. doi:10.1063/1.4881683
21. Roduit C, Saha B, Alonso-Sarduy L et al (2012) OpenFovea: open-source AFM data processing software. Nat Methods 9(8):774–775. doi:10.1038/nmeth.2112
22. Burnham NA, Chen X, Hodges CS et al (2003) Comparison of calibration methods for atomic-force microscopy cantilevers. Nanotechnology 14(1):1–6. doi:10.1088/0957-4484/14/1/301
23. Keely PJ, Fong AM, Zutter MM et al (1995) Alteration of collagen-dependent adhesion, motility, and morphogenesis by the expression of antisense α2 integrin mRNA in mammary cells. J Cell Sci 108(2):595–607. jcs.biologists.Org/content/108/2/595.Long
24. Graham HK, Hodson NW, Hoyland JA et al (2010) Tissue section AFM: in situ ultrastructural imaging of native biomolecules. Matrix Biol 29(4):254–260. doi:10.1016/j.matbio.2010.01.008
25. Lopez JI, Kang I, You WK et al (2011) In situ force mapping of mammary gland transformation. Integr Biol (Camb) 3(9):910–921. doi:10.1039/c1ib00043h
26. Laklai H, Miroshnikova YA, Pickup MW et al (2016) Genotype tunes pancreatic ductal adenocarcinoma tissue tension to induce matricellular fibrosis and tumor progression. Nat Med 22(5):497–505. doi:10.1038/nm.4082
27. Fuierer R (2009) Procedural operation 'Manualette', version 10.5. Accessed 1 Oct 2016
28. Asylum-Research (2010) Asylum research Cypher scanning probe microscope, version a, revision 548. https://support.asylumresearch.com/forum/content.php?25-Manuals. Accessed 6 Sept 2016
29. Asylum-Research (2013) Cypher user guide, version 13, revision: A-1714. http://user.physics.unc.edu/~lizimeng/share/Sharonda/Asylum_User_Guides_Ver_13A/02_Cypher_Guide_Ver_13A.pdf. Accessed 10 Sept 2016
30. JPK-Instruments (2009) Summary Notes – Force spectroscopy measurements and processing. http://www.jpk.com/jpk-note-force-spectroscopy1.download.cef677f9a5b-01de28d82caffde3d1ec2. Accessed 5 Oct 2016
31. Hertz H (1882) Ueber die Berührung fester elastischer Körper. Journal für die reine und angewandte Mathematik 1882(92):156–171. doi:10.1515/crll.1882.92.156
32. Hutter JL, Bechhoefer J (1993) Calibration of atomic-force microscope tips. Rev Sci Instrum 64(7):1868–1873. doi:10.1063/1.1143970
33. Sader JE, Chon JWM, Mulvaney P (1999) Calibration of rectangular atomic force microscope cantilevers. Rev Sci Instrum 70(10):3967–3969. doi:10.1063/1.1150021
34. Matthewson MJ (1981) Axi-symmetric contact on thin compliant coatings. J Mech Phys Solids 29(2):89–113. doi:10.1016/0022-5096(81)90018-1
35. Dimitriadis EK, Horkay F, Maresca J et al (2002) Determination of elastic moduli of thin layers of soft material using the atomic force microscope. Biophys J 82(5):2798–2810. doi:10.1016/S0006-3495(02)75620-8
36. Mahaffy RE, Park S, Gerde E et al (2004) Quantitative analysis of the viscoelastic properties of thin regions of fibroblasts using atomic force microscopy. Biophys J 86(3):1777–1793. doi:10.1016/S0006-3495(04)74245-9
37. Costa KD, Sim AJ, Yin FCP (2006) Non-Hertzian approach to analyzing mechanical properties of endothelial cells probed by atomic force microscopy. J Biomech Eng 128(2):176–184. doi:10.1115/1.2165690

Chapter 30

Spectral Unmixing Methods and Tools for the Detection and Quantitation of Collagen and Other Macromolecules in Tissue Specimens

Zachary T. Harmany, Farzad Fereidouni, and Richard M. Levenson

Abstract

Collagen and other components in the extracellular matrix are proving of increasing importance for the understanding of complex cell and tissue interactions in a variety of settings. Detection and quantitation of these components can still prove challenging, and a number of techniques have been developed. We focus here on methods in fluorescence-based assessments, including multiplexed immunodetection and the use of simpler histochemical stains, both complemented by linear unmixing techniques. Typically, differentiating these components requires the use of a set of optical filters to isolate each fluorescent compound from each other and from often bright background autofluorescence signals. However, standard fluorescent microscopes are usually only able to separate a limited number of components. If the emission spectra of the fluorophores are spectrally distinct, but overlapping, sophisticated spectral imaging or computational methods can be used to optimize separation and quantitation. This chapter describes spectral unmixing methodology and associated open-source software tools available to analyze multispectral as well as simple color (RGB) images.

Key words Multispectral imaging, Linear unmixing, Fluorescent imaging, Microscopy, Image analysis, Spectroscopy

1 Introduction

The studies of collagen and other connective tissues are proving of increasing importance for the understanding of disease as well as complex cell and tissue interactions. Accurate detection and quantitation of fluorescent signals from these components can still prove challenging, and a number of techniques have been developed. When studying such biological phenomenon or providing medical diagnoses, it is often desirable to image multiple aspects of the specimen simultaneously, especially if co-localization of different antigens is of interest. Multiple fluorescently labeled antibodies can be used simultaneously to measure such biomolecules, allowing direct visualization of the distribution of the various targets

Laure Rittié (ed.), *Fibrosis: Methods and Protocols*, Methods in Molecular Biology, vol. 1627, DOI 10.1007/978-1-4939-7113-8_30, © Springer Science+Business Media LLC 2017

throughout the sample. However, this multiplexing ability comes with additional analysis challenges. If only a few fluorescent labels are used, they can often be chosen to have non-overlapping spectra (either excitation, emission, or both). The signals from these fluorophores can then be separated using simple optical filters. In commercial microscopes, these filters may be packaged together with a dichroic mirror in filter cubes. Images of different fluorescent compounds can be acquired by simply switching among several preloaded filter cubes.

There is a current trend to push the multiplexing capability in fluorescent microscopy. This push necessitates the use of multiple fluorophores that have large spectral overlap. In this case, simple optical filtering is insufficient to separate the signals arising from such labels. To distinguish these components, additional spectral information is required in the form of multispectral image capture, which can be conveniently accomplished using tunable filters or multiposition filter wheels, and is usually followed by application of computational techniques, such as linear unmixing, in order to effectively separate fluorescent labels for further analysis and quantitation. It should be noted that color (red, green, and blue or RGB) imaging is simply a common special case of multispectral imaging. We show in this chapter how both multispectral and RGB data can be analyzed with spectral unmixing methods.

It is important to mention that collagen can be detected using a number of techniques beyond immunofluorescence. These include, of course, time-honored histochemical stains, such as Mallory's trichrome [1] or Masson's trichrome [2]. Typically collagen can be visualized with high contrast and appears distinct from other tissue components. However, it can be a challenge in some cases to isolate the collagen signal in trichrome- or hematoxylin and eosin (H&E)-stained tissue using just three-color information alone, and spectral imaging and unmixing can be used to assist [3, 4]. Intriguingly, it is possible to identify collagenous components directly in conventional H&E-stained specimens. The exact treatment and preparation necessary for collagen depends on the tissues and types of collagens under investigation [5–7]. Ordinarily, it would seem that the overall pink hue of stained stroma would be unlikely to yield collagen-specific spectral signals, but Batista and Yagi [8] demonstrated that there is sufficient signal in the absorbance spectrum of stained collagen vs other tissue components to allow this discrimination. This "virtual histochemistry" was performed directly on H&E-stained slides using spectral imaging and corresponded well with traditional histochemistry images, which served as ground truth.

Collagen is an optically active molecule—a property that persists even in formalin-fixed, paraffin-embedded preparations. Accordingly, it is possible to detect and quantitate collagen using techniques such as second harmonic generation [9], which is a robust but complex method requiring expensive instrumentation (*see* Chap. 27 for protocols and tips). However, it does require a certain amount of collagen fiber deposition to be present in order to generate a signal. Birefringence imaging, using Polscope technology [10], is a more sensitive and much less expensive method, but more sophisticated versions that go beyond the deployment of simple polarizing filters are still not widely available in commercial instrumentation (*see* [11] for additional information). An intriguing snapshot variant of this, the polychromatic polscope, was recently described [12]. Finally, collagen also demonstrates useful and distinct autofluorescence signals, which can be detected with appropriate methods. We will demonstrate the use of 280-nm excitation and color camera collection for the isolation of collagen signals from a complex tissue.

This chapter will describe the challenges of analyzing multispectral datasets (including the near-limiting case of simple three-channel color images) through linear unmixing and will provide software tools that permit the separation of fluorescent datasets into their constituent components.

2 Importance of Sample Preparation

Multispectral imaging has a wide variety of applications in medicine, such as cell biology, clinical pathology, and preclinical drug development [13]. Mansfield discusses a number of other applications in anatomic pathology where it has been used to study joints, liver, respiratory systems, transplantation, cardiovascular disease, cancer treatment, and aspects of neuroscience [14]. Given the vast number of applications, the details of how to properly prepare specimens for fluorescent imaging are obviously application specific. Immunofluorescence detection methods for collagen I, for example, can be technically challenging, as pointed out below.

Generally, examination of formalin-fixed, paraffin-embedded tissues via immunohistochemistry or immunofluorescence requires some antigen-retrieval steps for enabling access of antibodies to otherwise cross-linked protein targets [15, 16]. However, it turns out that collagen I can be a more challenging molecule to detect than many and for idiosyncratic reasons. While fixation and attendant cross-linking can contribute to the difficulty, another explanation may be found in the physicochemical state of collagen I, which is less a simple collection of collagen molecules than a complex mixture of several collagens and noncollagenous macromolecules.

Antigen retrieval may open up the structure and allow antibody binding, but it may require partial degradation via additional protease treatment to obtain a signal. A helpful discussion on this topic can be found online [17]. Other references provide early observations of the challenges encountered in antibody-based imaging studies [6, 7].

Tissue endogenous fluorescence or autofluorescence often poses challenges in the detection and quantitation of immuno-labeled signals. Different tissue processing steps may increase the intensity of the autofluorescent response, with formalin fixation being especially problematic [18]. While the linear unmixing methods described in this chapter can be used to overcome the presence of autofluorescence, a large amount of autofluorescence may mask weak signals.

Finally, the choice of fluorescent dyes must be carefully considered. Ideally, when multiplex labeling a biological specimen, the dyes used should have non-overlapping emission spectra, although a suboptimal choice in emission spectra may be worth the added sensitivity or specificity of a given labeled detection probe. Additional discussions of staining strategies for multiplexed images can be readily found in the literature [19, 20].

3 UnmixingGUI Software

3.1 Need for a Spectral Imaging and Unmixing Tool

Spectral imaging and unmixing techniques, including their semi-automated application to multispectral datasets of multiplexed immunofluorescently labeled samples, have been documented and are implemented in a number of commercially available platforms [18–20]. However, the principles behind these approaches can best be grasped by performing actual unmixing and redisplay on a simple synthetic dataset using freely available software that illustrates the principles involved. Unmixing is often the first step toward absolute quantitation. The initial unmixing results represent simply the intensity measured for each component and are not directly interpretable as the absolute abundances of a particular analyte. The relationship between measured intensity (which is a consequence of the labeling and imaging processes) and true abundance can only be established using some calibration strategy against some kind of relevant standard. The mathematics involved are outlined in [21, 22].

Suffice it to say that if the spectra used in the unmixing are not accurate, the unmixing will give erroneous values. If only pure spectra were present (imagine a sample composed of differently colored bright fluorescent beads, with inconsequential amounts of contaminating autofluorescence or stray light), then simply unmixing using the pure spectra from such beads would allow for accurate unmixing. On the other hand, if the signals are possibly spatially overlapping, or are weak relative to significant autofluorescence, then accurate spectra cannot be captured simply be sampling pixels in the image. Instead, some preprocessing, in which the contaminating spectral moieties are subtracted from the desired spectrum, is necessary before unmixing [23]. There are some automated software tools that estimate true spectral identities which include, among others, the pixel purity index (PPI) [24] and multivariate curve resolution (MCR) [25], but these are complex and their operation difficult to understand intuitively. A comprehensive review of some of these methods, along with various approaches to linear unmixing, can be found in Bioucas-Dias et al. [26]. Here, we demonstrate a straightforward approach, which seems to work in many instances quite satisfactorily.

3.2 The UnmixingGUI Software

We have developed a free and open-source software tool called "UnmixingGUI" for performing linear unmixing of multispectral images. The interface and algorithm code is written in MATLAB (MathWorks, Natick, MA). The MATLAB app is available on GitHub (https://github.com/UCDavisMUSE/unmixinggui). Stand-alone applications for Windows 64 bit and Mac OS are also available on the website (*see* **Note 1**). With this chapter, our goal is to provide a visual tutorial demonstrating the use of the UnmixingGUI software.

UnmixingGUI allows one to select spectral "endmembers" (spectral library components) directly from the image data by drawing regions of interest (ROIs) on the image. However, as noted above, these spectra may be a mixture of the pure spectral components required for accurate unmixing. Using the Spectral Calculator function, we can compute pure spectra that are then used to correctly unmix the fluorescence data. Currently, the operation is limited to an unscaled subtraction with a threshold to prevent negative values. However, a more advanced version of this software will be able to adjust the amount of spectra subtracted in the future (frequently, simple (unscaled) subtraction disproportionately removes too much of the background signal from the mixed data). In the following sections, we will demonstrate how the Spectral Calculator can be used to obtain pure components by showing a step-by-step example on a simulated dataset.

4 Unmixing Simulated Data

This example can serve as an illustration on how to unmix actual multispectral datasets of immunofluorescently labeled tissues—bearing in mind the caveats noted above about challenges in tissue preparation and fluorescent antibody labeling, plus counterstains.

4.1 File Naming and Nomenclature

A multispectral dataset can be imported from a series of TIFF files (*see* **Note 2**) as long as it follows a precise nomenclature. All the TIFF files of a series should share the same name at the start of their file name, but have different wavelengths appended to the name, i.e., named according to a "name_wavelength.tif" pattern, where "name" is the name of the dataset and "wavelength" is the wavelength of the spectral channel in nanometers. These wavelengths will be recognized by the UnmixingGUI. To display the hyperspectral image, UnmixingGUI uses RGB spectral response functions to simulate a true-color image. One can also use the Stack mode to show individual spectral bands as grayscale images. Different spectral bands can be explored by using either the mouse wheel or the scroll bar below the image.

4.2 Using the Spectral Calculator

To demonstrate how to use the UnmixingGUI, we will be utilizing a simulated dataset called "Blobs." This simulated dataset consists of ten 256 × 256 grayscale TIFF images, one for each spectral channel in the range 425–650 nm, collected every 25 nm. In accordance with the naming convention described above, these images are named Blobs_425.tif, Blobs_450.tif, and all the way through Blobs_650.tif.

1. Load the dataset in the UnmixingGUI by selecting Load Stack from the Stack menu, selecting the first image of the stack, and clicking on "open." UnmixingGUI will load all the images of the folder (*see* **Note 3**).
2. In this dataset, there are three fluorescent components as well as an omnipresent fluorescent background. These are meant to represent three fluorophores of interest as well as endogenous fluorescence (or autofluorescence) that must be removed from the sample for more accurate analysis and subsequent quantitation. Following the steps below will result in pure fluorescent signals devoid of corrupting background autofluorescence.
3. Draw small ROIs corresponding to each of the color components and background: Under Spectra (Fig. 1, left), click on

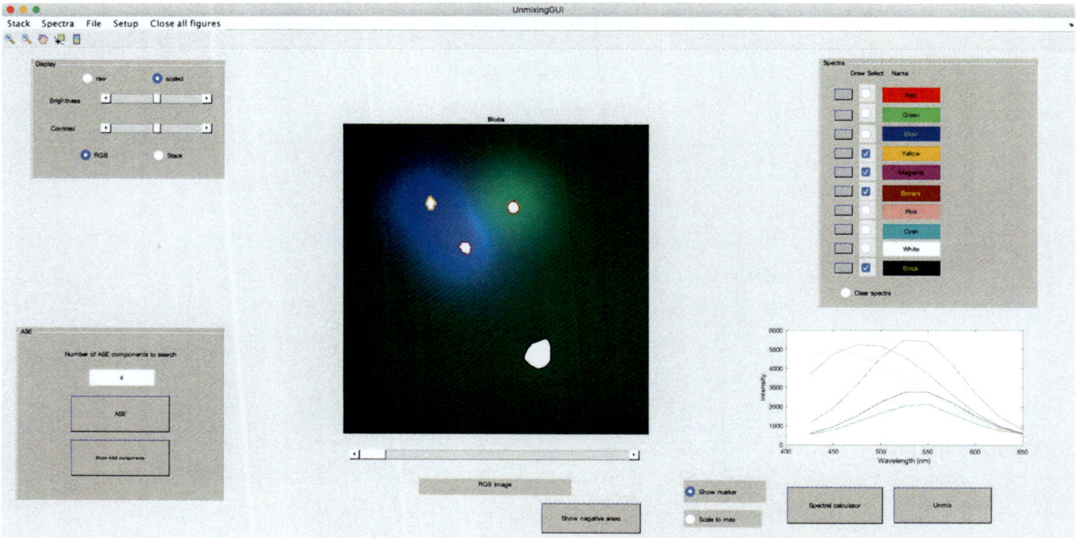

Fig. 1 UnmixingGUI screenshot with the Blobs dataset loaded with marked ROIs on each of the fluorescent components and the autofluorescent background

the rectangle to the left of the desired color component and draw the desired ROI on the main image. Choose a small ROI that contains as least overlap with other color components as possible. Start drawing by pressing the mouse button and moving the mouse while holding its button down. The ROI shape will automatically close and become visible upon releasing the mouse button, and a checkmark will appear next to the selected color under Spectra (*see* **Note 4**). Figure 1 shows ROIs respectively placed into the yellow, magenta, brown, and black channels.

4. Click on the Unmix button to perform a spectral unmixing into the four selected components. These components, as well as a remixed composite image, are shown in Fig. 2.
5. Examining the yellow, magenta, and brown components in Fig. 2a–c, these components are in line with our expectations: we see a well-localized fluorescent signal in each of the images. However, examining the background component in Fig. 2d, we see that there is a large heart-shaped dark area in the background, which does not reflect the reality that the background is roughly uniform in this dataset. This is due to the fact that each of the spectrum we measured for the yellow, magenta, and brown components contains a portion of the black background component. Therefore, when we unmix using these impure spectra, some of the background intensity is misallocated to the primary fluorescent components. To counter this effect, we must compute the pure spectra from the measured spectra using the Spectral Calculator tool.
6. In the main window menu, click on "Close all Figures" and answer Yes to closing the composite.
7. Click on the Spectral Calculator button (Fig. 1, lower right corner) to launch the window shown in Fig. 3a: by default, the window shows the measured spectra. Use this tool to remove the background spectrum from the spectra of each of the fluorescent components: In the example of Fig. 3a, selecting yellow as spectrum A and black as spectrum B, saving the result of A minus B as red, and clicking on "Calculate" removes the contribution of the simulated autofluorescence from the yellow fluorescent component. Likewise, remove the background from the magenta component (saved as green) and the brown component (saved as blue). These operations will produce pure fluorescent spectra, as shown in Fig. 3b.
8. Click on "Save and close" to return to the main UnmixingGUI interface (Fig. 1), and perform a second unmixing by clicking on the Unmix button. The results of unmixing with the pure computed spectra are shown in Fig. 2f–j. Notice that the updated black background component no longer has the

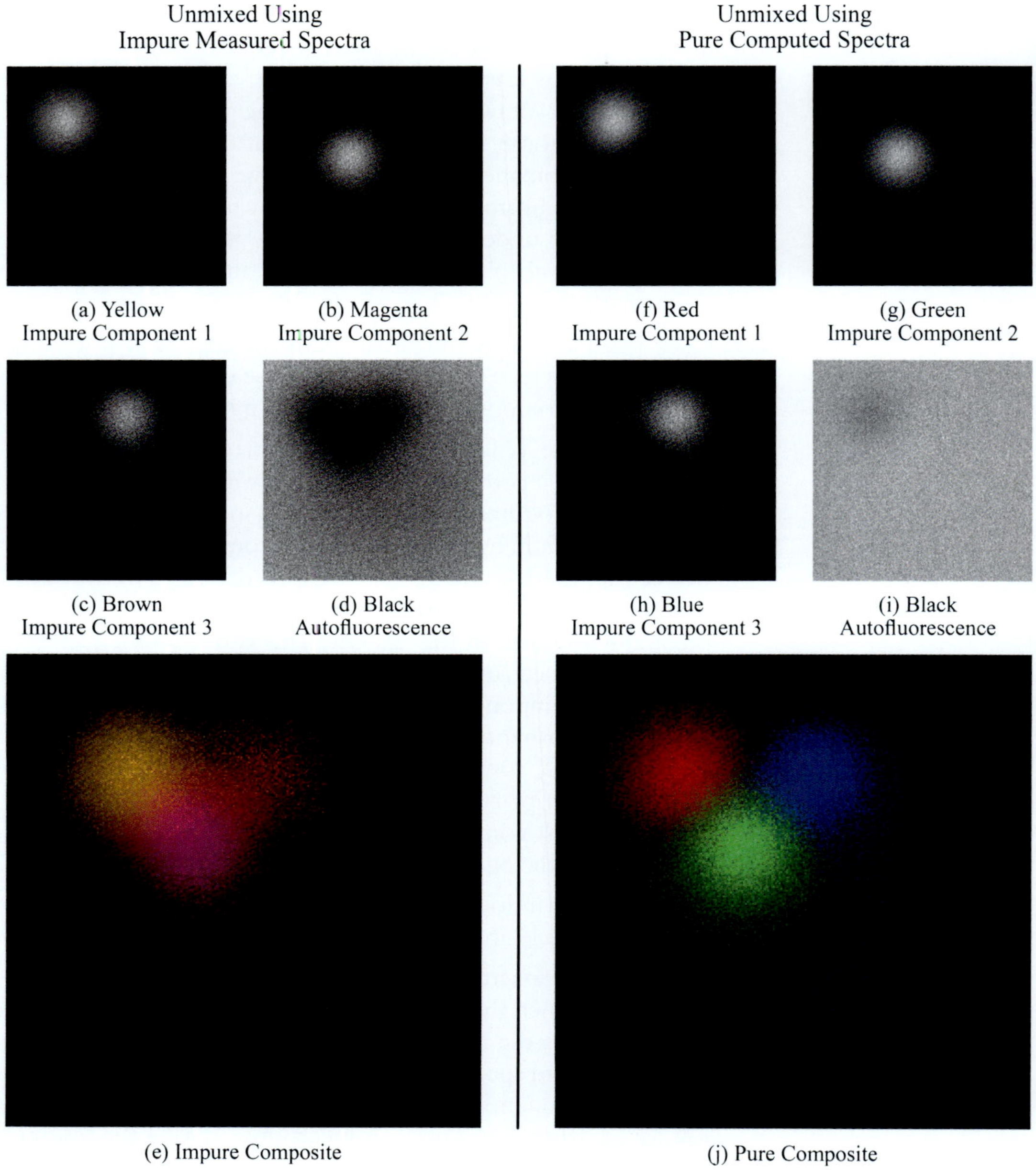

Fig. 2 Unmixing results on the Blobs dataset using first the impure measured spectra (**a**–**e**) and then using the pure computed spectra (**f**–**j**). All images have been brightened such that the maximum value of the image corresponds to *white* for the grayscale images or the most saturated color channel for the color composite images

heart-shaped missing intensity and appears roughly uniform. Additionally, the red, green, and blue components now represent just the contribution of fluorescent intensity due to the presence of the additional fluorophores in the image. Background removal is crucial for subsequent analysis and accurate quantitation (*see* **Note 5**). If the background is not

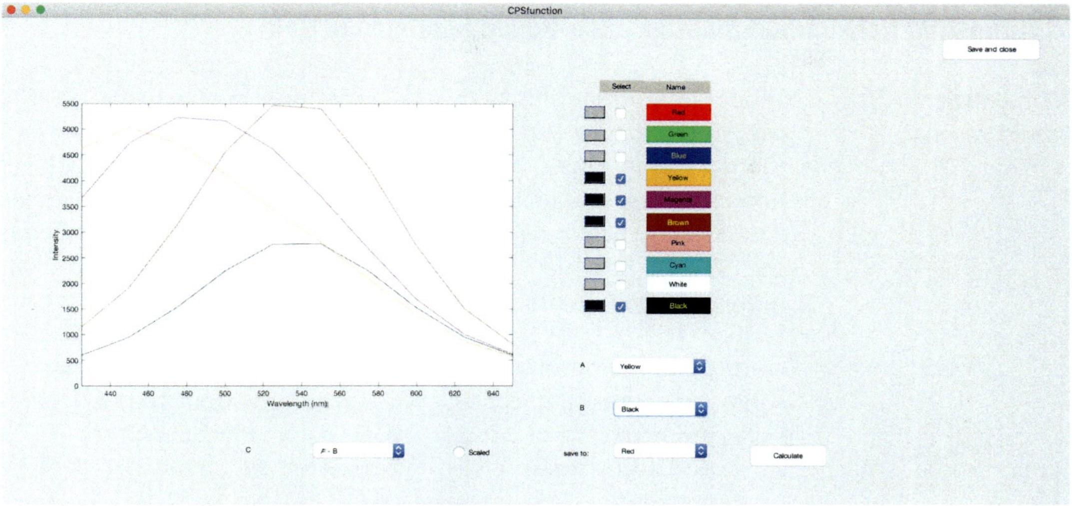

(a) Spectral Calculator Showing Impure Measured Spectra

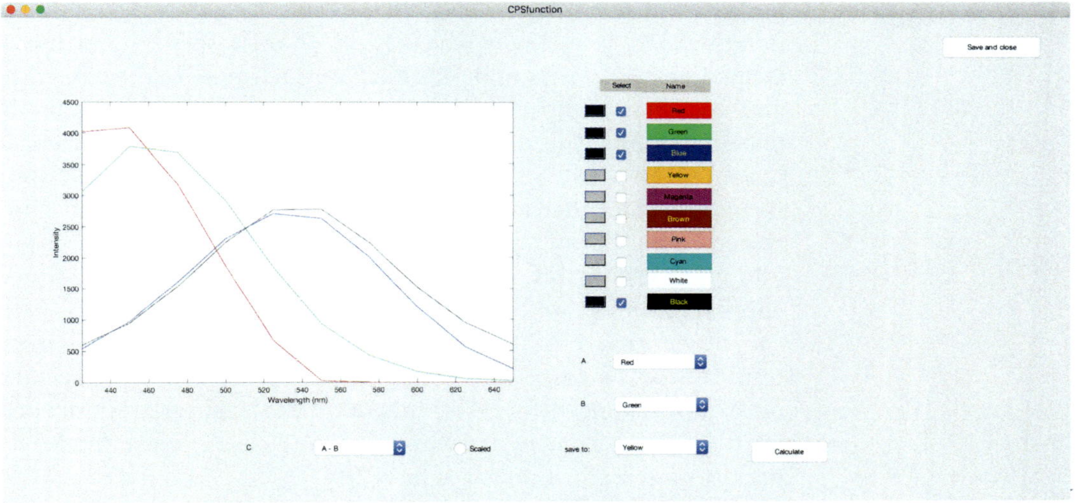

(b) Spectral Calculator Showing Pure Computed Spectra

Fig. 3 Spectral Calculator showing (**a**) the impure measured spectra and (**b**) the pure computed spectra resulting from subtracting the autofluorescence (*Black*) from each of the fluorescent components

nicely separated in your image, you may have to clear all the spectra and redraw the ROIs.

9. Save the unmixed image by clicking on the "Export components and composite" in the "Show Composite" window. The software will save one file for each of the unmixed color components (i.e., red, green, blue, and black in our example), plus one file of the composite image. The default format (TIFF 16-bit) can be changed to JPEG in the "Save components as" dialog box.

5 Unmixing Non-immunofluorescence-Based Microscopy Data

5.1 General Considerations

While immunofluorescence (or immunohistochemistry) is the usual approach to detecting multiple molecular species of interest, there are a number of other methods that are commonly used for fibrosis research, including conventional histochemical stains. These can generate complex colored images that can be challenging to split into their components. Multispectral imaging techniques can help in distinguishing the various signals, as has already been noted [4]. Even with simple one-color (brown with blue counterstain) immunohistochemical (bright-field) stains, there is some indication that multispectral imaging and analysis is technically preferable over simple RGB color image capture [27]. However, using these tools it is possible to obtain better-than-expected results even from just RGB images (which, of course, represent three-channel spectral data).

We will show here how it is possible to use the techniques described above, namely, calculation of pure spectra and linear unmixing, even with simple RGB datasets to improve the detection and quantitative separation of tissue components. As an example data source, we will use an image acquired using a color camera mounted on a MUSE (Microscopy with UV Surface Excitation) imaging system that takes advantage of autofluorescent and fluorescent signals from tissue dyes (not labeled antibodies) excited at 280 nm. While this is a special case, the same computational approach can be used for other three-channel color images, with the caveat that bright-field images need to be converted from transmission to absorbance mode first. The latter can be accomplished by taking the negative logarithm of the absorbance divided by the illumination light (which in most cases is just the white background regions on the slide) [28].

5.2 Data Description

Shown in Fig. 4 is data collected from a MUSE fluorescent imaging system [29]. MUSE uses a 280 nm UV excitation light in an oblique configuration and collects the emitted light using conventional microscope optics. Many commonly used fluorescent dyes can be excited at this wavelength, including such dyes as eosin, Hoechst, rhodamine, DAPI, acridine orange, and propidium iodide. These dyes then fluoresce at their usual emission wavelengths. When staining a tissue sample with several of these dyes, a single excitation wavelength is used to cause fluorescence in all the dyes. The excitation light can then be captured by a color or multispectral camera. Given the various binding properties of each dye, different structures in the tissue can be identified based on the color information in the captured data. And as alluded to above, linear unmixing methods can be used to accurately separate fluorescent components for further analysis and quantitation.

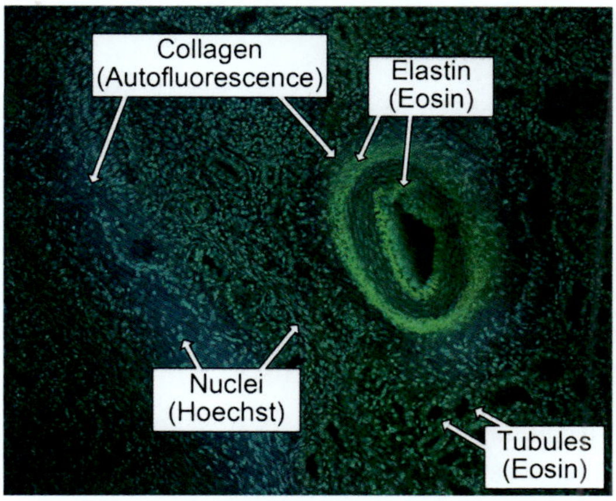

Fig. 4 Porcine kidney imaged with MUSE. Eosin has strongly stained the elastic laminae surrounding an artery. Hoechst, a nuclear dye, appears *bright blue*. Additionally, there is a strong autofluorescence signal from collagen. The kidney tubules have less eosin uptake and are also autofluorescent, giving rise to the *blue-green* hue versus the more *bright green* of the elastin

Returning to Fig. 4, this dataset shows an image of a porcine kidney that has been double-stained with Hoechst and eosin. First, the sample was placed in a 0.25 mg/ml solution of Hoechst for 10 s, placed in a 0.33 mg/ml solution of eosin for 20 s, rinsed for 30 s, and immediately imaged using a 10X NA 0.45 objective. The data was collected with a standard RGB charge-coupled device camera. The field of view shown is approximately 1 mm × 1 mm.

In Fig. 4, we see four dominant colored features: Eosin has strongly stained the internal and external elastic laminae of the blood vessel in green (visible on the right). Hoechst, a nuclear dye, appears with lilac hue, while the tubule cytoplasm is a darker blue-green. Additionally visible is a strong bluish autofluorescence signal from collagen, which did not pick up any eosin stain in this procedure. Analyzing this data is especially challenging since these fluorescent components change slightly based on their local environment, meaning that the green signal from the elastin is not simply just a brighter version of the green eosin signal from the tubule cytoplasm (*see* **Note 5**). However, as we will see, these slight variations allow us to separate these components in serial fashion even though we would typically require higher spectral resolution (i.e., more than just three bands) in order to simultaneously unmix them.

5.3 Data Preprocessing

1. It can be useful to preprocess an image prior to unmixing. However, one should be careful to not perform any processing steps that may negatively impact the linear unmixing step. For instance, linear unmixing interprets black pixels as not having any fluorescent signal. Therefore, it is crucial that any adjustment of brightness or contrast does not introduce or remove

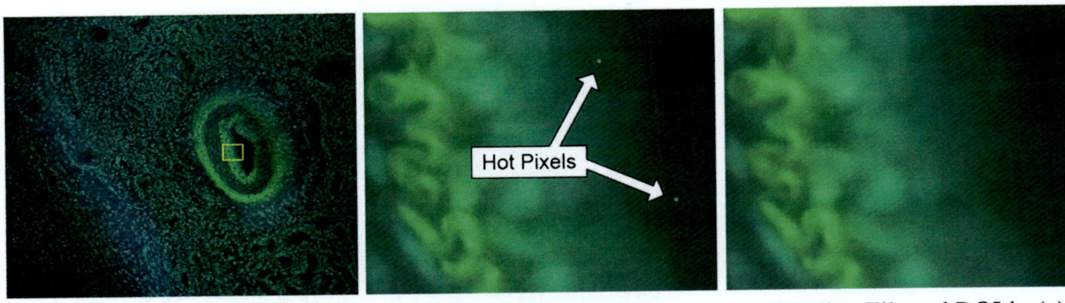

(a) Original RGB Image (b) ROI Indicated in (a) (c) Median Filtered ROI in (a)

Fig. 5 Porcine kidney image showing nominal preprocessing steps. (**a**) The original data collected from the CCD camera. (**b**) A close-up of the *yellow* ROI indicated in (**a**) showing the hot pixels. (**c**) Result of applying a 3 × 3 median filter to the data to remove hot pixels

black pixels in the image. Additionally, any nonuniform brightness enhancement may bias the results. Care should be taken to avoid saturating the image as well. To prepare the raw data for linear unmixing, we applied a 3 × 3 median filter to eliminate bright but spurious 'hot' pixels due to sensor imperfections (Fig. 5) (*see* **Notes 6** and 7).

2. To prepare this dataset for import into UnmixingGUI, create a grayscale TIFF series from the RGB image (*see* **Note 8**). In this example, we named the files Kidney_450.tif, Kidney_550.tif, and Kidney_650.tif for the blue, green, and red channels, respectively. These particular wavelengths were selected to correspond to the approximate peak intensity of the Bayer pattern RGB filters used in color cameras.
3. Proceed with linear unmixing.

5.4 Linear Unmixing

5.4.1 Principles of Serial Unmixing

Since the captured data is only an RGB image, we are limited in the number of components we can simultaneously separate. Ideally, we would want to isolate four distinct components: collagen, elastin, nuclei, and cytoplasm. Since there are only three color channels in the data, it is impossible to unmix four species simultaneously. From basic linear algebra, we essentially have three equations, but only four unknowns. In many cases, even unmixing three components is challenging if the spectra are similar. From a mathematical perspective, we would require the three components to be linearly independent. For example, since red and green together form yellow, it would be impossible to chromatically distinguish an overlapping mixture of two species that are stained purely red and purely green versus a single species stained yellow.

However, by performing unmixing steps serially, we can extract relevant components one at a time. This is possible if we expect one or more fluorophores to be present with the component of interest in the same relative amounts. This mixture can then be thought of as a simple background signal that we wish to eliminate.

In the example of the Kidney dataset, we show how to isolate both the collagen and elastin signals by performing two serial unmixing steps. These serial unmixing steps make use of our prior histological knowledge (because we know how components of the tissue react with each dye). As a result, an experimenter with such knowledge can interact with the UnmixingGUI in a way that capitalizes on this extra information in order to extract the pure spectra of interest. These spectra can then be used to unmix the images to obtain components that quantified for further analysis.

5.4.2 Example of Serial Unmixing to Separate Collagen from Elastin

1. Load the dataset in the UnmixingGUI as described in **step 1** of Subheading 4.2.
2. We will first focus on isolating the signal from the collagen (the blue signal shown in Fig. 4). To this end, we will draw three ROIs: from the collagen itself (green), from a nucleus within the collagen area (yellow), and finally some background signal arising from the cytoplasm outside the collagen area (magenta). The particular ROIs selected are shown in Fig. 6. The idea here is to now compute the pure nuclei spectrum (that we will store in red) in order to remove it from the collagen signal. This is done by using the Spectral Calculator (method described in Subheading 4.2) to subtract the measured collagen spectrum from the measured nuclear spectrum (i.e., yellow minus green equals red). At this point, we have three defined spectra (green, magenta, and red). The background signal (magenta) is present to eliminate some background signal that has a color

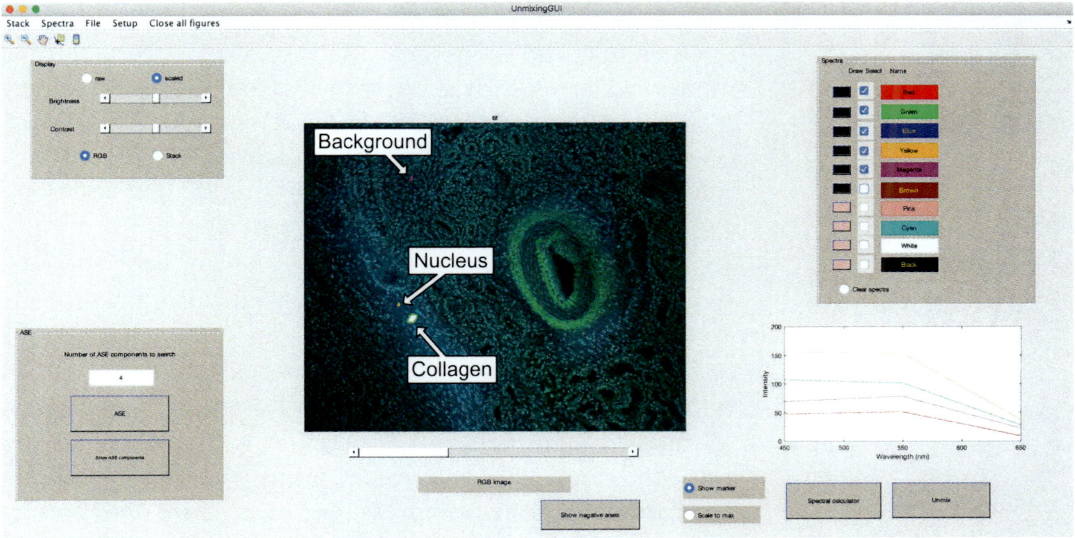

Fig. 6 UnmixingGUI screenshot with the kidney dataset loaded with marked ROIs on the measured fluorescent components used to isolate the collagen signal

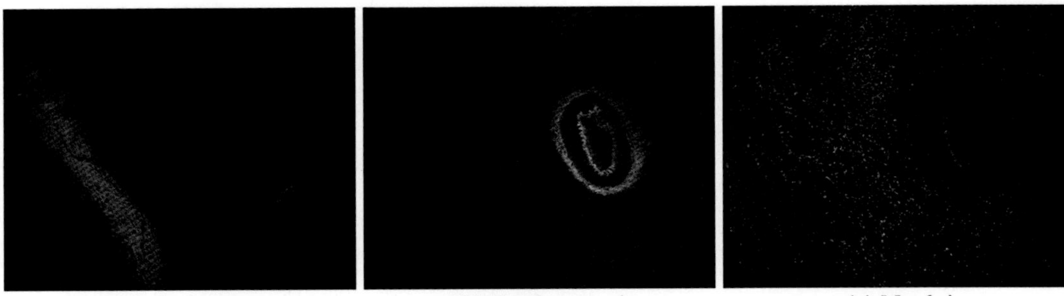

Fig. 7 Unmixing results demonstrating the separation of collagen. Shown here are (**a**) the desired collagen component, (**b**) the background component due to a mixture of eosin and tissue autofluorescence, and (**c**) the nuclei component due to Hoechst. The intensity of each component has been independently scaled to have its maximum intensity appear as *white*

that is very similar to the collagen itself. Figure 7 shows the output of this unmixing. We see that the collagen is well separated (Fig. 7a) from the background and nuclei components.

3. Next, we turn our attention to obtaining a pure signal of the elastin in and around the artery. Here, we will measure the signal in only two areas. The reason for this is that the elastin is well located spatially, unlike the collagen which has many overlapping signals with the nuclei. To this end, we will draw ROIs corresponding to a small portion of the internal elastic lamina (yellow) and some adjacent background signal (blue) (*see* **Note 9**). Shown in Fig. 8 are the selected regions. Purify the elastin component by again performing a subtraction (yellow minus blue) using the Spectral Calculator and store the result in the red component. The results of the unmixing shown in Fig. 9 clearly show the extracted elastin component as two concentric rings. Notice in Fig. 9b that there is no residual shadow or faint outline of the elastin on the background component, showing that we are capturing the just additional intensity due to the elastin component in Fig. 9a.
4. To create the composite fluorescence image with the pure spectra of collagen and elastin, select "scale components" and export the TIFF files as described in **step 9** of Subheading 4.2 (*see* **Note 10**).
5. While the UnmixingGUI can create a composite image, more advanced composite images can be created. Shown in Fig. 10 are composite images created using the output of the UnmixingGUI, one where we use the native fluorescence appearance of the images and the other where we mimic the appearance of standard bright-field microscopy. These procedures are outlined in the following steps:

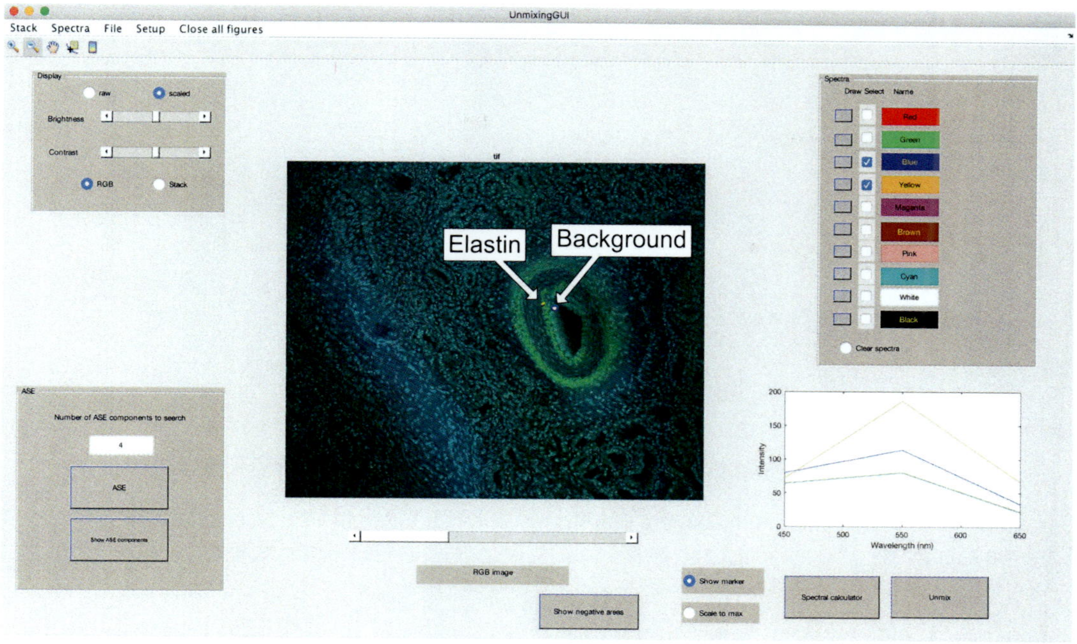

Fig. 8 UnmixingGUI screenshot with the kidney dataset loaded with marked ROIs on the measured fluorescent components used to isolate the elastin signal

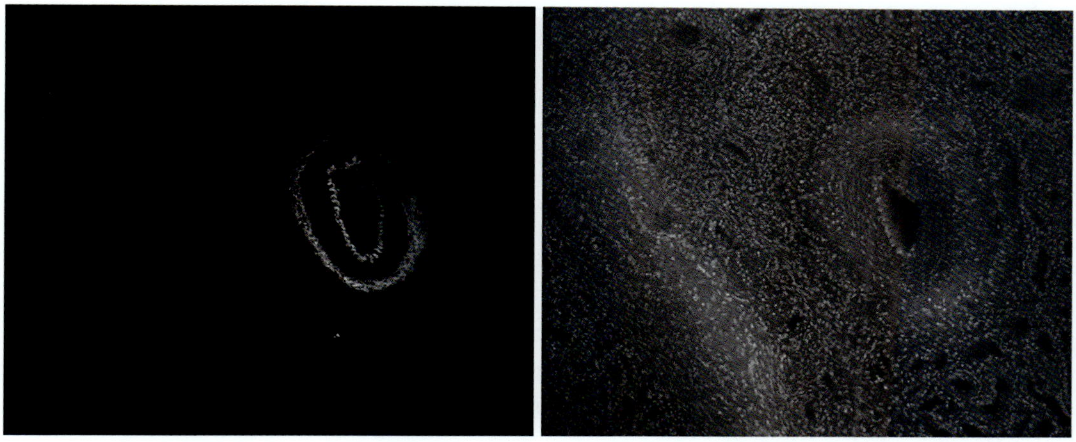

(a) Elastin (Red) Component (b) Background (Blue) Component

Fig. 9 Elastin unmixing results. Shown here are (**a**) the desired elastin component, (**b**) the background component due to a mixture of eosin, Hoechst, and tissue autofluorescence

6. Fluorescent composite:

   (a) Open an image manipulation app such as GIMP (*see* **Note 11**). Open the three images as layers. Rearrange the layers' order if needed so that they are, from back to front, the background component (Fig. 9b), the elastin component (Fig. 9a), and the collagen component (Fig. 7a).

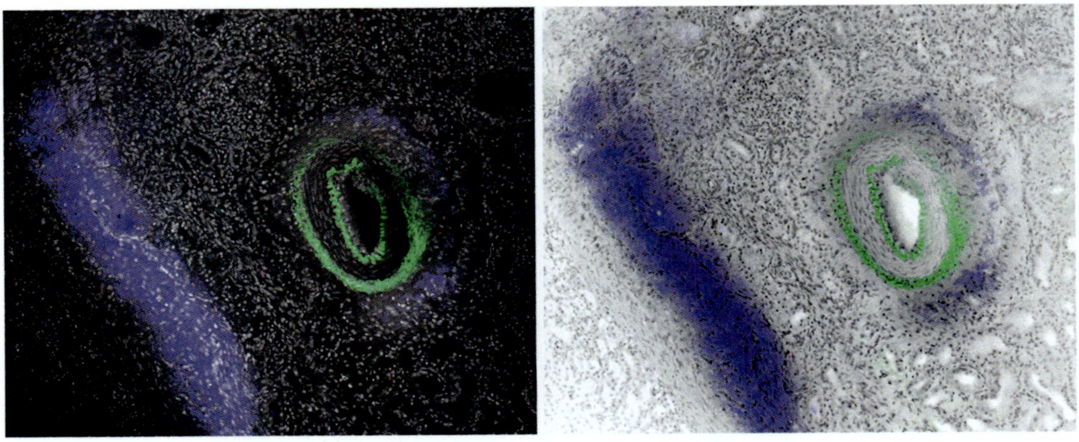

(a) Fluorescent Composite (b) Brightfield Composite

Fig. 10 Creation of a composite image. Both (**a**) fluorescent and (**b**) bright-field composites can be created. Here, we overlay the collagen (*blue*) and elastin (*green*) on a grayscale background image

(b) To combine these components in grayscale, the Screen blending mode should be used on the elastin and collagen layers: Select the elastin layer, and change the layer mode to Screen (*see* **Note 12**). Repeat with the collagen layer.

(c) Adjust the contrast of the background layer by selecting the background layer, and call the Brightness-Contrast option from the Colors menu. Adjust the Contrast to 30 and keep the Brightness at 0. Click on OK.

(d) The final step is to color the components in order to visually differentiate them. First, change the image mode to RGB using the Image menu. Then, color the layers one by one using the Colorize option from the Colors menu: Select the elastin layer and colorize it to a green color (Hue 120, Saturation 70, Lightness 0). Select the collagen layer and colorize to a blue color (Hue 240, Saturation 100, Lightness 0). Figure 10a shows the final fluorescent composite image.

7. Bright-field composite:

(a) Open the three images as layers as described in **steps 6a**.

(b) Invert each image using the Invert command found in the Colors menu. This inversion mimics the appearance of bright-field microscopy, which follows a subtractive or absorbance-based color model.

(c) Merge all components by applying a Multiply blending mode on the elastin and collagen layers (*see* **Note 12**).

(d) Color the components as described in **step 6d**. The bright-field composite result is presented in Fig. 10b.

6 Discussion

Like the UnmixingGUI and GIMP, there exist many free, open-source tools for analyzing multispectral data and combining the results for analysis and presentation. Using these, we have shown that linear unmixing can be a powerful tool for resolving overlapping fluorescent components in biological specimens from multispectral, or even color (RGB) datasets. The key to successful unmixing is the selection of spectral endmembers (i.e., areas of "pure" color). While isolated compounds can be used to generate a spectral library, accurate unmixing can be performed by directly selecting spectra from the image itself, provided these spectra are then purified by subtracting the mixed components. This approach can successfully extract signals from collagen and elastin in multiple stained tissue samples, even from an RGB image, which allows further quantitation and study to be performed without confounding background signals.

7 Notes

1. Stand-alone application requires prior installation of the free MATLAB runtime to be able to run without installing MATLAB. Details on how to install stand-alone applications are in the readme.txt file of the respective stand-alone folder (Windows or Mac OS) at https://github.com/UCDavisMUSE/unmixinggui.
2. TIFF is the abbreviation for Tagged Image File Format and corresponds to files that have the extension .tif or .tiff. The internal file format is the same between .tif and .tiff. Nomenclature difference stems from older file system that only accommodated three characters for the extension, vs newer systems that allow longer filenames.
3. What we refer to as a "stack" here is a series of TIFF files that contain one layer each. You will need to split the channels of multilayered TIFFs before loading them in UnmixingGUI. This can easily be done with ImageJ (https://imagej.nih.gov/ij/) (Image → Color → Split channels).
4. If a trace is misplaced, click on the checkmark next to the trace's color to remove the checkmark, and repeat the process (i.e., select the rectangle to the left of the color and draw). Check "Clear Spectra" under Spectra to erase all traces and start over.
5. It is important to note that even though the spectra of the Blue component and the autofluorescence are very similar (*see* Fig. 3b), these components can still be easily separated, even in this noisy data.

6. Median filter can be applied using ImageJ (Process → Filters → Median ...).
7. Other sources of noise, such as shot noise due to low photon counts or thermal sensor noise, may need to be removed prior to unmixing in order to obtain accurate results.
8. This can be accomplished in ImageJ (Image → Color → Split channels)
9. These areas will be in addition to the three existing spectra.
10. When the Scale components option is selected, the output will be scaled such that the maximum intensity for each component is white, rather than maintaining the relative intensities.
11. GIMP (GNU Image Manipulation Program, http://www.gimp.org) is a free and open-source image editing program similar to Adobe Photoshop. We will describe procedures using this app, but any other image manipulation program can be used.
12. On the top left portion of the layer window, below the Layers tab, the default Mode is Normal. Change the mode by clicking on Normal and select the desired blending mode.

Acknowledgments

We acknowledge Nenad Bozinovic for providing the MATLAB code for the UnmixingGUI.

References

1. Mallory FB (1936) The anilin blue collagen stain. Stain Technol 11(3):101–102. doi:10.3109/10520293609110505
2. Eroschenko VP, diFiore MSH (2013) diFiore's atlas of histology with functional correlations, 12th edn. Wolters Kluwer Health/Lippincott Williams & Wilkins, Philadelphia, PA
3. Tadrous PJ (2010) Digital stain separation for histological images. J Microsc 240(2):164–172. doi:10.1111/j.1365-2818.2010.03390.x
4. Turner NJ, Pezzone MA, Brown BN et al (2013) Quantitative multispectral imaging of Herovici's polychrome for the assessment of collagen content and tissue remodelling. J Tissue Eng Regen Med 7(2):139–148. doi:10.1002/term.508
5. von der Mark K, von der Mark H, Timpl R et al (1977) Immunofluorescent localization of collagen types I, II, and III in the embryonic chick eye. Dev Biol 59(1):75–85. doi:10.1016/0012-1606(77)90241-X
6. Hendrix MJC, Hay ED, von der Mark K et al (1982) Immunohistochemical localization of collagen types I and II in the developing chick cornea and tibia by electron microscopy. Invest Ophthalmol Vis Sci 22(3):359–375
7. Mendler M, Eich-Bender SG, Vaughan L et al (1989) Cartilage contains mixed fibrils of collagen types II, IX, and XI. J Cell Biol 108(1):191–197. doi:10.1083/jcb.108.1.191
8. Bautista PA, Yagi Y (2012) Multispectral enhancement towards digital staining. Anal Cell Pathol 35(1):51–55. doi:10.3233/ACP-2011-0038
9. Keikhosravi A, Bredfeldt JS, Sagar MAK et al (2014) Second-harmonic generation imaging of cancer. In: Waters JC, Wittman T (eds) Quantitative imaging in cell biology, Methods

in cell biology, vol 123. Academic Press, New York, NY, pp 531–546. doi:10.1016/B978-0-12-420138-5.00028-8

10. Oldenbourg R (1996) A new view on polarization microscopy. Nature 381(27):811–812. doi:10.1038/381811a0
11. Fuchs KO, Solis O, Tapawan R et al (2003) The effects of an estrogen and glycolic acid cream on the facial skin of postmenopausal women: a randomized histologic study. Cutis 71(6):481–488
12. Shribak M (2015) Polychromatic polarization microscope: bringing colors to a colorless world. Sci Rep 5(17340):1–10. doi:10.1038/srep17340
13. Zhou L, El-Deiry WS (2009) Multispectral fluorescence imaging. J Nucl Med 50(10):1563–1566. doi:10.2967/jnumed.109.063925
14. Mansfield JR (2014) Multispectral imaging: a review of its technical aspects and applications in anatomic pathology. Vet Pathol 51(1):185–210. doi:10.1177/0300985813506918
15. Shi S-R, Taylor CR (2014) Antigen retrieval in immunohistochemistry. In: McManus LM, Mitchell RN (eds) Pathobiology of human disease: a dynamic encyclopedia of disease mechanisms. Academic Press, New York, NY, pp 3817–3828. doi:10.1016/B978-0-12-386456-7.07404-9
16. Vinod KR, Jones D, Udupa V (2016) A simple and effective heat induced antigen retrieval method. MethodsX 3:315–319. doi:10.1016/j.mex.2016.04.001
17. Fukunaga-Kalabis M, Martinez G, Liu ZJ et al (2006) CCN3 controls 3D spatial localization of melanocytes in the human skin through DDR1. J Cell Biol 175(4):563–569. (see supp figures). doi:10.1083/jcb.200602132
18. Levenson RM, Mansfield JR (2006) Multispectral imaging in biology and medicine: slices of life. Cytometry A 69A(8):748–758. doi:10.1002/cyto.a.20319
19. Levenson RM, Lynch DT, Kobayashi H et al (2008) Multiplexing with multispectral imaging: from mice to microscopy. ILAR J 49(1):78–88. doi:10.1093/ilar.49.1.78
20. Stack EC, Wang C, Roman KA et al (2014) Multiplexed immunohistochemistry, imaging, and quantitation: a review, with an assessment of Tyramide signal amplification, multispectral imaging and multiplex analysis. Methods 70(1):46–58. doi:10.1016/j.ymeth.2014.08.016
21. Waters JC (2009) Accuracy and precision in quantitative fluorescence microscopy. J Cell Biol 185(7):1135–1148. doi:10.1083/jcb.200903097
22. Verdaasdonk JS, Lawrimore J, Bloom K (2014) Determining absolute protein numbers by quantitative fluorescence microscopy. In: Waters JC, Wittman T (eds) Quantitative imaging in cell biology, Methods in cell biology, vol 123. Academic Press, New York, NY, pp 347–365. doi:10.1016/B978-0-12-420138-5.00019-7
23. Mansfield JR, Gossage KW, Hoyt CC et al (2005) Autofluorescence removal, multiplexing, and automated analysis methods for in-vivo fluorescence imaging. J Biomed Opt 10(4):041207-041201–041207-041209. doi:10.1117/1.2032458
24. Boardman JW (1994) Geometric mixture analysis of imaging spectrometry data. Paper presented at the IEEE International Geoscience and Remote Sensing Symposium (IGARSS), Aug
25. Tauler R, Smilde A, Kowalski B (1995) Selectivity, local rank, three-way data analysis and ambiguity in multivariate curve resolution. J Chemometr 9(1):31–58. doi:10.1002/cem.1180090105
26. Bioucas-Dias J, Plaza A, Dobigeon N et al (2012) Hyperspectral unmixing overview: geometrical, statistical, and sparse regression-based approaches. IEEE J Sel Top Appl Earth Observ Remote Sens 5(2):354–379. doi:10.1109/JSTARS.2012.2194696
27. Liu W-L, Wang L-W, Chen J-M et al (2016) Application of multispectral imaging in quantitative immunohistochemistry study of breast cancer: a comparative study. Tumour Biol 37(4):5013–5024. doi:10.1007/s13277-015-4327-9
28. Ruifrok AC, Johnston DA (2001) Quantification of histochemical staining by color deconvolution. Anal Quant Cytol Histol 23(4):291–299
29. Levenson RM, Harmany ZT, Demos SG et al (2016) Slide-free histology via MUSE: UV surface excitation microscopy for imaging unsectioned tissue. Paper presented at the Proceedings of SPIE

Chapter 31

Simple Analysis of Deposited Gene Expression Datasets for the Non-Bioinformatician: How to Use GEO for Fibrosis Research

Yang Guo, Richard Townsend, and Lam C. Tsoi

Abstract

In the past decade, high-throughput techniques have facilitated the "-omics" research. Transcriptomic study, for instance, has advanced our understanding on the expression landscape of different human diseases and cellular mechanisms. The National Center for Biotechnology Center (NCBI) initialized Genetic Expression Omnibus (GEO) to promote the sharing of transcriptomic data to facilitate biomedical research. In this chapter, we will illustrate how to use GEO to search and analyze the public available transcriptomic data, and we will provide easy to follow protocol for researchers to data mine the powerful resources in GEO to retrieve relevant information that can be valuable for fibrosis research.

Key words RNA-seq, Microarray, Transcriptomic, GEO, Data analysis

1 Introduction

In the past decade, high-throughput techniques have facilitated the "-omics" research. Transcriptomic study, for instance, has advanced our understanding on the expression landscape of different human diseases and cellular mechanisms [1–4]. From the early studies utilizing microarray technology to the more recent work employing next-generation sequencing (NGS)-based technique (i.e., RNA-sequencing, also called RNA-seq), these high-throughput methods are able to profile gene expressions in time-efficient manner. These approaches generate large amount of data that can be overwhelming and troublesome to retrieve without an organized database. The National Center for Biotechnology Center (NCBI) initialized the Genetic Expression Omnibus (GEO) in 2000 to serve this purpose [5, 6]. GEO allows users to submit their gene expression datasets via file transfer protocol (FTP); the raw/processed data or associated results can then be retrieved or reanalyzed by the research community. In fact, most journals now

Laure Rittié (ed.), *Fibrosis: Methods and Protocols*, Methods in Molecular Biology, vol. 1627, DOI 10.1007/978-1-4939-7113-8_31, © Springer Science+Business Media LLC 2017

require authors to deposit the microarray or RNA-seq data to public databases (including GEO and ArrayExpress) for manuscripts describing new transcriptomic data. GEO datasets are submitted by their investigators and later organized by GEO curators. The original submitter-supplied dataset will each be assigned to GEO *Platform*, *Sample*, and *Series* records; biologically and statistically comparable GEO samples are curated by NCBI into GEO *DataSets* and analyzed to provide individual gene GEO *Profiles*. As of 2016, there are over 4300 GEO DataSets, consisting of over 72,000 Series and over 1.9 million Sample records.

Let us first start by defining some basic GEO record types. GEO *Platform* (GPL) provides information regarding the types, manufacturers, and other elements regarding the array or sequencer platforms for the experiments. GEO supplies template for the array-based platform in the GPL record. Each*DataSets*or *Series* record corresponds to one or more GPL record(s). GEO *Series* (GSE) summarizes research studies conducted by the submitter, and each *Series record* can include multiple GEO *Sample records*. Series record contains basic information for the study including title, aims, organism involved, experimental types and comparisons conducted, and overall experimental design. Published papers regarding the record are cited, and contact information of the data submitter is also provided. *Series* records can be searched through GEO *DataSets* interface and are referenced by corresponding*DataSets*and *Sample* records accession pages. GEO *Sample* (GSM) describes specific information for the experimental condition under which an individual sample was handled and processed, and the protocols of any specific manipulation are also provided. Each GSM record can only reference to one GPL but can be involved in multiple Series. GEO *DataSets* (GDS) is a study-based database consisting of curated records of biologically and statistically comparable Sample records. All Sample records from the same *DataSets*record were processed using the same Platform. Each *DataSets*record lists basic information of the studies included. Furthermore, analysis and bioinformatics tools such as cluster heat map, sample comparison tools, and information regarding phenotypic subsets are also available. Finally, GEO *Profiles* provides gene-level information and presents the expression level of a gene across all samples in a *DataSets* record. It includes percentile rank for a gene among all the genes expressed in each sample: the higher the ranking percentile, the higher level the gene was expressed in the sample.

GEO is one of the most organized and resourceful repositories for high-throughput gene expression data. While the examples we illustrate are microarray based, there is an increasing number of sequencing-based datasets deposited to GEO. There have been many researchers utilizing the GEO datasets to facilitate their research: replicating findings, meta-analysis, lookup gene(s) of interest, etc. Indeed, it is not surprising that we can retrieve additional knowledge from existing data when comparing the initial studies. Therefore, it is crucial to understand the fundamental queries to retrieve basic information from GEO. In this chapter, we will illustrate how to use GEO to search and analyze the public available transcriptomic data. There are more advanced data retrieval options, including download the raw microarray intensity or sequence files from GEO via file transfer protocol (most commonly known as FTP), but these advanced options require the users to be familiar with additional data processing procedures and analysis.

Here, we aim to provide an easy to follow protocol for researchers to data mine the powerful resources in GEO, to undergo basic analysis for fibrosis research, and to raise awareness for this valuable resource to facilitate the efficiency of scientific discovery.

2 Materials

2.1 Instruments

The queries and analysis we present do not require any special computational requirements. Users can use their desktops or laptops (both Windows and Mac operating systems are supported) which are connected to the Internet to undergo the exercise listed below. The GEO and GEO2R support different web browsers, including *Internet Explorer*, *Safari*, *Firefox*, and *Chrome*.

2.2 GEO and GEO2R

1. GEO (http://www.ncbi.nlm.nih.gov/geo/) is a web-based application that allows collecting the vast amount of transcriptomic data and comparing samples between different conditions as desired. GEO comes with built-in browser-based analytical software, GEO2R, for this purpose.
2. GEO2R (http://www.ncbi.nlm.nih.gov/geo/) is a tool that allows user to manually select data for comparison from a GEO Series (*see* **Note 1**). GEO2R is particularly useful if there is no curated *DataSets* record associated with the GEO Series record.

We provide below detailed explanation of the various configurations and functions of the NIH GEO search engine (*see* Subheading 3.1). We will first use a GEO *DataSets* record as an example to demonstrate how to construct standardized and advanced queries to refine search results. We will illustrate how to find gene of interest from GEO and retrieve its *Profile* records and will also provide an advanced example to show how to use GEO2R, a tool provided by GEO, to compare expression profiles in different conditions.

3 Methods

3.1 The GEO Search Engine: Definitions, Configurations, and Functions

3.1.1 Searching for DataSets

The simplest way to search for *DataSets* records is by their corresponding accession numbers (e.g., GDSXXX). This works best if users know exactly which set(s) of data they are looking for. Otherwise, users can search the database via keywords. This might not be trivial, however, due to the large volume and diversity of the deposited GEO *DataSets* records. Applying filters to search relevant records can be conducted by utilizing keywords or phrases to refine search results.

By combining search field descriptions, GEO advanced query is able to narrow down results based on over 20 fields [6]. Specifically, advanced queries can be achieved using search terms and/or the associated fields; for instances, users can search by organism involved [ORGANISM] (or [ORGN]), published date [Publication Date], author [Author], platform (e.g., GPL570), etc. In addition, different symbols can be used to construct advanced query, and their specific meanings are listed in Table 1.

Users can also construct advanced query via advanced search builder, and they can select different fields from drop-down menus, and the search engine will automatically generate the desired query. Advanced search builder also allows users to save their search history, and new searches can be made by incorporating several previous searches (e.g., "#1 NOT #2" will include search results from the search query in "#1" but exclude search results from query in "#2").

3.1.2 Navigating DataSets

Users can obtain different information in the *DataSet* browser page for a *DataSets* record. As an example, we here work with *DataSets* record GDS4268, a transcriptomic study of peripheral blood cells of patients with scleroderma-associated pulmonary hypertension deposited by Risbano et al. [7] (Fig. 1). This page lists the title, summary, organism involved, and platform used of the dataset (Fig. 1a). It also references the corresponding *Series* (Fig. 1b) and count of *Sample* records (Fig. 1c).

Table 1
Symbols used in advanced query

Symbol	Representation	Examples
" "	Indicates phrase to search	"atopic dermatitis"
( )	Combine multiple search terms	("atopic dermatitis") OR ("psoriasis")
WORD*	Search entries with prefix WORD	"atopic derm*"
:	Range for date in YYYY/MM format	2015/01:2016/05
[ ]	Indicates field	("atopic dermatitis"[Title]) OR ("psoriasis"[Title])

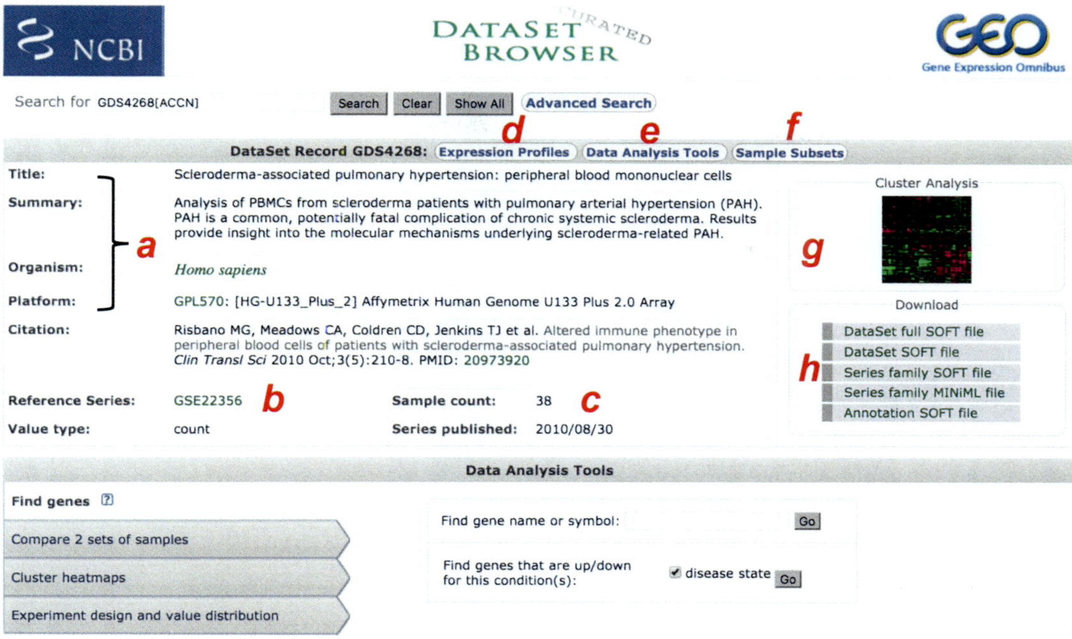

Fig. 1 DataSet browser pages for (**A**) general layout and (**B**) advanced search link. The link for browser page of DataSets GDS4268 is http://www.ncbi.nlm.nih.gov/sites/GDSbrowser?acc=GDS4268

1. By clicking on the *Series* accession number (Fig. 1b), users can go to the corresponding *Series* display page linked to this *DataSets* record. The citation provides the specific study related to the dataset. On the top of the DataSet browser page, "Expression Profile" (Fig. 1d), "Data Analysis Tools" (Fig. 1e), and "Sample Subsets" (Fig. 1f) provide in-depth information and analytical support for this dataset.
2. By clicking on the "Expression Profile" button, a new window that contains all Profiles of the genes related to the *DataSets* record will be opened.
3. By clicking on "Data Analysis Tools" button (linked to the bottom of the page), users arrive to several tools provided by GEO. There are four data analysis tools available on the Dataset browser page: "Find genes," "compare 2 sets of samples," "cluster heatmaps," and "Experiment design and value distribution." These tools allow users to find specific genes and compare gene expression and will be further explained below.
4. By clicking on the "Sample Subsets" tab, users can view subgroups that were phenotyped in the dataset. Users can further find cluster heatmap (Fig. 1g) and download options (Fig. 1h) on the upper right corner of the DataSet browser page. The different types of download options are summarized in Table 2.

Table 2
Download options of GEO database

File type	Description
Dataset Full SOFT[a]	Dataset info, experimental variables, expression value measurement, up-to-date gene annotation for the dataset platform (plain text)
Dataset SOFT[a]	Dataset info, experimental variables, expression value measurements, gene symbols (plain text)
Series Family SOFT[a]	Complete original submitter-supplied records (plain text)
Series Family MINiML[b]	Complete original submitter-supplied records (XML format)
Annotation SOFT[a]	Comprehensive up-to-date gene annotation for subset (plain text)

[a]*SOFT* Simple Omnibus Format in Text
[b]*MINiML* MIAME Notation in Markup Language

3.1.3 Focusing on a Gene

1. If users know what gene they are interested in, they can search this gene by name or symbol using the "Find Genes" tab (Fig. 2A-a) under "Data Analysis Tool" (Fig. 2A-b). The search yields gene Profile record(s) associated with that gene.
2. If users do not have a gene of interest, they can use "Find genes that are up/down for this condition(s)" tool (Fig. 2A-c) to search for genes that are differentially expressed under different conditions [6]. The tab "Compare 2 sets of samples" (Fig. 2B-a) further allows users to define two subgroups for comparison. By performing statistical tests for different expression analysis, users are able to identify genes that are dysregulated between two user-defined sample groups.
3. Users can also search expression profiles for the genes of interest directly in the GEO Profiles page (http://www.ncbi.nlm.nih.gov/geoprofiles/). By searching gene of interest in the database, different gene *Profiles* records are shown for that gene under different *DataSets* records (Fig. 3). This page includes or links to all the basic information of the gene (Fig. 3a, b) such as its function, genomic regions, transcripts, products, and phenotypes. In addition, the "GEO *DataSets*" button (Fig. 3c) links to the corresponding *DataSets* record(s) for each of the gene's *Profiles* records. Users can also find information and related/homologous genes (Fig. 3d). The expression profiling (i.e., profileGraph page) for the gene in the corresponding *DataSets* record is available as bar graph (Fig. 3e). We illustrate in Fig. 4

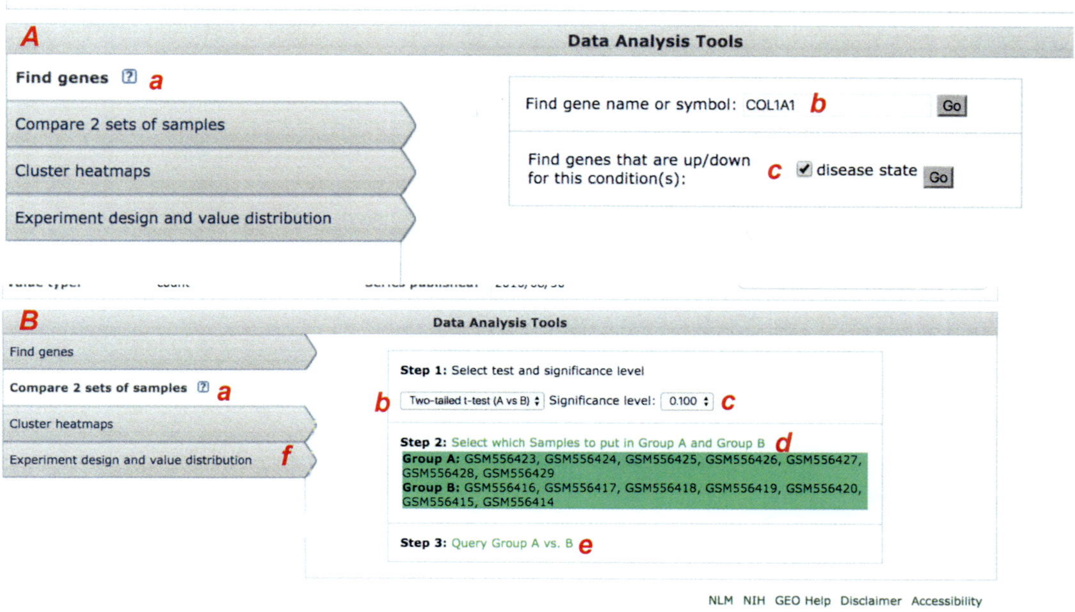

Fig. 2 Data analysis tools: (**A**) find genes tool; (**B**) compare two sets of samples tool

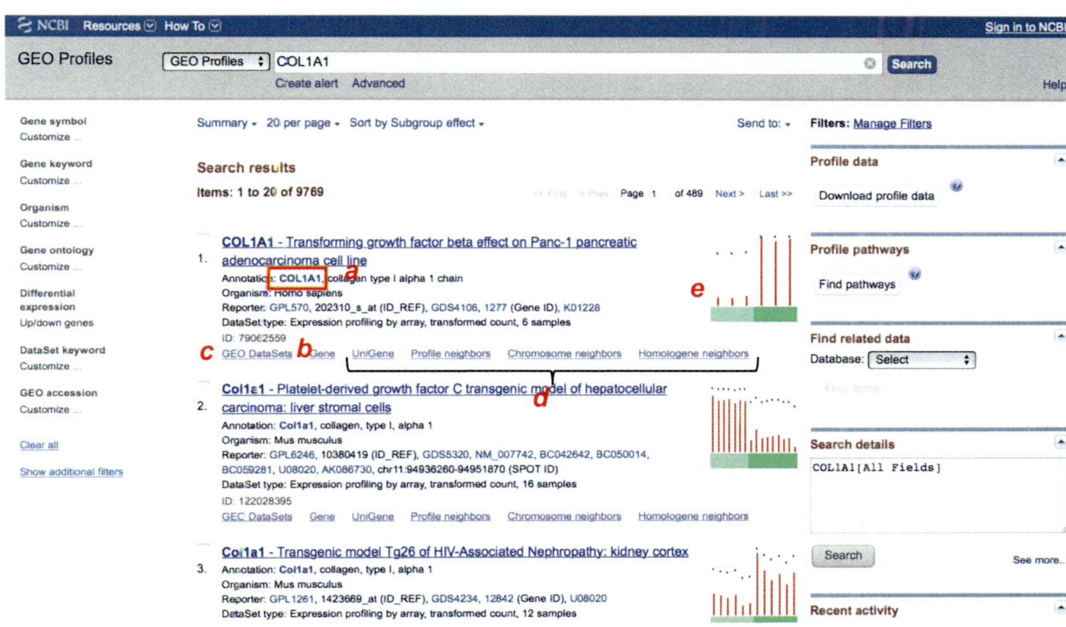

Fig. 3 GEO Profiles summary page

an example for the profileGraph page of *COL1A1* from probe-set 217430_x_at in *DataSets* GDS4268. The red bars (Fig. 4a) represent the expression values of the specific gene across the different samples. These values were extracted from the original submitter-supplied files, and the expression levels usually indi-

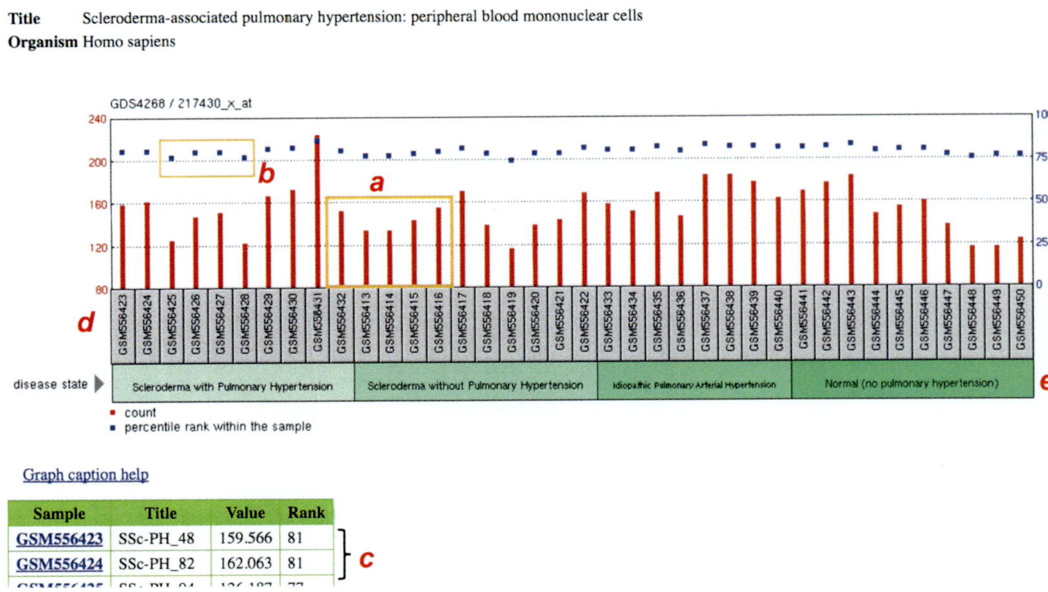

Fig. 4 GEO Profiles page for

cate normalized values, depending on the processing procedures conducted by the submitter. The blue squares (Fig. 4b) represent the percentile ranks of the specific gene in different samples: the higher the percentile rank, the higher the expression level when comparing with other genes within the sample. The actual expression values and percentile ranks are summarized in a table at the bottom of the page (Fig. 4c). In addition, the gray boxes (Fig. 4d) show the accession numbers for the GEO *Sample* records (i.e., GSM). The *Sample* records are grouped by phenotypes/conditions, which are indicated below the accession numbers (Fig. 4e).

3.2 Querying a GEO DataSets

In this session, we will continue to use GDS4268, introduced in Subheading 3.1.2, as an example to illustrate how to interrogate a *DataSets* record.

1. Go to GEO: http://www.ncbi.nlm.nih.gov/geo/.
2. Click "DataSets" under "Browser Content" (*see* **Note 2**).
3. Either of the following three strategies can be used to retrieve *DataSets* record GDS4268:
   (a) Enter "((scleroderma) AND homo sapiens [Organism]) AND hypertension[Title]" (without quotation marks) in the search box. This allows users to search scleroderma-related datasets with hypertension in its title and *Homo sapiens* as the organism (*see* **Note 3**).
   (b) Instead of the search entered in (**a**), users can build a query using advanced search builder: on the right of the search

box, click on the "Advanced Search" option (Fig. 1). Click on that will bring users to the GEO DataSet browser search page. Click on the "Advanced" link right below the search box will bring you to the advanced search builder page.

(c) Enter "scleroderma," "homo sapiens," and "hypertension" in search boxes as shown in Fig. 5a. Select Fields as shown in Fig. 5b. Select "AND" as shown in Fig. 5c to intersect the search queries. Index lists under the phrases entered can be seen by clicking "Show index list" button (Fig. 5d) (*see* **Note 4**).

4. After clicking search (Fig. 5e), it would yield two *DataSets*, four *Series*, and three *Platforms* records. Users can choose the record with title "Scleroderma-associated pulmonary hypertension: peripheral blood mononuclear cells" (*see* **Note 5**).
5. When users are at DataSet browser page for GDS4268, they are able to retrieve more gene-level data for this dataset (*see* **Note 6**).
6. Say users are interested in COL1A1, collagen type I alpha 1 chain, which codes for the pro-alpha1 chain of type I collagen, a protein typically overproduced in fibrotic diseases. Type "COL1A1" into the search box under the "Find genes" tab (Fig. 2A-b) and click on "Go." This search will yield five GEO *Profiles* of COL1A1 in the dataset. There are five different Profiles because the microarray platform used by this dataset contains five different probesets (i.e., 217430_x_at, 202312_s_at, 202310_s_at, 202311_s_at, 1556499_s_at). Refer to Subheading 3.1.3 for how to interpret gene *Profiles* records.

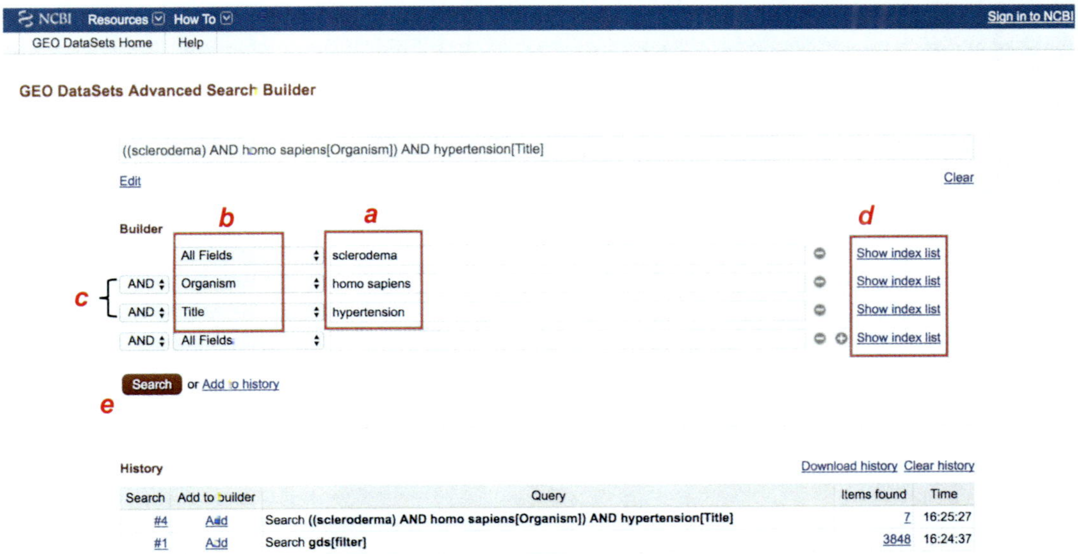

Fig. 5 GEO DataSets advanced search builder

7. To find genes that are differentially expressed in factor(s) evaluated in the *DataSets*, use the "Find genes that are up/down for this conditions(s)" under the "Find Genes" tab. Users can restrict the retrieval of data to certain factor(s) by selecting the corresponding box (Fig. 2A-c). The number of factors varies between *DataSets*, and there is only one factor (i.e., "disease state") in the GDS 4268 *DataSets* record.
8. Next, we will compare data based on customized subgroups.
9. Click on the tab "Compare 2 sets of samples" (Fig. 2B-a).
10. Select the desired type of statistical test and significance level using the drop-down menus (Fig. 2B-b, c, respectively).
11. Assign samples to various groups by clicking on "Select which samples to put in Group A and Group B" (Fig. 2B-d). A page similar to the one shown in Fig. 6 will pop out.
12. Select samples by clicking on the sample accession number (GSMXXXX) and assign them to either Group A or Group B; selected sample will become shaded. Deselect them by clicking on the sample accession number again. Samples selected on the left will be in group A (Fig. 6a) while samples selected on the right will be in group B (Fig. 6b).
13. Click OK (Fig. 6c).

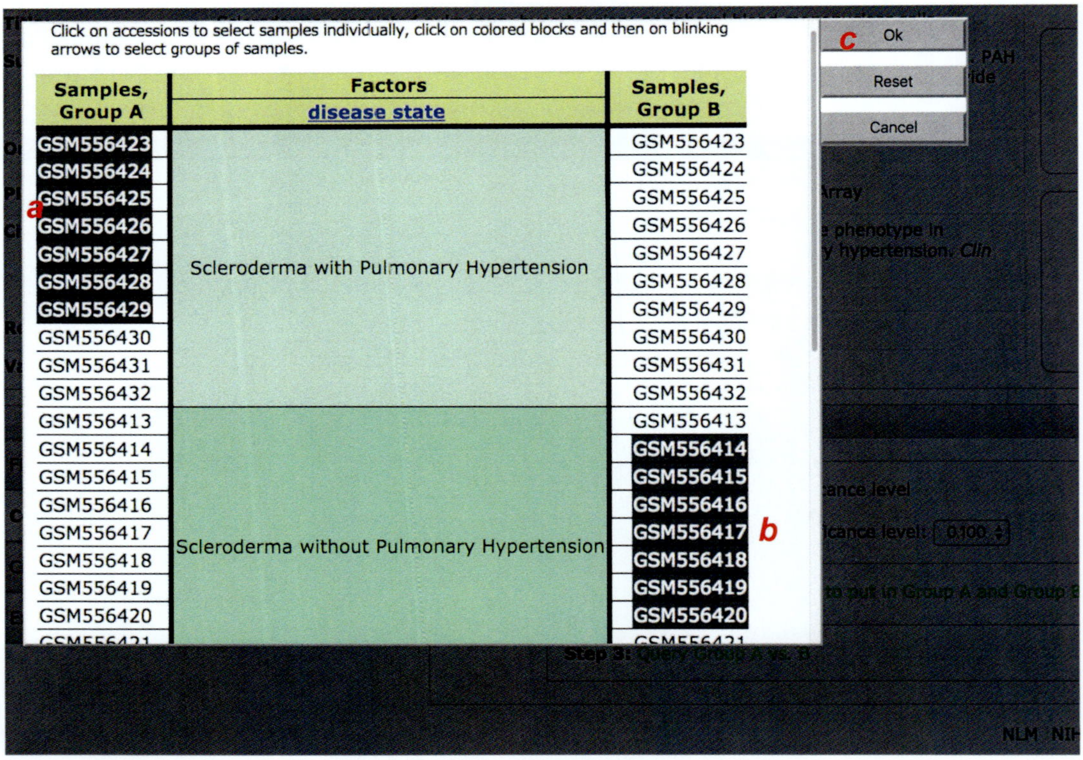

Fig. 6 Sample selection window for comparing two sets of samples tool

14. Finally, click on "Query Group A vs. B" (Fig. 2B-e) which will compute and identify genes expressed differentially between Group A and Group B samples.
15. To analyze the *DataSets* record utilizing heatmaps based on co-expression or chromosomal location, click on the "Cluster heat-maps" tab, which provides three clustering options to display. The three options available are unsupervised hierarchical clusters, K-means/K-median clusters, and heatmaps organized by location of genes on the chromosome. GEO also provides options to zoom in/out images or even to export selected data.
16. To view boxplots displaying all samples' expression values, click on the "Experiment design and value distribution" tab (Fig. 2B-f). This is a critical quality control and verification procedure to evaluate if the samples are normalized accordingly and comparable to each other; this will also be helpful to identify potential outliers, which should be excluded in the above analysis. The color bar at the bottom shows different subgroups of the samples.

3.3 Data Analysis Using GEO2R

In this session, we will use GSE71999 (*see* **Note 7**), a study that used mice model for scleroderma research, as an example to illustrate how to conduct more advanced data analysis data using GEO-developed tool GEO2R.

1. Starting from GEO's homepage (http://www.ncbi.nlm.nih.gov/geo/), type in the search bar: Scleroderma AND (Mus musculus [organism] NOT Homo sapiens [organism]) AND microarray AND "Comparative Genomics."
2. Click on the series named "Interspecies Comparative Genomics Identifies Optimal Mouse Models of Scleroderma" (*see* **Note 8**). The GEO search will provide any GEO records that match the query provided by users; they may select the "Entry type" on left side of the screen to filter down the search results. Otherwise, if users know the GSE number for the Series (i.e., GSE71999 in this case), they can type directly into the search bar to be brought directly to the Series page.
3. To analyze this *Series* record, go to the bottom of the page and click the blue link "Analyze with GEO2R" (*see* **Note 9**).
4. A large list of all the samples from this GEO *Series* should have appeared. If this is not the case, type in the accession number once more in the search box on the top left corner and click "Set." Click the blue button labeled "Define Groups," and now a drop-down box should appear (*see* **Note 10**).
5. We will analyze data on several of the samples used in this study, specifically the bleomycin-treated mice as compared between 5 and 21 days. Type into the drop-down box "Bleomycin Treated 5d" and click enter. The drop-down box

should just have extended downward with a category labeled "Bleomycin Treated 5d." This is the first group but it has no sample associated with it yet.

6. Assign the five samples GSM1849526 to GSM1849530 to the group: click on the desired samples (GSM1849526 to GSM1849530) to highlight them and click back "Bleomycin Treated 5d" in the drop-down box (*see* **Note 11**).
7. Create a second group named "Bleomycin Treated 21d" and add the samples GSM1849531 to GSM1849535 to this group as described in **step 6** (*see* **Note 12**).
8. Analyze the samples above by GEO2R. There are five tabs labeled "GEO2R," "Value Distribution," "Options," "Profile Graph," and "R script." We will go over the contents of each below (*see* **Note 13**):
9. The "GEO2R" tab displays the top 250 differentially expressed genes. The genes are separated by row and, by default, display statistical information (e.g., *p*-value, t-statistic, logarithmic value of Fold Change (logFC)) for each record. An identification number (ID) is given at the far left of the row that identifies this particular GEO Profiles record. Click on a row to get a drop-down profile of gene expression between the samples being compared. Comparisons are color-coded based the groups users have created. Click on the "Select columns" button above the table to change what is displayed in the result table. Check the box next to the desired information and click "set" to apply the change. Click "Save all results" to bring a new page with the full list created by GEO2R, past the top 250 differently expressed genes.
10. In the "Value distribution" tab, click "View" to display boxplots of the data being compared by GEO2R. This is intended to give the user an idea of how statistically comparable the samples are, as described above. Click on "Export" to open a new page with the statistics of the box plots displayed on the graph. The "Options" tab allows users to change parameters or arguments that determine how the differential expression analysis by GEO2R data was conducted. Importantly, if any changes are made here, users must go back to the "GEO2R" tab and click "Recalculate" before the desired changes take effect.
11. The "Profile graph" tab generates an expression profile graph of any gene tested, even if it is not in the top 250 differently expressed genes. Enter the accession ID of the gene of interest to generate a new browser tab displaying a text document of all the genes tested for by this platform (*see* **Notes 14–16**).
12. The "R script" tab displays the actual coding on how the data was calculated in GEO2R.

4 Notes

1. GEO2R can be accessed either from a link at the bottom of GEO Series page or at http://www.ncbi.nlm.nih.gov/geo/geo2r/. More detailed instruction by NCBI can be found in http://www.ncbi.nlm.nih.gov/geo/info/geo2r.html, or in a YouTube video created by NCBI [8].
2. Users can also click on "Series," "Platforms," and "Samples" to search for GEO records other than "*DataSets*." There are also links to tutorials and tools on this page.
3. Spelling of queries matters, as there is not auto-correction. Even space between words makes a difference. For instance, Homosapiens and Homo sapiens could yield different results. Make sure you have the correct spelling.
4. Users can select various fields from the down bar and enter the phrases in the search box (Fig. 5a, b). There is also a drop-down menu in front of each field down bar where users can select AND, OR, or NOT (Fig. 5c).
5. This is the result of the search as of September 2016. The number of search results will likely increase if additional relevant datasets are submitted after this date. Also note the searching history is automatically saved. You can search for datasets by combining two searches, e.g., #1 NOT #2.
6. The GDS4268 page is http://www.ncbi.nlm.nih.gov/sites/GDSbrowser?acc=GDS4268.
7. The GSE link for this GEO Series is http://www.ncbi.nlm.nih.gov/geo/query/acc.cgi?acc=GSE71999.
8. It should be noted that Series record (i.e., GSE71999) is a super Series record, which contains multiple Series records. The super Series record behaves like regular Series records with the only difference that it references other Series records as well as the constituted samples. If you explore the page, you can find various information such as contact of the submitter(s), citations with a link (the PMID link) to the associated article, organization/institution that submitted the information along with contact information, or links to each of the samples and series making up this record. At the bottom you can find the download links. We will use this page as the subject for analysis using GEO2R.
9. Alternatively, you may also start with the GEO2R page http://www.ncbi.nlm.nih.gov/geo/geo2r/ and type in the ascension number of this document (GSE71999) into GEO2R's search bar page.
10. Instead of clicking one sample by one sample, users can hold the control key to highlight all samples first, and then click

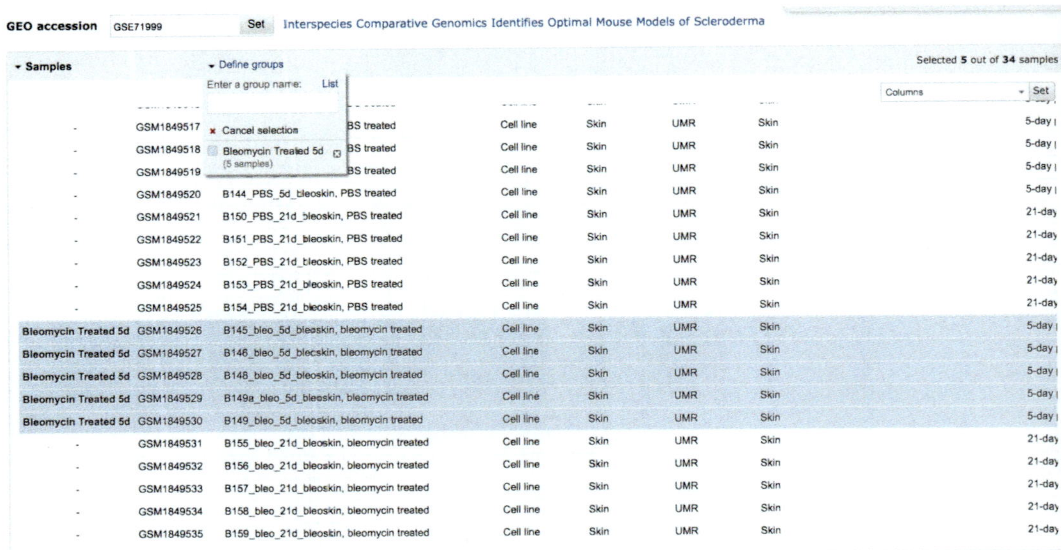

Fig. 7 Sample selection in GEO2R

back the "Bleomycin Treated 5d" in the drop-down box (Fig. 7).

11. This feature can also be used to create customized group name(s) for different groups for comparison.
12. A maximum of ten groups for comparison can be set using GEO2R.
13. Links can be found on top of the GEO2R webpage for a thorough description of GEO2R and the results it may give. The first link, labeled Full Instructions, gives you a full description of GEO2R and its purpose. The second link, a YouTube link, takes you to a video by NCBI on how to use GEO2R.
14. Note that the ID, not necessarily of the gene symbol, is required as input.
15. Note that within a microarray platform, there can be multiple probesets hybridizing different parts of the same gene (hence one ID, several hits).
16. Output the differential expression analysis results for all genes under the "GEO2R" tab to search the accession IDs for the gene(s) you are interested in. For example, COL1A1 would have IDs: "A_52_P658611," "A_52_P525107," "A_51_P377094." Entering one of the IDs to the "Enter ID" search box under "Profile graph" would generate expression graph for this gene under the selected samples.

Acknowledgments

LCT is supported by the University of Michigan Babcock Endowment Fund, the Dermatology Foundation, National Psoriasis Foundation, and the Arthritis National Research Foundation. The authors acknowledge the support from the Undergraduate Research Opportunity Program from the University of Michigan.

References

1. Chang JC, Wooten EC, Tsimelzon A et al (2003) Gene expression profiling for the prediction of therapeutic response to docetaxel in patients with breast cancer. Lancet 362(9381):362–369. doi:10.1016/S0140-6736(03)14023-8
2. Tsoi LC, Qin T, Slate EH et al (2011) Consistent Differential Expression Pattern (CDEP) on microarray to identify genes related to metastatic behavior. BMC Bioinformatics 12:438. doi:10.1186/1471-2105-12-438
3. Li B, Tsoi LC, Swindell WR et al (2014) Transcriptome analysis of psoriasis in a large case-control sample: RNA-seq provides insights into disease mechanisms. J Invest Dermatol 134(7):1828–1838. doi:10.1038/jid.2014.28
4. Tsoi LC, Iyer MK, Stuart PE et al (2015) Analysis of long non-coding RNAs highlights tissue-specific expression patterns and epigenetic profiles in normal and psoriatic skin. Genome Biol 16:24. doi:10.1186/s13059-014-0570-4
5. Edgar R, Domrachev M, Lash AE (2002) Gene Expression Omnibus: NCBI gene expression and hybridization array data repository. Nucleic Acids Res 30(1):207–210
6. Clough E, Barrett T (2016) The Gene Expression Omnibus Database. Methods Mol Biol 1418:93–110. doi:10.1007/978-1-4939-3578-9_5
7. Risbano MG, Meadows CA, Coldren CD et al (2010) Altered immune phenotype in peripheral blood cells of patients with scleroderma-associated pulmonary hypertension. Clin Transl Sci 3(5):210–218. doi:10.1111/j.1752-8062.2010.00218.x
8. NCBI (2012) GEO2R: Analyze GEO Data. https://youtu.be/EUPmGWS8ik0. Accessed on 23 October 2016

INDEX

Laure Rittié (ed.), *Fibrosis: Methods and Protocols*, Methods in Molecular Biology, vol. 1627, DOI 10.1007/978-1-4939-7113-8, © Springer Science+Business Media LLC 2017